Zannis

4th edition

obstetrics and gynecology

The National Medical Series for Independent Study

4th edition
obstetrics and gynecology

William W. Beck, Jr., M.D.

*Professor of Obstetrics and Gynecology
Associate Dean for Student and
  Housestaff Affairs
University of Pennsylvania School
  of Medicine
Hospital of the University of
  Pennsylvania
Philadelphia, Pennsylvania*

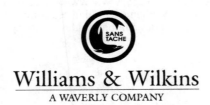

Williams & Wilkins
A WAVERLY COMPANY

BALTIMORE • PHILADELPHIA • LONDON • PARIS • BANGKOK
BUENOS AIRES • HONG KONG • MUNICH • SYDNEY • TOKYO • WROCLAW

Editor: Elizabeth A. Nieginski
Managing Editor: Amy G. Dinkel
Production Coordinator: Felecia R. Weber
Cover Designer: Cathy Cotter
Typesetter: Maryland Composition
Printer: Port City Press
Binder: Port City Press

Copyright © 1997 Williams & Wilkins

351 West Camden Street
Baltimore, Maryland 21201-2436 USA

Rose Tree Corporate Center
1400 North Providence Road
Building II, Suite 5025
Media, Pennsylvania 19063-2043 USA

Accurate indications, adverse reactions and dosage schedules for drugs are provided in this book, but it is possible that they may change. The reader is urged to review the package information data of the manufacturers of the medications mentioned.

Printed in the United States of America

Fourth Edition,

Library of Congress Cataloging-in-Publication Data
Obstetrics and gynecology / [edited by] William W. Beck, Jr. — 4th
  ed.
      p.   cm. — (The National medical series for independent study)
    Includes index.
    ISBN: 0-683-18015-0
    1. Gynecology—Outlines, syllabi, etc.   2. Obstetrics—Outlines,
syllabi, etc.   3. Gynecology—Examinations, questions, etc.
4. Obstetrics—Examinations, questions, etc.   I. Beck, William W.,
1939–   . II. Series.
RG112.O73   1996
618'.076—dc20
DNLM/DLC
for Library of Congress
                                                                        96-29165
                                                                          CIP

The publishers have made every effort to trace the copyright holders for borrowed material. If they have inadvertently overlooked any, they will be pleased to make the necessary arrangements at the first opportunity.

To purchase additional copies of this book, call our customer service department at **(800) 638-0672** or fax orders to **(800) 447-8438.** For other book services, including chapter reprints and large quantity sales, ask for the Special Sales department.

Canadian customers should call **(800) 268-4178,** or fax **(905) 470-6780.** For all other calls originating outside of the United States, please call **(410) 528-4223** or fax us at **(410) 528-8550.**

Visit Williams & Wilkins on the Internet: **http://www.wwilkins.com** or contact our customer service department at **custserv@wwilkins.com.** Williams & Wilkins customer service representatives are available from 8:30 am to 6:00 pm, EST, Monday through Friday, for telephone access.

                                                        97 98 99
                                          1 2 3 4 5 6 7 8 9 10

Contents

Contributors

Michelle Battistini, M.D.
Assistant Professor of Obstetrics and Gynecology
Director Penn Health for Women
University of Pennsylvania
Philadelphia, Pennsylvania

William W. Beck, Jr., M.D.
Professor, Department of Obstetrics and
    Gynecology
Associate Dean for Student and Housestaff
    Affairs
University of Pennsylvania School of Medicine
Philadelphia, Pennsylvania

Jane Fang, M.D.
Assistant Professor of Obstetrics and Gynecology
University of Pennsylvania Medical Center
Philadelphia, Pennsylvania

Kavita Nanda, M.D.
Women's Health Fellow
Division of Health Services Research
Duke University Medical Center
Staff Physician, Duke Women Veterans
    Comprehensive Health Center
Duke Veterans Administration Medical Center
Durham, North Carolina

Matthew F. Rhoa, M.D.
Assistant Professor
University of Pennsylvania School of Medicine
Philadelphia, Pennsylvania

Preface

As NMS *Obstetrics and Gynecology* has moved into its fourth edition, the mission has remained the same—to provide relevant and current information on a broad range of topics in obstetrics and gynecology for both students and residents as they review for whatever examination lies ahead. A group of new, young authors have assisted me on this edition, each of them either currently at or recently departed from the University of Pennsylvania School of Medicine. All of the chapters have been updated or revised; some nonrelevant material has been removed; and some new chapters have been written. Furthermore, there are five new case studies in clinical decision making to complement the four already in place. Those nine cases cover major clinical areas in the specialty that are confronted on a daily basis by providers interested in women's health care. The basic format of the book remains the same—information in an outline form that allows the reader to readily access any area of interest.

William W. Beck, Jr., M.D.

Chapter 1

Endocrinology of Pregnancy

William W. Beck, Jr.

I. INTRODUCTION

A. **Endocrine changes during pregnancy.** The most important endocrine changes are the production of human chorionic gonadotropin (hCG), human placental lactogen (hPL), prolactin, progesterone, and estrogens by the placenta. **Maternal hormone levels,** which differ from those in the nonpregnant state, are **dependent on:**

1. The **presence of a placenta,** a rich store of steroid and protein hormones

2. The **presence of a fetus,** whose endocrine structures—the pituitary gland, thyroid, adrenal cortex, pancreas, and gonads—function as early as the eleventh week of pregnancy
   a. In the **male fetus,** the testes, in response to placental gonadotropin, produce testosterone, which is necessary for normal male development.
   b. In the **female fetus,** although the ovaries are responsive to placental gonadotropins, normal development is not dependent on fetal ovarian steroid production. The ovaries in the fetus produce small but progressively greater amounts of estrogen.

3. The **presence of elevated levels of circulating estrogens,** which have the following effects:
   a. They increase the effects of binding proteins, such as thyroid-binding globulin (TBG) and cortisol-binding globulin (CBG). These proteins bind thyroxine and cortisol and falsely raise their levels in the maternal circulation. The free fraction, however, changes little, and, thus, the metabolic processes that are dependent on these hormones usually are unaltered.
   b. They **partially inhibit the enzyme 3-β-hydroxysteroid dehydrogenase.** This enzyme is necessary to convert steroid precursors with a Δ-5,3-hydroxyl configuration to a Δ-4,3-ketosteroid configuration. The latter steroids, which are active biologically and highly significant, include testosterone and corticosteroids.
   c. They **inhibit maternal pituitary gonadotropin synthesis** and release, thus making placental gonadotropins responsible for gonadotropic function.

4. The **ability of the placenta to regulate molecular transport** by permitting or restricting passage and transfer of oxygen and nutrients from the mother to the fetus and metabolic wastes and carbon dioxide from the fetus to the mother

B. **Hormones that are significant during pregnancy** are understood best in terms of the following four characteristics:

1. **Chemical nature**
   a. Steroids (e.g., progesterone, estrogen, fetal adrenal steroids)
   b. Protein hormones (e.g., hCG, hPL, prolactin, α-fetoprotein [AFP])

2. **Source**
   a. The **placenta** is an important source of sex steroids and protein hormones, including hCG and hPL.
   b. The **mother** is the exclusive source of certain hormones early in pregnancy; however, as the pregnancy progresses, the fetus (after the first trimester) produces thyroid substances, pituitary tropic hormones, and gonadal steroids; and the placenta (at the end of the first trimester) secretes large quantities of progesterone along with many releasing and inhibiting hormones, including gonadotropin-releasing hormone (GnRH), corticotropin-releasing hormone (CRH), and thyrotropin-releasing hormone (TRH)

1

    c. Occasionally, there are **multiple sources of hormones;** for example, estriol is produced by the mother, the placenta, and the fetus.

  3. Normal patterns. Recognizing normal patterns of hormone activity during pregnancy can help to distinguish abnormal pregnancies and fetal compromise.

  4. Significance. Understanding the function of a particular hormone may illuminate its role in reproductive physiology, particularly in maintaining pregnancy and fetal well-being; for example, hormone deficiencies that are deleterious to the pregnancy can be corrected by exogenous hormones, and the presence of certain hormones may serve as markers for gestational abnormalities.

    a. High levels of hCG suggest a trophoblastic neoplastic disease because hCG originates in trophoblastic tissue.

    b. Progesterone deficiency early in pregnancy suggests corpus luteum insufficiency because progesterone is produced by the corpus luteum in early pregnancy.

II. HUMAN CHORIONIC GONADOTROPIN (hCG)

A. **Chemical nature.** hCG is a glycoprotein composed of two side chains, the α- and β-subunits. This hormone has a molecular weight of approximately 35,000.

  1. The α-subunit is biochemically similar to:
    a. Luteinizing hormone (LH)
    b. Follicle-stimulating hormone (FSH)
    c. Thyroid-stimulating hormone (TSH)

  2. The β-subunit is relatively unique to hCG.

B. **Source.** hCG is an almost exclusive product of trophoblastic tissue, specifically the syncytiotrophoblast. hCG is produced by trophoblastic tissue in the following conditions.

  1. Normal placental tissue as early as 6 to 8 days postconception as shown by immunofluorescence

  2. Multiple placental development (multiple gestation)

  3. Hydatidiform moles by virtue of trophoblastic proliferation

  4. Choriocarcinoma cells

  5. Ectopic pregnancies

C. **Mode of determination.** hCG levels can be measured by biologic and immunologic assays and by radioreceptor assays on blood or urine. Immunologic assays are more specific and sensitive than are biologic assays and, thus, have replaced them for routine methods.

  1. Biologic assays are of historic note only; they are not used today because of the more specific and reliable immunologic tests.

    a. The **Friedman rabbit test** measures maternal hCG levels by its ability to cause ovulation in rabbits 12 hours after administration.

    b. The **male frog test** measures sperm release into the ejaculatory ducts in male frogs after administration of hCG.

    c. The **Aschheim-Zondek rat test** measures ovarian follicular development after exposure to hCG.

  2. Immunologic assays

    a. Agglutination, or the latex particle fixation test, determines hCG levels in urine. Several drops of the patient's urine are mixed with antibodies to hCG, then latex particles coated with hCG are added to the mixture. If hCG is in the urine, it binds the antibodies; if no hCG is present in the urine, the antibodies bind to the latex particles. This is a rapid assay and is positive in 95% of cases 28 days post-conception.

    b. Radioimmunoassay is used on blood specimens using antibodies to the β-sub-unit of hCG. It is positive 8 days postconception.

    c. Radioreceptor assay measures the amount of hCG in blood that competes with radiolabeled hCG for a given amount of receptor sites on bovine luteal cell membranes. It is a rapid assay, but it is not as specific as that of the hCG β-subunit radioimmunoassay.

D. Normal patterns

    1. hCG rises rapidly 8 days postconception, **doubling every 2 to 3 days** and reaching a peak at approximately 80 days, **then dropping** to a plateau for the remainder of pregnancy. hCG is detectable throughout pregnancy.

    2. hCG is increased in the presence of multiple gestation.

E. Significance

    1. hCG stimulates progesterone production by the corpus luteum. It maintains luteal function, which, in the absence of pregnancy, persists for approximately 14 days.

    2. hCG stimulates Leydig cells of the male fetus to produce testosterone in concert with fetal pituitary gonadotropins. It is, thus, involved indirectly in the development of fetal male external genitalia.

    3. hCG is used as a marker for pregnancy (pregnancy testing).
        a. Low values early in pregnancy suggest poor placental function and may predict abortion or ectopic pregnancy.
        b. Significantly high values suggest multiple gestation or trophoblastic neoplasia (e.g., hydatidiform mole and choriocarcinoma).

    4. hCG determinations are used to **follow the course of patients** treated for trophoblastic neoplasia.

    5. hCG is used clinically for induction of ovulation **to treat anovulation** based on its biologic similarities to that of LH.

    6. hCG has some **TSH-like activities.**

III. HUMAN PLACENTAL LACTOGEN (hPL)

A. Chemical nature.
hPL is a protein hormone with growth hormone and prolactin-like effects. Its molecular weight is 22,000.

B. Source.
hPL is formed by the placenta as early as 3 weeks postconception and can be detected in maternal serum as early as 6 weeks postconception. It is secreted by the syncytiotrophoblast and disappears promptly from the blood after delivery. It has a half-life of approximately 15 minutes.

C. Mode of determination.
hPL is measured by radioimmunoassay.

D. Normal patterns

    1. hPL can be detected in the serum of pregnant women as early as the sixth week of pregnancy. It rises steadily during the first and second trimesters, disappearing rapidly after delivery.

    2. hPL levels vary directly with fetal and placental weight; very high maternal levels are found in association with those of multiple gestations.

E. **Significance**

1. hPL, the "growth hormone" of the latter half of pregnancy, is a major force in the diabetogenic effects of pregnancy and has the following properties.
   a. It **induces lipolysis** and **elevates plasma free fatty acids,** which provide energy for the mother.
   b. It **induces insulin resistance** and **carbohydrate intolerance** in the mother.
   c. It **inhibits glucose uptake** and **gluconeogenesis** in the mother.
   d. It **has an insulinogenic action,** which elevates plasma insulin levels, favoring protein synthesis and ensuring a source of amino acids for the fetus.

2. hPL determinations have been used to **test placental function;** however, fetal heart rate monitoring techniques are more reliable and sensitive in assessing fetal well-being.

IV. PROLACTIN

A. **Chemical nature.** Prolactin is a protein hormone with a molecular weight of 22,000.

B. **Source.** Three potential sources of prolactin during pregnancy are the:

1. Anterior lobe of the maternal pituitary gland
2. Anterior lobe of the fetal pituitary gland
3. Decidual tissue of the uterus

C. **Mode of determination.** Prolactin is assayed by radioimmunoassay of blood or amniotic fluid.

D. **Normal patterns**

1. Prolactin levels in the normal nonpregnant female range between 8 and 25 ng/ml. Levels above this range are related to the following factors.
   a. Ingestion of certain drugs that elevate prolactin (e.g., phenothiazines)
   b. Hypothyroidism
   c. Pituitary adenomas
   d. Hypothalamic disease

2. During pregnancy, maternal prolactin levels rise to a maximum of 100 ng/ml near term as a result of increased maternal pituitary production.

3. Amniotic fluid levels of prolactin increase significantly during pregnancy. The source of amniotic fluid prolactin is neither the maternal nor the fetal pituitary gland but the uterine decidua.

E. **Significance**

1. Prolactin prepares the mammary glands for lactation.

2. Decidual prolactin is thought to be important for fluid and electrolyte regulation of the amniotic fluid.

3. Levels of prolactin in pregnancy should not be interpreted as indicative of pituitary adenoma growth. However, patients with prolactin-secreting adenomas who conceive should be monitored by visual field determinations for the possibility of enlargement.

V. α-FETOPROTEIN (AFP)

A. **Source.** A unique glycoprotein derived largely from the fetal liver and partially from the yolk sac.

1. In early pregnancy (5–12 weeks), amniotic fluid AFP is mainly from a yolk sac origin.

2. Maternal circulating AFP is mainly from the fetal liver.

3. Its function is unknown.

B. AFP is highly concentrated in the fetal central nervous system (CNS). Abnormal direct contact of CNS with the amniotic fluid (as with neural tube defects) results in elevated amniotic fluid and maternal blood levels.

C. Elevated levels also are seen with intestinal obstruction, omphalocele, congenital nephrosis, and multiple gestation.

VI. PROGESTERONE

A. **Chemical nature.** Progesterone is a Δ-4,3-ketosteroid hormone that contains 21 carbon atoms. It has two angular methyl groups at the 10 and 13 positions and a two-carbon side chain at the 17 position.

B. **Source**

1. **In the nonpregnant state,** progesterone is **produced by all steroid-forming glands,** including the ovaries, testes, and adrenal cortex. It serves as an intermediary and a precursor for other hormones (e.g., testosterone, corticosteroids, and 17-hydroxyl progesterone) and as an end-product when it is produced by the corpus luteum.

2. **In the pregnant state,** progesterone has a **dual source**—it is produced by the **corpus luteum** until the seventh to tenth week of pregnancy, after which the **placenta** assumes its production until parturition. This shift in production occurs at approximately the seventh week of pregnancy, and, by the ninth week, the corpus luteum becomes an insignificant source of progesterone. This point is clinically significant because progesterone produced by the corpus luteum is essential for pregnancy maintenance until the eighth week.

C. **Mode of determination**

1. Progesterone can be measured in the blood by **radioimmunoassay and competitive protein-binding assay.** There does not seem to be diurnal variation in blood levels.

2. Some laboratories may measure **pregnanediol,** the major metabolite of progesterone, by 24-hour analysis (full-day specimens), using **chromatographic techniques** after extraction; however, this assay is used infrequently today.

D. **Normal patterns**

1. Because progesterone originates initially from the corpus luteum, it is present at ovulation. In a nonconception cycle, the peak production of progesterone reaches 25 mg/day, and levels measure approximately 20 to 25 ng/ml in peripheral blood.

2. In the late luteal phase in a conception cycle, progesterone levels increase slowly as a result of hCG stimulation.

3. As a placental progesterone supplements corpus luteum progesterone, levels increase more rapidly.

4. A transient decline in peripheral blood progesterone levels has been described in the seventh to eighth weeks of pregnancy, the time of the luteoplacental shift; however, this subtle change can be appreciated only when daily measurements are made.

5. Progesterone concentrations in the blood continue to increase up until the time of parturition, at which time the placenta produces 250 mg/day; most of the progesterone produced enters the maternal circulation.

6. Progesterone is produced in large quantities in the presence of multiple gestation.

E. **Significance.** Progesterone has all of the following properties.

1. It **prepares the endometrium for nidation.**

2. It **maintains the endometrium.**

3. It **relaxes the myometrium.**

4. It is thought to be **instrumental in preventing the uterus from contracting,** and interference with its production or action on the myometrium is thought to result in the onset of parturition.

5. It has **natriuretic actions** and, thus, stimulates the increased production of aldosterone during pregnancy.

6. It serves as a major **precursor for critical fetal hormones** during pregnancy.
   a. The fetus has a relative deficiency in 3-β-hydroxysteroid dehydrogenase, which, as stated in I A 3 b, is an enzyme necessary to convert steroids to a Δ-4,3-keto-steroid configuration.
   b. Placental progesterone is, thus, used by the fetal adrenal cortex as a precursor for corticosteroids and by the testes as a precursor for testosterone.

VII. ESTROGENS

A. **Chemical nature**

1. Estrogens are phenolic 18-carbon steroids characterized by an aromatic A ring. Estrogens lack an angular methyl group at the 10 position.

2. There are three classic estrogens, which differ by the number of hydroxyl groups they contain.
   a. **Estrone,** a relatively weak estrogen, has one hydroxyl group at the 3 position.
   b. **Estradiol,** the most potent estrogen, contains two hydroxyl groups at positions 3 and 17.
   c. **Estriol,** a very weak estrogen, contains three hydroxyl groups at positions 3, 16, and 17. Estriol is produced in very large quantities during pregnancy (1000 times more than in the nonpregnant state). More estriol is produced than all of the other estrogens.

B. **Source**

1. **Production of estriol.** Estriol accounts for 90% of the estrogens produced during pregnancy. Its synthesis involves integration of metabolic steps in the mother, the placenta, and the fetus; is complex; and is dependent on **two important biochemical principles.**
   a. Ample levels of precursor are necessary to produce a specific steroid.
   b. Tissues involved in converting a precursor to a specific steroid must possess the appropriate enzymes to carry out the conversion.
      (1) The fetus is able to produce the following enzymes, which cannot be produced by the placenta.
         (a) Cholesterol-synthesizing enzyme
         (b) 16-hydroxylase
         (c) Sulfokinase
      (2) The placenta is able to produce the following enzymes, which cannot be produced by the fetus.
         (a) Sulfatase
         (b) 3-β-hydroxysteroid dehydrogenase
      (3) The placenta, unlike the fetus and the mother, is virtually unable to manufacture cholesterol.

2. **Steps in estriol synthesis** are as follows.
   a. **Cholesterol,** mainly of maternal origin, is converted by the placenta to pregnenolone and then to progesterone.
   b. **Placental pregnenolone** enters the fetal circulation where, together with pregnenolone synthesized by the fetal adrenal glands, it is converted in part to pregnenolone sulfate.
   c. **Pregnenolone sulfate** is converted by the fetal adrenals to $DHEASO_4$, the most important precursor of placental estrone and estradiol. Estrone and estradiol are produced in the placenta from $DHEASO_4$ by reactions involving hydrolysis of the sulfate, conversion of dehydroepiandrosterone (DHEA) to androstenedione, and aromatization.
   d. **$DHEASO_4$,** formed by the fetal adrenal glands, is converted to 16-α-hydroxy $DHEASO_4$ mainly in the fetal liver.
   e. **16-α-hydroxy $DHEASO_4$** is converted by two steps to estriol by the placenta.
      (1) **Sulfatase activity,** which removes the sulfate radical
      (2) **Aromatase activity,** which converts the A ring to the phenolic structure characteristic of estrogens
   f. The **estriol molecule** enters the maternal circulation.

C. **Mode of determination.** Estriol is measured by radioimmunoassay of peripheral blood specimens. Although results can be obtained rapidly (i.e., there is no 24-hour delay from onset of collection to onset of assay), there is a distinct diurnal variation, with levels peaking early in the morning.

D. **Normal patterns**

1. **Significant amounts** of estriol are produced early in the second trimester, and levels continue to rise until parturition, increasing 1000-fold over the nonpregnant levels.

2. **Extremely low levels or no estriol** may be associated with:
   a. Fetal demise
   b. Anencephaly
   c. Maternal ingestion of corticosteroids
   d. Congenital adrenal hypoplasia
   e. Placental sulfatase deficiency

3. **The decline in estriol production or the failure of estriol levels to increase** may be because of:
   a. Maternal renal disease
   b. Hypertensive disease during pregnancy
   c. Preeclampsia and eclampsia
   d. Intrauterine growth retardation

E. **Significance**

1. Estriol is an **index of normal function of the fetus.**

2. Estriol is an **index of normal placental function.**

3. When estriol levels are reduced below normal or fail to increase during pregnancy, fetal and placental well-being should be studied by supplemental tests, including ultrasonography, fetal heart rate testing, and biophysical profile.

▌ STUDY QUESTIONS

DIRECTIONS: The numbered item in this section is followed by answers or by completions of the statement. Select the ONE lettered answer or completion that is BEST.

1. The source of α-fetoprotein (AFP) in maternal blood at 18 weeks' gestation is which of the following?

(A) Fetal adrenal glands
(B) Placenta
(C) Yolk sac
(D) Fetal liver
(E) Maternal liver

DIRECTIONS: Each of the numbered items or incomplete statements in this section is negatively phrased, as indicated by a capitalized word such as NOT, LEAST, or EXCEPT. Select the ONE lettered answer or completion that is BEST in each case.

2. Which of the following hormones is NOT a product of placental synthesis or production?

(A) Human chorionic gonadotropin (hCG)
(B) Human placental lactogen (hPL)
(C) Prolactin
(D) Progesterone
(E) Estriol

3. Which is NOT a characteristic of human placental lactogen, the growth hormone of pregnancy?

(A) It elevates free fatty acids
(B) It elevates plasma insulin levels
(C) It induces lipolysis
(D) It inhibits gluconeogenesis in the mother
(E) It stimulates glucose uptake in the mother

4. Which of the following is NOT a characteristic of progesterone?

(A) It is an intermediary product in steroid metabolism
(B) It contains 21 carbon atoms
(C) Its main source during early pregnancy is the corpus luteum of pregnancy
(D) It is a precursor of testosterone
(E) Its ovarian source is important after the first 9 weeks of pregnancy

DIRECTIONS: The set of matching questions in this section consists of a list of lettered options (some of which may be in figures) followed by several numbered items. For each numbered item, select the ONE lettered option that is most closely associated with it. To avoid spending too much time on matching sets with large numbers of options, it is generally advisable to begin each set by reading the list of options. Then, for each item in the set, try to generate the correct answer and locate it in the option list, rather than evaluating each option individually. Each lettered option may be selected once, more than once, or not at all.

Questions 5–8

Match each major action of hormones in pregnancy with the appropriate placental hormone.

(A) Human chorionic gonadotropin (hCG)
(B) Prolactin
(C) Human placental lactogen (hPL)
(D) Progesterone
(E) Estriol

5. Pregnancy maintenance

6. Diagnosis of pregnancy

7. Index of health of the maternal-fetal-placental unit

8. Regulation of carbohydrate and protein metabolism

ANSWERS AND EXPLANATIONS

1. The answer is D [V A 1–2]. α-Fetoprotein (AFP) is derived totally from the fetus. It is derived mainly from the fetal liver, especially after the first trimester. There is a small contribution of AFP from the yolk sac in the first 5 to 12 weeks of pregnancy. The fetal adrenal glands are not involved in the secretion of AFP.

2. The answer is C [IV B 1–3]. Human chorionic gonadotropin (hCG) and human placental lactogen (hPL) are manufactured totally by the placenta during pregnancy. hCG appears early and declines to low levels after the first trimester; hPL rises during the first and second trimesters and declines rapidly after delivery. During pregnancy, progesterone is produced in large quantities by the placenta after the ninth week; before that time, progesterone is produced by the corpus luteum of pregnancy. Estriol synthesis is a complex process that involves the mother, the placenta, and the fetus; the placenta does not have all the enzymes necessary to synthesize estrogen and depends on the fetus for some of the intermediate metabolites. Prolactin is not produced by the placenta; for the most part, it is a product of the anterior lobe of both the maternal and fetal pituitary glands.

3. The answer is E [III E 1 a–c]. Human placental lactogen (hPL) induces changes in the maternal physiology that encourage growth of the fetus. It induces lipolysis, elevating free fatty acids, which provide energy for the mother. It elevates plasma insulin levels, which favor protein synthesis, ensuring a source of amino acids for the fetus. And, it inhibits gluconeogenesis and glucose uptake in the mother, which allows for the transfer of materials to the fetus, thus contributing to fetal growth.

4. The answer is E [VI A, B]. Progesterone, a steroid hormone that contains 21 carbon atoms, is produced in all steroid-forming glands and serves as an intermediary and a precursor for other steroid hormones, such as testosterone and the corticosteroids. The main source of progesterone during the first 6 to 7 weeks of pregnancy is the corpus luteum of pregnancy; this structure ensures adequate progesterone for implantation and maintenance of the early pregnancy. The placenta is the main source of progesterone during the major part (9–40 weeks) of pregnancy.

5–8. The answers are: 5-D [VI B 2], **6-A** [II E 3], **7-E** [VII B, E], **8-C** [III E]. Progesterone in pregnancy promotes the development and maintenance of the decidua, which is the endocrine and structural support for the pregnancy. Human chorionic gonadotropin (hCG) is secreted from the trophoblastic tissue. It is the basis for the biochemical detection of pregnancy. Before the placenta is developed, hCG stimulates the corpus luteum to continue to produce progesterone until the placenta can assume that role for the pregnancy. hCG also stimulates the Leydig cells in the fetal testis to produce testosterone and, thus, is involved indirectly with the development of the external genitalia of the male fetus. It is an excellent marker to observe the regression or recurrence of trophoblastic disease, because the hormone is secreted by choriocarcinomas and hydatidiform moles. The increase in estrogens in the pregnancy, particularly in the third trimester, is 1000-fold more than in the nonpregnant state. The placenta cannot synthesize estrogens independently of the mother and fetus. A fetus must be healthy with an intact circulation and the placenta must be viable to produce this steroid. The estriol precursors are produced by the maternal liver and fetal adrenal glands. Consequently, normal levels of estriol reflect the health of the maternal-fetal-placental unit. Human placental lactogen (hPL) is a "growth hormone." It regulates carbohydrate and protein metabolism, which are determinants of growth, in the placental–fetal unit. It is synthesized solely by the placenta and exhibits lactogenic and luteotrophic activities as well.

Chapter 2

Normal Pregnancy, the Puerperium, and Lactation
William W. Beck, Jr.

I. DIAGNOSIS OF PREGNANCY

A. Presumptive symptoms

1. **Cessation of menses.** The abrupt cessation of spontaneous, cyclic, and predictable menstruation is strongly suggestive of pregnancy. Because ovulation can be late in any given cycle, the menses should be **at least 10 days late** before their absence is considered a reliable indication.

2. **Breast changes.** In very early pregnancy, women report tenderness and tingling in the breasts. Breast enlargement and nodularity are evident as early as the second month of pregnancy. The nipples and areolae enlarge and become more deeply pigmented.

3. **Nausea (with or without vomiting). Morning sickness of pregnancy** usually begins early in the day and lasts for several hours. Gastrointestinal disturbances begin at 4 to 6 weeks' gestation and usually last no longer than the first trimester. Excessive nausea and vomiting (i.e., **hyperemesis gravidarum**) can result in dehydration, weight loss, electrolyte imbalance, and the need for hospitalization; intravenous hyperalimentation may be indicated in severe cases.

4. **Disturbances in urination.** Early in pregnancy, the enlarging uterus puts pressure on the bladder, causing **frequent urination.** This condition improves as the uterus grows and moves up into the abdomen but returns late in pregnancy when the fetal head settles into the pelvis against the bladder.

5. **Fatigue.** Tiredness is one of the earliest symptoms of pregnancy. Fatigue usually persists into the second trimester, with the woman getting back to normal by the sixteenth to eighteenth week.

6. **Sensation of fetal movement.** Between the sixteenth and twentieth week after the last menstrual period (LMP), a woman begins to feel movement in the lower abdomen, described as a fluttering or gas bubbles. This is known as quickening.

B. Clinical evidence

1. **Enlargement of the abdomen.** By the end of the twelfth week of pregnancy, the uterus can be felt above the symphysis pubis. By the twentieth week, the uterus should be at the level of the umbilicus.

2. **Uterine and cervical changes.** The uterus enlarges and softens early in pregnancy (at approximately 6 weeks' gestation), and lateral uterine vessel pulsations are palpable by vaginal examination. Because of the softening between the cervix and the uterine fundus, there is the sensation that these are two separate structures (**Hegar's sign**). The cervix has a bluish color within the first 6 to 8 weeks of pregnancy (**Chadwick's sign**).

3. **Endocrine tests for pregnancy** depend on **human chorionic gonadotropin (hCG)** levels in maternal plasma and excretion of hCG in the urine, which are identified by a number of immunoassays and bioassays.

   a. **Urine pregnancy tests** detect the presence of hCG. This is dependent on the recognition of hCG or its β-subunit by an antibody to the hCG molecule or the β-subunit.

   b. **Serum pregnancy tests** quantify the β-subunit of hCG, thus providing greater sensitivity than the urine tests and allowing serial determinations to observe increases and decreases in the level of hCG.

C. **Confirming the diagnosis of pregnancy**

1. **Identification of a heart beat.** The diagnosis of pregnancy is confirmed with the identification of the fetal heart beat, which ranges from 120 to 160 beats per minute. The fetal heart can be identified at 12 to 14 weeks by an ultrasound fetal heart monitor and at 17 to 19 weeks by auscultation with a stethoscope.

2. **Ultrasonographic recognition of the fetus.** The small, white gestational ring can be seen by vaginal ultrasound probes after 5 weeks of amenorrhea and by abdominal ultrasound after 6 weeks of amenorrhea. The embryo can be shown within the gestational ring after 8 weeks of amenorrhea. Fetal heart action is seen by real-time ultrasonography after 7 to 8 weeks of gestation.

D. **Pregnancy dating.** The estimated date of delivery (EDD), or due date, is based on the assumption that a woman has a 28-day cycle, with ovulation on day 14 or 15. Pregnancy lasts for 280 days (40 weeks) from the LMP. The EDD is therefore 9 months plus 7 days from the start of the LMP (Naegele's rule). Because ovulation does not always occur at midcycle (the postovulatory phase in any cycle lasts for 14 days), the EDD must be adjusted accordingly. For example, ovulation in a woman with a 35-day cycle occurs on approximately day 21; therefore, the EDD in such a woman must be pushed back 1 week.

II. PREGNANCY

A. **The first trimester** extends from the LMP through the first 12 to 13 weeks of pregnancy.

1. **Signs and symptoms**
   a. Nausea
   b. Fatigue
   c. Breast tenderness
   d. Frequent urination
   e. Minimal abdominal enlargement (the uterus is still in the pelvis)

2. Bleeding occurs in the first trimester of approximately 25% of all pregnancies; spontaneous abortion occurs in half of these pregnancies, and the other half continue without problems. Uterine cramping with bleeding in the first trimester is more suggestive of impending abortion than is either bleeding or cramping alone.

B. **The second trimester** extends from 14 weeks of pregnancy through 27 weeks of pregnancy.

1. **Signs and symptoms**
   a. **General well-being.** The second trimester is often the most comfortable time for a pregnant woman because the symptoms of the first trimester are gone, and the discomfort of the last trimester is not yet present.
   b. **Pain.** As the uterus grows, there is a certain amount of pulling and stretching of pelvic structures. Round ligament pain, which results from the stretching of the round ligaments that are attached to the top of the uterus on each side and the corresponding lateral pelvic wall, is very common. Round ligament pain usually does not last past 22 weeks.
   c. **Contractions.** Palpable uterine contractions (**Braxton Hicks contractions**) that are painless and irregular can begin during the second trimester.

2. **Bleeding.** A low-lying placenta that causes bleeding at this stage usually moves away from the cervix as the uterus grows.

3. **Fetus.** The fetus attains a size of almost 1000 g (more than 2 lbs) by the twenty-eighth week.
   a. **Motion.** Quickening (see I A 6) begins between the sixteenth and twentieth week.
   b. **Viability.** There is an 80% to 90% chance of survival for infants born at the end

of the second trimester. If death occurs, it is usually from respiratory distress due to lung immaturity.

4. **Complications of second-trimester pregnancies** include an incompetent cervix (i.e., the premature dilation of the cervix in the second trimester), which can result in either premature labor or rupture of the membranes.
   a. **Premature rupture of the membranes** can occur without labor or an incompetent cervix and can result in serious bacterial infections in both the mother and fetus.
   b. **Premature labor** can occur without an incompetent cervix. When dilation or effacement of the cervix occurs, tocolytic agents are necessary to prevent delivery.

C. **The third trimester** extends from 28 weeks of pregnancy until term, or 40 weeks' gestation.

1. **Symptoms**
   a. **Braxton Hicks contractions** (see II B 1 c) become more apparent in the third trimester.
   b. **Pain in the lower back and legs** is often caused by pressure on muscles and nerves by the uterus and fetal head, which fills the pelvis at this time.
   c. **Lightening** is the descent of the fetal head to or even through the pelvic inlet due to the development of a well-formed lower uterine segment and a reduction in the volume of amniotic fluid.

2. **Fetus**
   a. **Weight.** The fetus gains weight at a rate of approximately 224 g (0.5 lb) per week for the last 4 weeks and weighs an average of 3300 g (7.0–7.5 lbs) at term.
   b. **Motion.** A decrease in fetal motion is usually because of the size of the fetus and lack of room within the uterus. However, some decreased fetal activity may be an indication of fetal compromise due to uteroplacental insufficiency.

3. **Bleeding**
   a. **Bloody show,** a discharge of a combination of blood and mucus caused by thinning and stretching of the cervix, is a sure sign of the approach of labor.
   b. **Heavy bleeding** suggests a more serious condition, such as **placenta previa** (the placenta developing in the lower uterine segment and completely or partially covering the internal os) or abruptio placentae (premature separation of the normally implanted placenta).

4. **Rupture of membranes** is either a sudden gush or a slow leak of amniotic fluid that can happen at any time without warning.
   a. **Brownish or greenish fluid** may represent meconium staining of the fluid, the sign of a **fetal bowel movement** that may or may not represent fetal stress.
   b. **Labor** usually begins within 24 hours after rupture of membranes.
   c. **Induction of labor** is indicated if there is no labor within 48 hours of rupture or if there is any evidence of infection (**chorioamnionitis**).

5. **Labor.** Contractions that occur at decreasing intervals with increasing intensity cause the progressive dilation and effacement of the cervix.

III. STATUS OF THE FETUS

A. **Growth and development**

1. **Weight.** A normal fetus weighs approximately 1000 g (more than 2 lbs) at 26 to 28 weeks, 2500 g (5.5 lbs) at 36 weeks, and 3300 g (7.0–7.5 lbs) at 40 weeks.

2. **Lung maturity**
   a. Normal fetal lung maturity is indicated by measuring **surface-active lipid components of surfactant (i.e., lecithin and phosphatidyglycerol),** which are secreted by the **type II pneumocytes of fetal lung alveoli** and which are essential for normal

respiration immediately after birth. These measurements are made by laboratory examination of amniotic fluid.

    b. Lecithin to sphingomyelin (L/S) ratio. Studies have shown that when the level of lecithin in amniotic fluid increases to at least twice that of sphingomyelin (at approximately 35 weeks), the risk of respiratory distress is very low.

    c. Phosphatidylglycerol. The presence of phosphatidylglycerol in the amniotic fluid has been shown to provide even more definite assurance of lung maturity.

    d. Respiratory distress syndrome. Infants born before phosphatidylglycerol appears in surfactant, even with an L/S ratio of 2:1, may be at risk for respiratory distress syndrome.

    e. Early fetal lung maturation (from 32 to 35 weeks) is seen with maternal hypertension, premature rupture of membranes, and intrauterine growth retardation, all of which are stressful to the fetus. This stress, before 35 weeks, increases **fetal cortisol secretion,** which, in turn, accelerates fetal lung maturation.

    f. Administration of glucocorticoids to mothers between the twenty-ninth and thirty-third week of pregnancy effects an increase in the rate of maturation of the human fetal lung and is associated with a reduced rate of respiratory distress in their prematurely born infants.

B. **Lie of the fetus** is the relation of the long axis of the fetus to the long axis of the mother and is either longitudinal or transverse.

    1. Longitudinal lie. In most labors (more than 99%) at term, the fetal head either is up or down in a longitudinal lie.

    2. Transverse lie. The fetus is crosswise in the uterus in a transverse lie.

    3. Oblique lie. This indicates an unstable situation that becomes either a longitudinal or transverse lie during the course of labor.

C. **Fetal presentation** is determined by the portion of the fetus that can be felt through the cervix.

    1. Cephalic presentations are classified according to the position of the fetal head in relation to the body of the fetus.

    a. Vertex. The head is flexed so that the chin is in contact with the chest, and the occiput of the fetal head presents. A vertex presentation occurs in 95% of all cephalic presentations.

    b. Face. The neck is extended sharply so that the occiput and the back of the fetus are touching, and the face is the presenting part.

    c. Brow. The fetal head is extended partially but converts into a vertex or face presentation during labor.

    2. Breech presentations are classified according to the position of the legs and buttocks, which present first. Breech presentations occur in 3.5% of all pregnancies.

    a. In a frank breech, the thighs are flexed, and the legs are extended.

    b. In a complete breech, the legs are flexed on the thighs, and the thighs are flexed on the abdomen.

    c. In a footling breech, one or both feet or knees present.

IV. **THE PUERPERIUM.** is a period of 4 to 6 weeks that starts immediately after delivery and is completed when the reproductive tract has returned to its nonpregnant condition.

A. **Involution of the uterus.** The uterus regains its usual nonpregnant size within 5 to 6 weeks, shrinking from 1000 g immediately postpartum to 100 g. This rapid atrophy is because of the marked decrease in size of the muscle cells rather than the decrease in their total number. Breast-feeding (nursing) accelerates involution of the uterus because stimulation of the nipples releases oxytocin from the neurohypophysis; the resulting contractions of the myometrium facilitate the involution of the uterus.

1. **Afterpains.** The uterus contracts throughout the period of involution, which produces afterpains, especially in multiparous women and nursing mothers. In primiparous women, the uterus tends to remain contracted tonically, whereas in multiparous women, the uterus contracts vigorously at intervals.

2. **Lochia** is the uterine discharge that follows delivery and lasts for 3 or 4 weeks. Foul-smelling lochia suggests infection.
   a. **Lochia rubra** is blood-stained fluid that lasts for the first few days.
   b. **Lochia serosa** appears 3 to 4 days after delivery; it is paler than lochia rubra because it is admixed with serum.
   c. **Lochia alba.** After the tenth day, because of an admixture with leukocytes, the lochia assumes a white or yellow-white color.

B. **Clinical aspects**

1. **Urine.** The puerperal bladder has an increased capacity and a relative insensitivity to intravesical fluid pressure.
   a. **Incomplete emptying,** resulting in excessive residual urine, and overdistension may facilitate the occurrence of a postpartum urinary tract infection.
   b. **Diuresis** usually occurs between the second and fifth postpartum day.

2. **Blood.** A marked **leukocytosis** occurs during and after labor. The leukocytosis, primarily a granulocytosis, may be as high as 30,000/mm³.
   a. By 1 week postpartum, the increased blood volume of pregnancy returns to the usual nonpregnant level.
   b. Pregnancy-induced changes in **blood coagulation factors** persist for variable periods of time after delivery. The elevated plasma fibrinogen level is maintained at least through the first week of the puerperium. The gradual decline of the increased blood coagulation factors explains the occurrence of phlebitis of the lower extremities, which is more common in the puerperium than during pregnancy.

3. **Menstruation**
   a. **Nonlactating women.** The first menstrual flow usually returns within 6 to 8 weeks after delivery, with ovulation occurring at 2 to 4 weeks postpartum.
   b. **Lactating women.** Ovulation has been detected as early as 10 weeks postpartum, so nursing mothers must understand that the contraception afforded by lactation lasts absolutely for only 8 to 9 weeks, after which ovulation and pregnancy are possible.

C. **Postpartum hemorrhage** is defined as a blood loss in excess of 500 ml during the first 24 hours after delivery.

1. **Causes**
   a. **Trauma to the genital tract** as a result of:
      (1) Episiotomy
      (2) Lacerations of the cervix, vagina, or perineum
      (3) Rupture of the uterus
   b. **Failure of compression of blood vessels at the implantation site** of the placenta as a result of:
      (1) **A hypotonic myometrium** due to general anesthesia; overdistension of the uterus from a large fetus, hydramnios (excess amniotic fluid), or multiple fetuses; prolonged labor; very rapid labor; high parity; or a labor vigorously stimulated with oxytocin
      (2) **Retention of placental tissue,** as seen in placenta accreta, a succenturiate placental lobe, or a fragmented placenta
   c. **Coagulation defects,** either congenital or acquired, as seen in hypofibrinogenemia or thrombocytopenia

2. **Management** includes:
   a. **Vigorous massage** of the uterine fundus
   b. **Use of uterine contracting agents,** such as intramuscular or intravenous ergono-

vine (0.2 mg), intravenous oxytocin (20 U in 1000 ml of lactated Ringer's solution), or intramuscular or intramyometrial prostaglandin (75 mg)

   c. Manual exploration of the uterine cavity for retained placental fragments or uterine rupture

   d. Inspection of the cervix and vagina for lacerations

   e. Curettage of the uterine cavity

   f. Hypogastric artery **ligation, embolization** of the uterine vessels, and, rarely, **hysterectomy**

D. Puerperal infection is defined as any infection of the genital tract during the puerperium accompanied by a temperature of **100.4°F (38°C) or higher** that occurs for at least 2 of the first 10 days postpartum, **exclusive of the first 24 hours.** Prolonged rupture of the membranes accompanied by multiple vaginal examinations during labor is a major predisposing cause of puerperal infection.

  1. Pelvic infections

    a. Endometritis (childbed fever), the most common form of puerperal infection, involves primarily the endometrium and the adjacent myometrium.

    b. Parametritis, infection of the retroperitoneal fibroareolar pelvic connective tissue, may occur by:

      (1) Lymphatic transmission of organisms

      (2) Cervical lacerations that extend into the connective tissue

      (3) Extension of pelvic thrombophlebitis

    c. Thrombophlebitis results from an extension of puerperal infection along pelvic veins.

  2. Urinary tract infections are quite common during the puerperium as a result of:

    a. Trauma to the bladder from a normal vaginal delivery

    b. A **hypotonic bladder** from conduction anesthesia

    c. Catheterization

  3. Management begins with taking a culture of the urine, endometrial cavity tissue, and blood and determining the sensitivity of each.

    a. Antibiotics should be administered according to the sensitivity of the infecting organism to the drug. Broad-spectrum antibiotics, which include anaerobic coverage, are recommended for those pelvic infections in which identification of the offending organism is impossible. **Common organisms include:**

      (1) Aerobic (group B *Streptococcus, Enterococcus,* and *Escherichia coli*)

      (2) Anaerobic (*Peptococcus, Peptostreptococcus, Bacteroides,* and *Clostridium*)

    b. Heparin should be administered when thrombophlebitis is suspected and a spiking temperature does not respond to intravenous antibiotics.

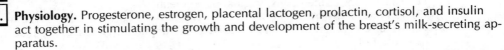

V. LACTATION

A. Physiology. Progesterone, estrogen, placental lactogen, prolactin, cortisol, and insulin act together in stimulating the growth and development of the breast's milk-secreting apparatus.

  1. Prolactin, which is released from the anterior pituitary gland, stimulates milk production.

    a. Initiation of lactation. The delivery of the placenta causes a sharp decrease in the levels of estrogens and progesterone, which, in turn, leads to the release of prolactin and the consequent stimulation of milk production.

    b. Continued prolactin production. A stimulus from the breast (i.e., a suckling infant) curtails the release of prolactin-inhibiting factor from the hypothalamus, thus inducing a transiently increased secretion of prolactin.

  2. Oxytocin is responsible for the **let-down reflex** and the subsequent release of breast milk. Stimulation of the nipples during nursing causes oxytocin to be released from the posterior pituitary gland.

B. **Nursing.** Breast milk is ideal for the newborn because it provides a balanced diet. It contains protective maternal antibodies, and the maternal lymphocytes in breast milk may be important to the infant's immunologic processes. Most drugs given to the mother are secreted in low concentrations in the breast milk. Water-soluble drugs are excreted in high concentrations into colostrum, whereas lipid-soluble drugs are excreted in high concentrations into breast milk.

C. **Mastitis** is parenchymatous inflammation of the mammary glands that can present at some point after lactation has begun.

1. **Symptoms.** Engorgement of the breasts is accompanied by a temperature increase, chills, and a hard, red tender area on the breast.

2. **Etiology.** The most common offending organism is *Staphylococcus aureus* from the infant's nose and throat, which usually enters the breast through the nipple at the site of a fissure or abrasion during nursing.

3. **Therapy**
   a. **Gram-positive antibiotic coverage** (e.g., penicillin, ampicillin) is recommended; erythromycin is recommended for penicillin-resistant organisms.
   b. **Heat** should be applied to the breast.
   c. **Nursing** from the affected breast should continue to decrease engorgement.
   d. **The abscess should be drained** if the mastitis has progressed to suppuration.

4. **Prevention.** The use of an emollient cream is recommended to help prevent cracking of the nipple.

STUDY QUESTIONS

1. A complete breech presentation is best described by which of the following statements?

(A) The legs and thighs of the fetus are flexed
(B) The legs are extended, and the thighs are flexed
(C) The arms, legs, and thighs are flexed completely
(D) The legs and thighs are extended
(E) None of the above

2. Which of the following statements about birth control after delivery is correct?

(A) It is not important until after the first menses
(B) It is not necessary in a woman who is nursing
(C) It should begin immediately in a nonlactating woman
(D) It is not necessary for 1 month after a cesarean section

3. Fetal lung maturation is ensured by the presence of

(A) lecithin
(B) prostaglandin
(C) sphingomyelin
(D) phosphatidylglycerol
(E) cortisol

4. A woman reports to the physician's office on June 12, 1995, with a positive pregnancy test. She reports regular 35-day cycles and a last menstrual period that began on April 1, 1995, and ended April 4, 1995. Her estimated due date is

(A) January 1, 1996
(B) January 8, 1996
(C) January 15, 1996
(D) January 22, 1996
(E) January 29, 1996

5. Which of the following signs or symptoms are NOT present in a 12-week pregnancy?

(A) Chadwick's sign
(B) Quickening
(C) Ultrasonographic fetal heart action
(D) Amenorrhea
(E) Hegar's sign

6. Which of the following complications is NOT characteristic of the second trimester of pregnancy?

(A) Premature labor
(B) Cervical incompetence
(C) Premature rupture of membranes
(D) Abruptio placentae
(E) Round ligament pain

7. Which of the following is NOT a characteristic of a 28-week pregnancy?

(A) Viability
(B) A fetal weight of 1000 g (over 2 lbs)
(C) Lecithin to sphingomyelin (L/S) ratio of
less than 2:1
(D) The absence of type II fetal lung alveoli
cells
(E) the presence of phosphatidylglycerol

DIRECTIONS: The set of matching questions in this section consists of a list of lettered
options (some of which may be in figures) followed by several numbered items. For each
numbered item, select the ONE lettered option that is most closely associated with it. To
avoid spending too much time on matching sets with large numbers of options, it is
generally advisable to begin each set by reading the list of options. Then, for each item in
the set, try to generate the correct answer and locate it in the option list, rather than
evaluating each option individually. Each lettered option may be selected once, more than
once, or not at all.

Questions 8–11

For each of the following postpartum conditions, select the substance that is released during or is responsible for the event.

(A) Estrogen
(B) Progesterone
(C) Oxytocin
(D) Prostaglandin
(E) Prolactin

8. Let-down reflex

9. Delivery of the placenta

10. Initiation of lactation

11. Involution of the uterus

ANSWERS AND EXPLANATIONS

1. The answer is A [III C 2]. In a complete breech presentation of the fetus, the legs are flexed on the thighs, and the thighs are flexed on the abdomen. In a frank breech, the legs are extended, and in a footling breech, both the thighs and the legs are extended. The arms have nothing to do with the description of a breech presentation.

2. The answer is C [IV B 3]. Because a nonlactating woman can ovulate as early as 2 to 4 weeks postpartum, she must use birth control with her first coitus, which is usually permitted 4 weeks postpartum. Ovulation after delivery can occur at 10 to 12 weeks in a lactating woman. A woman should not delay birth control until after the first menses, because ovulation may have occurred by then. The method of delivery does not influence ovulation.

3. The answer is D [III A 2 a–e]. The presence of phosphatidylglycerol in the amniotic fluid is assurance of lung maturity. Fetal lung maturity is assessed by measuring the surface active lipids (i.e., lecithin and phosphatidylglycerol), which are secreted by fetal lung alveoli. For example, the lecithin to sphingomyelin (L/S) ratio usually measures 2:1 at 35 to 36 weeks' gestation. However, lecithin and sphingomyelin are present in both immature and mature fetal lungs, so neither by itself is an assurance of lung maturity. Prostaglandin is involved with the initiation of labor and has nothing to do with fetal lung maturity. Cortisol accelerates fetal lung maturation but is not measured as a test of lung maturity.

4. The answer is C [I D]. The calculated due date of 9 months plus 7 days from the last menstrual period is based on the assumption that a woman has 28-day cycles with ovulation on day 14. The calculation is made from the first day of the last menstrual period, assuming that a woman ovulates 14 days before her menses. In a 35-day cycle, ovulation occurs on about day 21 instead of day 14. Thus, 7 days must be added to the regular calculation, making the due date of this patient January 15, 1996.

5. The answer is B [I A 1, 6, B 2, C 2]. Quickening, the woman's sensation of fetal movement, occurs sometime between 16 and 20 weeks of pregnancy and, therefore, is not present in a 12-week pregnancy. Chadwick's and Hegar's signs occur as early as 6 weeks' gestation and are associated with changes in the cervix and the lower uterine segment. Real-time ultrasonographic fetal heart action can be seen at approximately 7 to 8 weeks. Amenorrhea is an ongoing sign of pregnancy.

6. The answer is D [II B 1 b, 4, C 3 b]. Abruptio placentae (i.e., premature separation of a normally implanted placenta) rarely occurs before 28 weeks' gestation, making it atypical in a second-trimester pregnancy. Because the viability occurs by 28 weeks' gestation, it is possible to salvage the fetus from this emergency situation. Although cervical incompetence, premature labor, premature rupture of membranes, and round ligament pain all may occur in the second trimester, cervical incompetence is more serious than the others. Not only can each of these complications occur separately, but cervical incompetence also may be accompanied by premature labor or premature rupture of the membranes, or both. Round ligament pain occurs between 16 and 22 weeks' gestation.

7. The answer is E [II B 3 b; III A 1, 2]. At 28 weeks' gestation, the normal fetal weight is approximately 1000 g, which is a little more than 2 lbs. There is an 80% to 90% survival rate of infants born at the beginning of the third trimester. Because of fetal lung immaturity, one would expect a lecithin to sphingomyelin (L/S) ratio of 1:1 or lower and an absence of type II fetal lung alveoli cells, which secrete increasing quantities of lecithin and phosphatidylglycerol at 35 to 36 weeks. Therefore, the presence of phosphatidylglycerol would not be expected at 28 weeks' gestation.

8–11. The answers are: 8-C [V A 2], **9-E** [V A 1 a], **10-E** [V A 1 a], **11-C** [IV A]. Stimulation of the nipples during breast-feeding causes the release of oxytocin and the release of milk (i.e., the let-down reflex) from the breast. The delivery of the placenta causes a sharp drop in circulating estrogen and progesterone levels, which stimulates the release of prolactin from the anterior pituitary. With the accompanying decrease in prolactin-inhibiting factor, the secretion of prolactin initiates the lactation process. The oxytocin released during breast-feeding induces contractions of the myometrium, which accelerate the involution of the uterus and often cause afterpains.

Chapter 3

Antepartum Care
William W. Beck, Jr.

I. **INTRODUCTION.** Pregnancy is a normal physiologic state, not a disease state. It is important for physicians to be familiar with the normal as well as the abnormal changes caused by pregnancy. The **objective of prenatal care** is the delivery of a healthy infant and maintenance of the health of the mother.

A. Components of antepartum care

1. **Preconceptional counseling**
   a. **Identify medical conditions** (e.g., diabetes) and **personal behaviors** (e.g., alcohol abuse) associated with poor pregnancy outcome.
   b. **Focus on the total health and well-being** of the family to include medical, psychological, social, and environmental variables affecting health.

2. **Periodic assessment,** which begins with a **comprehensive history** and **physical examination** to identify risk factors and abnormalities, should continue at regular intervals.

3. **Patient education** fosters optimal health, good dietary habits, and proper hygiene.

4. **Psychosocial support** is important during an emotional experience as profound as pregnancy.

B. **Definitions of parity.** The number of pregnancies reaching viability, not the number of fetuses delivered, determines parity.

1. A **nulligravida** is a woman who is not and has never been pregnant.

2. A **gravida** is a woman who is or has been pregnant irrespective of the pregnancy outcome. With the first pregnancy, she becomes **primigravida** and with subsequent pregnancies, a **multigravida.**

3. A **nullipara** is a woman who has never completed a pregnancy to the stage of viability; she may or may not have aborted previously.

4. A **primipara** is a woman who has completed one pregnancy (single or multiple gestation) to the stage of viability.

5. A **multipara** is a woman who has completed two or more pregnancies to the stage of viability.

II. **HISTORY**

A. Estimated date of delivery (EDD)

1. **Calculation.** The estimated date of delivery (EDD) is calculated by adding 9 months plus 7 days (**Naegele's rule**) to the date of the last menstrual period (LMP). This calculation assumes a 28- to 30-day menstrual cycle with ovulation around the fourteenth day of the cycle.

2. **Irregular cycles.** This calculation is unreliable in women with irregular menstrual cycles (4–6 weeks apart) because the day of ovulation could range from the fourteenth to the twenty-eighth day of the cycle. In such women, the calculated EDD would be earlier than the true biologic EDD.

3. Birth control pills. This calculation is unreliable in women using birth control pills for contraception who get pregnant in the first postpill cycle. Ovulation may have occurred later than 2 weeks after the onset of the LMP.

B. **Review of past pregnancies** should include:

1. A history of full-term and premature deliveries, including the route of each delivery

2. A history of repeated spontaneous or induced abortions

3. A history of high parity because of the increased risk for puerperal hemorrhage (see Chapter 2 IV C), multiple gestation, and placenta previa (i.e., the placenta developing in the lower uterine segment, completely or partially covering the internal os)

4. The length of each previous pregnancy as well as the sex and weight of the fetus or neonate

5. The indication for a previous cesarean section

6. Complications of previous pregnancies and deliveries, such as premature labor, premature rupture of membranes, shoulder dystocia, postpartum hemorrhage, fetal or neonatal deaths, perinatal morbidity, diabetes, and hypertension

C. **Identification of risk factors,** such as maternal health problems, alcohol consumption, substance abuse, cigarette smoking, hypertension, and exposure to environmental and occupational hazards (e.g., radiation, heat, anesthesia, or chemicals) must be undertaken. Consultation and counseling may be helpful when there has been exposure to possible teratogenic agents.

D. **Review of patient and family health histories** should include:

1. Information on metabolic disorders (e.g., diabetes), cardiovascular disease, malignancy, mental retardation, and multiple births

2. The family history of congenital anomalies to identify a fetus at risk for an inherited disease, and the birth of a previous child with congenital anomalies, indicating the need for prenatal genetic counseling and studies

III. PHYSICAL EXAMINATION

A. **General examination.** A general examination should include an evaluation of height, weight, blood pressure, eye fundus, breasts, heart, lungs, abdomen, rectum, extremities, and current nutritional status (e.g., obesity or malnutrition).

1. **A systolic flow murmur** at the left sternal border in pregnancy is within normal limits.

2. **Edema**
   a. **Normal.** Edema of the feet and ankles during the day is normal.
   b. **Abnormal.** Generalized edema of the face, hands, abdomen, and ankles is abnormal.

B. **Pelvic examination**

1. **Vagina and cervix**
   a. The **speculum examination** permits visualization of the vagina and the cervix.
      (1) **The blue-red passive hyperemia (Chadwick's sign)** of the cervix is characteristic of pregnancy.
      (2) **A dilated cervix** may show membranes at the internal os.
   b. **Evaluation of cervical and vaginal lesions** can be accomplished by performing a Pap smear (Papanicolaou's test), biopsy, or culdoscopic examination.
   c. **Discharge**

(1) **Normal.** A moderate amount of white mucoid discharge in pregnancy is normal.

(2) **Abnormal**

    (a) A foamy white liquid in the vagina is suggestive of a ***Trichomonas* infection.**

    (b) A white curd-like discharge is consistent with a ***Candida* infection.**

2. **Pelvis and uterus.** Bimanual examination permits the evaluation of the pelvis and the uterus.

    a. The configuration and capacity of the bony pelvis should be evaluated.

    b. Because the uterus is usually in the pelvis until 12 weeks' gestation, early pregnancy is the best time to correlate accurately uterine size and duration of gestation.

C. **Abdominal examination** allows the ongoing evaluation of the growth and status of the fetus.

1. **Estimating weeks of gestation.** Between 18 and 30 weeks, there is an excellent correlation between the size of the uterus and the gestation by weeks. The measurement in centimeters from the symphysis pubis to the top of the fundus should approximate the weeks of gestation. At midpregnancy (20 weeks' gestation), the fundus of the uterus is at the level of the umbilicus.

2. **Fetal heart tones** can be identified by a Doppler (sonar) device at 12 to 14 weeks and by a fetoscope at 18 to 20 weeks.

3. **Use of real-time ultrasonography**

    a. The **vaginal probe** can detect fetal viability at human chorionic gonadotropin (hCG) levels of 1500 to 2000 mIU/ml, or 5 to 6 weeks from the LMP.

    b. **Fetal heart activity** can be seen by the abdominal probe at hCG levels of 5000 to 6000 mIU/ml or 6 to 7 weeks from the LMP.

IV. ANTEPARTUM MANAGEMENT

A. **Laboratory tests**

1. **Initial screening** should include the following studies.

    a. Hemoglobin or hematocrit levels

    b. Urinalysis for protein and glucose

    c. Blood group and Rh type

    d. Irregular antibody screening

    e. Rubella and rubeola titers and hepatitis antigen titers if immunity has not been established by previous blood tests

    f. Cervical cytologic analysis

    g. Serologic testing for syphilis

2. **Additional screening.** The following evaluations should be performed if indicated by ethnic, racial, social, or health histories.

    a. Urine culture

    b. Cervical culture for gonorrhea and chlamydia

    c. One-hour glucose tolerance test, particularly for women with a positive family history of diabetes, a history of glucosuria or gestational diabetes, or a history of delivery of large neonates (more than 4000 g) or of a stillbirth

    d. Sickle cell test

    e. Skin test for tuberculosis

3. Maternal serum α-fetoprotein (MSAFP) levels are measured at 16 weeks, and values are reported as the **multiple of the mean (MOM).**

    a. **Elevated MSAFP (2.5 MOM and above)** may indicate:

    (1) Open neural tube defects (e.g., anencephaly, spina bifida, meningomyelo-cele)

    (2) Omphalocele

    (3) Multiple gestation

    (4) Duodenal atresia

  b. Depressed MSAFP (0.5 MOM and below). The mothers of 15% to 20% of infants with Down syndrome have these low values while pregnant.

  c. The MSAFP can be either high or low without any obvious reason and with a normal fetus.

  d. Some cases of high MSAFP have been associated with placental abnormalities that are nonspecific.

4. The **triple screen examination** is a screening test for Down syndrome performed at 16 weeks' gestation in women younger than 35 years of age; it measures MSAFP, hCG, and estriol.

  a. The mothers of 60% of infants with Down syndrome will have abnormal triple screen test results.

  b. Abnormal results should be followed up with a genetic amniocentesis for chromosomes.

5. Third-trimester routine testing should include the following studies.

  a. Repeat hemoglobin or hematocrit level

  b. Diabetes screening with a 1-hour glucose tolerance test

  c. Repeat antibody testing in unsensitized patients who are Rh negative at 28 to 32 weeks

  d. Prophylactic Rh_o (anti-D) immune globulin administration (300 μg) to reduce the incidence of Rh isoimmunization in an Rh-negative woman when her antibody screen is negative and the father of the fetus is Rh positive

B. **Office visits**

1. Frequency

  a. In an **uncomplicated pregnancy,** a woman should be seen every 4 to 6 weeks for the first 28 to 30 weeks of pregnancy, every 2 weeks until 36 weeks, and weekly thereafter until delivery.

  b. High-risk pregnancies. Women with medical or obstetric problems require close surveillance at intervals determined by the nature and severity of the problems.

2. Monitoring

  a. Mother

    (1) Blood pressure with notation of any change

    (2) Weight and notation of any change

    (3) Presence of headache, altered vision, abdominal pain, nausea, vomiting, bleeding, fluid from the vagina, and dysuria

    (4) Height of the uterine fundus above the symphysis pubis

    (5) Position, consistency, effacement, and dilation of the cervix (late in pregnancy)

  b. Fetus

    (1) Fetal heart rate

    (2) Size of fetus (actual and rate of change)

    (3) Amount of amniotic fluid

    (4) Fetal activity

    (5) Presenting part and station (late in pregnancy)

C. **Special instructions.** Patients are instructed about the following danger signals, which should be reported immediately whenever they occur.

1. Any vaginal bleeding

2. Swelling of the face or fingers

3. Severe or continuous headache

4. Blurring of vision

5. Abdominal pain

6. Persistent vomiting

7. Chills or fever

8. Dysuria

9. Escape of fluid from the vagina

10. Marked change in frequency or intensity of fetal movements

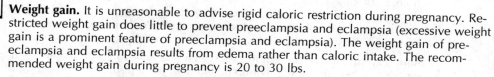

V. NUTRITION

A. **Weight gain.** It is unreasonable to advise rigid caloric restriction during pregnancy. Restricted weight gain does little to prevent preeclampsia and eclampsia (excessive weight gain is a prominent feature of preeclampsia and eclampsia). The weight gain of preeclampsia and eclampsia results from edema rather than caloric intake. The recommended weight gain during pregnancy is 20 to 30 lbs.

1. **Pregnancy-induced changes** account for 20 lbs of weight gain in normal conditions in the following approximate distribution.
   a. Fetus—7.5 lbs
   b. Placenta plus membranes—1.5 lbs
   c. Amniotic fluid—2 lbs
   d. Weight of the uterus increases—2.5 lbs
   e. Blood volume increases—3.5 lbs
   f. Breasts—2 lbs
   g. Lower extremity fluid increases—2 to 3 lbs

2. **Failure to gain weight** may be a dangerous sign; every pregnant woman should gain at least 15 to 20 lbs. If there has been less than a 10-lb weight gain by the twentieth week of gestation, dietary habits should be reviewed.

B. **Calories.** The pregnant woman of average weight requires approximately 2400 calories daily during pregnancy. This represents an increase of 300 calories daily above her nonpregnant requirements.

1. **Inadequate caloric intake** may be associated with an increased risk of fetal difficulties in utero and in low-birthweight neonates who have problems in the intrapartum and postpartum periods.
   a. Whenever caloric intake is inadequate, protein may be metabolized as a source of energy rather than being spared for growth and development.
   b. Inadequate caloric intake seems to have its greatest effect in women who are of low weight before pregnancy.

2. All patients, especially those who are obese, should be reminded that they should not begin a weight-reduction program during pregnancy.

C. **Protein.** Cell growth requires protein. Animal studies suggest that inadequate intake during pregnancy can lead to suboptimal growth of the fetus, a decrease in size of various fetal organs, and an increase in perinatal morbidity and mortality.

1. Most mothers store an additional 200 to 350 g of protein in preparation for losses that occur during labor and parturition.

2. During pregnancy, an adult woman needs approximately 1.3 g/day/kg of body weight, and an adolescent needs 1.5 g/day/kg.

3. Most of the protein should come from animal sources, such as meat, milk, eggs, cheese, poultry, and fish, because these sources furnish sufficient amino acids for protein synthesis.

D. **Minerals**

1. **Iron**
   a. **Iron depletion.** Many women have inadequate iron stores because of blood loss during menses. During pregnancy, iron stores may be depleted even further.
      (1) Supplemental iron is needed for both the fetus and the expanded maternal blood volume.
      (2) The fetus maintains normal hemoglobin levels at the mother's expense, and this may leave her severely anemic.
   b. **Recommended intake.** Elemental iron (30–60 mg) should be given daily to supplement the diet. Iron is found in liver, red meat, dried beans, green leafy vegetables, whole grain cereal, and dried fruits.

2. **Calcium**
   a. The **recommended intake** of calcium is 1200 mg daily, which can be met by a mother drinking a quart of milk (preferably skim) every day. Other sources of calcium are tofu (soybean curd) and dairy foods, including cheese and yogurt.
   b. **Leg cramps** (especially those occurring at night) are the classic symptom of calcium deficiency in a pregnant woman.

3. **Sodium.** A restriction of sodium intake, which was advocated in the past, is no longer advised because of the natriuretic effect of progesterone. There is no justification for the use of diuretics in pregnancy.

E. **Vitamins.** The practice of prescribing supplemental vitamins is common among obstetricians, although there is little evidence that vitamins benefit either the mother or the fetus. Vitamins should not be regarded as a substitute for food.

1. **Folic acid.** Folic acid is required in the formation of **heme,** the iron-containing protein of hemoglobin. Deficiencies in folic acid can affect red cell formation and cause megaloblastic anemia.
   a. Approximately **1 mg folic acid daily** is required during pregnancy. Folic acid can be found in many of the foods that provide iron and protein.
   b. Studies have implicated maternal folate deficiencies in a variety of reproductive problems, including abruptio placentae and pregnancy-induced hypertension, and fetal abnormalities, such as neural cord defects (e.g., spina bifida, anencephaly, encephalocele).
   c. For women with a **history of infant or fetal neural cord defect,** 4 mg folic acid daily should be taken for 1 month before conception and for the first 3 months of pregnancy.
   d. All fertile women should consume 0.4 mg folic acid daily.

2. **Vitamin B$_{12}$.** This vitamin occurs naturally only in foods of animal origin (meat or fish). Because vegetarians may produce infants whose B$_{12}$ stores are low, pregnant vegetarians should be identified so that B$_{12}$ supplements (i.e., pills) can be provided.

3. **Vitamin C.** During pregnancy, 80 mg daily of vitamin C is recommended, and a reasonable diet should provide this amount. Large doses (1 g or more) of vitamin C taken for common cold prophylaxis may be harmful to the fetus.

VI. LIFESTYLE ADAPTATIONS

A. **Exercise.** It is not necessary for a pregnant woman to limit her exercise, provided she does not become excessively tired. Severe restrictions may be necessary in situations such as suspected or actual cervical incompetence, pregnancy-induced hypertension, premature labor, and multiple gestation.

B. **Travel.** No harmful effects have been ascribed to travel; pressurized aircraft present no risk. A pregnant woman should move around every 2 hours to guard against lower extremity venous stasis and thrombophlebitis.

C. **Bowel habits.** Bowel habits during pregnancy tend to become irregular because of the progesterone-induced gastrointestinal smooth muscle relaxation and the pressure of the enlarging uterine mass. A woman may avoid constipation with liberal fluid intake, exercise, mild laxatives, stool softeners, and bulk-producing substances.

D. **Coitus.** Sexual intercourse does no harm at any time during pregnancy unless there is a pregnancy complication, such as ruptured membranes, premature labor, or cervical incompetence. Prostaglandins in the seminal plasma and female orgasm may be responsible for the occasional transient contractions that occur with coitus.

E. **Smoking.** Mothers who smoke often have smaller (by an average of 250 g) infants with increased perinatal mortality. Mothers should be encouraged to quit smoking completely during pregnancy. The adverse effects due to smoking are thought to be a function of:

1. Carbon monoxide and its functional inactivation of fetal and maternal hemoglobin

2. The vasoconstrictor action of nicotine, causing reduced perfusion of the placenta

3. Reduced appetite and reduced caloric intake by women who smoke

F. **Alcohol.** The current recommendation is that no alcohol be consumed during pregnancy. The fetal abnormalities associated with heavy drinking during pregnancy are known as **fetal alcohol syndrome** and include craniofacial defects, limb and cardiovascular defects, prenatal and postnatal growth retardation, and mental retardation.

G. **Medication.** Any drug administered during pregnancy will cross the placenta and reach the fetus; therefore, if a drug must be used, its advantages must outweigh the risks.

1. The possibility of long-term adverse effects of a medication on a developing fetus (e.g., diethylstilbestrol) must be remembered.

2. Because of the adverse effects of aspirin on the hemostatic mechanism of the fetus and its displacement of bilirubin from protein-binding sites, aspirin use, especially late in pregnancy, is contraindicated.

STUDY QUESTIONS

DIRECTIONS: Each of the numbered items or incomplete statements in this section is followed by answers or by completions of the statement. Select the ONE lettered answer or completion that is BEST in each case.

1. A pregnant vegetarian is likely to be deficient in which of the following substances?

(A) Calcium
(B) Folic acid
(C) Iron
(D) Protein
(E) Vitamin B_{12}

2. A woman in her first pregnancy reports that she smokes one pack of cigarettes a day. An ultrasound is ordered in the thirty-second week of the pregnancy to evaluate for which of the following?

(A) Amniotic fluid volume
(B) Fetal size
(C) Fetal abnormalities
(D) Fetal motion
(E) Fetal respiratory motion

DIRECTIONS: Each of the numbered items or incomplete statements in this section is negatively phrased, as indicated by a capitalized word such as NOT, LEAST, or EXCEPT. Select the ONE lettered answer or completion that is BEST in each case.

3. Which of the following is NOT a basis in Naegele's rule for estimating a woman's due date?

(A) Regular monthly menstrual cycles
(B) A pregnancy of 280 days
(C) Ovulation about day 14
(D) Cycle regulation with birth control pills before conception
(E) Conception at midcycle

4. Which of the following is NOT a usual screening test in an early, uncomplicated pregnancy?

(A) Repeat human chorionic gonadotropin (hCG) levels
(B) Hemoglobin
(C) Serology
(D) Cervical cytology
(E) Blood type and Rh factor

5. Which of the following dietary instructions is NOT appropriate for a pregnant woman?

(A) Restrict salt intake
(B) Take 1200 mg calcium daily
(C) Take 800 mg folic acid daily
(D) Take supplemental iron
(E) Gain at least 15 lbs during the pregnancy

6. A woman who is 16 weeks pregnant has a maternal serum α-fetoprotein (MSAFP) level of 2.8 multiple of the mean (MOM). Which of the following conditions is NOT an explanation of this abnormal finding?

(A) Anencephaly
(B) Down syndrome
(C) Duodenal atresia
(D) Omphalocele
(E) Twins

DIRECTIONS: The set of matching questions in this section consists of a list of lettered options (some of which may be in figures) followed by several numbered items. For each numbered item, select the ONE lettered option that is most closely associated with it. To avoid spending too much time on matching sets with large numbers of options, it is generally advisable to begin each set by reading the list of options. Then, for each item in the set, try to generate the correct answer and locate it in the option list, rather than evaluating each option individually. Each lettered option may be selected once, more than once, or not at all.

Questions 7–8

Match each of the following clinical situations with the correct parity.

(A) Nullipara
(B) Primipara
(C) Multipara

7. A woman who has had a first trimester abortion, an ectopic pregnancy, and a term twin gestation

8. A woman who has had two elective abortions, a 22-week spontaneous abortion, and a cesarean section for fetal distress

ANSWERS AND EXPLANATIONS

1. The answer is E [V E 2]. A vegetarian eats no meat, and vitamin B_{12} occurs naturally only in foods of animal origin (meat and fish). Thus, a physician should assume a lack of vitamin B_{12} in the diet of a vegetarian. If a vegetarian drinks milk and eats cheese, beans, fruits, green leafy vegetables, and whole grain cereal, she should not have folic acid, protein, calcium, or iron deficiencies.

2. The answer is B [VI E 1–3]. When a pregnant woman smokes, it is important to identify the small, or growth-retarded, fetus early in the third trimester so that bed rest and fetal testing can be instituted. Smoking is not associated with fetal abnormalities or amniotic fluid problems. Decreased fetal activity and respiratory motion might be a factor in severe intrauterine growth retardation, but initially, a size determination of the fetus would be important.

3. The answer is D [II A 1–3]. The estimated date of delivery (EDD) is calculated by adding 9 months plus 7 days to the date of the last menstrual period (LMP), which is a total of 280 days. This calculation assumes a 28- to 30-day cycle, with ovulation and conception around midcycle, or day 14. This calculation would not be accurate in a woman with regular 35-day cycles because her ovulation occurs around day 21, which then affects the true due date. Because of an occasional delay in ovulation in the cycle after stopping birth control pills, ovulation may occur later than 2 weeks after the last pill period, and the calculation once again is unreliable.

4. The answer is A [IV A 1 a–g]. With a previous positive pregnancy test, there is no need to repeat it under normal conditions. If the uterus is too small on examination or if there is bleeding, a repeat human chorionic gonadotropin (hCG) would be advisable to diagnose a threatened abortion with inappropriately rising hCG levels. Screening tests for hemoglobin, serologic analysis, cervical cytologic analysis, blood type, and Rh factor are indicated in an early, uncomplicated pregnancy.

5. The answer is A [V A 2, D, E 1]. Because of the natriuretic effect of progesterone, it is unwise to restrict the sodium intake of a pregnant woman. Thus, the use of diuretics in pregnancy can be harmful, leading to a hyponatremic state. Although it is not necessary to be restrictive about weight gain during pregnancy, the usual weight gain is 20 to 30 lbs. A weight gain of less than 15 lbs, even in an obese woman, is cause for concern. Daily supplements of iron, calcium (1200 mg), and folic acid (800 mg) are recommended.

6. The answer is B [IV A 3 a–b]. Maternal serum α-fetoprotein (MSAFP) levels are measured at 16 weeks and are reported as the multiple of the mean (MOM). Approximately 15% to 20% of cases of Down syndrome are associated with very low (0.5 MOM and below) α-fetoprotein levels. Elevated levels (above 2.5 MOM) can be associated with neural tube defects (e.g., spina bifida, anencephaly), omphalocele, multiple gestation, and duodenal atresia.

7–8. The answers are: 7-B, 8-B [I B 1–5]. A primipara is a woman who has had one pregnancy that reached viability and who delivered a fetus (single gestation) or fetuses (multiple gestation). The number of fetuses delivered in that one pregnancy does not change the parity. The route of delivery, such as a cesarean section, also does not change the parity.

Chapter 4

Labor and Delivery
William W. Beck, Jr.

I. THEORIES OF THE CAUSES OF LABOR

A. **Oxytocin stimulation.** Oxytocin is known to cause uterine contractions when administered late in pregnancy; therefore, it would seem that endogenously produced oxytocin may play a role in the spontaneous onset of labor.

1. Levels of oxytocin in maternal blood in early labor are higher than before the onset of labor, but there is no evidence of a sudden surge.

2. Oxytocin influence must therefore rely on the presence of oxytocin receptors.
   a. Receptors are found in the nonpregnant uterus.
   b. There is a 6-fold increase in receptors at 13 to 17 weeks and an 80-fold increase at term.
   c. In preterm labor, there are receptor levels two to three times higher than would be expected at the same stage in the absence of labor.

B. **Fetal cortisol levels.** It is possible that fetal cortisol levels and the proper functioning of the **fetal adrenal gland** influence the spontaneous onset of labor.

1. In pregnant sheep, hypophysectomy, adrenalectomy, or transection of the hypophyseal portal vessels in the fetus results in prolonged gestation.

2. Infusion of either cortisol or adrenocorticotropic hormone into a sheep fetus with an intact adrenal gland causes premature labor.

3. In humans, a naturally prolonged gestation results in an anencephalic fetus with faulty brain-pituitary-adrenal function.

C. **Progesterone withdrawal.** Although the withdrawal of progesterone is followed by the prompt evacuation of the contents of the pregnant uterus in rabbits, there is **no decrease in the human maternal blood levels of progesterone at term.** The progesterone level at the placental site, however, may decrease before the onset of labor and assist in the synthesis of prostaglandin.

D. **Prostaglandin release** seems to be involved in the spontaneous onset of labor. Prostaglandins are known to cause uterine contractions; for example, vaginally administered prostaglandins induce contractions in second-trimester therapeutic abortions. Also, stimuli known to cause the release of prostaglandins (e.g., cervical manipulation and rupture of the membranes) augment or induce uterine contractions.

1. **Site of production. Prostaglandin synthetase** is found in **fetal membranes** and **decidua vera,** both of which produce prostaglandins.

2. **Synthesis.** Nonesterified arachidonic acid is an absolute precursor of prostaglandins. There is a 6-fold increase of nonesterified arachidonic acid in the amniotic fluid during labor.
   a. The esterified form of **arachidonic acid** is thought to be stored in the fetal membranes.
   b. **Phospholipase** liberates arachidonic acid from its esterified form in the fetal membranes.
   c. There is a 6-fold increase in **nonesterified arachidonic acid** in the amniotic fluid during labor.

3. **Oxytocin** stimulates prostaglandin synthesis, which occurs in the decidua.
   a. There is an **increase in oxytocin receptors** in the decidua.
   b. Oxytocin stimulates the **release of $PGF_2\alpha$**.

    c. $PGF_2\alpha$ seems to be essential for **progressive labor.**

    d. The dual role of oxytocin **stimulates uterine contractions and prostaglandin synthesis.**

II. DEFINITION AND CHARACTERISTICS OF LABOR

A. **Definition.** Labor is characterized by contractions that occur at decreasing intervals with increasing intensity, causing dilation of the cervix.

B. **Myometrial physiology**

1. **Contraction of uterine smooth muscle** is caused by the interaction of the proteins **actin** and **myosin.**
   a. The interaction of actin and myosin is regulated by the enzymatic phosphorylation of myosin light chains.
   b. The phosphorylation of myosin light chains is catalyzed by the enzyme myosin light-chain kinase, which is activated by calcium ion (Ca^{2+}).

2. **Gap junctions** are important cell-to-cell contacts that facilitate communication between cells via electrical or metabolic coupling.
   a. Uterine gap junctions, which are virtually absent during pregnancy, increase in size and number before and during labor.
   b. Gap junctions facilitate synchronization of the contraction of individual cells, which permits the simultaneous recruitment of large numbers of contractile units during excitation.
   c. **Progesterone** appears to prevent and estrogen appears to promote gap-junction formation.
   d. **Prostaglandins** are believed to be important stimulators of gap-junction formation. If prostaglandins are inhibited, then so is gap-junction formation.
   e. Gap-junction formation is not stimulated by oxytocin.

3. **Substances that interfere with the physiology of the myometrium** can inhibit contractions. Tocolysis occurs with the following agents:
   a. **Antiprostaglandin agents,** such as indomethacin and acetylsalicylic acid, inhibit the synthesis of prostaglandin, which, in turn, decreases uterine contractions and inhibits gap-junction formation. If the drugs are discontinued by 34 weeks' gestation, premature closure of the fetal ductus arteriosus does not occur.
   b. **Calcium channel blockers** (e.g., nifedipine, magnesium sulfate) inhibit calcium influx.
   c. **Beta mimetic agonists** stimulate cyclic adenosine monophosphate (cAMP) generation; an increase in intracellular cAMP stimulates **calcium uptake** in various cellular organelles, including the sarcoplasmic reticulum, thereby **lowering intracellular-free calcium.**

C. **Stages of labor**

1. **First stage.** The first stage of labor entails effacement and dilation. It begins when uterine contractions become sufficiently frequent, intense, and long to initiate obvious effacement and dilation of the cervix.

2. **Second stage.** The second stage of labor involves the expulsion of the fetus. It begins with the complete dilation of the cervix and ends when the infant is delivered.

3. **Third stage.** The third stage of labor involves the separation and expulsion of the placenta. It begins with the delivery of the infant and ends with the delivery of the placenta.

Table 4-1. True Versus False Labor

	True Labor	**False Labor**
Contractions	Regular intervals 2–4 minutes apart; intensity gradually increases and can last for 1 minute	Irregular intervals; no pattern; intensity remains steady
Discomfort	Back and abdomen	Lower abdomen
Dilation	Progressive	No change in cervix
Effect of sedation	Contractions are not affected	Contractions are relieved or stopped

D. **True labor and false labor** are compared in Table 4-1.

E. **Characteristics of uterine contractions**

1. Effective uterine contractions last for 30 to 90 seconds, create 20 to 50 mm Hg of pressure, and occur every 2 to 4 minutes.

2. The **pain of contractions** is thought to be caused by one or more of the following:
   a. Hypoxia of the contracted myometrium
   b. Compression of nerve ganglia in the cervix and lower uterus by the tightly inter-locking muscle bundles
   c. Stretching of the cervix during dilation
   d. Stretching of the peritoneum overlying the uterus

3. During labor, contractions cause the uterus to differentiate into two parts.
   a. The **upper segment of the uterus** becomes thicker as labor progresses and con-tracts down with a force that expels the fetus with each contraction.
   b. The **lower segment of the uterus** passively thins out with the contractions of the upper segment, promoting effacement of the cervix.

F. **Changes of the cervix before or during labor**

1. Effacement of the cervix is the shortening of the cervical canal from a structure of ap-proximately 2 cm in length to one in which the canal is replaced by a more circular orifice with almost paper-thin edges. Effacement occurs as the muscle fibers in the vi-cinity of the internal os are pulled upward into the lower uterine segment.

2. Dilation of the cervix involves the gradual widening of the cervical os. For the head of the average fetus at term to be able to pass through the cervix, the canal must di-late to a diameter of approximately 10 cm. When a diameter is reached that is suffi-cient for the fetal head to pass through, the cervix is said to be **completely or fully di-lated.**

III. NORMAL LABOR IN THE OCCIPUT PRESENTATION

A. **Occiput (vertex) presentations** (Figure 4-1) occur in approximately 95% of all labors. The occiput may present in the transverse, anterior, or posterior position. **Position** refers to the relation of an arbitrarily chosen portion of the fetus (in this case, the **occiput of the fetal head**) to the right or left side of the maternal birth canal. Positions of the occi-put presentation include the following:

1. **Occiput transverse.** On vaginal examination, the sagittal suture (in the midline front to back) of the fetal head occupies the transverse diameter of the pelvis more or less midway between the sacrum and the symphysis.
   a. In the **left occiput transverse positions,** the smaller posterior fontanelle is to the

A

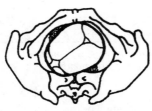
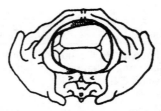
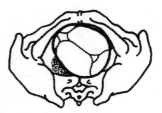

Left occiput anterior   Left occiput transverse   Left occiput posterior

B

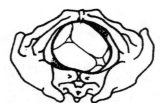
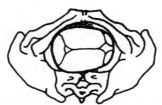
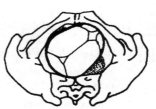

Right occiput anterior   Right occiput transverse   Right occiput posterior

C

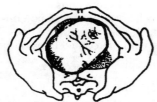
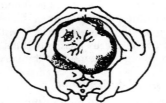
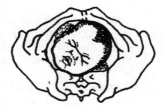

Left face anterior   Right face anterior   Right face posterior

FIGURE 4-1. Occiput and face presentations in labor. *(A)* Left positions in occiput presentations, with the fetal head viewed at a cross-section of the pelvis from below. *(B)* Right positions in occiput presentations. *(C)* Left and right positions in face presentations. (Reprinted with permission from Pritchard JA, MacDonald PC, Gant NF: *Williams Obstetrics,* 17th edition. East Norwalk, CT, Appleton & Lange, 1980, pp 237–239.)

    left in the maternal pelvis, and the larger anterior fontanelle is directed toward the opposite side.
    b. In the **right occiput transverse positions,** the reverse is true.

  2. Occiput anterior. The head either enters the pelvis with the occiput rotated 45 degrees anteriorly from the transverse position, right occiput anterior or left occiput anterior, or subsequently does so.

  3. Occiput posterior. The incidence of posterior positions is approximately 10%. The right occiput posterior position is more common than is the left occiput posterior position. The posterior positions often are associated with a narrow forepelvis.
    a. In the **right occiput posterior position,** the sagittal suture occupies the right oblique diameter. The small posterior fontanelle is directed posteriorly to the right of the midline, whereas the large anterior fontanelle is directed anteriorly to the left of the midline.
    b. In the **left occiput posterior position,** the reverse holds true.

B. **The seven cardinal movements in labor and delivery.** A process of positional adaptation of the fetal head to the various segments of the pelvis is required for the completion of childbirth. These positional changes of the presenting part constitute the mechanism of labor and delivery and involve seven cardinal movements (Figure 4-2), which **occur sequentially** in the following order:

1. **Engagement.** This is the mechanism by which the biparietal diameter of the fetal head, the greatest transverse diameter of the head in occiput presentations, passes through the pelvic inlet. When engagement occurs, the lowest point of the presenting part is, by definition, at the level of the ischial spines, which is designated as **0 station.** Levels 1, 2, and 3 cm above the spines are designated as **−1, −2, and −3 station,** respectively; levels 1, 2, and 3 cm below the spines are designated as **+1, +2, and +3 station,** respectively. At +3, the presenting part is on the perineum.
   a. Engagement may take place during the last few weeks of pregnancy, or it may not do so until labor begins. It is more likely to happen before the onset of labor in a primigravida than in a multigravida.
   b. When the fetal head is not engaged at the onset of labor, and the fetal head is freely movable above the pelvic inlet, the head is said to be **floating.**

2. **Descent.** The first requirement for the birth of an infant is descent. When the fetal head is engaged at the onset of labor in a primigravida, descent may not occur until the start of the second stage. In a multiparous woman, descent usually begins with engagement.

3. **Flexion.** When the descending head meets resistance from either the cervix, the walls of the pelvis, or the pelvic floor, flexion of the fetal head normally occurs.
   a. The chin is brought into close contact with the fetal thorax.
   b. This movement causes a smaller diameter of fetal head to be presented to the pelvis than would occur if the head were not flexed.

4. **Internal rotation.** This movement always is associated with descent of the presenting part and usually is not accomplished until the head has reached the level of the ischial spines (0 station). The movement involves the gradual turning of the occiput from its original position anteriorly toward the symphysis pubis.

5. **Extension** of the fetal head is essential during the birth process. When the sharply flexed fetal head comes in contact with the vulva, the occiput is brought in direct contact with the inferior margin of the symphysis.
   a. Because the vulvar outlet is directed upward and forward, extension must occur for the head to pass through it.
   b. The expulsive forces of the uterine contractions and the patient's pushing, along with the resistance of the pelvic floor, result in the anterior extension of the vertex in the direction of the vulvar opening.

6. **External rotation.** After delivery of the head, **restitution** occurs. In this movement, the occiput returns to the oblique position from which it started and then to the transverse position, left or right. This movement corresponds to the rotation of the fetal body, bringing the shoulders into an anteroposterior diameter with the pelvic outlet.

7. **Expulsion.** After external rotation, the anterior shoulder appears under the symphysis and is delivered. The perineum soon becomes distended by the posterior shoulder. After delivery of the shoulders, the rest of the infant's body is extruded quickly.

IV. CONDUCT OF LABOR

A. **Detection of ruptured membranes.** Ruptured membranes are signified at any time during pregnancy by either a sudden gush or a steady trickle of clear fluid from the vagina. In a term pregnancy, labor usually follows within 24 hours of membrane rupture. There is a real possibility of intrauterine infection (**chorioamnionitis**) if the patient has ruptured membranes for longer than 24 hours, with or without labor.

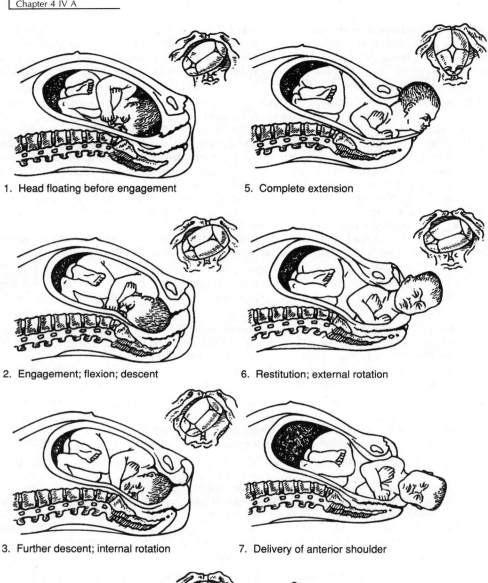

1. Head floating before engagement
2. Engagement; flexion; descent
3. Further descent; internal rotation
4. Complete rotation; beginning extension
5. Complete extension
6. Restitution; external rotation
7. Delivery of anterior shoulder
8. Delivery of posterior shoulder

FIGURE 4-2. Principal movements in labor and delivery, left occiput anterior position. (Reprinted with permission from Cunningham FG, MacDonald PC, Gant NF: *Williams Obstetrics*, 18th edition. East Norwalk, CT, Appleton & Lange, 1989, p 228.)

1. **Nitrazine test.** Nitrazine paper changes color, depending on the pH of the fluid being tested. Amniotic fluid, which is alkaline, turns nitrazine paper deep blue.

2. **Ferning.** Amniotic fluid, like many body fluids, has a high sodium content, which causes a ferning pattern when the fluid is air dried on a slide. Other vaginal secretions do not have such a ferning pattern. A positive fern test confirms ruptured membranes, because the nitrazine paper can turn blue with alkaline cervical mucus or blood in the absence of ruptured membranes.

B. **First stage of labor.** On the average, the first stage lasts for approximately **12 hours in the primigravida** and approximately **7 hours in the multigravida,** although there is great variability from patient to patient.

1. **Fetal monitoring.** The fetal heart tones should be monitored by any device immediately after a uterine contraction because a sudden drop to less than 120 beats per minute (bpm) or an increase to above 180 bpm may be an indication of fetal distress.

2. **Amniotomy.** Artificial rupture of the membranes permits the observation of the color of the amniotic fluid (whether or not it is stained by **meconium,** a sticky, dark-green substance found in the intestine of the full-term fetus) and often shortens the length of labor if a woman is already contracting regularly.

3. **Latent phase of labor.** During the latent phase, the uterine contractions typically are infrequent, somewhat uncomfortable, and, in some cases, irregular, but they generate sufficient force to cause slow dilation and some effacement of the cervix. A **prolonged latent phase** is longer than 20 hours in the primigravida and longer than 14 hours in the multigravida.

4. **Active phase of labor.** The active phase, or clinically apparent labor, follows the latent phase and is characterized by progressive cervical dilation. A prolonged active phase is seen in the primigravida who dilates at less than 1.2 cm/hr and in the multigravida who dilates at less than 1.5 cm/hr.

5. **Dysfunctional labor patterns.** Uterine dysfunction in any phase of cervical dilation is characterized by lack of progress, because one of the cardinal features of normal labor is its progression.
   a. In **hypotonic uterine dysfunction,** the uterine contractions have a normal gradient pattern but a pressure increase during a contraction of less than 15 mm Hg. This type of dysfunction usually is corrected by stimulating the contractions with an **intravenous infusion of oxytocin.**
   b. In **hypertonic uterine dysfunction,** the uterine contractions have an abnormal gradient, possibly because of contraction of the uterus midsegment with more force than the fundus. The result is painful contractions that result in little or no cervical dilation. Oxytocin is not indicated in a hypertonic uterus. **Sedation with morphine** relieves the pain, relaxes the patient, and usually results in a normal labor pattern.

C. **Second stage of labor.** On the average, the second stage lasts for approximately 50 minutes in the primigravida and approximately 20 minutes in the multigravida. However, second stages lasting 2 hours, especially in the primigravida, are not uncommon. This stage is characterized by intense pushing on the part of the patient.

1. **Spontaneous vaginal delivery**
   a. **Delivery of the head.** With each contraction, the vulvar opening is dilated by the head. The encirclement of the largest diameter of the fetal head by the vulvar ring is known as **crowning.** The head then is delivered slowly with the base of the occiput rotating around the lower margin of the symphysis pubis.
   b. **Delivery of the shoulders.** In most cases, the shoulders appear at the vulva just after external rotation and are delivered spontaneously. If the shoulders are not delivered spontaneously, gentle traction is used to engage and deliver the anterior and then the posterior shoulders. Excessive traction with extension of the infant's

Table 4-2. Types of Episiotomy

	Advantages	Disadvantages
Median	Ease of repair Rare faulty healing Rare dyspareunia Good anatomic result Small blood loss	Extension through anal sphincter and into rectum is relatively common
Mediolateral	More space at vaginal outlet for breech or shoulder dystocia Rare extension through anal sphincter	Difficulty of repair Common faulty healing Occasional dyspareunia Occasional faulty anatomic result Greater blood loss than with median episiotomy

neck can result in temporary or permanent **injury to the brachial plexus,** known as **Erb's palsy.**

   2. Episiotomy (Table 4-2) is the most common operation in obstetrics. It is an incision in the perineum that is either in the midline (a **median episiotomy**) or begun in the midline but directed laterally away from the rectum (a **mediolateral episiotomy**). The episiotomy substitutes a straight, clean surgical incision for the ragged laceration that may otherwise result. An episiotomy is easier to repair and heals better than a tear; it shortens the second stage of labor; and it spares the infant's head from prolonged pounding against the perineum.

D. **Third stage of labor.** The placenta usually is delivered within 5 minutes of the delivery of the infant.

   1. Signs of placental separation
      a. The uterus becomes globular and firmer.
      b. There often is a sudden gush of blood.
      c. The uterus rises in the abdomen because the placenta, having separated, passes down into the lower uterine segment and vagina, where its bulk pushes the uterus upward.
      d. The umbilical cord protrudes farther out of the vagina, indicating that the placenta has descended.

   2. Uterine hemostasis. The mechanism by which hemostasis is achieved at the placental site is **vasoconstriction,** produced by a well-contracted myometrium. Intravenous or intramuscular **oxytocin** (10 U intramuscularly or 20 U in a 1000-ml intravenous bottle) or **ergonovine** (0.2 mg intramuscularly or intravenously) helps the uterus to contract and decreases blood loss. These medications are administered after the placenta has been delivered.

E. **Lacerations of the birth canal.** There are four types of vaginal or perineal lacerations, all of which are less likely to occur with an appropriate episiotomy.

   1. First-degree lacerations involve the fourchette, the perineal skin, and vaginal mucosa, but not the fascia and muscle.

   2. Second-degree lacerations involve the skin, the mucosa, the fascia, and muscles of the perineal body, but not the anal sphincter.

   3. Third-degree lacerations extend through the skin, mucosa, perineal body, and involve the anal sphincter.

   4. Fourth-degree lacerations are extensions of the third-degree tear through the rectal mucosa to expose the lumen of the rectum.

STUDY QUESTIONS

DIRECTIONS: Each of the numbered items or incomplete statements in this section is followed by answers or by completions of the statement. Select the ONE lettered answer or completion that is BEST in each case.

1. The cardinal movements of labor and delivery involve a sequence of events that occurs in an orderly fashion. Which of the following sequences is correct?

(A) Descent, internal rotation, flexion
(B) Engagement, flexion, descent
(C) Engagement, internal rotation, descent
(D) Engagement, descent, flexion
(E) Descent, flexion, engagement

2. Engagement is said to have occurred when which of the following events takes place?

(A) The infant's head is within the pelvis
(B) The biparietal diameter of the infant's head is through the plane of the inlet
(C) The presenting part is just above the level of the ischial spines
(D) The vertex is in the transverse position
(E) The infant's head is flexed

3. A woman delivers a 9-lb infant with a midline episiotomy and suffers a third-degree tear. Inspection shows that which of the following structures is intact?

(A) Anal sphincter
(B) Perineal body
(C) Perineal muscles
(D) Fascia
(E) Rectal mucosa

DIRECTIONS: Each of the numbered items or incomplete statements in this section is negatively phrased, as indicated by a capitalized word such as NOT, LEAST, or EXCEPT. Select the ONE lettered answer or completion that is BEST in each case.

4. Which of the following is NOT characteristic of arachidonic acid?

(A) The nonesterified form is a precursor of prostaglandin
(B) The esterified form is stored in the decidua vera
(C) It is found in high levels in the amniotic fluid
(D) It is liberated from the esterified form by phospholipase
(E) It combines with prostaglandin synthetase to produce prostaglandin

5. Which of the following is NOT involved with the synthesis of prostaglandin?

(A) Fetal membranes
(B) Phospholipase
(C) Esterified arachidonic acid
(D) Prostaglandin synthetase
(E) Progesterone

6. Which of the following is NOT a characteristic of a mediolateral episiotomy?

(A) Difficulty of repair
(B) Common faulty healing
(C) Occasional dyspareunia
(D) Relatively common extension through anal sphincter and into rectum
(E) Occasional faulty anatomic result

7. Which of the following is NOT characteristic of active-phase uterine contractions?

(A) They create 40 mm Hg of pressure
(B) They cause dilation of the cervix
(C) They cause thickening of the lower uterine segment
(D) They occur every 2 to 4 minutes
(E) They last for 45 seconds

DIRECTIONS: The set of matching questions in this section consists of a list of lettered options (some of which may be in figures) followed by several numbered items. For each numbered item, select the ONE lettered option that is most closely associated with it. To avoid spending too much time on matching sets with large numbers of options, it is generally advisable to begin each set by reading the list of options. Then, for each item in the set, try to generate the correct answer and locate it in the option list, rather than evaluating each option individually. Each lettered option may be selected once, more than once, or not at all.

Questions 8–10

For each activity listed below, select the substance that is most likely to be responsible for it.

(A) Oxytocin
(B) Prostaglandin
(C) Indomethacin
(D) Magnesium sulfate
(E) Progesterone

8. Stimulates gap-junction formation

9. Influences calcium ion (Ca^{2+}) flux in the treatment of premature labor

10. Prevents gap-junction formation directly

ANSWERS AND EXPLANATIONS

1. The answer is D [III B 1–7]. There are seven cardinal movements in labor and delivery, and they occur sequentially. In order, they are engagement, descent, flexion, internal rotation, extension, external rotation, and expulsion.

2. The answer is B [III B 1 a, b]. During labor, engagement occurs when the biparietal diameter of the infant's head is at or through the plane of the inlet. At this moment, the presenting part of the infant is at or below the ischial spines, which is 0 station. The head is within the pelvis at station −1 or −2, but it is not engaged at that point. Neither the position of the infant's head nor its degree of flexion has anything to do with the definition of engagement.

3. The answer is E [IV C 2, E 1–4]. Each of the first-, second-, third-, and fourth-degree lacerations involves progressively more of the structures of the perineum. The third-degree tear goes through vaginal mucosa, fascia, the perineal body, the transverse perineal muscles, and the anal sphincter. Inspection of the third-degree tear would show an intact rectal mucosa. A tear in the rectal mucosa would make the laceration a fourth-degree tear.

4. The answer is B [I D 1–2]. The esterified form of arachidonic acid is stored in the fetal membranes, not the decidua vera, and it is liberated from its esterified form by phospholipase. The nonesterified form is an absolute precursor of prostaglandin. Prostaglandin synthetase is stored in the fetal membranes and the decidua vera, and it catalyzes the synthesis of prostaglandin.

5. The answer is C [I D 1, 2 a, b]. The synthesis of prostaglandin is possible because prostaglandin synthetase is stored in the fetal membranes. The enzyme phospholipase liberates arachidonic acid from its stored esterified form to a nonesterified form. Thus, the nonesterified form of arachidonic acid, not the ester-

ified form, is involved in the synthesis of prostaglandin. Progesterone also assists in the synthesis of prostaglandin.

6. The answer is D [Table 4-2]. Extension through the anal sphincter and into the rectum is a relatively common disadvantage of a median, not a mediolateral, episiotomy. Disadvantages of a mediolateral episiotomy are its difficulty of repair, common faulty healing, occasional dyspareunia, occasional faulty anatomic result, and a greater blood loss than that which occurs with a median episiotomy.

7. The answer is C [II E; Table 4-1]. Uterine contractions in the active phase of labor cause progressive effacement and dilation of the cervix, occur every 2 to 4 minutes, last 30 to 90 seconds, and attain pressures of 20 to 50 mm Hg. During the active phase, the uterus differentiates into two parts. The active upper segment, or uterine fundus, thickens and contracts down. The passive lower uterine segment thins out with the contractions, thus promoting effacement.

8–10. The answers are: 8-B [II B 2 c], **9-D** [II B 3 b], **10-E** [II B 2 b]. Gap junctions are important cell-to-cell contacts that facilitate communication between coupled cells. These junctions, which are absent during pregnancy, increase in size and number before and during labor. Prostaglandins appear to be important stimulators of gap-junction formation. Progesterone seems to prevent the formation of gap junctions directly, and oxytocin appears to have no effect. Indomethacin indirectly prevents the formation of gap junctions by inhibiting the synthesis of prostaglandin, in whose absence gap-junction formation is not possible. Magnesium sulfate affects calcium ion (Ca^{2+}) metabolism by antagonizing Ca^{2+}, which prevents the activation of myosin light-chain kinase, which, in turn, inhibits the phosphorylation of myosin light chains. Uterine contractions are, thus, inhibited, which is the goal of the treatment of premature labor.

Chapter 5

Intrapartum Fetal Monitoring
William W. Beck, Jr.

I. FETAL MONITORING

A. **Fetal distress** is defined in terms of the manifestations of the **fetal hypoxia** (i.e., by changes in the **fetal heart rate [FHR] or fetal blood pH**).

  1. Adequate fetal oxygenation is essential for a healthy neonate. Assessment of the fetus during labor is essential in detecting the hypoxia that underlies fetal distress.

  2. The **extent and cause of fetal distress** can be predicted reliably by either of two methods.

  a. Continuous FHR monitoring to record the variability of, baseline of, and any changes in the FHR

  b. Fetal scalp capillary blood sampling to record fetal blood pH

B. **Significance of hypoxia.** Hypoxic damage to the fetus is difficult to quantify, but the effects can be devastating.

  1. **Neurologic abnormalities.** Cerebral palsy and mental retardation represent the sublethal effects of asphyxia that may not be observed at birth.

  2. **Fetal death** can result from severe intrapartum asphyxia.

II. PATHOPHYSIOLOGY OF FETAL HYPOXIA

A. **Nonstressed fetus.** In the absence of stress, the fetus is neither acidotic nor hypoxic. An adequate delivery of oxygen to the fetal tissues occurs despite the low fetal arterial partial pressure of oxygen (Po_2). The transfer of oxygen across the placenta to the fetus is enhanced by the following mechanisms:

  1. Fetal cardiac output and systemic blood flow rates that are considerably higher than those of the adult

  2. The affinity of fetal blood for oxygen and the fetal oxygen-carrying capacity, both of which are greater than those of an adult

B. **Stressed fetus.** When perfusion is decreased because of impaired uterine or umbilical blood flow, the transfer of oxygen to the fetus is diminished, and the result is an accumulation of carbon dioxide in the fetus.

  1. **Increased carbon dioxide** causes an increase in the partial pressure of carbon dioxide (Pco_2) and a concomitant fall in pH, analogous to adult respiratory acidosis.

  2. **Continued hypoxia** deprives the fetus of sufficient oxygen to perform the aerobic reactions of intermediary metabolism, resulting in a buildup of organic acids.

  3. With the **accumulation of pyruvic and lactic acids,** there is a further drop in fetal pH, resulting in **metabolic acidosis.**

  4. **Transient decreases in fetal or uterine perfusion** usually cause a short-lived respiratory acidosis, whereas **more prolonged or profound decreases** result in a combined respiratory and metabolic acidosis.

  5. **Fetal oxygen deprivation** usually results in a decrease in the FHR or fetal bradycardia. Bradycardia appears to be an adaptive response to hypoxia, which allows the fetal myocardium to work more efficiently than it does at higher rates.

III. **FETAL HEART RATE (FHR) MONITORING.** Either an external ultrasound device (using the ultrasound Doppler principle) or an internal electrode attached to the fetal scalp is used to monitor the FHR in conjunction with uterine contractions.

A. **Elements of the FHR pattern**

1. The **baseline FHR** is the steady rate that occurs during and between contractions in the absence of accelerations or decelerations. The normal baseline FHR is 120 to 160 beats per minute (bpm).
   a. At 16 weeks, the average baseline is 160 bpm.
   b. The baseline FHR decreases approximately 24 bpm from 16 weeks to term.

2. The **beat-to-beat variability** represents the continuous interaction of the sympathetic and parasympathetic nervous systems in adjusting the FHR to fetal metabolic or hemodynamic conditions.
   a. **Decreased variability** may signify loss of fine autonomic control of the FHR.
   b. **Good variability** usually predicts a good fetal outcome.

3. **Reactivity.** When a healthy fetus is stimulated, there is a transient increase in baseline acceleration (10–15 bpm for 15–20 seconds). The stimulation can be external (e.g., sound or scalp stimulation) or internal (e.g., spontaneous fetal movement).

B. **Abnormal FHR changes.** There are many reasons for variability and baseline FHR changes.

1. **Causes of decreased variability**
   a. Asphyxia
   b. Drugs (e.g., atropine, scopolamine, tranquilizers, narcotics, barbiturates, anesthetics)
   c. Prematurity
   d. Tachycardia
   e. Physiologic fetal "sleep states"
   f. Cardiac and central nervous system abnormalities
   g. Arrhythmias

2. **Causes of fetal tachycardia** (i.e., rates above 160 bpm)
   a. Asphyxia (early)
   b. Maternal fever
   c. Fetal infection
   d. Prematurity
   e. Drugs (e.g., ritodrine and atropine)
   f. Fetal stimulation
   g. Arrhythmias
   h. Maternal anxiety
   i. Maternal thyrotoxicosis
   j. Unknown causes (idiopathic)

3. **Causes of fetal bradycardia** (i.e., rates below 120 bpm)
   a. Asphyxia (sudden or profound)
   b. Drugs
   c. Reflex (e.g., to pressure on fetal head)
   d. Arrhythmias
   e. Hypothermia
   f. Unknown causes (idiopathic)

C. **FHR decelerations.** Periodic changes in the FHR assume importance in defining the mechanism and intensity of asphyxial insults. There are three patterns of periodic decelerations based on the configuration of the waveform and the timing of the deceleration in relation to the uterine contraction.

1. **Early decelerations** (Figure 5-1A):
   a. Are not caused by systemic hypoxia
   b. Do not appear to be associated with poor fetal outcome
   c. Occur with fetal head compression
   d. Begin with the onset of uterine contractions
   e. Reach their lowest point at the peak of the contraction
   f. Return to baseline as the contraction ends

2. **Late decelerations** (Figure 5-1B):
   a. Usually are found in association with acute or chronic fetoplacental vascular insufficiency
   b. Occur after the peak of and extend past the length of the uterine contraction, often with a slow return to the baseline
   c. Are precipitated by hypoxemia (which slows the FHR as a result of central nervous system asphyxia), direct myocardial depression, or both
   d. May be associated with a mixed respiratory and metabolic acidosis
   e. Are found with increased frequency in patients with preeclampsia, hypertension, diabetes mellitus, intrauterine growth retardation, or other disorders associated with chronic placental insufficiency
   f. Occur in situations in which there is an acute decrease in the intervillous space flow, such as abruptio placentae, maternal hypotension from conduction anesthesia, or excessive uterine activity, often associated with hyperstimulation during an oxytocin infusion

3. **Variable decelerations** (Figure 5-1C):
   a. Are inconsistent in configuration
   b. Have no uniform temporal relationship to the onset of the contraction
   c. Usually are the result of transient compression of the umbilical cord between fetal parts or between the fetus and surrounding maternal tissues
   d. Often are associated with oligohydramnios, with or without ruptured membranes
   e. Cause a short-lived respiratory acidosis if they are mild
   f. May be associated with profound combined acidosis if they are prolonged and recurrent

IV. FETAL SCALP BLOOD SAMPLING

A. **Rationale.** Information about fetal acid–base balance can be obtained by sampling blood from the fetal scalp. There is generally good agreement among scalp blood pH, cord pH, and Apgar scores.

1. **Normal fetal capillary pH** is 7.25 to 7.35 in the first stage of labor.

2. **Fetal scalp pH** is lower than maternal pH by approximately 0.10 to 0.15.

B. **Interpretation of fetal scalp pH**

1. Most authorities consider **pH values less than 7.20** indicative of significant asphyxia and **values between 7.20 and 7.24** as preacidotic and warranting further evaluation. The scalp pH test should be repeated in 20 to 30 minutes if the result is low or low-normal.

2. Because a pathologic fetal pH may reflect a severe maternal acidosis, fetal acidemia does not necessarily reflect an asphyxial insult.

C. **Predictive value of fetal scalp pH**

1. **Accuracy.** The accuracy of predicting Apgar scores is only about 80% using fetal capillary pH alone.
   a. **False-normal pH values** are found in 6% to 20% of infants tested.
   b. **False-low pH values** are found in 8% to 10% of infants tested.

A. Early deceleration
(uniform shape; early timing)

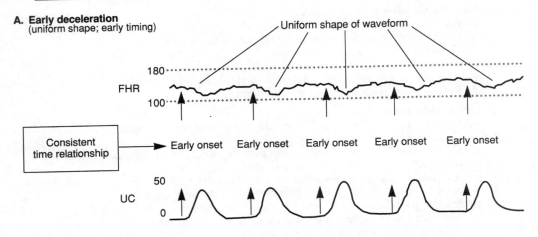

B. Late deceleration
(uniform shape; late timing)

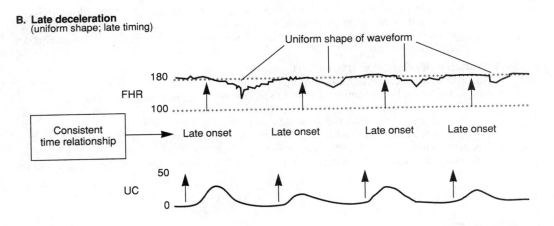

C. Variable deceleration
(variable shape; variable timing)

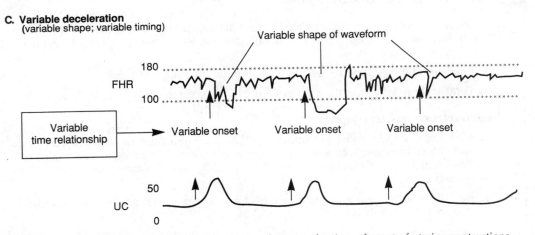

FIGURE 5-1. Fetal heart rate *(FHR)* deceleration in relation to the time of onset of uterine contractions *(UC)*. *(A)* Early deceleration; *(B)* late deceleration; *(C)* variable deceleration. (Reprinted with permission from Hon EH: *Atlas of Fetal Heart Rate Patterns.* New Haven, Harty Press, 1968, p 283.)

    2. **False normal pH values in the presence of low Apgar scores** usually result from:
      a. Sedatives, analgesics, or general anesthesia, resulting in poor respiratory effort and flaccidity at birth but normal pH in utero
      b. Prematurity, fetal infection, or any traumatic insult or meconium that occurs at delivery
      c. A hypoxic episode that occurs between the sampling period and the delivery period, such as abruptio placentae just before delivery

    3. **False-low pH values** may be related to:
      a. Maternal acidosis
      b. Local scalp edema or vasoconstriction
      c. Fetal recovery in utero from an episode of documented acidosis before delivery

V. IATROGENIC CAUSES OF FETAL DISTRESS

A. Maternal position

    1. When a pregnant woman lies in the **supine position,** her uterus obstructs blood flow through the abdominal aorta and the inferior vena cava.
      a. Resultant **supine hypotension** accompanied by decreased cardiac output occurs 10% of the time.
      b. Supine hypotension can lead to decreased placental perfusion and **consequent fetal distress.**

    2. Placing the woman in a **lateral recumbent position** causes the uterus to fall away from the great vessels, thus improving fetal oxygenation and relieving hypotension.

B. **Oxytocin stimulation.** Use of uterotonic agents has been associated with an increased incidence of late decelerations and decreased placental perfusion. These occurrences result from hyperstimulation and incomplete relaxation of the uterus after a contraction. Hyperstimulation with oxytocin can be minimized with the use of an infusion pump and an internal (intrauterine) pressure catheter.

C. **Peridural anesthesia.** The use of epidural or caudal anesthesia creates a sympathetic blockade, which may result in decreased venous return, consequent diminished cardiac output, maternal hypotension, decreased uteroplacental perfusion, and late decelerations. When peridural anesthesia is used, women in labor should be:

    1. **Well hydrated** so that there is a normal intravascular volume and less likelihood of hypotension

    2. **Lying in the lateral position** so that the potential effects of the sympathetic blockade are not compounded by pressure of the uterus on the great vessels

VI. INTRAUTERINE RESUSCITATION. Fetal distress occasionally may demand immediate delivery either vaginally or by cesarean section. However, there is usually time to attempt intrauterine resuscitation.

A. **Improvement of uterine blood flow.** Late decelerations usually are related to impaired intervillous space blood flow. Fetal hypoxia and late decelerations may be improved by maneuvers that maximize uterine blood flow.

    1. **Maternal position.** All patients with suspected fetal distress should be placed in one of the lateral recumbent positions.

    2. **Maternal hydration.** It is not unusual for women in labor to have been without oral intake for long periods. This can result in a total body water deficit. Although mater-

nal pulse and blood pressure may be stable, blood flow may be diverted from the uterus to maintain flow in vital organs.

   a. When **signs of fetal distress** are evident, an **infusion of intravenous fluids** should be given. If an intravenous infusion is in place, the infusion should be increased.

   b. **In the presence of late decelerations,** an infusion of **lactated Ringer's** or **physiologic saline** to replace depleted intravascular volume is sometimes curative.

3. **Uterine relaxation.** If oxytocin is being used to stimulate labor, it should be discontinued. Further attempts at tocolysis (relaxation of uterine contractions) with agents such as **intravenous ritodrine** or **subcutaneous terbutaline** may allow the fetus to recover before delivery and be in a more favorable physiologic state than if it had been delivered at the height of its distress.

B. **Improvement in umbilical blood flow.** Attempts to improve severe variable decelerations should include all of the measures for improving uterine blood flow with additional attention paid to the following.

1. **Maternal position.** Changing the mother's position by moving her from side to side, to the Trendelenburg position, or even the knee–chest position frequently corrects the patterns.

2. **Fetal head position.** When overt cord prolapse has occurred, manual elevation of the fetal head out of the pelvis to take pressure off the cord is an effective method of postponing delivery while preparations are being made for a cesarean section.

C. **Improvement of fetal oxygenation.** Increasing the concentration of inspired oxygen to the mother results in a small increase in fetal P_{O_2} and may be a useful measure in treating fetal distress. Although fetal P_{O_2} may increase by a small degree, fetal oxygen content may increase considerably because of the affinity of fetal blood for oxygen.

D. **Amnioinfusion** involves the infusion of fluid into the amniotic cavity through the dilated cervix to expand the cavity and relieve the pressure on a compressed umbilical cord.

STUDY QUESTIONS

DIRECTIONS: Each of the numbered items or incomplete statements in this section is followed by answers or by completions of the statement. Select the ONE lettered answer or completion that is BEST in each case.

1. A 16-year-old primigravida presents with severe preeclampsia. She has meconium-stained amniotic fluid. Contractions occur every 3 minutes, and there is a late deceleration with each contraction. Fetal changes would include which of the following?

(A) Decreased lactic acid
(B) Increased pH
(C) Increased P_{CO_2}
(D) Decreased bicarbonate
(E) Increased P_{O_2}

2. A woman arrives at the hospital in active labor stating that her membranes ruptured 2 hours earlier. The fetal heart rate (FHR) monitor shows decelerations that do not seem related to any point in the contraction and quickly return to baseline with good variability. Which of the following is characteristic of these decelerations?

(A) They are associated with fetal head compression
(B) They are caused by uteroplacental insufficiency
(C) They are indications of fetal metabolic acidosis
(D) They are associated with a rise in fetal pH
(E) They are influenced by the ruptured-membrane status

3. A patient in the active phase of labor is 5-cm dilated, and the fetal heart monitor shows decreased variability. The monitor shows a baseline fetal rate of 125 beats per minute (bpm), with occasional late decelerations. A fetal scalp pH of 7.22 is obtained. This situation indicates which of the following conditions or actions?

(A) Significant fetal metabolic acidosis
(B) The need to repeat the fetal scalp pH test in 20 minutes
(C) The need for immediate cesarean section
(D) Chorioamnionitis with maternal fever
(E) The need for an intrauterine pressure catheter

4. A 31-year-old woman has been pushing in the second stage of labor for 2 hours. The vertex is at the +2 station. Each contraction is associated with a fetal bradycardia as low as 100 beats per minute (bpm) that lasts for 30 seconds. This clinical scenario suggests which of the following situations?

(A) Systemic fetal hypoxia
(B) Poor fetal outcome
(C) An association with oligohydramnios
(D) Fetal head compression
(E) A depressed fetal pH

5. A woman with prolonged rupture of membranes at term is being stimulated with oxytocin. She has progressed to 6-cm dilation and 0 station when late decelerations occur after each of her contractions, which are occurring every 90 seconds. Which of the following would be an appropriate therapy at this point?

(A) Cesarean section
(B) Shift to the left lateral position
(C) Subcutaneous terbutaline
(D) Amnioinfusion
(E) Intrauterine pressure catheter

DIRECTIONS: Each of the numbered items or incomplete statements in this section is negatively phrased, as indicated by a capitalized word such as NOT, LEAST, or EXCEPT. Select the ONE lettered answer or completion that is BEST in each case.

6. Which of the following fetal mechanisms does NOT compensate for the normal low fetal arterial partial pressure of oxygen (PO_2)?

(A) Increased fetal cardiac output
(B) Increased fetal systemic blood flow rates
(C) Increased fetal pulmonary blood flow
(D) Increased affinity of fetal blood for oxygen
(E) Increased fetal oxygen-carrying capacity

7. Which of the following explanations is NOT an explanation for decreased variability to the fetal heart rate (FHR) tracing?

(A) Fetal "sleep state"
(B) Prematurity
(C) Barbiturate ingestion
(D) Fetal stimulation
(E) Asphyxia

8. Which of the following is NOT a characteristic or associated finding with late decelerations?

(A) They are seen in patients with pre-eclampsia
(B) They may be associated with respiratory alkalosis
(C) They are associated with a decreased uteroplacental blood flow
(D) They usually are accompanied by a decrease in partial pressure of oxygen (PO_2)
(E) They usually are accompanied by an increase in partial pressure of carbon dioxide (PCO_2)

9. A woman with ruptured membranes is in the active phase of labor and is 5-cm dilated with sustained, deep variable decelerations. The decision is made to perform a cesarean section. Which of the following would NOT be an appropriate intrauterine resuscitative measure done before the cesarean section?

(A) Increase the intravenous fluids
(B) Place the patient in the supine position
(C) Start nasal oxygen
(D) Start amnioinfusion
(E) Administer subcutaneous terbutaline

10. A 25-year-old pregnant woman presents to the labor floor reporting extreme abdominal pain and heavy vaginal bleeding. The fetal heart monitor shows a fetal bradycardia with late decelerations. Which of the following acid–base characteristics would NOT be present in the fetus?

(A) Respiratory alkalosis
(B) An increased partial pressure of carbon dioxide (PCO_2)
(C) A drop in fetal pH
(D) Accumulation of lactic acid
(E) Metabolic acidosis

ANSWERS AND EXPLANATIONS

1. The answer is C [II B 1–4; III C 2 a–f]. Late decelerations usually reflect uteroplacental insufficiency, which is seen in severe pre-eclampsia. With uteroplacental insufficiency, fetal hypoxia can develop, resulting in a decrease in fetal partial pressure of oxygen (PO_2). At first, a respiratory acidosis develops in the fetus, which means that partial pressure of carbon dioxide (PCO_2) and bicarbonate rises; there is a concomitant decrease in fetal pH. As the hypoxia continues, a metabolic acidosis develops with a rise in lactic and pyruvic acids.

2. The answer is E [III C 1–3]. The decelerations in the fetal heart rate (FHR) in this clinical scenario are variable decelerations, which have no temporal relationship to the onset of a contraction. Early and late decelerations are associated with fetal head compression and uteroplacental insufficiency, respectively. When variable decelerations are mild, as in this case, they may be associated with mild respiratory acidosis, but not metabolic acidosis; in either case, the pH would fall and not rise. Variable decelerations are associated with cord compression, which is a finding consistent with that of ruptured membranes and the consequent loss of the fluid buffer between the fetus and the uterus.

3. The answer is B [IV A 1, B 1–2]. A fetal scalp pH of 7.20 to 7.24 is worrisome but is not indicative of severe distress, asphyxia, or metabolic acidosis in the fetus; there is no need for immediate cesarean section delivery. The scalp pH measurement, however, must be repeated in 20 to 30 minutes. A chorioamnionitis with a maternal temperature elevation would produce a fetal tachycardia of greater than 160 beats per minute (bpm). An intrauterine pressure catheter is used to monitor the intensity of the uterine contractions, not fetal pH.

4. The answer is D [III C 1–3]. With the vertex deep in the pelvis, there is considerable compression of the fetal head with the pushing during each contraction. Fetal heart rate (FHR) decelerations associated with fetal head compression are early decelerations and are benign. Because the decelerations are mirror images of the contractions, beginning at the onset of the contraction and lasting for 30 seconds, they are not associated with fetal hypoxia, decreased fetal pH, or poor fetal outcome. It is variable decelerations that are associated with oligohydramnios.

5. The answer is C [VI A 1–3, B 1–2, D]. This patient is being stimulated with oxytocin and is hyperstimulated, with contractions occurring every 90 seconds. As a result, the uterus does not relax between contractions, and uteroplacental insufficiency (i.e., late decelerations) develops. To correct the situation acutely, the oxytocin stimulation is withdrawn and subcutaneous terbutaline is given to relax the hyperstimulated uterus. Shifting position is important, but not effective in this case. Cesarean section is not yet necessary, and amnioinfusion would not help. An intrauterine pressure catheter would be indicated after the hyperstimulation of the uterus has been corrected.

6. The answer is C [II A 1, 2]. Despite the normal low fetal arterial partial pressure of oxygen (PO_2), the nonstressed fetus is neither hypoxic nor acidotic. It compensates with a physiology that exhibits increased cardiac output, increased fetal systemic blood flow rates, increased affinity of fetal blood for oxygen, and increased fetal oxygen-carrying capacity, but not an increased pulmonary blood flow. In fact, there is very little pulmonary blood flow because there is no oxygenation of blood in the lungs of the fetus; the blood bypasses the lungs and is shunted into the general circulation through the patent ductus arteriosus.

7. The answer is D [III B 1 a–g]. Decreased fetal heart rate (FHR) variability can be seen in a number of benign and ominous situations during labor, such as fetal "sleep states," prematurity, drug ingestion, asphyxia, tachycardia, arrhythmias, and fetal anomalies. With fetal stimulation in a healthy fetus, there is a transient tachycardia and no change in the FHR variability.

8. The answer is B [III C 2 d, e]. Late decelerations are indications of a decreased uteroplacental blood flow and often reflect hypoxemia or acidosis in the fetus. Preeclampsia is one of the several clinical entities that may have a decreased uteroplacental blood flow. The pathophysiology involves a fetal respiratory acidosis (not alkalosis) and metabolic acidosis, which means there is a decreased partial pressure of oxygen (PO_2) and an increased partial pressure of carbon dioxide (PCO_2).

9. The answer is B [VI A 1–3, B 1, C, D]. The patient should be placed in a lateral recumbent position, not in the supine position; the supine position may lead to decreased venous return and cardiac output due to compression of the vena cava by the pregnant uterus. In an effort to get the fetus in the best possible condition before delivery, it is advisable to perform some intrauterine resuscitative measures before the cesarean section. Increasing intravenous fluids increases the intravascular volume, which ensures maximum blood flow to the uterus. Nasal oxygen to the patient can result in small increases in fetal partial pressure of oxygen (PO_2). Amnioinfusion takes the pressure off the compressed cord, and tocolysis, the use of subcutaneous terbutaline, decreases contractions and allows maximal placental blood flow.

10. The answer is A [II B 1–5]. This clinical situation represents a classic case of placental abruption, which is the ultimate condition of uteroplacental insufficiency. In this situation, there is a decreased transfer of oxygen to the fetus with a decreased partial pressure of oxygen (PO_2) and an increased partial pressure of carbon dioxide (PCO_2). Because the fetus is unable to sustain aerobic metabolism, there is a shift to an anaerobic metabolism, with an accumulation of organic acids (e.g., lactic and pyruvic) and a drop in fetal pH. This is analogous to adult respiratory or metabolic acidosis, not alkalosis.

Chapter 6

Postterm Pregnancy
Matthew Rhoa

I. **INTRODUCTION.** Postterm pregnancy is a **gestation of 42 weeks or more** (294 days or more from the last menstrual period). The frequency is declining because of better dating of pregnancies early in gestation. This early dating of pregnancies results from the increasing use of ultrasound in early gestations. Because the group of patients carrying the diagnosis of postterm pregnancy has decreased, those that remain in the category are at even higher risk for complications associated with postterm pregnancy. Perinatal mortality increases after 40 weeks' gestation and doubles by 42 weeks' gestation. Approximately 80% of all pregnancies last between 38 and 42 weeks, 10% are delivered preterm, and 10% extend beyond 42 weeks. This chapter examines the significance of postterm pregnancies, the risk to the fetus and mother, and the management of postterm pregnancy.

A. **The average duration of a pregnancy** is 280 days from the first day of the last menstrual period (LMP) or 266 days from ovulation, based on a 28-day cycle. The estimated date of delivery (EDD) can be calculated by subtracting 3 months from the first day of the LMP and adding 7 days (Naegele's rule). The length of gestation increases approximately 1 day for each day the menstrual cycle is more than 28 days.

B. **The exact duration of pregnancy** is of foremost importance and can be determined in a number of ways at various stages of pregnancy. The clinician must begin by obtaining an accurate history and examination. A woman's LMP and a menstrual history provide the first EDD. Clinical data can be used to confirm or amend an EDD based solely on an LMP.

1. **Clinical data** that can assist the physician in dating a pregnancy include:
    a. Quickening (maternal perception of fetal movement) occurs at about 16 to 20 weeks.
    b. By 18 to 20 weeks, the fetal heart can be heard using a nonelectric fetal stethoscope.
    c. The fetal heart can be heard starting at 11 weeks with Doppler ultrasound.
    d. The date of the first pregnancy test can assist in determining the LMP date.
    e. The size of the uterus at an early examination in the first trimester should be consistent with dates.
    f. **First- and second-trimester ultrasound** has proven helpful in accurately dating pregnancies.
        (1) First-trimester scans are accurate to within 3 to 5 days. The crown–rump length is most accurate in the first trimester; by 12 weeks, the fetus begins to curve and this measurement becomes less accurate.
        (2) After 12 weeks the biparietal diameter becomes more accurate. During the second trimester the accuracy of ultrasound is within 1.5 weeks.
        (3) Bone growth rate decreases in the third trimester and the accuracy falls to within only 3 to 4 weeks.

2. **Inaccurate pregnancy dating** can result from a first visit late in pregnancy, erroneous LMP date, oligoovulation, ultrasound late in pregnancy, recent pregnancy, recent abortion, oral contraceptive use without resumption of menses, acute illness, intrauterine growth retardation, and drug use.

C. **Cause of postterm pregnancy.** Animal experiments have suggested that the cause of postmaturity stems from a combination of maternal, fetal, and genetic factors, all of which are predetermined.

1. **Potential causative factors.** A deficiency of adrenocorticotropic hormone in the fetus and placental sulfatase deficiency have been hypothesized as potential causative factors.

2. **The exact mechanism of spontaneous onset of labor** is unclear (see Chapter 4 I), but the fetus, placenta, and mother are all involved. The longest pregnancy on record is 1 year and 24 days, ending in a liveborn anencephalic infant. Central nervous system abnormalities, such as anencephaly, are associated with prolonged pregnancy.

II. CLINICAL SIGNIFICANCE OF POSTTERM PREGNANCY

A. **Incidence.** Postterm pregnancies occur more frequently in primigravidas who are younger or older than average childbearing age and in grandmultiparas (women who have had six or more pregnancies resulting in viable fetuses). The fetal mortality for all groups is:

1. 40 to 41 weeks' gestation: 1.1%

2. 43 weeks' gestation: 2.2%

3. 44 weeks' gestation: 6.6%

B. **Dysmaturity syndrome.** Normally, there is little growth of the fetus postterm (after 40 weeks); the little growth that does occur plateaus at 42 weeks. Dysmaturity syndrome is observed in 30% of postterm infants and in 3% of term infants. The **clinical features of the syndrome** include:

1. Loss of subcutaneous fat

2. Dry, wrinkled, and cracked skin

3. Meconium staining of the skin, membranes, and umbilical cord

4. Long nails

5. An unusual degree of alertness

C. **Fetal compromise secondary to placental insufficiency,** resulting from placental aging, or senescence, which critically reduces the metabolic and respiratory support to the fetus, is the major concern in postterm pregnancy. **Asphyxia** is frequently responsible for the perinatal morbidity and mortality in postterm pregnancy. Findings at autopsy of postterm infants suggestive of **hypoxia** include:

1. Petechiae of the pleura and pericardium

2. Amniotic debris in the lung

D. **Histology.** There is no pathognomonic histologic picture for postterm pregnancy. However, because placental insufficiency is the major concern, **placental changes** have been noted histologically and may correlate with insufficiency. These changes, which may be simply physiologic, can reduce the placental surface area available for nutritional and endocrine support to the fetus; they include the following:

1. Calcification

2. Edema of villi

3. Syncytial pseudohyperplasia

4. Syncytial knots

5. Fibroid degeneration of villi

6. Placental microinfarction

III. ANTEPARTUM ASSESSMENT OF THE POSTTERM FETUS.
Assessment techniques include biophysical profile, fetal heart rate (FHR) testing, and ultrasound (see I B 1 f).

A. FHR testing

1. The **nonstress test (NST)** is a noninvasive test of fetal activity that correlates with fetal well-being. Fetal heart rate accelerations are observed during fetal movement. An external monitor is used to record the FHR, and the mother participates by indicating fetal movements.

   a. A **reactive test** requires **two fetal heart rate accelerations** of at least 15 beats' amplitude of 15 seconds' duration in a 20-minute period.

   b. In one study, 99% of oxytocin challenge tests were negative for signs of fetal distress when performed after a reactive NST.

   c. The most common cause for a nonreactive NST is a period of fetal inactivity or sleep. Studies have shown the longest interval of fetal inactivity in the healthy fetus is 40 minutes.

   d. If the test is nonreactive after 40 minutes, a contraction stress test (CST) is performed.

   e. Approximately 25% of those fetuses that have a nonreactive NST have a positive CST.

2. The **contraction stress test** is a test of the FHR in response to uterine contractions that indirectly measures placental function. An intravenous infusion of oxytocin is used to stimulate uterine contractions. The nipple stimulation test is an endogenous means of releasing oxytocin in response to manual stimulation of the patient's nipples. It is a noninvasive CST. A CST is performed when the NST is nonreactive.

   a. Criteria for a negative CST consist of three uterine contractions of moderate intensity lasting 40 to 60 seconds over a 10-minute period with no late decelerations in the FHR tracing. A positive CST has late decelerations associated with greater than 50% of the uterine contractions. A CST with inconsistent late decelerations is considered suspect.

   b. More often, a favorable outcome follows a negative CST, but as many as 25% of fetuses may experience intrapartum fetal distress after a negative CST.

   c. CSTs have a **25% false-positive rate.**

   d. Studies have shown the incidence of perinatal death within 1 week of a negative CST to be less than 1/1000. Most of these deaths are caused by cord accidents or abruptions.

   e. A positive CST has been associated with an increased incidence of intrauterine death, late decelerations in labor, low 5-minute Apgar scores, intrauterine growth retardation, and meconium-stained amniotic fluid. The overall perinatal death rate after a positive CST is between 7% and 15%.

   f. A suspect CST should be repeated in 24 hours.

B. Biophysical profile
(see also Chapter 12 IV A 9). This is a composite of tests designed to identify a compromised fetus during the antepartum period (Table 6-1).

Table 6-1. Management Based on Biophysical Profile Score

Score	Interpretation	Management
10	Normal	Repeat testing
8	Normal	Repeat testing
6	Suspect chronic asphyxia	If ≥36 weeks, deliver Repeat testing in 4–6 hours
4	Suspect chronic asphyxia	If ≥32 weeks, deliver Repeat testing in 4–6 hours
0–2	Strongly suspect chronic asphyxia	Extend testing to 120 minutes, if score ≤4, deliver at any gestational age

1. **Components of the profile**
   a. NST
   b. Fetal breathing
   c. Fetal tone
   d. Fetal motion
   e. Quantity of amniotic fluid
2. **Scoring of the profile.** Each test is given either 2 or 0 points, for a maximum of 10 points. An important feature in the postterm profile is the amniotic fluid component. Oligohydramnios is an ominous sign signifying placental insufficiency.

IV. MANAGEMENT OF THE POSTTERM PREGNANCY

A. **Expectant.** Because the induction of labor can be accompanied by higher incidences of uterine inertia, long labor, trauma, forceps delivery, and cesarean delivery, expectant management is warranted in many instances. Cervical examinations should be performed weekly starting at 39 weeks to assess cervical ripening. An attempt should be made at estimating fetal weight. In instances of suspected macrosomia, an ultrasound should be performed.

1. **Spontaneous labor.** Because 60% of patients go into labor spontaneously between 40 and 41 weeks and 80% by 43 weeks, the pregnancy managed expectantly should be monitored carefully using the testing methods described previously.
2. The **ability of antepartum testing to accurately identify the fetus at risk** is far from ideal. Because no single test is adequate, a combination of tests is desirable. Testing should be performed twice weekly starting at 41 weeks.

B. **Active.** Regardless of the status of the cervix, delivery is indicated for the fetus identified as at risk. In spite of sophisticated testing, the postterm group has more induced labors, prolonged labors, and uterine inertia; higher incidences of intrapartum fetal distress; and higher cesarean birth rates. Nonetheless, with careful antepartum, intrapartum, and neonatal monitoring, the perinatal mortality for the postterm infant can approach that of the term population.

C. **Methods of induction.** In the postterm pregnancy, delivery is indicated if the cervix is ripe based on a Bishop score, there is evidence of deteriorating fetal well-being, there is suspected macrosomia, or the pregnancy is beyond 42 weeks.

1. **Oxytocin infusion.** This method may or may not be successful because of the condition of the cervix. An uneffaced, unripe cervix may not respond to oxytocin stimulation, resulting in an increased cesarean section rate.
2. **Prostaglandin gel.** Prostaglandin gel ripening has proved useful in postterm pregnancies because 80% of patients reaching 42 weeks have an unripe cervix. Application of prostaglandin gel to the cervix produces softening, shortening, and dilation of the cervix. The time in labor as well as the failed induction rate is reduced.

D. **Intrapartum management.** The major complications in the intrapartum period include macrosomia, fetal intolerance to labor, and meconium staining.

1. **Meconium staining** is four times more common in postterm pregnancies. The use of amnioinfusions and suctioning of the neonate before delivery of the shoulders has decreased the incidence and severity of meconium aspiration syndrome.
2. When **macrosomia** is suspected, an ultrasound should be performed to estimate the fetal weight. The clinician should always be prepared to deal with a potential shoulder dystocia.
3. **Intrapartum asphyxia** is more common in postterm labors, and careful monitoring should be instituted when this is suspected.

V. CONCLUSION. The most important first step in managing postterm pregnancies is to ensure appropriate dating. The mother and infant are at increased risk for complications. With appropriate fetal testing, and intervention when indicated, a satisfactory outcome can be achieved.

STUDY QUESTIONS

DIRECTIONS: Each of the numbered items or incomplete statements in this section is followed by answers or by completions of the statement. Select the ONE lettered answer or completion that is BEST in each case.

1. The first step in the assessment of the post-term gestation is

(A) ultrasound examination
(B) determination of the true length of gestation
(C) measurement of fetal heart rate (FHR)
(D) determination of amniotic fluid volume
(E) contraction stress test

2. The perinatal mortality rate at 44 weeks' gestation is

(A) less than 1%
(B) 1% to 2%
(C) 2% to 3%
(D) 4% to 5%
(E) 6% to 7%

3. After having identified a fetus at risk in prolonged pregnancy, management should consist of

(A) amniocentesis for maturity studies
(B) delivery regardless of the status of the cervix
(C) fetal sampling of scalp pH
(D) measurement of human chorionic somato-mammotropin
(E) repeat antepartum studies in 1 week

DIRECTIONS: Each of the numbered items or incomplete statements in this section is negatively phrased, as indicated by a capitalized word such as NOT, LEAST, or EXCEPT. Select the ONE lettered option or completion that is BEST in each case.

4. Which of the following factors has NOT been associated with a postterm pregnancy?

(A) Fetal macrosomia
(B) Meconium-stained fluid
(C) Placental sulfatase deficiency
(D) Insufficient oxytocin level
(E) Increased incidence of cesarean section

5. Which of the following is NOT included in the biophysical profile for the risk assessment of a postterm fetus?

(A) Fetal breathing
(B) Amniotic fluid volume
(C) Fetal tone
(D) Contraction stress test (CST)
(E) Fetal motion

DIRECTIONS: The set of matching questions in this section consists of a list of lettered options (some of which may be in figures) followed by several numbered items. For each numbered item, select the ONE lettered option that is most closely associated with it. To avoid spending too much time on matching sets with large numbers of options, it is generally advisable to begin each set by reading the list of options. Then, for each item in the set, try to generate the correct answer and locate it in the option list, rather than evaluating each option individually. Each lettered option may be selected once, more than once, or not at all.

Questions 6–8

For each of the following biophysical profile scores, select the appropriate management.

(A) Repeat testing twice weekly
(B) Repeat testing in 12 hours
(C) Extend testing and deliver if less than 4

6. 8

7. 9

8. 10

ANSWERS AND EXPLANATIONS

1. The answer is B [I A, B]. Before embarking on postterm testing, it is essential to determine the true length of the pregnancy. A seemingly postterm pregnancy may, in fact, not be postterm because of uncertain dating of the last menstrual period (LMP) or an irregular menstrual cycle in which the pregnant woman ovulated later than the usual day 14 of the cycle. Review of such features as quickening, uterine size at first visit and serial measurements thereafter, and the date of the first detectable fetal heart tones can be helpful in establishing the due date.

2. The answer is E [II A 1–3]. As pregnancy progresses beyond 40 weeks, perinatal morbidity and mortality increase. The perinatal mortality at term is 1.1%, and, by 44 weeks' gestation, there is a sixfold increase (6%–7%).

3. The answer is B [IV B]. Delivery of a fetus at risk in postterm pregnancy should be accomplished without regard to the status of the cervix. Delivery can, however, be accomplished through induction of labor, which is always accompanied by electronic intrapartum monitoring. One week is commonly the interval used for repetitive testing, but only if testing remains negative. Fetal scalp testing cannot be done with intact membranes.

4. The answer is D [I C]. There is no evidence to support the theory that oxytocin may be insufficient in prolonged pregnancy. The absence of placental sulfatase and the high incidence of central nervous system abnormalities, particularly anencephaly, with prolonged pregnancy are well documented.

5. The answer is D [III A 2, B 1]. The biophysical profile for risk assessment of a postterm fetus evaluates fetal breathing, tone, and motion; fetal heart rate, using the nonstress test (NST); and amniotic fluid volume. The contraction stress test (CST) could be used as a substitute for the NST, but only if the NST is nonreactive.

6–8. The answers are: 6-A, 7-C , 8-A [Table 6-1].

Chapter 7

Medical Complications of Pregnancy

Kavita Nanda

I. **DIABETES.** Diabetes is a medical disease that is made worse by pregnancy and that increases the risks of pregnancy complications. Diabetes affects **2% to 3% of pregnant women. Ninety percent of these cases are gestational diabetes.**

A. Diagnosis of diabetes during pregnancy

1. **Diabetes should be strongly suspected** in women who have:
   a. A strong family history of diabetes
   b. Previously given birth to large (i.e., macrosomic) infants
   c. Persistent glucosuria
   d. A history of unexplained stillbirth or miscarriage

2. **Persistent glucosuria** during pregnancy should be investigated, although the presence of glucosuria does not always reflect hyperglycemia from impaired glucose tolerance but may reflect a lower renal threshold for glucose, which may be induced by a normal pregnancy.

3. **Glucose testing.** Screening may be based on risk factors or be universal, depending on the patient population. Selective screening will miss cases of gestational diabetes, so **many authorities recommend universal screening.**
   a. The **1-hour glucose tolerance test** is a good screening test and is performed after a 50-g glucose load. An abnormal test necessitates a standard glucose tolerance test. Abnormalities are reflected by a 1-hour value of 140 mg/dl or higher.
   b. The **standard glucose tolerance test** is a 3-hour test with periodic blood determinations after a 100-g glucose load is ingested. **Class A diabetes (gestational diabetes)** is diagnosed when two or more plasma glucose levels equal or exceed:
      (1) 105 mg/dl (fasting)
      (2) 190 mg/dl (1 hour)
      (3) 165 mg/dl (2 hours)
      (4) 145 mg/dl (3 hours)

4. Diabetes in pregnant women is generally categorized as either gestational or pregestational diabetes. The **White classification** may be useful for further delineation:
   a. **Class A:** gestational diabetes
   b. **Class B:** maturity-onset diabetes; age at onset older than 20 years and duration of less than 10 years
   c. **Class C_1:** age at onset of 10 to 19 years
   d. **Class C_2:** duration of 10 to 19 years
   e. **Class D_1:** age at onset of less than 10 years
   f. **Class D_2:** duration of more than 20 years
   g. **Class D_3:** benign retinopathy
   h. **Class D_4:** peripheral vascular disease
   i. **Class D_5:** hypertension
   j. **Class F:** nephropathy
   k. **Class R:** proliferative retinopathy

B. Effects of pregnancy on glucose tolerance

1. The diabetogenic properties of pregnancy are reversible but still may induce abnormalities in glucose tolerance in women who have no evidence of diabetes.

a. **Insulin antagonism** is caused by the action of human placental lactogen and the steroids estrogen and progesterone.

b. **Placental insulinase** accelerates insulin degradation.

2. **Control of diabetes** may be more difficult in pregnancy.

a. **Insulin shock** can result from nausea and vomiting (because of the patient's lack of sustenance).

b. **Insulin resistance** and **ketoacidosis** can result from infection.

3. **Insulin requirements in patients with diabetes** decrease rapidly after delivery because of the disappearance of human placental lactogen and insulinase, as well as the reduction in estrogen and progesterone.

C. **Gestational diabetes mellitus (GDM)**

1. **Definition**

a. With the onset or recognition of glucose intolerance during pregnancy, there is a 15% to 20% chance of developing diabetes mellitus within the first year.

b. GDM is diagnosed by **two or more abnormal values on a 3-hour** glucose tolerance test.

2. **Management**

a. Nutritional consultation and dietary adjustment

b. Fasting and postprandial glucose monitoring at least weekly

(1) **Fasting glucose level** should be **less than 105 mg/dl**

(2) A **2-hour postprandial glucose level** should be **less than 120 mg/dl**

c. If plasma glucose is persistently elevated, insulin therapy is recommended. Patients on insulin need daily monitoring of blood glucose.

3. **Outcome**

a. There is a **risk of fetal macrosomia,** especially with poor glycemic control.

b. **Ultrasonography** may be used to assess fetal growth and aid in the timing and mode of delivery.

c. **Uncomplicated patients** with GDM **who are well controlled are at low risk for fetal death.** If the patient has gestational diabetes and does not require insulin, her fetus can be delivered at term; there is no need for early delivery.

d. **Patients with gestational diabetes who use insulin or those who are not well controlled should be managed as patients with preexisting diabetes,** as should patients with hypertension or previous stillbirth (see next sections).

4. **Follow-up.** A 2-hour, 75-g glucose postpartum tolerance test, especially if the patient is insulin dependent, should be administered.

D. **Effects of preexisting diabetes on pregnancy:**

1. **Mother.** There is an increased likelihood of:

a. **Mortality,** the rate of which is 0.11%

b. **Preeclampsia** and **eclampsia**

c. **Infection,** which can be severe

d. A **macrosomic infant,** which can present problems with delivery, such as shoulder dystocia

e. **Cesarean section delivery** because of the macrosomia of the infant

f. **Polyhydramnios**

g. **Postpartum hemorrhage**

h. **Diabetic ketoacidosis**

2. **Fetus.** There is an increased likelihood of:

a. **Perinatal mortality,** especially when the pregnant patient with diabetes is not managed appropriately. **In the past, the perinatal mortality rate was 14% to 35%; it is now 3% to 5%.**

b. **Perinatal morbidity from birth injury** (often because of macrosomia with accompanying shoulder dystocia and brachial plexus injury)

c. **Neonatal hypocalcemia, hypoglycemia, polycythemia,** and **hyperbilirubinemia**

    d. Congenital abnormalities, such as cardiac and neural tube defects
    e. Respiratory distress syndrome
    f. Diabetes in the offspring
    g. Intrauterine growth restriction

E. **Preconception and prenatal care of patients with pregestational diabetes**

1. **Hemoglobin A_{1c} determination** at the patient's first visit provides an assessment of her prior diabetic regulation. **A hemoglobin A_{1c} level of greater than 10% has been associated with increased risk of congenital malformations.**

2. **Strict glucose control before and during early pregnancy is thought to reduce the risk of severe malformations** such as cardiac and neural tube defects, which are seen in fetuses of women with poorly controlled diabetes. The maternal glucose level should be kept as close to normal as possible. **This may involve one or more antepartum hospitalizations for glucose control.**

3. **Determination of the precise fetal age is important in a woman with diabetes.**
    a. Early ultrasound evaluation is used in conjunction with the last menstrual period to date the pregnancy.
    b. A well-established estimated date of delivery is necessary to be able to assess the following accurately:
        (1) Macrosomia
        (2) Polyhydramnios
        (3) Fetal growth restriction, which is seen in women with diabetes with vascular disease

4. **Evaluation for congenital malformations** should be offered.
    a. Ultrasound evaluation of fetal anatomy at 16 to 20 weeks will detect many major anomalies.
    b. Screening for neural tube defects is possible by analysis of maternal serum α-fetoprotein (AFP) at 16 to 20 weeks. An elevated AFP greater than 2.5 multiples of the median indicates a possible neural tube defect and should be further evaluated by targeted ultrasound and assessment of amniotic fluid AFP and acetylcholinesterase.
    c. Fetal echocardiography at 20 to 22 weeks will detect most major structural cardiac malformations.

5. **Determination of the degree of vascular involvement** by renal, ophthalmologic, and cardiac evaluation is recommended.

6. **Nutrition counseling** should be offered to the patient.

7. **Insulin requirements** should be calculated based on the previous insulin dosage and the patient's weight and given in two or three divided doses. Insulin requirements may increase as gestation progresses. **Required doses cannot be gauged by the degree of glucosuria.**
    a. Glucosuria may be present because of an increase in the glomerular filtration of glucose without increased tubular reabsorption.
    b. Significant hypoglycemia could develop if the insulin dosage is manipulated because of the glucosuria rather than because of the blood glucose levels.
    c. The **goals of therapy** are as follows.
        (1) Fasting blood glucose level of 60 to 90 mg/dl
        (2) Prelunch, dinner glucose level of 60 to 105 mg/dl
        (3) 2-hour postprandial glucose level of less than 120 mg/dl

F. **Third trimester and delivery management**

1. **Surveillance** for fetal well-being should begin **between 28 and 32 weeks.**
    a. Methods of fetal surveillance, which are described in Chapter 6, may include fetal kick counts, the nonstress test (NST), the contraction stress test (CST), and the biophysical profile. The NST should be reactive and the CST should be negative if the fetus is healthy. Signs of fetal compromise include the following:

(1) Decreased fetal movement

(2) A nonreactive NST

(3) A positive CST

(4) A poor biophysical profile

  b. The frequency and timing of fetal surveillance depend on the severity of the disease and the degree of glycemic control.

  c. Frequent (every 4 to 6 weeks) ultrasound examinations to assess fetal growth should be performed.

2. Admission to the hospital at 34 to 36 weeks is indicated only for those patients with poor control or other complicating factors, such as hypertension or evidence of other vascular diseases, so that the fetus can be monitored closely to prevent sudden fetal demise.

3. The **timing of delivery** depends on the health and maturity of the fetus. In a woman with well-controlled diabetes with normal fetal testing, it may be prudent to await the onset of labor up to 40 weeks' gestation. If induction is considered at less than 39 weeks, assessment of fetal lung maturity is recommended.

  a. In a diabetic woman, the lecithin to sphingomyelin (L/S) ratio may take longer to show fetal lung maturity than in a nondiabetic. **The goal is an L/S ratio of 2:1 (or 2:0)** or greater, an event that usually occurs at approximately 35 to 36 weeks' gestation in most normal pregnancies. **The L/S ratio may not be truly reflective of fetal lung maturity in a diabetic woman, and the phosphatidylglycerol also should be measured.**

  b. Lung maturity at 37 to 38 weeks in the fetus of a woman with insulin-dependent diabetes cannot, therefore, be assumed without measuring amniotic fluid levels of lecithin, sphingomyelin, and phosphatidylglycerol.

4. Method of delivery

  a. Induction of labor may be attempted if the fetus is not excessively large and if the cervix is capable of being induced (i.e., if the cervix is soft, appreciably effaced, and somewhat dilated).

  b. The possibility of shoulder dystocia in the macrosomic infant of a mother with diabetes must be considered; **cesarean section may be indicated to avoid the trauma of a delivery of a large infant (> 4000 g) in a patient with diabetes.**

  c. Euglycemia should be maintained during labor.

II. ANEMIAS

A. Acquired anemias

1. Iron deficiency. The iron requirements of pregnancy are considerable, and in most women iron stores are low.

  a. A pregnant woman needs **an additional 800 mg of elemental iron,** of which 300 mg goes to the fetus and 500 mg is used to expand the maternal red cell mass.

  b. There is a natural decrease in the level of hematocrit during the second half of pregnancy because the newly formed hemoglobin and red cell mass do not keep pace with the expansion of the maternal blood volume. **Anemia exists with a hemoglobin of less than 10 g** during pregnancy. This is usually a hypochromic, microcytic anemia.

  c. Daily elemental iron (200 mg) is necessary to correct the anemia and maintain adequate stores.

  d. Because of the normal transfer of iron from the mother to the fetus, **the fetus does not suffer from iron deficiency anemia even in a severely anemic mother.**

2. Megaloblastic anemia is usually caused by a folic acid deficiency; women with this anemia are usually also iron deficient.

a. This anemia is found in pregnant women who consume neither fresh vegetables nor foods with a high content of animal protein.

b. Women with megaloblastic anemia during pregnancy may develop:

    (1) Nausea

    (2) Vomiting

    (3) Anorexia

c. Treatment includes:

    (1) A well-balanced diet

    (2) Oral iron

    (3) Folic acid (1 mg/day)

B. **Congenital anemias,** which are characterized by the hemoglobinopathies (i.e., sickle cell anemia, sickle cell–hemoglobin C disease, and α- and β-thalassemia), result in increased maternal morbidity and mortality rates, spontaneous abortion, and perinatal mortality. The impact of the hemoglobinopathy on the fetus parallels the severity of the anemia.

1. **Sickle cell anemia–hemoglobin SS disease (SS disease) occurs when an individual receives the gene for the production of hemoglobin S, an abnormal variant of hemoglobin, from each parent.** Because the sickle cell trait commonly appears in one of twelve black individuals, **the theoretical incidence of SS disease is one in five hundred seventy-six.** The actual rate among pregnant women is somewhat lower because of the high mortality rate among individuals with SS disease, especially during early childhood.

    a. **Pregnancy is a serious burden** on both the woman and the fetus in women with SS disease.

        (1) The anemia becomes more intense. Prophylactic transfusions to keep the hematocrit above 25% were used in the past, but current recommendations are to transfuse only in those patients with serious morbidity.

        (2) Seventy percent of patients experience painful vaso-occlusive crises. These are treated with hydration, oxygen, analgesics, blood transfusion, and antibiotics for concurrent infection.

        (3) Infection and pulmonary dysfunction are seen frequently.

            (a) Common infections include pyelonephritis, pneumonia, cholecystitis, and skin infections.

            (b) Asymptomatic bacteriuria should be treated.

            (c) Pneumococcal vaccine is recommended.

        (4) Preterm labor may occur.

        (5) Fetal growth restriction may occur, and fetuses should be followed up with serial sonography.

        (6) Preeclampsia is more common.

        (7) Death of the woman or the fetus may occur. Antepartum fetal surveillance from 32 to 34 weeks is recommended.

    b. There is intense erythropoiesis because of the shortened life span of the red blood cells containing abnormal hemoglobin. Because of this, the folic acid needs of a pregnant woman with SS disease are considerable (i.e., 1 mg/day).

    c. Labor is managed with:

        (1) Adequate hydration and oxygen to prevent sickling

        (2) Analgesia

        (3) Packed cell transfusion if a cesarean section is considered and the hemoglobin is very low.

2. **Sickle cell–hemoglobin C disease (SC disease) occurs in 1 in 2000 pregnant black women.** Hemoglobin C also may be seen in those of West African or Sicilian descent.

    a. **During pregnancy, maternal morbidity and mortality rates are higher in SC disease than in SS disease;** however, there is a lower perinatal mortality rate in SC disease as compared with SS disease.

    b. In the past, one in eight pregnancies ended in maternal death, abortion, stillbirth, or neonatal death. Current reports show improved outcome, however.

    c. There is a high incidence of severe pain and pulmonary dysfunction, the latter resulting from embolization of necrotic bone marrow, both the fat and cellular components.

    d. Early ambulation and observation for infection postpartum is recommended because of the risk of thromboembolism.

3. Sickle cell/β-thalassemia disease has a perinatal mortality and morbidity rate similar to that of SC disease, with somewhat less maternal morbidity and mortality.

4. Sickle cell trait is characterized by the inheritance of the gene for the production of hemoglobin S from one parent and hemoglobin A from the other. The trait occurs in 8.5% of black individuals. It also may be seen in patients of Mediterranean, Caribbean, Latin American, North African, Indian, and Southeast Asian descent.

    a. Most patients have only a mild anemia.

    b. Sickle cell trait does not influence the frequency of spontaneous abortion, perinatal mortality, low birth weight, or pregnancy-induced hypertension.

    c. Urinary tract infection and asymptomatic bacteriuria are twice as common in patients with sickle cell trait as in those without the trait and should be treated promptly to avoid pyelonephritis.

    d. Paternal testing is important to determine the risk of a fetus with SS or SC disease. Prenatal diagnosis is available to detect SS fetuses.

5. Thalassemias. The normal adult hemoglobins are A, A_2, and F. Hemoglobin A, which accounts for 95% or more of adult hemoglobin, is made up of two α-chains and two β-chains. Most individuals also have small amounts of hemoglobin A_2, which consists of two α-chains and two Δ-chains. The remainder is made up of hemoglobin F, which comprises two α-chains and two γ-chains. Patients with the thalassemias may be initially detected by a screening complete blood count that shows a mean corpuscular volume of less than 70.

    a. α-Thalassemia. The α-thalassemias are characterized by a deletion of one or more of the four genes for the α-chain.

        (1) Deletion of one α-gene does not cause anemia.

        (2) Deletion of two genes causes α-thalassemia trait, characterized by mild anemia.

        (3) Deletion of three genes (hemoglobin H) causes moderate anemia, with rare need for transfusion or splenectomy.

        (4) Deletion of four genes (Bart's hemoglobin) causes severe intrauterine anemia with fetal hydrops and death, and maternal preeclampsia and postpartum hemorrhage.

    b. β-Thalassemia. The β-thalassemias occur because of point mutations in the genes for β-chain production, leading to a decrease in β-chain formation. This decrease leads to a decrease in hemoglobin A production and a relative increase in the percentage of hemoglobin A_2 ($> 4.0\%$), which can be noted on hemoglobin electrophoresis.

        (1) β-thalassemia trait occurs when β-globin production is decreased by 50%. This causes a mild anemia with hypochromic microcytosis and occasional hepatosplenomegaly.

        (2) β-thalassemia intermedia occurs when production is decreased by 75%, leading to moderate anemia with occasional need for transfusion, hepatosplenomegaly, and iron overload.

        (3) β-thalassemia major occurs with no production of the β-chain, causing severe anemia, transfusion dependency, iron overload, bone deformities, and death in early adulthood.

    c. Women with the most severe forms of α- or β-thalassemia do not usually survive until childbearing age.

    d. During pregnancy, women with β-thalassemia intermedia may experience a drop in hemoglobin and hematocrit levels. The red blood cell mass does not expand normally because of deficient hemoglobin production.

        (1) Folic acid supplementation is recommended to keep up with the accelerated red blood cell turnover.

(2) **Iron therapy is indicated** only for patients with demonstrable iron deficiency because of the risk of iron overload and hepatotoxicity.

e. Patients with α- or β-thalassemia trait tolerate pregnancy very well. **Paternal testing should be considered** to predict the risk of severe fetal disease in the fetus. Prenatal diagnosis is also available.

III. **URINARY TRACT INFECTION.** Pregnancy, with its functional and anatomic changes of the urinary tract, predisposes women to the development of urinary tract infections. **Five percent of pregnant women have bacteriuria at the first prenatal visit.**

A. **Cystitis** is characterized by dysuria, particularly at the end of urination, as well as the urgent and frequent need to urinate, accompanied by a urine culture positive for bacterial growth with at least 100 colonies/ml. If cystitis is not treated, the upper urinary tract may become involved in an ascending infection.

B. **Acute pyelonephritis** is one of the most common medical complications of pregnancy. **It complicates late pregnancy and the puerperium in 2% of women** and usually results from an ascending infection of the bladder. When unilateral, the disease usually is right-sided.

1. **Characteristics of acute pyelonephritis**
   a. The abrupt onset of fever
   b. Shaking chills
   c. Aching pain in one or both lumbar regions
   d. Anorexia
   e. Nausea
   f. Vomiting
   g. Preterm labor

2. *Escherichia coli* is the organism most commonly cultured from the urine.

3. **Factors that predispose the pregnant woman to pyelonephritis** include the following.
   a. **Compression of the ureter** at the pelvic brim by the enlarging uterus and by the enlarged ovarian vein, which leads to a progressive dilation of the renal calyces, pelves, and ureters
   b. **Decrease in tone and peristaltic action of the ureters** secondary to the increased levels of progesterone, which is known to relax smooth muscle
   c. **Decreased bladder sensitivity to volume in the puerperium** secondary to spinal or epidural anesthesia, which may lead to overdistension of the bladder and the need for catheterization, resulting in the seeding of bacteria

4. **Therapy**
   a. **Inpatient treatment** is recommended in pregnancy.
   b. **Intravenous hydration** is needed.
   c. **Intravenous antibiotic therapy,** usually with a first-generation cephalosporin, should be continued until the patient is afebrile for 24 to 48 hours. Treatment should be completed with a course of oral antibiotics for at least 10 to 14 days total.
   d. Patients who do not respond should be evaluated by ultrasonography for stones and abscesses.
   e. Antibiotic suppression for the remainder of gestation should be considered.

5. **Complications**
   a. Bacteremia and septic shock
   b. Preterm delivery
   c. Adult respiratory distress syndrome
   d. Renal dysfunction

C. **Asymptomatic bacteriuria (ASB)** is the presence of actively multiplying bacteria within the urinary tract without the symptoms of a urinary tract infection. The commonly accepted definition is $\geq 10^5$ colonies of a bacterial organism per milliliter of urine on a clean-catch, midstream specimen.

1. The highest incidence is in black multiparas with sickle cell trait.

2. Twenty percent to 40% of women with untreated ASB during pregnancy subsequently develop acute pyelonephritis.

3. Untreated bacteriuria also may be a factor in the genesis of low birthweight and prematurity; this risk can be reduced by screening and treating all pregnant women with ASB.

4. Treatment involves one of the following:
   a. **Nitrofurantoin,** 100 mg daily for 10 days, which may precipitate a hemolytic crisis in patients with glucose-6-phosphate dehydrogenase deficiency
   b. **Trimethoprim/sulfamethoxazole,** one double-strength tablet twice a day for 10 days
      (1) **Should not be used in the first trimester** because trimethoprim is a folate antagonist.
      (2) **Use with caution in the third trimester** because sulfonamides may cause hyperbilirubinemia in the newborn.
   c. **Ampicillin,** 500 mg four times a day for 10 days. Many isolates of *E. coli* are resistant.
   d. **A follow-up culture** should be obtained post-treatment.

IV. THYROID DISEASE

A. **Hyperthyroidism.** Signs and symptoms of normal pregnancy may mimic the hyperthyroid state. In addition, normal pregnancy is accompanied by an increase in the thyroid-binding globulin, which leads to a slight increase in total thyroxine (T_4) and total triiodothyronine (T_3) levels. The free levels of T_4 and T_3 remain relatively unchanged.

1. **Diagnosis.** Hyperthyroidism during pregnancy can be identified by:
   a. Tachycardia that exceeds the increase caused by normal pregnancy (> 100 beats per minute at rest)
   b. An enlarged thyroid gland
   c. Exophthalmos
   d. Failure to gain weight normally
   e. Severe hyperemesis gravidarum
   f. Elevated plasma-free T_4 levels as compared with normal values in the nonpregnant state, or a suppressed thyroid stimulating hormone

2. **Treatment.** Treatment of thyrotoxicosis during pregnancy is recommended to prevent complications such as preterm delivery and perinatal mortality. Hyperthyroidism can almost always be controlled with antithyroid medication without any threat to the mother. Treatment may be medical or surgical.
   a. **Medical therapy**
      (1) **Propylthiouracil** prevents both the synthesis of thyroid hormone in the thyroid gland and the peripheral conversion of T_4 to T_3. The drug readily crosses the placenta and may induce fetal hypothyroidism and goiter. The goal is, therefore, a maternal T_4 level that is high–normal.
      (2) **Methimazole** prevents only the release of thyroid hormone and has been associated with aplasia cutis, a reversible developmental disorder of the fetal scalp.
      (3) **β-blockers** may be used to control symptoms of hyperthyroidism.
      (4) **Radioactive iodine** is contraindicated in pregnancy because it crosses the placenta and can ablate the fetal thyroid gland.

b. Surgical therapy. Thyroidectomy may be necessary in cases of thyrotoxicosis refractory to medical therapy. Surgery is most properly timed during the second trimester.

B. Hypothyroidism

1. **Unique features**
   a. Hypothyroidism is often associated with infertility.
   b. If pregnancy occurs, there is an apparent increased risk of spontaneous abortion, preeclampsia, placental abruption, and low birth weight.
   c. If hypothyroidism is treated inadequately, stillbirth may result.
   d. Infants of well-controlled hypothyroid mothers are healthy and without evidence of thyroid dysfunction.

2. **Diagnosis** of hypothyroidism in pregnancy is made by a high-thyroid stimulating hormone or low free T_4.

3. **Treatment** is with supplemental thyroid hormone. For the woman already undergoing thyroid replacement therapy, the dosage usually does not have to be increased. Serum thyroid function tests should be monitored, however.

V. HEART DISEASE

A. Incidence of heart disease in pregnancy

1. **Heart disease occurs in 1% of all pregnancies.** Because of the decreased incidence of rheumatic fever, fewer women are seen with rheumatic heart disease. Corrective surgery has enabled more women with congenital heart disease to reach childbearing age.

2. **There is a 38% incidence of fetal death in the pregnancies of women with severe hypoxic congenital heart disease.** Severe maternal hypoxia results in:
   a. Abortion
   b. Premature delivery
   c. Intrauterine demise
   d. Intrauterine growth restriction

3. **The risk of maternal mortality is considerable and depends on the specific cardiac lesion.** Patients with pulmonary hypertension, Eisenmenger's syndrome, coarctation of the aorta with valvular involvement, or Marfan's syndrome with aortic involvement have a mortality rate in pregnancy of 25% to 50%. Other conditions such as small septal defects, patent ductus arteriosus, and corrected tetralogy of Fallot have a maternal mortality rate of less than 1%. Preconceptual counseling is recommended for all patients with heart disease who are considering pregnancy.

B. Diagnosis of heart disease during pregnancy

1. **Symptoms** that occur in normal pregnancies **that can be confused with symptoms of heart disease** include:
   a. Functional systolic murmurs
   b. Accentuated respiratory effort, which sometimes represents dyspnea
   c. Edema, especially in the lower extremities during the last half of pregnancy

2. **Symptoms and signs of heart disease** in pregnancy include:
   a. Severe dyspnea
   b. Syncope with exertion
   c. Chest pain related to exertion
   d. Paroxysmal nocturnal dyspnea
   e. Unequivocal cardiac enlargement
   f. A diastolic, presystolic, or continuous heart murmur
   g. A loud, harsh systolic murmur, especially if associated with a thrill

     h. Cyanosis and clubbing
     i. Arrhythmias

C. **Classification of heart disease.** The woman's functional status before or in early pregnancy is an important prognosticator. The New York Heart Association classification is useful.

1. **Class I:** asymptomatic
2. **Class II:** symptoms with greater than normal activity
3. **Class III:** symptoms with normal physical activity
4. **Class IV:** symptoms at bed rest

D. **Management of pregnant cardiac patients**

1. **Class I and II cardiac patients.** Patients generally have a favorable prognosis during pregnancy. They must be aware constantly of the signs of developing cardiac failure. Forty-four percent of patients with cardiac disease will first develop pulmonary edema in the third trimester of pregnancy.

2. **Class III cardiac patients**
    a. One third of class III patients will decompensate during pregnancy. When such patients cannot or do not want to be hospitalized or stay in bed for most of their pregnancy, a therapeutic abortion is sometimes considered.
    b. The method of delivery is vaginal.
       (1) The sick cardiac patient withstands major surgical procedures poorly.
       (2) Severe heart disease is a contraindication for cesarean section.

3. **Class IV cardiac patients** must be treated for cardiac failure in pregnancy, labor, and the puerperium. Delivery by any method carries a high maternal mortality rate.

4. **Recommended prenatal care** for all pregnant patients with cardiac disease includes:
    a. Team approach to medical care with a cardiologist and an obstetrician
    b. Limitation of physical activity
    c. Intensive maternal and fetal monitoring to assess potential cardiac and obstetric complications
    d. Avoidance of foods rich in sodium
    e. Fetal echocardiography in patients with congenital heart defects
    f. Drug therapy as indicated

5. **Hospitalization before delivery** is common, either for congestive heart failure or optimal management of labor.
    a. Labor
       (1) The patient must be placed in the lateral recumbent position.
       (2) The maternal pulse and respiratory rate must be monitored. A pulse of greater than 100 beats per minute or a respiratory rate of greater than 24/min is a sign of possible cardiac compromise.
       (3) Continuous epidural anesthesia is appropriate for most patients for relief of pain and apprehension. Avoidance of hypotension is important.
       (4) Careful management of fluid status is essential, and management may be guided by invasive hemodynamic monitoring
       (5) Delivery should be accomplished vaginally unless there is an obstetrical reason for a cesarean section. Morbidity and mortality rates are lower with vaginal deliveries than with cesarean section.
       (6) Endocarditis prophylaxis where appropriate should be given.
    b. Congestive heart failure. The onset may be subtle, so observation must be constant.
       (1) Signs and symptoms include:
          (a) Increasing dyspnea
          (b) Increasing fatigue, with inability to carry out normal household chores
          (c) Cough with rales on physical examination

      (2) Before labor or full dilation of the cervix:
         (a) The failure must be treated before there can be any attempt at delivery. Although the fetus can be severely distressed by cardiac failure, the mother will be compromised if delivery is effected before therapy.
         (b) Treatment includes:
            (i) Morphine
            (ii) Oxygen
            (iii) Digitalization
            (iv) Diuresis
      (3) After complete dilation of the cervix and fetal descent, forceps or vacuum-extraction delivery is recommended to reduce the stress of pushing in the second stage of labor.

   c. Postpartum
      (1) The autotransfusion that occurs after delivery of the placenta can cause a marginally compensated woman to go into heart failure.
      (2) Postpartum infection and hemorrhage are potential problems in women with heart disease.

VI. THROMBOEMBOLIC DISEASE

A. Epidemiology

1. Thromboembolic disease is the leading cause of death in pregnant and postpartum women.

2. It occurs in 0.02% to 0.3% of pregnant patients and in 0.1% to 1.0% of postpartum patients.

3. Untreated deep vein thrombosis (DVT) in pregnancy causes pulmonary embolism (PE) in as many as 24% of patients.
   a. The mortality rate is 15%.
   b. If patients are treated adequately, the risk of PE is 4.5%, with a risk of mortality of less than 1%.

B. Pathophysiology

1. Pregnancy is a hypercoagulable state.

2. The gravid uterus may cause venous stasis.

C. Diagnosis

1. DVT
   a. Possible signs and symptoms
      (1) Calf pain
      (2) Palpable cord
      (3) Tenderness
      (4) Unilateral edema of the leg
      (5) Homan's sign
      (6) Dilated superficial veins
   b. Doppler ultrasound. Venous dopplers have a sensitivity of only 50% to 80% for calf vein DVT.
   c. Venography
      (1) This procedure is considered the gold standard for diagnosis of DVT.
      (2) The dose of radiation is minimal, and the fetus can be protected by abdominal shielding.
      (3) This procedure is invasive and expensive.
   d. ^{125}**I radioisotope scanning** should **not** be used in pregnancy.

    e. Impedance plethysmography is safe, but sensitivity and specificity have not been well studied in pregnancy.

  2. PE

    a. Clinical findings

      (1) Tachypnea

      (2) Dyspnea

      (3) Pleuritic pain

      (4) Apprehension

      (5) Cough

      (6) Tachycardia

      (7) Hemoptysis

    b. Arterial blood gas analysis

      (1) An arterial partial pressure of oxygen (PaO_2) of more than 80 mm Hg on room air makes the diagnosis unlikely. If signs and symptoms persist, further evaluation is recommended.

      (2) An increased alveolar–arterial gradient may indicate PE.

    c. Ventilation/perfusion scan

      (1) Most patients with a PE will have an abnormal ventilation/perfusion scan. Sensitivity = 98%.

      (2) Many patients without emboli also will have an abnormal scan. Specificity = 10%.

      (3) The degree of abnormality is graded low, intermediate, or high probability, with further intervention and therapy guided by clinical suspicion.

    d. Pulmonary angiogram

      (1) The gold standard for diagnosis of PE

      (2) Indicated for anticoagulation failures when caval interruption is considered, to distinguish between recurrent embolization and fragmentation of the original clot

      (3) Minimal risk to fetus

      (4) Safe in pregnancy

D. **Treatment**

  1. DVT

    a. Bed rest with extremity elevation

    b. Application of moist heat

    c. Therapeutic anticoagulation. **Heparin is the anticoagulant of choice during pregnancy.**

      (1) The initial goal is an activated partial thromboplastin time of 2.0 to 2.5× control.

      (2) There are some known risks when heparin is used.

        (a) Bleeding is the most common adverse effect of heparin. If major bleeding occurs, discontinue heparin. The administration of 10 to 20 mg of protamine sulfate intravenously (over at least 5 minutes) may be used to neutralize heparin's effects.

        (b) Osteoporosis is a serious, but less common side effect associated with prolonged use of high doses of heparin. Three months of heparin treatment with moderate doses (20,000 U/24 hrs) will most likely not be associated with clinically significant osteoporosis.

        (c) A small percentage of patients treated with heparin develop serious idiosyncratic thrombocytopenia, which usually begins between 3 and 15 days after commencing therapy.

    d. Coumadin is a known teratogen and should be avoided in pregnancy. It may be used postpartum, even if the mother is nursing.

  2. PE

    a. Oxygen to maintain maternal PaO_2 more than 70 mm Hg

    b. Bed rest for 5 to 7 days

    c. Therapeutic anticoagulation with heparin for 6 to 12 months, including labor and delivery and the puerperium

3. **DVT and PE management.** The management of pregnant women who have previously had a DVT or PE is controversial. Heparin 5000 to 10,000 U every 12 hours subcutaneously throughout pregnancy is recommended by some authorities.

VII. SEIZURE DISORDERS

A. **Epidemiologic analysis.** Between 0.3% and 0.6% of pregnant women have epilepsy.

B. **Effects of pregnancy on seizures**
1. The seizure frequency may increase.
2. Anticonvulsant dosage requirements may increase.

C. **Effects of epilepsy on pregnancy**
1. **Mother.** There is no significant increase in maternal complications.
2. **Fetus**
   a. There is an increased risk of stillbirth, especially with uncontrolled maternal seizures.
   b. There is an increased risk of epilepsy in the child, especially with idiopathic epilepsy in the mother.
   c. There is an increased risk of hemorrhagic disease of the newborn in fetuses exposed to anticonvulsants in utero.
   d. There is an increased risk of congenital anomalies, two times the increase over baseline.
      (1) Fetuses of mothers with epilepsy have a 4% to 6% risk of major congenital anomalies, most commonly cleft lip and palate and congenital heart defects.
      (2) It is unclear whether this risk is because of the seizure disorder itself or because of anticonvulsant therapy.
      (3) The risk increases with the number of anticonvulsant medications the mother is taking at the time of organogenesis.
   e. **Specific anticonvulsants and the associated problems:**
      (1) Phenytoin–microcephaly, dysmorphic facies, mental deficiency
      (2) Carbamazepine—craniofacial defects, nail hypoplasia, neural tube defects
      (3) Valproic acid—neural tube defects
      (4) Trimethadione—multiple malformations and mental retardation in more than 50% of exposed fetuses
      (5) Phenobarbital—neonatal withdrawal syndrome

D. **Therapeutic approach to the pregnant woman with seizures**
1. Monotherapy; begin preconceptually if possible
2. Compliance with taking medication
3. Monitoring of anticonvulsant levels
4. Folic acid supplements; begin preconceptually if possible
5. Screening for anomalies with targeted ultrasound and maternal serum AFP analysis
6. Vitamin K supplementation in the last month of pregnancy
7. Vitamin K administered to the newborn

VIII. Rh ISOIMMUNIZATION

A. **Definition.** Rh isoimmunization is caused by maternal antibody production in response to exposure to fetal red blood cell antigens of the Rh group, including Cc, Dd, and Ee (the Rh alleles).

B. **Epidemiology**

1. Approximately 1.5% of all pregnancies are complicated by red blood cell sensitization. The incidence of Rh isoimmunization in the United States has fallen since the 1960s because of Rho (anti-D) immune globulin use.

2. Native Americans and Asians are almost all (99%) Rh positive. Seven percent of African Americans and 13% of whites are Rh negative.

C. **Hemolytic disease of the fetus and newborn is synonymous with erythroblastosis fetalis.** There are three classifications.

1. **Mild hemolytic disease**
   a. Half of all affected infants are classified as mild cases.
   b. No prenatal or neonatal treatment is required.
   c. Infants are mildly anemic at birth.

2. **Moderate hemolytic disease**
   a. Twenty-five to thirty percent of affected infants are classified as moderate.
   b. Prenatal treatment may include transfusions, but usually only one neonatal transfusion is required.
   c. Moderate anemia with hemoglobin levels from 7 to 12 g/dl is found.
   d. In the neonatal period, treatment with exchange transfusions and phototherapy for hyperbilirubinemia is essential.

3. **Severe hemolytic disease**
   a. Twenty to twenty-five percent of affected fetuses become severely anemic.
   b. Prenatal treatment by transfusion is usually necessary to prolong the pregnancy until fetal maturity.
   c. Cord hemoglobin levels of less than 7 to 12 g/dl are found.
   d. In utero, total body edema (i.e., hydrops fetalis) occurs if the fetus is not transfused. Hydrops fetalis occurs when the hemoglobin level decreases by more than 7 g/dl below the normal hemoglobin level (which is 12–18 g/dl, depending on gestational age) and is characterized by the following.
      (1) Generalized edema
      (2) Congestive heart failure
      (3) Extramedullary hematopoiesis
      (4) Enlarged, edematous placental villi with poor placental perfusion

D. **Pathology of erythroblastosis fetalis**

1. **Fetal red blood cell destruction.** Rh-positive fetal red blood cells are hemolyzed by maternal Rh antibody (IgG anti-D), and fetal anemia develops. The anemia stimulates erythropoietin production via extramedullary hematopoiesis in the fetal liver, spleen, adrenal gland, kidneys, placenta, and intestinal mucosa, causing:
   a. Portal and umbilical vein obstruction, simulating portal hypertension
   b. Cessation of normal hepatic function
   c. Decreased colloid osmotic pressure in blood vessels, resulting in edema
   d. **Fetal anemia**
      (1) The severity of fetal anemia is not necessarily proportional to the presence of hydrops fetalis.
      (2) Some fetuses with very low hemoglobin levels are not very edematous.

2. **Bilirubin excretion**
   a. Amniotic fluid is stained with bilirubin in proportion to the degree of fetal red blood cell hemolysis.
   b. Although the maternal liver can metabolize the excess bilirubin products, transfer across the placenta from the fetus to the mother is slow, allowing the fetal blood and urine bilirubin levels to increase.

E. **Evaluation of the immunized patient**

1. The **history** and **physical examination** can help to **predict the severity of Rh hemolytic disease.** A detailed history should include:

a. The maternal blood type and antibody screen. **If the mother is Rh negative, the blood type of the father must be determined.**

    (1) If both the mother and father are Rh negative, there is no need to obtain further antibody screens for Rh disease.

    (2) If the Rh-negative mother has an Rh-positive partner and a positive antibody screen, the antibody should be identified.

        (a) An IgM antibody does not place the pregnancy at risk for erythroblastosis fetalis (i.e., Lewis antigen).

        (b) An IgG antibody such as anti-C, -D, or -E may cause erythroblastosis fetalis; therefore, once it is identified, it should be titered to determine the antibody level.

b. Previous episodes of possible sensitization such as:

    (1) Ectopic pregnancy

    (2) Spontaneous or elective abortion

    (3) Previous blood transfusions with Rh-positive blood

    (4) Previous delivery of an Rh-positive infant by an Rh-negative mother. If the fetus is ABO compatible, 16% of women in this situation become sensitized, as opposed to 2% if the fetus is ABO incompatible.

c. Previously affected fetuses

    (1) Severity of hemolytic disease

    (2) Information about the delivery of previously affected infants also is important, including the gestational age at which delivery and hydrops fetalis occurred. Generally, hydrops develops in a subsequent pregnancy at the same time or earlier than in a previous pregnancy.

    (3) The type of delivery and events surrounding delivery that may increase the risk of Rh isoimmunization, such as cesarean section, placental abruption, preeclampsia, manual placental removal, external version, amniocentesis, and chorionic villus sampling.

d. Knowledge of previous titers

2. **Diagnosis of affected fetuses.** Maternal antibody titers and obstetric history help predict the severity of erythroblastosis fetalis in the current pregnancy in approximately 62% of cases. If amniocentesis and ultrasound are added to the regimen, the predictability is increased to 89%. A critical titer is that antibody level above which the possibility of stillbirth is significant.

    a. Once the titer of maternal antibody reaches a level greater than 1:16, the fetus has a 10% risk of dying in utero. Antibody titers should be repeated every 2 to 4 weeks beginning at 16 to 18 weeks, until the critical titer is reached. Once this occurs, intervention depends on the gestational age.

    b. With amniocentesis, the amniotic fluid surrounding a fetus suffering from hemolytic anemia has elevated levels of bilirubin. Amniotic fluid bilirubin reflects the degree of hemolysis. In normal, unsensitized pregnancies, amniotic fluid bilirubin rises in early pregnancy, reaches a plateau at approximately 25 weeks' gestation, and decreases steadily to term. Amniocentesis should be performed to determine the severity of the fetal anemia if the antibody titer equals or exceeds the critical titer.

        (1) Spectrophotometry is used to measure the optical density (OD) reading at 450 nm (wave length). Because bilirubin products show maximal deviation from the curve at 450 nm, the difference between test fluid and the control is measured as the delta (Δ) OD450.

        (2) Contaminants such as blood and meconium may render the curve inaccurate.

    c. The Liley curve (Figure 7-1) was designed to provide a means to predict the severity of hemolytic disease in the third trimester. A single value is only predictive if it is very high or low. Generally, the trend of serial values must be followed. A falling trend is predictive of a mildly affected or unaffected fetus, and a rising trend may predict a fetus at risk of dying in utero. The upward trend of OD450 is drastic. The Liley curve is divided into three prognostic zones.

        (1) Zone I (lowest zone) fetuses are usually unaffected and have a cord hemo-

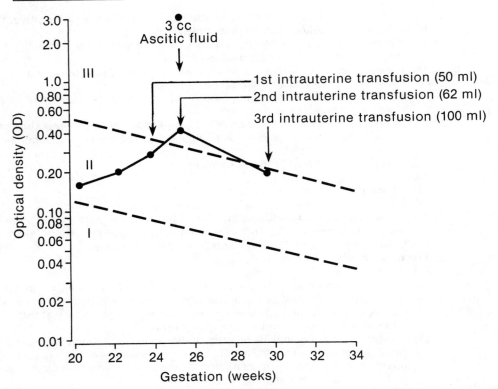

FIGURE 7-1. Liley curve showing readings from serial amniocenteses in a patient who eventually had three intrauterine transfusions. (Reprinted with permission from Creasy R, Resnick R: *Maternal-Fetal Medicine: Principles in Practice.* Philadelphia, WB Saunders, 1984, p 576.)

globin greater than 12 g/dl. Normal hemoglobin at term is 16.5 g/dl. Patients with zone I fetuses are usually allowed to deliver at term.

(2) **Zone II (midzone)** fetuses may be carried in utero until the amniotic fluid bilirubin level increases or until the pregnancy reaches 32 weeks' gestation, in which case delivery is advised. The cord hemoglobin is usually 8 to 12 g/dl. Early delivery is indicated in the following cases.

    (a) The L/S ratio is mature, and phosphatidyglycerol is present.

    (b) A previous intrauterine demise occurred at about the same time.

(3) **Zone III (highest zone)** fetuses are in jeopardy of dying in utero within 7 to 10 days.

    (a) They must be transfused or delivered.

    (b) Cord hemoglobin is usually less than 8 g/dl.

  d. Timing of amniocentesis depends on the antibody titers and the history of previously affected fetuses.

    (1) Because intrauterine transfusions are usually unsuccessful before 18 to 20 weeks' gestation, there is rarely a need for amniocentesis until 18 weeks' gestation, if the critical titer is reached before that time. However, if there is a history of a fetal or neonatal death, fetal transfusion, or birth of a severely affected infant, the first amniocentesis is generally performed 10 weeks before the time of the expected event.

    (2) If the critical titer is reached after 18 weeks' gestation, then the initial amniocentesis is performed immediately after that titer is reached.

    (3) Amniocentesis is repeated at 1- to 4-week intervals, depending on the previous values and history of hydrops fetalis or stillbirths.

    (4) A downward trend in the ΔOD450, after a second or third amniotic fluid

determination, is a good prognostic sign. If the ΔOD450 falls into zone I, no further intervention is required.

e. **Percutaneous umbilical blood sampling (PUBS).** Sampling blood from the umbilical cord is performed using ultrasound-directed needle aspiration, which provides direct assessment of fetal blood, including:

   (1) Hemoglobin and hematocrit levels; during the second trimester, obtaining fetal blood to test for hematocrit level may be preferable to using the Liley curve to estimate the degree of fetal anemia.

   (2) Blood group and Rh type; if the fetus proves to be Rh negative, no further evaluation is required for the remainder of the gestation.

   (3) Direct Coombs' titer (antibodies attached to fetal red cells)

   (4) Bilirubin level

   (5) Reticulocyte count

   (6) Serum protein levels

f. **Real-time ultrasound.** Several studies have shown that serial ultrasound is not an accurate method of assessing the degree of fetal anemia. Polyhydramnios may be the earliest sign of significant fetal anemia, but it is not always present. When the other sonographic signs of hydrops appear, the fetus is already extremely anemic. Ultrasound should therefore be used as an adjunctive tool and cannot replace amniocentesis or PUBS.

F. Treatment of erythroblastosis fetalis

1. **Timing.** If, after 34 weeks' gestation, the patient's ΔOD450 is in zone III or the fetal hematocrit level is below 30%, the fetus should be delivered. At less than 34 weeks' gestation, an intrauterine transfusion should be performed because there are fewer risks associated with a transfusion than there are with a premature delivery. Transfusions may be performed as early as 18 weeks' gestation, via either intraperitoneal or direct intravascular transfusion.

2. **Complications of transfusion:**
   a. Fetal death
   b. Laceration of fetal organ (e.g., liver, bowel, bladder)
   c. Premature labor
   d. Bradycardia
   e. Bleeding from the puncture site with intravascular transfusion
   f. Amnionitis
   g. Preterm rupture of membranes

G. Prevention of D-isoimmunization

1. **Mechanism of action.** When an antigen and its antibody are injected together, there is no immunologic response, provided the dose of antibody is adequate. By this same principle, D-immunoglobulin (the antibody) protects against an immunologic reaction when an Rh-negative woman is exposed to Rh-positive (D-positive) fetal cells (the antigen).

2. **Indications for protection.** Rh immune globulin should be given to unsensitized, D-negative women as follows:
   a. At 28 weeks' gestation to an Rh-negative, nonimmunized woman (negative anti-D titer) when the father of the fetus is Rh positive
   b. Postpartum if the woman remains nonimmunized and delivers an Rh-positive fetus (a Du-positive fetus who is D-negative should be treated as D-positive because the Du antigen is capable of immunizing an Rh-negative woman)
   c. After amniocentesis, chorionic villus sampling, PUBS, external version, or fetal surgery
   d. After evacuation of a molar pregnancy
   e. After an ectopic pregnancy
   f. After a spontaneous or elective abortion
   g. After an accidental transfusion of Rh-positive blood to an Rh-negative premenopausal woman

  h. After a platelet transfusion

  i. After a clinical situation associated with a spill of fetal cells into the maternal circulation, such as:

   (1) Placental abruption or undiagnosed uterine bleeding

   (2) Maternal trauma (e.g., automobile accident)

3. Administration of Rh immune globulin

  a. Standard dose. A 300-μg dose of Rh immune globulin covers a fetomaternal hemorrhage of 30 ml fetal whole blood or 15 ml red cells. This is sufficient after most deliveries. A dose of 50 μg is sufficient if the pregnancy was less than 13 weeks' gestation.

  b. Correct dose. Determination of the correct dose is by the Kleihauer–Betke test, which estimates the quantity of fetal red blood cells that have entered the maternal circulation. This is especially helpful in suspected large fetomaternal hemorrhage, such as may occur with abruption, or after the administration of mismatched blood.

4. Failure of Rh immune globulin prophylaxis may result from the following:

  a. The dose given may have been too small.

  b. The dose may have been given too late. Rh immune globulin is most effective if given within 72 hours of delivery or of exposure to Rh-positive cells.

  c. The patient may already be immunized, but the level of antibody is lower than can be measured by the laboratory.

  d. The Rh immune globulin dose may have been substandard (i.e., deficient in strength) to cover the amount of fetal red blood cells transferred to the mother.

5. The risk of HIV transmission from D-immunoglobulin is estimated to be minimal to absent, because of the fractionation process that is involved in preparation. All plasma used to make D-immunoglobulin has been tested for HIV since 1985.

STUDY QUESTIONS

DIRECTIONS: Each of the numbered items or incomplete statements in this section is followed by answers or by completions of the statement. Select the ONE lettered answer or completion that is BEST in each case.

1. A pregnant woman with the sickle cell trait is at risk for an increased incidence of which of the following?

(A) Perinatal mortality
(B) Low-birthweight infants
(C) Pregnancy-induced hypertension
(D) Urinary tract infection
(E) Spontaneous abortion

2. Which of the following is a sign of heart disease in pregnancy?

(A) Lower extremity edema
(B) Systolic murmur
(C) Increased respiratory effort
(D) Arrhythmia
(E) Dyspnea

3. A 1-hour glucose tolerance test in a woman with a previous stillborn infant resulted in the following value: 1-hour blood sugar = 140. Follow-up for this patient should include which of the following?

(A) Nothing further
(B) A 2000-calorie diet
(C) Standard glucose tolerance test
(D) Home glucose urine testing
(E) A 2-hour postprandial blood sugar

4. The incidence of Rh isoimmunization after a full-term delivery in a D-positive infant to an Rh-negative mother when no Rh immune globulin prophylaxis has been undertaken is

(A) 1%
(B) 5%
(C) 6%
(D) 40%
(E) 90%

5. Which of the following has been associated with methimazole for the treatment of hyperthyroidism in pregnancy?

(A) Cleft lip and palate
(B) Congenital cardiac anomalies
(C) Stillbirth
(D) Aplasia cutis
(E) Neural tube defects

6. An epileptic pregnant woman is noted to have an elevated maternal serum α-fetoprotein (AFP), and subsequent evaluation shows the suspected congenital anomaly. Which of the following anticonvulsants is she most likely to be taking?

(A) Phenytoin
(B) Trimethadione
(C) Phenobarbital
(D) Primidone
(E) Valproic acid

DIRECTIONS: Each of the numbered items or incomplete statements in this section is negatively phrased, as indicated by a capitalized word such as NOT, LEAST, or EXCEPT. Select the ONE lettered answer or completion that is BEST in each case.

7. The infant of a diabetic mother is NOT at risk for which of the following?

(A) Increased perinatal death rate
(B) Hypocalcemia
(C) Hyperglycemia
(D) Neural tube defects
(E) Macrosomia

8. Which of the following factors does NOT contribute to an acute urinary tract infection during pregnancy, delivery, and the puerperium?

(A) Compression of the ureter by the large uterus at the pelvic brim
(B) Increased ureteral tone and peristalsis
(C) Symptomatic bacteriuria
(D) Decreased bladder sensitivity after epidural anesthesia
(E) Bladder catheterization following delivery

9. Which of the following maternal antibodies does NOT cause erythroblastosis fetalis in the fetus?

(A) Anti-C
(B) Anti-E
(C) Anti-D
(D) Anti-Lewis

10. Which of the following characteristics and complications of pregnancy does NOT increase the risk of Rh sensitization?

(A) Type of delivery
(B) Vaginal bleeding
(C) Preeclampsia
(D) Maternal age

11. Which of the following is NOT likely in a patient with acute pulmonary embolism?

(A) Tachycardia
(B) Tachypnea
(C) Increased alveolar–arterial gradient
(D) $Pao_2 > 80$ mm Hg
(E) Pleuritic chest pain

DIRECTIONS: The set of matching questions in this section consists of a list of lettered options (some of which may be in figures) followed by several numbered items. For each numbered item, select the ONE lettered option that is most closely associated with it. To avoid spending too much time on matching sets with large numbers of options, it is generally advisable to begin each set by reading the list of options. Then, for each item in the set, try to generate the correct answer and locate it in the option list, rather than evaluating each option individually. Each lettered option may be selected once, more than once, or not at all.

Questions 12–14

For each clinical presentation listed below, select the hematologic condition that is most likely to be associated with it.

(A) Iron-deficiency anemia
(B) Megaloblastic anemia
(C) β-Thalassemia intermedia
(D) Sickle cell–hemoglobin C (SC) disease
(E) Sickle cell trait

12. A woman presents at 33 weeks' gestation, reporting severe chest pain and difficulty breathing. When her abdomen is auscultated, there are no fetal heart tones. Ultrasound examination confirms a fetal demise.

13. A woman with a hemoglobin of 9.0 g before becoming pregnant has a hemoglobin of 8.0 g during her pregnancy, despite supplemental oral iron and folic acid. The anemia is noted to be microcytic, and a hemoglobin electrophoresis shows an elevated hemoglobin A_2 level.

14. A woman at 32 weeks' gestation presents for the second time in 6 weeks with premature uterine contractions. Bacteriuria was found in the urine and treated each time, and the contractions stopped on both occasions after the treatment.

ANSWERS AND EXPLANATIONS

1. The answer is D [II B 4 a–d]. Sickle cell trait occurs in one in twelve blacks, or 8.5%. It is important to know if a woman has sickle cell trait because of the increased incidence of asymptomatic bacteriuria and urinary tract infection in these women. However, sickle cell trait does not influence the frequency of abortion, perinatal mortality, pregnancy-induced hypertension, or birth weight.

2. The answer is D [V B 1, 2]. Arrhythmias are one of the diagnostic signs of heart disease in pregnancy. Lower extremity edema, however, occurs in most pregnancies because of the pressure of the large uterus on the inferior vena cava and is not indicative of heart disease. Similarly, functional systolic or flow murmurs are common in pregnancy. Increased respiratory effort and dyspnea also are common and are caused by the elevation on the diaphragm secondary to the pressure upward from the intraabdominal contents (i.e., the enlarged pregnant uterus and the bowel).

3. The answer is C [I A 1, 3 a–b]. The screening 1-hour glucose tolerance test was ordered because of the woman's history of a stillborn infant. In a woman with a history of unexplained fetal death, there should be a high index of suspicion of diabetes. Although the 1-hour test results were abnormal, a diagnosis of gestational diabetes cannot be made on that value alone; therefore, there is no immediate need for dietary control or postprandial blood sugar monitoring. However, the abnormal 1-hour test results should be followed up by a standard 3-hour glucose tolerance test. If two or more of the four results are abnormal, the patient is diagnosed as having gestational diabetes. In addition, even if the patient is diagnosed as diabetic, the degree of glycosuria in a patient with diabetes does not reflect plasma glucose values.

4. The answer is C [VIII E 1 b–c]. The incidence of Rh isoimmunization after a full-term delivery (i.e., no Rh immune globulin prophylaxis) in a D-positive infant to an Rh-negative mother is 10% to 20%. There is a significant risk of sensitization after a term delivery be-

cause a large fetomaternal hemorrhage occurs during the actual delivery process. Antibodies may appear either postpartum or after exposure to the Rh antigen in the next pregnancy. ABO incompatibility between the mother and infant confers very mild protection against Rh sensitization.

5. The answer is D [IV A 2 a]. Medical treatment of hyperthyroidism in pregnancy usually involves the thionamide drugs propylthiouracil (PTU) and methimazole. Both drugs prevent the synthesis of thyroid hormone by inhibiting the iodination of thyroglobulin. PTU has the added benefit of inhibiting the conversion of T_4 to T_3. Neither drug is highly teratogenic, but methimazole fell into disfavor because of reports of fetal aplasia cutis, a reversible scalp defect.

6. The answer is E [I E 4 b; VII C 2 d, e (3)]. A neural tube defect is the most likely congenital anomaly to be diagnosed after an elevated serum α-fetoprotein (AFP) level. An elevated maternal serum AFP level is seen in 85% of pregnancies with this defect, and the diagnosis is confirmed by analysis of amniotic fluid AFP and acetylcholinesterase. Pregnant women with seizures are at increased risk for congenital anomalies in general, but specific anticonvulsants are associated with specific defects. Of the drugs listed, only valproic acid has been shown to have a significant risk of neural tube defects in the fetus.

7. The answer is C [I D 2 a–d]. The effects of diabetes on the fetus and infant can be considerable, especially in uncontrolled diabetes. There is an increase in fetal abnormalities such as neural tube defects. Macrosomia is common, and the perinatal death rate is higher than normal. The newborn may show hypocalcemia and hypoglycemia (not hyperglycemia). The insulin secretion that has been stimulated in the fetus by the high levels of glucose from the mother continues after birth and can drop the newborn blood glucose to dangerously low levels.

8. The answer is B [III B 3 a–c, C 1, 2]. There are a number of factors that contribute to the increased incidence of urinary tract infection during pregnancy, delivery, and the puerperium. Because progesterone is a smooth muscle relaxant, for example, the increase in progesterone during pregnancy leads to a decrease in ureteral tone and peristalsis (not the reverse), and this predisposes a woman to urinary tract infection. Asymptomatic bacteriuria leads to acute urinary tract infection in 20% to 40% of untreated women. Conduction anesthesia can temporarily denervate the bladder, leading to overdistension and stasis. Catheterization effectively seeds the bladder with bacteria. The large uterus can compress the ureter, leading to dilation of the renal calyces, pelves, and ureters.

9. The answer is D [VIII A, E 1 a]. Only IgG antibodies are able to cross the placenta and attack fetal red blood cells, producing red cell destruction from hemolysis, as well as increased red blood cell production in the fetal bone marrow initially, followed by production in extramedullary sites. All of the Rh alleles (Cc, Dd, and Ee) on the surface of the red blood cell stimulate an IgG antibody response in the mother; however, only IgM is produced against the Lewis antigen. Therefore, the fetus of a mother with anti-Lewis antibodies is not at risk for anemia.

10. The answer is D [VIII E 1 b–c]. Maternal age does not increase the risk of sensitization; however, certain events that can occur during pregnancy and delivery are known to increase the risk of severe transplacental hemorrhage, resulting in maternal sensitization. These include antepartum hemorrhage, preeclampsia, eclampsia, cesarean section, manual removal of the placenta, and external version (an external maneuver performed by the physician to change a fetus's presentation). The incidence and amount of transplacental hemorrhage increase as pregnancy progresses. By the third trimester, 10% to 15% of women may have evidence of fetomaternal hemorrhage. At least 0.1 ml of fetal blood must enter the maternal circulation for sensitization to occur. After either spontaneous or therapeutic abortion, there is a 5% to 25% incidence of transplacental hemorrhage. If the abortion occurs

after 30 days' gestation, the Rh (D) antigen has been well enough developed to result in sensitization.

11. The answer is D [VI C 2 a–b]. Clinical findings in a patient with an acute pulmonary embolism (PE) may include tachypnea, tachycardia, dyspnea, pleuritic chest pain, cough, and hemoptysis. The patient also may experience a feeling of generalized apprehension. Arterial blood gas analysis is helpful when PE is suspected. If an arterial partial pressure of oxygen (Pao_2) of more than 80 is seen, the diagnosis is unlikely. If the alveolar–arterial gradient is increased, the diagnosis is likely and further studies are indicated.

12–14. The answers are: 6-D [II B 2 a–c], **7-A** [II B 5 a–d], **8-E** [II B 4 a–d]. One of the congenital hemoglobinopathies should be suspected as the cause of the death of the fetus in the woman at 33 weeks' gestation. Neither sickle cell trait nor α-thalassemia trait is accompanied by an increase in perinatal morbidity or mortality. In addition, the chest pain and difficulty breathing in the woman could be caused by a pulmonary embolus of necrotic bone marrow, which is characteristic of sickle cell disease.

The woman with a hemoglobin of 9.0 g entered pregnancy with a mild to moderate anemia that is characteristic of the minor forms of thalassemia. The anemia became worse in pregnancy because of the relative increase in plasma volume, with the inability of the red cell mass to keep up. Because the anemia became worse despite the administration of oral iron and folic acid, it is not likely to be either a megaloblastic anemia or iron deficiency anemia. Microcytosis may be seen in either iron deficiency or in the thalassemias, but only the β-thalassemias are accompanied by an increase in hemoglobin A_2.

A clue to the origin of the problem of the women with premature contractions is the bacteriuria. Urinary tract infection and asymptomatic bacteriuria are common in patients with sickle cell trait. Also, urinary tract infections are a common reason for premature uterine contractions, which usually disappear with treatment of the infection.

Chapter 8

Hypertension In Pregnancy

Kavita Nanda

I. **INTRODUCTION.** Hypertensive disease complicates 8% to 11% of all pregnancies. Hypertension rates second only to embolism as a cause of maternal mortality. It is responsible for 15% of maternal deaths in the United States.

II. **DEFINITIONS.** There are two main categories of hypertension in pregnancy, chronic hypertension and pregnancy-induced hypertension.

A. **Chronic hypertensive disease** is characterized by the presence of persistent hypertension **greater than 140/90 mm Hg** before the twentieth week of pregnancy.

B. **Pregnancy-induced hypertension (PIH)**

1. PIH may coexist with chronic hypertension; risk of PIH is increased in women with chronic hypertension.

2. PIH is a **multiorgan system disease,** involving much more than the blood pressure.

3. **Subsets**
   a. **Preeclampsia** occurs when renal involvement leads to proteinuria.
   b. **Eclampsia** occurs when central nervous system involvement causes seizures.
   c. **HELLP syndrome** is characterized by **h**emolysis, **e**levated **l**iver enzymes, and **l**ow **p**latelets.

4. PIH usually develops after 20 weeks' gestation, but may develop before 20 weeks in patients with gestational trophoblastic disease.

5. PIH may be classified as **mild** or **severe.** Characteristics of **severe disease** include one or more of the following:
   a. Blood pressure (BP) greater than 160 mm Hg systolic or 110 mm Hg diastolic
   b. Proteinuria in excess of 5 g/24 hours
   c. Elevated serum creatinine
   d. Grand mal seizures
   e. Pulmonary edema
   f. Oliguria of less than 500 ml/24 hours
   g. Microangiopathic hemolysis
   h. Thrombocytopenia
   i. Hepatic dysfunction
   j. Oligohydramnios
   k. Intrauterine growth restriction
   l. Symptoms suggesting significant end-organ involvement (e.g., headache, visual changes, epigastric pain)

III. **EPIDEMIOLOGY**

A. PIH complicates 6% to 8% of all pregnancies in the United States, and is principally a disease of the first pregnancy.

B. **Independent risk factors for PIH** include the following:

1. Nulliparity
2. Age older than 40 years
3. African-American race
4. Family history of PIH
5. Chronic hypertension
6. Chronic renal disease
7. Antiphospholipid syndrome
8. Diabetes
9. Multiple gestation

IV. **ETIOLOGY.** The etiology of PIH is unknown, but a **propensity to vasospasm** is established.

A. A number of **etiologic theories** have been proposed.

1. An imbalance between platelet-derived thromboxane, a potent vasoconstrictor, and endothelium-derived prostacyclin, a vasodilator

2. Alterations in the synthesis of endothelium-derived relaxing factor, endothelin-1, and nitric oxide

3. Incomplete invasion of the trophoblasts into the maternal spiral arteries in the uteroplacental bed during placental development

B. The resulting **generalized vasoconstriction** leads to:

1. **Poor placental perfusion,** which results in potential fetal hypoxia, growth restriction, and death

2. **Decreased renal blood flow,** which results in hypoxia of the glomerulus with resultant proteinuria, retention of sodium and water, and edema

V. **CLINICAL MANIFESTATIONS**

A. **Cardiovascular effects**

1. Hypertension is a sustained BP reading of at least 140/90 mm Hg with a proper-sized cuff while the patient is sitting.

2. Hypertension may be caused by an elevation of systemic vascular resistance or an increase in cardiac output.

B. **Renal effects** include the following:

1. Decreased glomerular filtration

2. Decreased clearance of uric acid

3. Proteinuria (greater than 300 mg/24 hours); results of a random dipstick analysis may not accurately reflect degree of proteinuria

4. Sodium retention

5. Glomerular endotheliosis (classic pathologic lesion)

6. Possible nondependent peripheral edema

C. **Hematologic effects** include the following:

1. Plasma volume contraction

2. Decreased colloid oncotic pressure

3. Thrombocytopenia

4. Microangiopathic hemolysis

5. Consumptive coagulopathy (usually seen with coexistent abruption or thrombocytopenia)

6. HELLP syndrome (blood pressures may be normal with this syndrome)

D. **Neurologic function** can be affected.

1. **Hyperreflexia** may be seen.
   a. The degree of hyperreflexia does not correlate with the severity of the disease process.
   b. Hyperreflexia may be noted in normal pregnancy.

2. **Grand mal seizures (eclampsia)**
   a. Grand mal seizures may cause **maternal death.**
   b. Origin of seizures is not well understood.
   c. If seizures occur more than 24 hours postpartum, consider cerebral imaging for other causes (e.g., intracranial mass, infarct, bleed, or thrombosis). Magnetic resonance imaging may demonstrate lesions with eclampsia alone.

3. **Other neurologic symptoms** may include **persistent, severe headache** or **visual changes.**

E. **Other organ involvement**

1. **Pulmonary edema** is related to decreased oncotic pressure, pulmonary capillary leak, fluid overload, or left heart failure.

2. **Liver involvement**
   a. **Elevated transaminases** reflect hepatocellular damage.
   b. Effects range from focal periportal necrosis and hemorrhage to infarction, subcapsular hematoma, and rupture.
   c. Symptoms may include epigastric or right upper quadrant pain.

VI. **FETAL EFFECTS.** The decreased placental perfusion that accompanies maternal vascular spasm causes increased perinatal morbidity and mortality.

A. **Uteroplacental insufficiency** occurs, which may cause:

1. Fetal death

2. Intrauterine growth restriction (IUGR), especially in women with superimposed PIH

B. **Placental abruption** is common.

VII. **MANAGEMENT**

A. **Prevention**

1. **Low-dose aspirin** has been studied in several randomized, controlled trials to prevent the development of PIH. Low doses of aspirin preferentially inhibit platelet cyclooxygenase, leading to an increase in the prostacyclin:thromboxane ratio.

2. Low-dose aspirin may be appropriate in women at high risk for development of PIH, but is not recommended for prophylaxis in unselected, normotensive, nulliparous or multiparous women.

B. **Treatment.** The goals of treatment are termination of the pregnancy with the least possible trauma to the mother and fetus and the birth of an infant who ultimately thrives.

1. **Delivery is the only definitive treatment.** It is usually indicated for PIH of any severity at term, or in preterm women with severe disease. The few exceptions include:

   a. Women at term with an unfavorable cervix and with only mild blood pressure elevation, minimal proteinuria, and no evidence of maternal or fetal compromise. In these patients, delivery may be delayed until 40 weeks.

   b. Delivery is usually recommended in women who have signs and symptoms of severe PIH preterm, but some patients may respond to **conservative management.**

      (1) **28 to 32 weeks.** Some patients may improve after observation and treatment with magnesium sulfate and antihypertensives. In these women, continued observation and administration of steroids to accelerate fetal lung maturity is reasonable in tertiary care centers.

         (a) Women with oliguria, renal failure, or HELLP syndrome should **always be delivered.**

         (b) Women who have continued symptoms or whose signs do not improve with observation should be delivered.

      (2) **Greater than 32 weeks.** There is marginal benefit from conservative management at this gestation, and all patients with severe PIH should be delivered.

      (3) **Less than 28 weeks.** Conservative management of women with severe disease at these early gestations often leads to an increase in both perinatal and maternal morbidity and mortality. Delivery should be accomplished to reduce maternal morbidity, although fetal morbidity and mortality are high.

   c. **Preterm patients with mild PIH**

      (1) **Conservative management with close monitoring.** Patients may be admitted to the hospital with weight, urinary protein, blood pressure, serum creatinine, and platelets monitored daily. Twenty-four–hour urine collection for assessment of protein and creatinine clearance should be obtained. Patients diagnosed as having severe disease by further evaluation should in general be delivered. Stable patients with only mildly elevated blood pressures, minimal proteinuria, and an uncompromised fetus may be managed as outpatients with bed rest and close follow-up.

      (2) **Regular assessment of fetal well-being,** with frequent nonstress tests and serial ultrasound evaluations of fetal growth and amniotic fluid, is essential to ensure an uncompromised fetus.

2. **Labor and delivery**

   a. **Induction of labor** with intravenous oxytocin or intravaginal prostaglandins is often successful when fetal test results are reassuring and the cervix is favorable. **Vaginal delivery** is the preferred mode of delivery.

   b. **Cesarean section** may be considered in cases of severe preeclampsia remote from term, especially in a severely ill patient with a cervix that is not favorable.

   c. Parenteral **magnesium sulfate** should be given during labor and delivery to prevent the development of eclamptic seizures. Magnesium sulfate is also the anticonvulsant of choice for patients already diagnosed with eclampsia, but additional medications may be necessary for refractory cases.

   d. **Antihypertensives** such as intravenous hydralazine and labetalol are used to treat diastolic pressure greater than 110 mm Hg or systolic pressure greater than 180 mm Hg during labor.

   e. **Invasive hemodynamic monitoring** may be needed in severely ill patients with oliguria or pulmonary edema.

   f. **Anesthesia**

    (1) In patients without significant thrombocytopenia or coagulopathy, **epidural anesthesia** is appropriate and indicated for either vaginal or cesarean delivery.

    (2) **General anesthesia** may be associated with significant elevations in blood pressure during induction and awakening.

  g. **Postpartum.** There is usually rapid improvement in hypertension after delivery, although it may transiently worsen.

    (1) Eclampsia may develop any time during the first 24 hours postpartum.

    (2) Magnesium sulfate instituted before or during delivery should be continued for 24 hours postpartum.

    (3) Oral calcium channel blockers may be used in the postpartum period for persistently elevated BP.

    (4) Diuresis should occur within 72 hours postpartum

    (5) PIH usually disappears by 2 weeks postpartum.

VIII. CHRONIC HYPERTENSION

A. Degrees of hypertension

1. **Mild:** BP greater than 140/90 mm Hg

2. **Moderate:** BP 150/100 to 170/110 mm Hg

3. **Severe:** BP greater than 170/110 mm Hg

B. Therapy and management

1. **Preconception counseling**

  a. The woman should be counseled with regard to risk of superimposed preeclampsia, IUGR, and abruption.

  b. Avoid medications such as **diuretics** and **angiotensin-converting enzyme (ACE) inhibitors.**

    (1) **ACE inhibitors** have been associated with fetal hypocalvaria, renal failure, oligohydramnios, and fetal and neonatal death when used beyond the first trimester.

    (2) **Diuretics** cause volume restriction and may have adverse fetal effects.

2. The **first prenatal visit** should include the following:

  a. Documentation of hypertension

  b. Complete blood count, urinalysis, serum creatinine

  c. Careful physical examination, including heart size and funduscopic examination

  d. If the hypertension is moderate to severe, **additional studies** are recommended:

    (1) Electrocardiogram

    (2) Chest radiograph for cardiac contour

    (3) Electrolytes

    (4) Twenty-four–hour urine collection for protein, creatinine clearance

    (5) Ophthalmologic evaluation for retinopathy

  e. **Establish accurate estimated date of delivery** based on last menstrual period or ultrasound examination.

  f. Recommend **low-salt diet** (i.e., less than 4 g/day).

3. Prenatal visits should be made every 2 weeks.

4. Consider home BP monitoring.

5. Encourage **frequent periods of bed rest in left lateral lie** to improve uteroplacental perfusion.

6. If diastolic BP is persistently greater than 100 mm Hg, consider **antihypertensive therapy** to prevent maternal morbidity and mortality.

    a. The drug of choice in pregnancy is *α*-**methyldopa.**

    b. Treatment of mild to moderate hypertension does not improve fetal morbidity.

   7. Serial sonography should be performed for evaluation of growth and amniotic fluid.

   8. Be alert for **superimposed PIH**.

   9. Be alert for signs or symptoms of **abruption** (four- to eightfold increased incidence).

  10. Assess fetal well-being, usually by nonstress test, from 28 to 32 weeks, along with daily fetal kick counts.

C. **Labor and delivery**

   1. Delivery should be accomplished by 40 weeks to avoid complications such as IUGR and superimposed PIH.

   2. Epidural anesthesia with avoidance of hypertension is appropriate.

   3. Treat hypertension as needed.

STUDY QUESTIONS

DIRECTIONS: Each of the numbered items or incomplete statements in this section is followed by answers or by completions of the statement. Select the ONE lettered answer or completion that is BEST in each case.

1. Which of the following is most likely to be seen on a urinalysis in a patient with pre-eclampsia?

(A) Proteinuria
(B) Hematuria
(C) Glycosuria
(D) Ketonuria

2. Eclampsia is defined by

(A) severe, unremitting headache
(B) hyperreflexia
(C) grand mal seizures
(D) petit mal seizures
(E) visual scotomata

DIRECTIONS: Each of the numbered items or incomplete statements in this section is negatively phrased, as indicated by a capitalized word such as NOT, LEAST, or EXCEPT. Select the ONE lettered answer or completion that is BEST in each case.

3. Which of the following is NOT an independent risk factor for pregnancy-induced hypertension (PIH)?

(A) Multiple gestation
(B) Chronic hypertension
(C) African-American race
(D) Age younger than 20 years
(E) Diabetes

4. Which of the following is NOT a sign of severe pregnancy-induced hypertension?

(A) Oligohydramnios
(B) Proteinuria in excess of 3 g/24 hours
(C) Thrombocytopenia
(D) Elevated serum creatinine
(E) Elevated transaminases

DIRECTIONS: The set of matching questions in this section consists of a list of lettered options (some of which may be in figures) followed by several numbered items. For each numbered item, select the ONE lettered option that is most closely associated with it. To avoid spending too much time on matching sets with large numbers of options, it is generally advisable to begin each set by reading the list of options. Then, for each item in the set, try to generate the correct answer and locate it in the option list, rather than evaluating each option individually. Each lettered option may be selected once, more than once, or not at all.

Questions 5 and 6

For each of the following cases, select the most appropriate management option.

(A) Immediate cesarean section
(B) Induction of labor
(C) Admission to hospital for observation
(D) Outpatient observation

5. A 38-year-old African-American woman gravida 1 presents for a routine visit at 39 weeks' gestation. Blood pressure is noted to be persistently 140/90 mm Hg, and urine protein is +2. She is completely asymptomatic and her physical examination is otherwise unremarkable. Cervix is 2 cm dilated, 90% effaced, with the fetal vertex at 0 station.

6. A 25-year-old Asian woman gravida 2 para 0 presents at 33 weeks' gestation for a routine visit. In the office, her blood pressure is noted to be 150/100 mm Hg, and urine protein is +3. She is otherwise asymptomatic.

ANSWERS AND EXPLANATIONS

1. The answer is A [II B 3; V B 3]. Pregnancy-induced hypertension is a multiorgan system disease, and commonly involves the cardiovascular, renal, neurologic, and hematologic systems. When renal involvement leads to proteinuria, the disease is called preeclampsia. Ketones, blood, or glucose are not commonly seen in the urine of preeclamptic women, unless accompanying other conditions.

2. The answer is C [II B 3; V D 2]. Eclampsia is a subset of pregnancy-induced hypertension that is defined by the occurrence of grand mal seizures. Symptoms and signs of impending neurologic instability may include headache, visual changes, or hyperreflexia, but the disease is defined only when a grand mal seizure occurs. Petit mal seizures do not occur with this disease.

3. The answer is D [III B 1–9]. Many studies have evaluated risk factors for the development of pregnancy-induced hypertension (PIH). These include nulliparity, multiple gestation, medical conditions such as chronic hypertension, renal disease, or diabetes, and age older than 40 years. Additional risk factors are African-American race, family history of PIH, and antiphospholipid syndrome. Although young maternal age was previously considered a risk factor, studies have not consistently demonstrated that it has an independent effect on the risk for PIH.

4. The answer is B [II B 5 a–l]. Significant proteinuria is a sign of pregnancy-induced hypertension. Mild preeclampsia is diagnosed when a 24-hour urine collection reveals more than 300 mg of protein. The disease is not categorized as severe unless there are more than 5 g of protein in 24 hours. Other features of severe disease include blood pressure greater than 160 mm Hg systolic or 110 mm Hg diastolic, elevated creatinine, grand mal seizures, pulmonary edema, oliguria, microangiopathic hemolysis, thrombocytopenia, hepatic dysfunction, oligohydramnios, or intrauterine growth restriction. Symptoms that suggest significant end-organ involvement such as headache, epigastric pain, or visual changes also qualify as evidence of severe disease.

5 and 6. The answers are 5-B [VII B 1, 2 a] **and 6-C** [VII B 1 c]. The first patient has a diagnosis of mild pregnancy-induced hypertension (PIH) at term. Because she does have proteinuria, she may be further classified as preeclamptic. The indicated treatment of PIH of any severity at term is delivery. Because her cervix is favorable, induction of labor is the preferred method of delivery. Induction can be started with intravenous oxytocin, and parenteral magnesium sulfate should be used for seizure prophylaxis.

The second patient presents with a more difficult problem because she is preterm. She appears to have PIH on examination, but does not at this point meet criteria for severe disease. With mild disease in a preterm patient, observation and evaluation for severe disease is indicated. Because of the serious complications that can occur, the patient is best managed in the hospital until sufficient evaluation to exclude severe PIH is completed. If further evaluation reveals severe disease, delivery is indicated.

Chapter 9

Fetal Physiology

William W. Beck, Jr.

INTRODUCTION

A. **Placenta.** The placenta consists of blood vessels, vascular spaces, and a small amount of supporting connective tissue. **Placental implantation** occurs predominantly on the posterior aspect of the fundus, the area with the most satisfactory blood supply.

1. Major **placental** functions
   a. Metabolism of glycogen, cholesterol, and fatty acids
   b. Transfer of substances by simple and facilitated diffusion, and active transport
   c. Secretion of protein and steroid hormones

2. The **maternal surface of the placenta** is divided into 12 to 20 cotyledons and appears dark, resembling venous blood. The circulation originates in the endometrial arterioles, and blood is propelled into the cotyledons by the maternal systole, and into the intervillous space.

3. The **fetal surface of the placenta** is shiny and smooth, with large blood vessels coursing through the membranous surface. The membrane covering this surface is the **chorion,** which is next to the **amnion** (innermost fetal membrane); the chorion and amnion are separated only by a small amount of connective tissue.

B. **Fetal and maternal circulations**

1. Substances that pass from the maternal blood to the fetal blood must traverse:
   a. **The trophoblast,** specifically the syncytiotrophoblast
   b. **Stroma** of the intervillous space
   c. **Fetal capillary wall,** which becomes thinner as pregnancy progresses

2. This unit is the site of exchange of water, carbon dioxide, oxygen, electrolytes, amino acids, sugars, vitamins, hormones, and antibodies for the maintenance of fetal biochemical homeostasis, nutrition, and growth.

3. **Harmful substances** (e.g., drugs, poisons, and infectious agents) also pass into the placenta.

4. **The intervillous space** contains 150 ml of blood, which is replenished three to four times per minute.

C. **Umbilical structures**

1. **Characteristics of umbilical arteries on the fetal side**
   a. They originate from the aorta.
   b. They divide and attach to the membranes.
   c. They subdivide continuously.
   d. They supply arterial blood to all portions of the placenta.

2. The **umbilical cord** is semirigid, and, through it, blood circulates from the placenta to the fetus. Blood is propelled by the fetal heart. The total umbilical cord blood flow is 125 ml/kg/min, or 500 ml/min. Uterine contractions cause a reduction of blood into the intervillous space.

II. HEMODYNAMICS OF THE FETUS (Figure 9-1)

A. Oxygenated, nutrient-bearing blood is carried from the placenta to the fetus through the abdominal wall by the umbilical vein. **Shunts,** which divert oxygenated blood to the arterial circulation, particularly to the brain, are characteristic of blood flow in the fetus.

1. The **ductus venosus** connects the portal sinus to the inferior vena cava and allows a portion of the umbilical and portal blood (by a sphincteric mechanism) to bypass the liver (60%). This blood going into the right ventricle is not as well oxygenated as blood coming directly from the placenta.

2. The **foramen ovale** is a right-to-left intracardiac (atrial) shunt. The inferior vena cava communicates with both atria by the foramen ovale.

3. The **ductus arteriosus** is an anastomosis between the left pulmonary artery and the arch of the aorta. The high vascular resistance in the pulmonary tree, which is secondary to increased vasomotor tone and collapsed lungs, is five times the total systemic resistance. The pulmonary artery pressure is greater than the aortic pressure directing blood into the ductus and the aorta, and bypassing the lung.

4. **Blood in the right atrium** is received from the coronary sinus (5%), superior vena cava (20%), and inferior vena cava (75%). A portion (45%) is shunted into the left atrium, and the remainder (55%) enters the right ventricle. From the right ventricle, blood flows into the lungs (10%) and the ductus arteriosus (90%). Blood from the ductus arteriosus flows into the descending aorta, hypogastric arteries, and the umbilical arteries.

5. **Blood in the left atrium** enters the left ventricle, ascending aorta, and the carotid arteries (see Figure 9-1).

B. **Cardiac output of the fetal heart** is 200 ml/kg/min, which is higher than the cardiac output of the adult. The cardiac output of the right ventricle is greater than that of the left ventricle, resulting in a right ventricular preponderance as recorded on the fetal electrocardiogram.

C. **Arterial blood pressure** increases progressively throughout gestation to 75/55 mm Hg at term. The umbilical venous pressure is 22 to 34 mm Hg, and a significant decrease results in death of the fetus. The fetal heart rate is 120 to 160 beats per minute.

III. REGULATION OF BLOOD FLOW AND PRESSURES. The placenta lacks autonomic innervation but acts as a damper to the effects of nervous stimulation from the maternal circulation. Ultimate regulation of fetal blood flow and pressures is by **vascular smooth muscle tone, autonomic nervous stimulation, sympathetic amines,** and **vasodilator metabolites.** Muscular contractions, gravity, and respiratory movement have no effect.

A. **Stimuli that affect umbilical circulation**

1. **Mild fetal hypoxia.** The arterial blood pressure and umbilical blood flow are increased without a change in umbilical venous resistance.

2. **Severe fetal hypoxia.** The umbilical blood flow is decreased, and the umbilical venous resistance is increased.

B. The **dynamics of the ductus arteriosus** are affected by various drugs and stimuli.

1. **Prostaglandins,** especially the E family, and intrauterine and neonatal asphyxia sustain patency. The increased sensitivity of the ductus arteriosus to prostaglandin E_2 suggests a role by this prostanoid in regulating or maintaining patency. Infusions of prostaglandin E_1 and E_2 have been shown to dilate the ductus arteriosus.

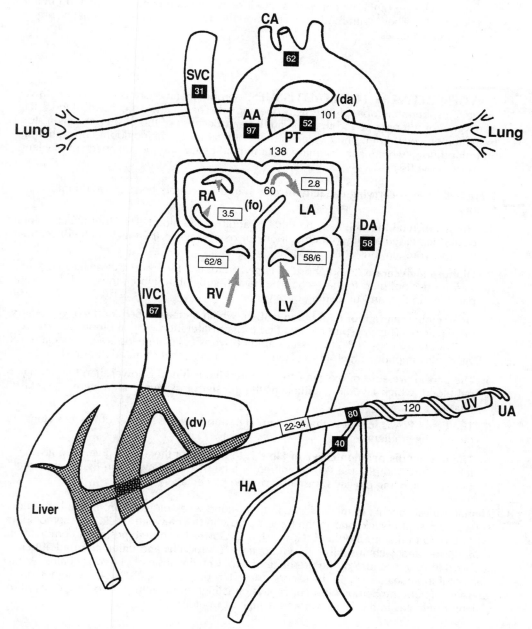

FIGURE 9-1. Hemodynamics of the fetus (in utero). *Black boxed numbers* = O$_2$ saturation (%); *white boxed numbers* = pressures (mm Hg); *unboxed numbers* = blood flow (ml/kg/min); *AA* = ascending aorta; *CA* = coronary arteries; *DA* = descending aorta; *(da)* = ductus arteriosus; *(dv)* = ductus venosus; *(fo)* = foramen ovale; *HA* = hypogastric artery; *IVC* = inferior vena cava; *LA* = left atrium; *LV* = left ventricle; *PT* = pulmonary trunk; *RA* = right atrium; *RV* = right ventricle; *SVC* = superior vena cava; *UA* = umbilical artery; *UV* = umbilical vein.

2. **Prostaglandin inhibitors, acetylcholine, histamine,** and **catecholamines promote closure.** Indomethacin is a potent prostaglandin synthetase inhibitor. The efficacy of non-surgical closure of the patent ductus arteriosus with indomethacin in preterm infants is well established, with morbidity and mortality at least as satisfactory as in surgically treated cases.

IV. **OXYGEN DELIVERY TO FETAL TISSUES.** Aerobic metabolism is the usual pathway in the fetus, but anaerobic glycolysis is operational. The fetal heart can withstand a lack of oxygen for a longer period than the adult heart because of the greater glycogen stores in the fetal myocardium. The oxygen content of fetal blood, hemoglobin concentration, and blood flow (which is the primary determinant) determine the adequacy of oxygen delivery to the tissues.

A. **Increased oxygen-carrying capacity of fetal blood** is possible because of a number of factors.

1. **The pH of fetal blood** is less than that of adult whole blood. The Bohr effect is applicable (decreased affinity of hemoglobin for oxygen when there is a high concentration of hydrogen ions).

2. **Diphosphoglycerate** (2,3-diphospho-D-glycerate) is a by-product of anaerobic glycolysis. It does not bind to the γ-chains of fetal hemoglobin (Hb F); thus, it does not impair the binding and unloading of oxygen.

3. **Hemoglobin content of fetal blood** is high, which increases the blood's oxygen-carrying capacity. Thus, despite the fact that oxygen saturation of fetal blood (see Figure 9-1) rarely exceeds 70%, the tissues are not hypoxic. Fetal needs are met because oxygen consumption is high (4 mg/kg/min)—as high as that of an adult at rest.

4. **The partial pressure of oxygen (Po_2) in intervillous blood** is lower than that in maternal blood, which favorably influences the transfer of oxygen from maternal to fetal blood.

5. **The tissue Po_2 is low** (less than 15 mm Hg), allowing the transfer of oxygen along a decreasing gradient.

6. **The oxygen dissociation curve of Hb F** is to the left of the adult curve. At a given temperature and pH, the Po_2 saturation of fetal blood is lower than that of maternal blood, enhancing oxygen transfer across the placenta.

B. **Hematopoiesis** occurs in the yolk sac in the second week of gestation, in the liver and spleen in the fifth week, and in the bone marrow in the eleventh week. The hemoglobin types that form first are Portland, Gower I, and Gower II. These types are a combination of α-, ζ-, ϵ-, and γ-chains. Hb F ($\alpha_2\gamma_2$) appears at 3 months and differs from adult hemoglobin (Hb AA), because of the presence of two γ-chains instead of two β-chains. Adult hemoglobin appears early in the second trimester, but, at term, 70% of the hemoglobin present is fetal. The hemoglobin concentration is high in the fetus, 16 to 18 g/dl. Erythropoietin originates in the fetal liver and is highest in utero.

V. **FETAL AND NEONATAL METABOLISM**

A. **Fetus**

1. As growth proceeds, extracellular water decreases. Early in gestation, 90% to 95% of body weight is water. At term, 70% to 75% of body weight is water. Fat deposition begins at a fetal weight of 800 g and increases toward term, while extracellular fluid decreases.

2. The fetus synthesizes its own **protein** from amino acids from maternal blood, transferred by diffusion.

3. The **principal sugar** in fetal blood is **glucose;** it is a major nutrient for growth and energy in the fetus.

   a. Fetal level is determined by maternal level.

   b. **Human placental lactogen,** a maternal hormone, blocks the peripheral uptake and utilization of glucose by maternal tissues while promoting the mobilization and utilization of free fatty acids.

   c. It crosses the placenta by facilitated diffusion.

4. **Calcium** and **phosphorus** are actively transported across the placenta from mother to fetus.

5. **Immunocompetence**

   a. In the absence of a direct antigenic stimulus in the fetus, such as infection, the immunoglobulins in the fetus consist almost totally of **immunoglobulin G (IgG).**

   b. IgG is **synthesized by the mother** and transferred across the placenta.

   c. **Antibodies** in fetus and newborn reflect the immunologic experiences of the mother.

B. **Neonate.** At birth, the following events occur, which change the fetal circulation to that of a normal adult.

1. The lungs become aerated, and pulmonary vascular resistance decreases. With the closure of the ductus arteriosus, the lung is no longer bypassed.

2. Pulmonary blood flow increases, allowing for the necessary oxygen–carbon dioxide exchange.

3. The left atrial pressure exceeds right atrial pressure, and the foramen ovale closes.

4. Bradykinin from the aerated lungs constricts the ductus arteriosus, ductus venosus, and umbilical vein. These are no longer functional and are known as the ligamentum arteriosum, ligamentum venosum, and the ligamentum teres, respectively.

5. The intraabdominal portion of the umbilical arteries becomes the lateral umbilical ligaments.

STUDY QUESTIONS

DIRECTIONS: Each of the numbered items or incomplete statements in this section is followed by answers or by completions of the statement. Select the ONE lettered answer or completion that is BEST in each case.

1. The approximate percentage saturation of fetal blood going to the heart, head, and upper limbs is

(A) 40%
(B) 50%
(C) 60%
(D) 70%
(E) 80%

2. Contraction of the sphincter of the ductus venosus results in increased blood flow in which of the following ways?

(A) Through the portal sinus to the portal veins into the hepatic sinusoids
(B) Through the ductus venosus into the right atrium
(C) Reversed through the umbilical vein
(D) By a sphincter mechanism, which is more theoretical than functional

3. Which of the following statements best describes the foramen ovale?

(A) It shunts blood from right to left
(B) It connects the pulmonary artery with the aorta
(C) It shunts deoxygenated blood into the left atrium
(D) It is an extracardiac shunt
(E) It is functional after birth

DIRECTIONS: The set of matching questions in this section consists of a list of lettered options (some of which may be in figures) followed by several numbered items. For each numbered item, select the ONE lettered option that is most closely associated with it. To avoid spending too much time on matching sets with large numbers of options, it is generally advisable to begin each set by reading the list of options. Then, for each item in the set, try to generate the correct answer and locate it in the option list, rather than evaluating each option individually. Each lettered option may be selected once, more than once, or not at all.

Questions 4–6

For each circulatory condition listed below, select the stimuli with which it is most likely to be associated.

(A) Severe fetal hypoxia
(B) Neonatal asphyxia
(C) Autonomic nervous stimulation
(D) Mild fetal hypoxia

4. Umbilical blood flow is elevated

5. The ductus arteriosus is closed

6. Umbilical venous resistance is increased

ANSWERS AND EXPLANATIONS

1. The answer is C [II A 1; Figure 9-1]. The blood returning from the placenta is very well oxygenated, although the level of oxygenation is somewhat reduced by the time the blood reaches the head and neck, secondary to mixing of oxygenated (umbilical vein, inferior vena cava) and deoxygenated (superior vena cava) blood. Consequently, the blood going to the head and neck by the carotid artery is approximately 60% saturated, which is still entirely adequate.

2. The answer is A [II A 1]. The sphincter of the ductus venosus is muscular. Contraction diverts blood to the liver, and relaxation allows more blood to pass through the ductus into the inferior vena cava and into the heart. During hypoxia and fetal distress, ductal flow decreases. The ductus venosus may also help to maintain umbilical venous pressure.

3. The answer is A [II A 2]. The foramen ovale is an intracardiac shunt that shunts oxygenated blood to the left atrium from the right atrium to increase delivery of oxygenated blood to the head, neck, and upper limbs. Like all shunts in the fetal circulation, it is not normally functional after birth.

4–6. The answers are: 4-D [III A 1], **5-C** [III B 2], **6-A** [III A 2]. Hypoxia is a major regulator of blood in the fetus. In the early stages of hypoxia or in mild cases, the blood pressure and the umbilical blood flow increase with no effect on umbilical venous resistance. As the hypoxia worsens, umbilical venous resistance increases, followed by a decrease in blood flow, which could eventually lead to the death of the fetus. Closure of the ductus arteriosus is promoted by drugs that act on the autonomic nervous system (i.e., acetylcholine and catecholamines). Prostaglandin inhibitors, however, are more potent, and therefore have greater therapeutic usefulness if the ductus remains patent in the neonatal period.

Chapter 10

Identification of the High-Risk Patient

Kavita Nanda

I. **INTRODUCTION. The goals of perinatal care are a healthy mother and a normal infant.** Thus, the necessity of identifying the patient at risk cannot be overemphasized. Early identification and management of risk factors are essential so that long-term sequelae can be averted. If possible, the initial evaluation for risk factors should be performed before conception. In addition, pregnancy is a dynamic state during which continuous surveillance is required and adjustment of management plans is common.

II. **MATERNAL MORTALITY**

A. **Definitions**

1. **Maternal death** is death that occurs either during pregnancy or within 42 days of the termination of pregnancy.

2. **Maternal mortality rate** is the number of maternal deaths per 100,000 live-births. In the late 1980s, the maternal mortality rate in the United States was 9/100,000 live-births—a dramatic improvement over the rate of 21.5 in 1972.

B. **Major causes of maternal death** in nonabortive pregnancies (excluding ectopic pregnancies) are, in order:

1. Pulmonary embolism

2. Hypertensive disorders of pregnancy

3. Obstetric hemorrhage

4. Sepsis

C. **Risk factors for maternal mortality**

1. **Advanced maternal age.** Women in their forties are seven times more likely to die in pregnancy than are women in their twenties.

2. **General anesthesia.** Increased mortality is associated with:
   a. An inability to intubate, particularly in women with short necks or women with anatomic airway distortion
   b. Aspiration of gastric contents due to the relative incompetence of the lower esophageal sphincter and delayed gastric emptying characteristic of pregnant women (which is further delayed by both labor and narcotics)

3. **Race.** The maternal mortality rate for nonwhite women is threefold greater than it is for whites.

4. **Hypertensive disease**
   a. When preeclampsia progresses to frank convulsions (**eclampsia**), the patient may lapse into a coma from the convulsions or may experience a cerebrovascular accident and die. Maternal **deaths from eclampsia** accounted for 7% to 17% of maternal deaths in the 1970s and 0.4% of maternal deaths in 1984.
   b. **Maternal deaths from severe chronic hypertension** range from 0.5% to 2%. There are more hypertensive deaths in African-American than in white gravidas.

5. **Cesarean delivery.** The risk of maternal mortality from a cesarean section is less than 1%; however, there is a higher risk of maternal death from a cesarean section than from a vaginal delivery because of general anesthesia complications, severe

sepsis, and thromboembolic events. In general, the maternal mortality rate from a cesarean section is six times higher than from a vaginal delivery.

6. **Cyanotic heart disease.** The prognosis for a pregnancy in women with Eisenmenger's syndrome and other causes of pulmonary hypertension is poor; there is a 30% to 50% incidence of maternal mortality associated with this syndrome.

III. **HISTORY.** The first task in risk identification and management is a thorough historical assessment. Continuous assessment for acute problems is imperative because many disease states can be unmasked by pregnancy. One study showed that even healthy women had at least six preconception risk factors. Risk assessment is most important before conception, when early intervention may affect outcome.

A. **General history**

1. **Socioeconomic status** is defined by an interrelated, complex group of factors—educational level, marital status, income, and occupation—all of which play an important role in maternal and fetal morbidity and mortality. **Low socioeconomic status** is related to an increased risk for perinatal morbidity and mortality.

2. **Age** is an identifiable risk factor.
   a. **Maternal age younger than 20 years** increases the risk for:
      (1) Premature births
      (2) Late prenatal care
      (3) Low birth weight
      (4) Uterine dysfunction
      (5) Fetal deaths
      (6) Neonatal deaths
   b. **Maternal age older than 35 years** increases the risk factor for:
      (1) **First-trimester miscarriage.** The miscarriage rate for women older than 40 years of age has been found to be three times higher than for women younger than 30.
      (2) **Genetically abnormal conceptuses.** The risk of fetal chromosomal anomalies increases in direct proportion to maternal age. (This increase may also explain in part the increase in first-trimester miscarriages.) **Trisomy 21** represents 90% of the chromosomal abnormalities, but the incidence of other autosomal trisomies (i.e., 13 and 18) and sex chromosomal anomalies also increases with advancing age.
      (3) **Maternal death**
      (4) **Medical complications**
         (a) **Hypertension.** In pregnant women older than age 35 years, there is a 6.2% incidence of hypertension (versus 1.3% in those 20–25 years of age).
         (b) **Diabetes.** In pregnant women older than age 35 years, there is a 6.8% incidence of diabetes (versus 1.6% in younger age groups).
         (c) **Preeclampsia.** The incidence of preeclampsia rises with age, from 6% at age 25 years, to 9% at age 35 years, to 15% at age 40 years.
      (5) **Multiple gestation.** The incidence of multiple gestation rises with age. For example, the rate of dizygotic twins is:
         (a) 3/1000 live-births in women younger then 21 years of age
         (b) 14/1000 live-births in women 35 to 40 years of age
      (6) **Antepartum complications**
         (a) **Bleeding.** There is a risk for increased bleeding, such as that associated with abruptio placentae and placenta previa.
         (b) **Preterm labor.** Controversy surrounds the association of preterm labor and advanced maternal age. One British study found a fourfold increase in preterm delivery in women older than 35 years of age, compared to those 20 to 25 years of age.

(c) **Premature rupture of the membranes.** There may be a trend toward increased premature rupture of the membranes with advanced maternal age, increasing the delivery rate of low-birthweight infants.

(d) **Intrauterine fetal demise**

(7) **Labor problems,** including:

(a) Increased breech presentations

(b) Abnormal progress in labor, especially slow cervical dilation and a prolonged second stage

(c) A high cesarean section rate. In a 1986 study, the rate rose from 16% for women 20 to 30 years of age to over 35% for women older than 40. Part of the increase may be attributed to a greater incidence of:

(i) Placenta previa

(ii) Abnormal presentations

(iii) Multiple gestations

(iv) Medical complications

(8) **Fetal morbidity and mortality.** A recent study showed that women older than 35 years of age had twice the stillbirth rate of their younger counterparts. Another study reported increased admissions to the neonatal intensive care unit.

3. **Addiction**

a. **Tobacco.** There is a dose–response relationship between heavy cigarette smoking and increased fetal morbidity and mortality. Although the physiologic mechanism is unclear, there is an increased risk for:

(1) Abruptio placentae

(2) Placenta previa

(3) Bleeding during pregnancy

(4) Premature rupture of membranes

(5) Prematurity

(6) Spontaneous abortion

(7) Sudden infant death syndrome

(8) Low birth weight

(9) A reduction in the supply of breast milk

(10) Respiratory illness

b. **Drugs.** The maternal and fetal consequences of drug addiction in pregnancy depend on the drug ingested.

(1) **Cocaine.** Cocaine use has been associated with increased risk of:

(a) Placental abruption

(b) Low birth weight

(c) Preterm labor

(d) Neonatal withdrawal

(e) Neurobehavioral abnormalities in the neonate

(2) **Opiates.** Opiate use during pregnancy increases the risk of:

(a) Neonatal withdrawal syndrome

(b) Low birth weight

(c) Fetal death

(3) **Marijuana.** A few inconclusive studies have associated prenatal marijuana use with low birth weight and congenital anomalies.

c. **Alcohol.** Not only does alcohol abuse undermine maternal health, but a pattern of abnormalities known as the **fetal alcohol syndrome** manifests in varying degrees of severity in the fetus.

(1) The severity of fetal involvement is usually related to the quantity of alcohol ingested and the gestational age at which the fetus is exposed; however, the relationship between alcohol and fetal effects is not a dose–response one.

(2) Because the effects of the occasional use of alcohol on the fetus are not known, most authorities recommend abstinence from alcohol during pregnancy.

d. Caffeine. Caffeine-containing beverages, including coffee, are frequently consumed by pregnant women. There is no increased risk of congenital anomalies or spontaneous abortion with caffeine intake, but there may be an association of low birth weight with excessive caffeine ingestion.

4. Employment may be associated with an increased incidence of preterm labor, especially for women in physically demanding or stressful jobs. This is a controversial issue.

5. Environmental risks
   a. Noxious chemicals may cause unpleasant symptoms in the mother (e.g., headache, nausea, lightheadedness).
   b. Radiation and radioactive compounds have been associated with spontaneous abortion, birth defects, and childhood leukemia.
   c. Infectious agents
      (1) For example, **Lyme disease** is a tick-borne infection caused by a spirochete (*Borrelia burgdorferi*).
      (2) Lyme disease is associated with the following findings.
         (a) Maternal multisystem effects
            (i) Erythema migrans, a bull's-eye skin lesion
            (ii) Flu-like symptoms
            (iii) Neurologic abnormalities
            (iv) Cardiac abnormalities
            (v) Arthritis of a large joint
         (b) Fetal effects
            (i) Most pregnancies associated with maternal Lyme disease have a positive outcome.
            (ii) The risk for congenital anomalies is controversial. Maternal infection in the first trimester may be associated with fetal cardiac malformations.

6. Domestic violence. Victims of domestic violence are more likely to be abused while pregnant. Such assaults may lead to placental abruption, fetal fractures, rupture of the uterus, spleen, or liver, and preterm labor. It is estimated that 37% of obstetric patients are physically assaulted while pregnant. All pregnant women should be asked about abuse, and assistance with available resources should be given to the abused.

B. **Obstetric history.** Maternal reproductive history has a strong predictive correlation to the development of future sequelae. Therefore, the following information should be obtained so that appropriate management plans can be made to ameliorate any risk factors (Table 10-1).

1. Parity
   a. Nullipara. Nulliparous women are at high risk for development of specific problems, including:
      (1) Pregnancy-induced hypertension
      (2) Physiologic changes and stresses heretofore never experienced and disease states that could be unmasked
      (3) Possible complications due to relative lack of knowledge and pregnancy state
   b. Multipara. Grand multiparous women (five or more pregnancies resulting in viable fetuses) seem to be at increased risk for:
      (1) Placenta previa
      (2) Postpartum hemorrhage secondary to uterine atony
      (3) Increased incidence of dizygotic twins (which may occur because grand multiparas are usually of advanced age)

2. Second-trimester elective abortion. Cervical trauma from elective dilation of the cervix may place a woman at increased risk for:
   a. Spontaneous abortion
   b. Incompetent cervix

Table 10-1. Risk Factors Identifiable at the First Prenatal Visit that Are Associated with Unfavorable Outcomes of Pregnancy

Risk Factor	Odds of Unfavorable Outcome
Information concerning previous pregnancies	
Stillbirth or neonatal death	1.8
Infant <1500 g	2.1
Eclampsia	1.7
Premature labor	2.2
Cervical suture	3.3
Current information about the mother	
Maternal antibodies	<1.0
Diabetes	1.3
Hemoglobinopathy	3.0
Daily alcohol consumption	<1.0
Drug use	<1.0

The data are derived from a study on 994 unselected pregnancies (470 primiparas, 524 multiparas). The odds were calculated as: frequency in cases with unsatisfactory fetal outcome/frequency in cases with satisfactory outcome. In cases where the odds are recorded as <1.0, the actual number of cases in this database was too small for a meaningful calculation. [Adapted with permission from Chard T: Obstetric risk scores. *Fetal Medicine Review* 3(1):2, 1991.]

    c. Preterm delivery
    d. Low-birthweight infant

3. Preterm delivery. The incidence of preterm delivery correlates well with past reproductive performance (Table 10-2).
    a. It increases with each subsequent preterm delivery. The recurrence rate for preterm labor is 25% to 40%.
    b. It decreases with each birth that is not preterm.

4. A large infant (4000 g or more) may indicate a previously undetected or uncontrolled glucose intolerance and may be associated with subsequent intrapartum complications, such as:
    a. Difficult vaginal delivery due to shoulder dystocia
    b. Cesarean section for arrest of dilation or descent
    c. Postpartum complications for the neonate, such as hypoglycemia

5. Perinatal death (stillborn or neonatal). A pregnancy that follows a perinatal death should be followed closely so that a similar outcome can be avoided. Perinatal death may be an indication of an underlying problem that may or may not have been detected previously, such as:
    a. Glucose intolerance
    b. Collagen vascular disease
    c. Congenital anomalies
    d. Preterm delivery
    e. Obstetric injury
    f. Hemolytic disease
    g. Abnormal labor
    h. Antiphospholipid syndrome (APS) [see III C 17]

6. Congenital anomalies. If a woman has previously given birth to a child with congenital anomalies, there is an increased risk of her having another child with congenital anomalies. Evaluation is necessary for future management decisions (e.g., amniocentesis or early termination).

7. Ectopic pregnancy. A woman with a history of ectopic pregnancy has an increased risk for development of another ectopic pregnancy; thus, it is imperative that she be evaluated by 6 weeks' gestation by pelvic examination or vaginal ultrasound so that the site of pregnancy can be confirmed immediately.

Table 10-2. System for Determining Risk of Spontaneous Preterm Delivery

Points Assigned	Socioeconomic Factors	Previous Medical History	Daily Habits	Aspects of Current Pregnancy
1	Two children at home Low socioeconomic status	Abortion × 1 Less than 1 year since last birth	Works outside home	Unusual fatigue
2	Maternal age younger than 20 years or older than 40 years Single parent	Abortion × 2	Smokes more than 10 cigarettes per day	Gain of less than 10 lbs by 32 weeks
3	Very low socioeconomic status Height less than 150 cm Weight less than 100 lbs	Abortion × 3	Engages in heavy or stressful work Takes long, tiring trip	Breech at 32 weeks Weight loss of 5 lbs Head engaged at 32 weeks Febrile illness
4	Maternal age younger than 18 years	Pyelonephritis		Bleeding after 12 weeks Effacement Dilation Uterine irritability
5		Uterine anomaly Second-trimester abortion Exposure to diethylstilbestrol Cone biopsy		Placenta previa Hydramnios
10		Preterm delivery Repeated second-trimester abortions		Twins Abdominal surgery

The score is computed by adding the number of points given any item. The score is computed at the first visit and again at 22–26 weeks' gestation. A total score of 10 or more places the patient at high risk for spontaneous preterm delivery. (Reprinted with permission from Creasy RK, Gummer BA, Liggins GC, et al: A system for predicting spontaneous preterm birth. *Obstet Gynecol* 55:692, 1980.)

8. **Cesarean section**
   a. A woman who has had a **previous cesarean section** should be encouraged to attempt a vaginal delivery with a subsequent pregnancy, provided there are no medical or surgical contraindications, such as:
      (1) Classical uterine incision
      (2) An active herpes infection at term
      (3) Myomectomy with penetration into the endometrium
   b. **Labor in a successive pregnancy** is usually safe.
      (1) **Transverse incision.** Patients with one or two previous transverse cesarean scars should be offered a trial of labor. They have less than a 1% chance of uterine rupture.

       (2) Classical incision. A trial of labor is contraindicated in patients with a known classical incision because of the high risk of catastrophic uterine rupture (12%).

   c. Repeat cesarean section is usually associated with a favorable outcome but carries the following risks.

       (1) Major abdominal surgery, including:

          (a) Wound infection and dehiscence

          (b) Major bleeding requiring transfusion, with the associated risks of human immunodeficiency virus (HIV) or hepatitis B virus (HBV) transmission

          (c) Damage to internal organs (i.e., inadvertently opening the bladder or bowel)

          (d) Anesthesia complications, including death

       (2) Placenta accreta, which is potentially lethal (incidence increases with repetitive cesarean sections)

9. Hemorrhage. Women with a history of hemorrhage have an increased risk of hemorrhage with subsequent pregnancies regardless of the cause (i.e., abruptio placentae, placenta previa, or postpartum hemorrhage). Bleeding during the pregnancy increases the risk of prematurity.

10. Pregnancy-induced hypertension (preeclampsia and eclampsia)

   a. There appears to be a familial tendency.

   b. Women with a history of preeclampsia or eclampsia have an increased risk for development of it in subsequent pregnancies.

   c. Some studies indicate that in women with pregnancy-induced hypertension, essential hypertension is likely to develop in the future, which may complicate a subsequent pregnancy.

C. **Medical history**

   1. Chronic hypertension (140/90 mm Hg or higher). Essential hypertension may be present at the first prenatal visit, or it may develop during the course of the pregnancy. The prognosis for a successful obstetric outcome in the well controlled hypertensive patient is very good. However, there does appear to be an association with development of:

      a. Preeclampsia

      b. Abruptio placentae

      c. Perinatal loss

      d. Maternal mortality

      e. Myocardial infarction

      f. Uteroplacental insufficiency

      g. Cerebrovascular accident

   2. Cardiac disease has both maternal and fetal implications.

      a. In the **mother,** heart disease may develop or worsen. Because of the hemodynamic changes associated with pregnancy, some cardiac lesions are particularly dangerous, such as Eisenmenger's syndrome, primary pulmonary hypertension, Marfan's syndrome, and hemodynamically significant mitral or aortic stenosis.

      b. Fetal growth and development depend on an adequate supply of well oxygenated blood. If this supply is limited, as it appears to be with certain cardiac lesions, then the fetus is at risk for abnormal development and even death.

      c. Offspring of parents with cardiac disease have an increased risk for development of cardiac disease in their lifetimes. This is sometimes identified in utero with fetal echocardiography.

      d. The various **medications** used to control cardiac disease have potential fetal complications.

   3. Pulmonary disease. Maternal respiratory function and gas exchange are affected by the associated biochemical and mechanical alterations that occur in a normal pregnancy. The effect of pregnancy on pulmonary disease is often unpredictable. Thus, when pulmonary disease affects maternal well-being or compromises the supply of well oxygenated blood to the fetus, there is need for concern.

4. Renal disease
   a. In a normal pregnancy, the renal system undergoes certain physiologic, anatomic, and functional changes that may cause stress to it; therefore, **continuous assessment is necessary** in patients with preexisting or developing renal disease.
   b. Under proper medical supervision and control of blood pressure, most women with underlying renal disease can have an **uneventful pregnancy** without adverse effects on either the primary disease or the ultimate prognosis, provided the woman's creatinine level is below 2 mg/100 ml.
   c. **Fetal mortality is increased,** and it is imperative that the patient understand the need for frequent prenatal visits and antepartum testing. Patients should also be aware of the potential complications of antihypertensive medication on the fetus.

5. Diabetes. The cornerstone of management for the pregnant diabetic is rigid metabolic control to make the patient as consistently euglycemic as possible. Ideally, these efforts should begin before conception and continue throughout the pregnancy. Many maternal and fetal problems may complicate the pregnancy of a diabetic, including:
   a. Maternal mortality (rare)
   b. Fetal mortality
   c. Hydramnios
   d. Congenital anomalies
   e. Chronic hypertension
   f. Preeclampsia
   g. Maternal edema
   h. Maternal pyelonephritis
   i. Neonatal mortality (congenital anomalies being the major cause)
   j. Neonatal morbidity, including:
      (1) Respiratory distress syndrome
      (2) Macrosomia
      (3) Hypoglycemia
      (4) Hyperbilirubinemia
      (5) Hypocalcemia

6. Thyroid disease. Pregnancy, with its associated hormonal and metabolic changes, makes the evaluation of thyroid function very complex. Untreated hypothyroidism or hyperthyroidism may profoundly alter pregnancy outcome. The fetal thyroid is autonomous and is unaffected by maternal thyroid hormone; however, treatment of thyroid disease during pregnancy can be complicated because the fetal thyroid responds to the same pharmacologic agents as does the maternal thyroid.

7. Collagen vascular disease. Many rheumatic diseases are common in women, especially during the reproductive years. The effect of pregnancy is unpredictable; precipitation, aggravation, or amelioration of the disease may occur. Collagen vascular disease may affect the outcome of the pregnancy (e.g., with systemic lupus erythematosus, there is an increased risk of abortion, premature labor, and intrauterine fetal death), and the particular pharmacologic agents used in the treatment of the disease may adversely affect the fetus.

8. Hematologic disorders
   a. Physiologic alterations and metabolic demands associated with pregnancy may result in anemias secondary to iron or folic acid deficiency.
   b. Hemoglobinopathies (e.g., sickle cell disease) may be severely affected by pregnancy, with the development of serious complications in both the mother and the child.
   c. Disorders of blood coagulation and platelets may not only affect antepartum management through their maternal and fetal effects, but may play a role in intrapartum, delivery, and postpartum management because of the possibility of hemorrhage.

d. Some hematologic disorders have a genetic component; therefore, genetic counseling and management decisions should be discussed before conception or in the early stages of pregnancy, if possible.

9. **Genetic disorders**
   a. **A genetic disorder of the mother** must be evaluated before pregnancy or in early pregnancy because the associated changes of pregnancy may so stress the genetic problem as to threaten her health, or the disease itself may compromise the intrauterine growth of the fetus. For example, infants born to mothers with **phenylketonuria** (serum levels of phenylalanine greater than 20 mg/dl) are at risk for microcephaly, mental retardation, congenital heart defects, and growth restriction. Dietary restriction of phenylalanine is recommended during the early weeks of gestation.
   b. **Historical factors** that may help to identify the **high-risk couple** include the following.
      (1) **Consanguinity.** Marriage between close relations results in a large pool of identical genes, thereby increasing the possibility of sharing similar mutant genes, resulting in:
         (a) An increased risk of miscarriage
         (b) An increased risk of rare recessive genetic disease in offspring
      (2) **Ethnicity.** Specific ethnic groups are more prone to specific diseases:
         (a) Tay-Sachs disease in Eastern European Jews and French Canadians
         (b) Thalassemias in Mediterranean, Southeast Asian, Indian, or African patients
         (c) Sickle cell anemia in African, Mediterranean, Caribbean, Latin American, or Indian patients
         (d) Cystic fibrosis in whites
      (3) **Parental age** (maternal and paternal)
         (a) There is an increased risk for Down syndrome with advanced maternal age (older than 35 years).
         (b) There is an increased risk of de novo single gene mutation with advanced paternal age (older than 55 years).
   c. **Once a high-risk couple is identified,** the following steps can lead to **wise reproductive planning** or the relief of anxiety in high-risk couples.
      (1) **Genetic counseling** should be undertaken to evaluate risks.
      (2) **Carrier testing** should be performed if the fetus is at risk for a recessive disorder.
      (3) **Chorionic villi sampling** or **amniocentesis** should be offered, where applicable, for reasons such as the following:
         (a) For biochemical analysis of the fetus at risk for a hemoglobinopathy or enzyme deficiency
         (b) For analysis of the fetal chromosomes in women who will be older than age 35 years at the time of delivery
         (c) For diagnosis of a neural tube defect

10. **Pituitary disorders.** Pregnancy is uncommon in women with pituitary abnormalities because pituitary integrity is necessary for conception. However, some pituitary disorders carry an increased health risk during pregnancy (e.g., prolactinoma).

11. **Adrenal disorders.** Gestational changes in adrenal function do occur, and it is important that adrenal homeostasis be preserved because some complications of inadequate adrenal function may be life threatening (e.g., acute adrenocortical insufficiency).

12. **Parathyroid disorders.** Parathyroid homeostasis is essential for maternal and fetal well-being, and serum calcium concentration is the key value in evaluating parathyroid function. Calcium requirements increase to 1200 mg during pregnancy and usually are maintained by a normal diet, although supplements may be added to ensure adequate intake.

13. **Liver disease.** Like most organ systems, the liver undergoes anatomic, physiologic, and functional changes during pregnancy; and liver disease, like most other disease

entities, may be aggravated or may become difficult to follow when it occurs in a pregnant patient. If a woman has liver disease, it is essential that it be identified, a baseline established, and the patient followed closely. Liver disease may have deleterious effects on the fetus (e.g., viral hepatitis).

14. **Neurologic disorders.** The effects of pregnancy on preexisting or concurrent neurologic disorders can be diverse. Treatment often involves a therapeutic dilemma common to the treatment of many other disorders in pregnancy—that is, assessing the risk of pharmacologic therapy, with its associated fetal effects, versus the risk of uncontrolled disease to the mother and the fetus.

15. **Venous thromboembolic disorders.** Pregnancy and the immediate postpartum period can predispose women to venous thrombosis. It is important to identify the women at high risk because many thromboembolic events can be prevented.

16. **Infectious diseases.** In addition to rubella and syphilis, for which pregnant women are routinely screened, certain viral and parasitic infectious agents are capable of crossing the placenta and producing serious problems for the fetus and the newborn. The following infections during pregnancy place the mother and her child at high risk for potential morbidity and mortality (see Chapter 14 for detailed information).
    a. **Cytomegalovirus (CMV)**
        (1) In the pregnant woman who acquires CMV as a primary infection, there is an increased risk for fetal congenital anomalies, chiefly in the central nervous system.
        (2) Neonatal death from disseminated disease may occur.
        (3) Postnatal infection may also occur, but is usually without sequelae.
    b. **Herpes simplex virus (HSV)**
        (1) This is a sexually transmitted virus.
        (2) Primary infection during pregnancy increases the risk of fetal loss and prematurity.
        (3) Most neonatal infections are acquired either during passage through an infected birth canal or as an ascending spread of the virus from the cervix after the membranes have ruptured.
        (4) A neonatal infection may go undetected without sequelae, or it may cause fatal disseminated disease. Survivors may manifest ophthalmologic or neurologic sequelae.
        (5) It is important to identify women with a history of HSV or newly acquired HSV so that appropriate management decisions, particularly regarding delivery, can be made.
    c. **Hepatitis B virus (HBV)**
        (1) **Maternal infection**
            (a) Maternal infection occurring in the first trimester is not associated with fetal disease.
            (b) Acute third-trimester infections, however, have been associated with an increased risk of prematurity (often resulting in fetal morbidity and mortality) and a 67% incidence of transmission of the hepatitis infection to the infant.
        (2) **Maternal chronic carriers.** Vertical transmission of HBV can occur from mothers who are chronic carriers of the hepatitis B surface antigen (HBsAg). If such mothers also carry the E antigen, the rate of transmission is 80% to 90%.
        (3) **Transmission of HBV to neonates** can result in infants who:
            (a) Are asymptomatic
            (b) Develop fulminant disease, cirrhosis, or hepatocellular carcinoma, resulting in death
            (c) Become chronic carriers
        (4) **Prevention**
            (a) **Measures required after maternal exposure.** Pregnant women exposed to HBV should receive both the hepatitis vaccine and hepatitis B im-

mune globulin (HBIG). Administration of HBIG should be repeated in 1 month, and the vaccination should be repeated in 1 and 6 months.

(b) Measures required after presumed fetal transmission. If the mother is a chronic carrier or has acute third-trimester disease, efforts to prevent the disease in the neonate must be initiated at birth. These efforts include:

(i) Nasogastric aspiration to remove secretions

(ii) Administration of hyperimmune serum globulin

(iii) Hepatitis vaccine and HBIG prophylaxis

(c) Identification of HBsAg-positive pregnant women is essential because vertical transmission of HBV is an important cause of acute and chronic hepatitis.

(i) First-trimester screening programs should be instituted to identify seropositive women (0.01%–5% of pregnant patients are seropositive). The neonates of women who test positive can then be treated with passive and active immunoprophylaxis.

(ii) Groups at high risk for HBV seropositivity include intravenous drug abusers, HIV-positive women, and Southeast Asian women.

(d) Universal immunization of **all** neonates, even those of HBsAg-negative mothers, has been recommended by the American Academy of Pediatrics. Immunizations should be given three times:

(i) At birth

(ii) At 1 month of age

(iii) At 6 months of age

d. Toxoplasmosis

(1) Toxoplasmosis is a parasitic infection that produces clinically vague maternal symptoms but can infect the fetus in utero.

(2) Fetal risk is related to the gestational age at which maternal infection occurs, which may be a reflection of the immune status of the fetus; for example, there is a greater risk of transmission to the fetus in the third trimester, but it is usually without significant sequelae. There is less frequent transmission in the first trimester, but the sequelae are usually more severe.

(3) There is increased risk for:

(a) Abortion

(b) Stillbirth

(c) Severe congenital infections in the fetus

(4) Because cats serve as reservoirs for toxoplasmosis, the physician should:

(a) Inquire about the patient's exposure to cats and alert the patient to the potential risks

(b) Encourage the patient to limit her contacts with cats and especially to avoid cleaning the litter box

(c) Consider serologic tests for toxoplasmosis if the patient is exposed to cats. This is most important preconceptually to detect susceptible individuals.

e. Parvovirus infection

(1) This is a single-stranded DNA virus that causes a wide spectrum of **maternal illness,** including:

(a) Asymptomatic infection

(b) Erythema infectiosum (also called fifth disease), a macular rash that often occurs in school-age children and is preceded by fever, myalgias, and respiratory or gastrointestinal symptoms

(c) Arthritis or arthralgias

(d) Aplastic crises, especially in women with a variety of chronic hemolytic anemias

(2) The **fetal effects** include the following.

(a) Hydrops fetalis can occur because of a severe nonimmune hemolytic anemia.

(b) Congenital anomalies. Although one aborted fetus was reported to have eye abnormalities, the incidence of abnormalities after maternal parvovirus infection is very rare.

    (c) Miscarriage

    (d) Fetal death. In cases of documented maternal infection, the incidence of fetal death is 15%. The highest rate of incidence occurs when the mother is infected during the first 18 weeks of pregnancy. Fetal deaths have been reported to occur from 1 to 10 weeks after clinical illness in the mother.

    (e) Asymptomatic infection. Infants born to infected women have had serologic evidence of infection without adverse effects.

f. Human immunodeficiency virus (HIV)

    (1) The rate of mother-to-infant transmission perinatally has been estimated to be 20% to 30%, regardless of maternal symptoms. Infants born to mothers with HIV infection may become infected:

        (a) In utero

        (b) During delivery

        (c) After birth, from contaminated breast milk

    (2) Zidovudine (AZT) given to HIV-positive women during pregnancy and delivery has been shown to reduce perinatal transmission to 8.3%.

    (3) Although certain "high-risk" groups have been identified, such as intravenous drug users, Haitians, prostitutes, people receiving blood products (e.g., hemophiliacs), and women whose partners have had a homosexual experience, over half of all pregnant women infected with HIV do not belong to any of these "high-risk" groups. The Centers for Disease Control and Prevention (CDC) recommends that all pregnant patients be offered HIV testing.

    (4) Women at risk for HIV infection may be infected through:

        (a) Blood products

        (b) Sexual intercourse

        (c) Contaminated needles

    (5) Women who are infected with the virus may show no symptoms of the disease and may feel well. In one study, asymptomatic women, identified because HIV-related disease developed in their children, were followed for 2 years postpartum. Symptoms developed in between 50% to 75% of women.

    (6) Women shown to be infected with HIV should be evaluated for:

        (a) Gonorrhea and syphilis

        (b) Chlamydia

        (c) HBV

        (d) Tuberculosis

        (e) CMV

        (f) Toxoplasmosis

    (7) Important guidelines to follow during labor and delivery of all potentially infected parturients are as follows.

        (a) Consider all patients infected until testing for HIV is proven negative.

        (b) Use the following protective clothing or techniques:

            (i) Protective eye wear

            (ii) Water-repellent gowns

            (iii) Gloves

            (iv) Frequent hand washing

            (v) Wall suction or bulb suction

        (c) Avoid direct exposure to maternal or neonatal secretions.

        (d) To avoid a contaminated needle puncture, never resheath needles.

        (e) Avoid early amniotomy because duration of membrane rupture may increase likelihood of fetal infection.

        (f) Avoid scalp sampling for fetal pH or scalp electrodes for monitoring fetal heart rate.

        (g) Discourage breast-feeding of the infant.

Table 10-3. Perinatal Effects of Drugs Used in Women with Human Immunodeficiency Virus (HIV)

Illness	Treatment and Dosage	Reported Risks in Pregnancy*
Pneumocystis carinii pneumonia	Sulfamethoxazole, 100 mg/kg/day, and trimethoprim, 20 mg/kg/day (folate antagonist)	Kernicterus and congenital malformations (rare) [Category C]
	Pentamidine, 4 mg/kg/day intravenously	Unknown (Category C)
Herpes simplex	Acyclovir (purine nucleoside analogue), 200 mg five times per day	Unknown (Category C)
Toxoplasmosis	Sulfadiazine, 1 g orally four times per day, and pyrimethamine, 25–50 mg/day	One case of gastroschisis, kernicterus; most reports show no effect (Category C)
Candidiasis	Ketoconazole, 400 mg/day, for 14 days, then for 5 days per month for 6 months	No known risks (Category C)
Symptomatic HIV (low T-cell count)	Zidovudine (AZT), 200 mg every 4 hours (thymidine analogue, inhibits reverse transcriptase)	Unknown

Reprinted with permission form Minkoff H: Care of pregnant women infected with human immunodeficiency virus. *JAMA* 258:2716, 1987.

* Category C indicates either that studies in animals have revealed adverse effects on the fetus (teratogenic, embryocidal, or other) and there are no controlled studies in women or that studies in women and animals are not available. Drugs should be given only if the potential benefit justifies the potential risk to the fetus.

    (8) Pregnant women with HIV infection are also at increased risk for:
      (a) Premature rupture of membranes
      (b) Low-birthweight infants
    (9) The perinatal effects of drugs used in pregnant women with HIV are listed in Table 10-3.
  g. Varicella zoster virus infection
    (1) Most women of childbearing age have a history of previous varicella (chickenpox) infection. More than 75% of women without a history of chickenpox also have varicella antibodies and are immune.
    (2) Varicella infection occurs in 1/10,000 to 5/10,000 pregnancies.
    (3) Maternal effects. Pregnant women have an increased risk for severe varicella infection, including varicella pneumonia.
      (a) In the past, the maternal mortality rate reached 40%.
      (b) With the use of acyclovir, the maternal mortality rate has dropped to 5%.
    (4) Fetal effects
      (a) Abortion and stillbirth may occur.
      (b) Fetuses exposed in the first 20 weeks of pregnancy have a 1% to 3% risk for congenital infection. Affected fetuses may have cutaneous cicatrices (scars), limb hypoplasia, microcephaly, chorioretinitis, or cortical atrophy.
      (c) When maternal infection occurs either 5 days before delivery or within 2 days of delivery, 10% to 20% of neonates contract the infection.
        (i) Infection occurs because of absence of passively acquired antibody.
        (ii) Neonatal mortality rate approaches 30%.
    (5) Pregnant women exposed to varicella who are found to be nonimmune should receive varicella zoster immunoglobulin (VZIG).
      (a) If given within 96 hours, this may prevent infection in the mother.

(b) VZIG does not prevent congenital infection.

(c) The cost of VZIG is $470.

(6) Susceptible women identified preconceptually may receive the varicella vaccine. This is contraindicated in pregnancy because it contains a live attenuated virus.

17. Autoimmune disorders include **antiphospholipid syndrome (APS),** an autoimmune syndrome caused by the lupus anticoagulant and the anticardiolipin antibody.

   a. Expression. The syndrome may be expressed as one or more of the following:

   (1) Recurrent fetal loss, such as miscarriage or stillbirth

   (2) Placental infarction

   (3) Preeclampsia

   (4) Arterial or venous thrombosis, including neurologic disease

   (5) Autoimmune thrombocytopenia

   b. Although controversial, **treatment** may improve the chances of a successful pregnancy outcome in a patient with a poor past pregnancy history.

   (1) Initially, **low-dose aspirin** (81 mg; the equivalent of baby aspirin) is administered daily.

   (2) Heparin or **corticosteroids** may be administered as well.

   (a) Heparin is the preferred choice because it has fewer side effects and is usually more effective than corticosteroids. Patients receiving heparin should be monitored closely with partial thromboplastin times, platelet counts, and other screening for bleeding abnormalities.

   (b) Using corticosteroids may predispose a patient to pregnancy-induced hypertension, cataracts, aseptic necrosis of the femur, and gestational diabetes.

D. **Family history.** There seems to be a familial tendency for the development of the following risk factors:

   1. Maternal

   a. Hypertension

   b. Multiple births

   c. Diabetes

   d. Hemoglobinopathy

   e. Uterine fibroids

   f. Eclampsia

   2. Maternal or paternal

   a. Mental retardation

   b. Congenital anomalies

   c. Congenital hearing loss

   d. Allergies

E. **Medications.** Various medications have adverse effects on the fetus, and it is imperative that the risks and benefits to the mother and fetus be evaluated and discussed with the patient before starting, continuing, or stopping the use of medications (see Chapter 14).

IV. **PHYSICAL EXAMINATION.** The obstetric patient should undergo a thorough physical examination so that her general health can be assessed.

A. **General examination.** Maternal size, which may reflect socioeconomic and nutritional status, has become an important predictive index.

   1. Mothers who are **short in stature** or **underweight** are at increased risk for:

   a. Perinatal morbidity and mortality

   b. Low-birthweight infants

   c. Preterm delivery

2. **Obesity** presents a medical hazard to the pregnant woman and her fetus. Complications that are more likely to develop in an obese woman include:
   a. Hypertension
   b. Diabetes
   c. Aspiration of gastric contents during the administration of anesthesia
   d. Wound complications
   e. Thromboembolism

B. **Pelvic examination**

1. The **perineum, vulva, vagina, cervix,** and **adnexa** should be examined and any abnormalities noted that may affect future management (e.g., adnexal masses or cervical lesions).

2. **Clinical pelvimetry** should also be done to assess adequacy of the maternal pelvis to facilitate vaginal delivery.

3. **Presentation** may also affect management and therefore must be assessed continually, especially in the later stages of the pregnancy.

C. **Evaluation of the uterus.** The size of the uterus is evaluated continuously throughout the course of the pregnancy. The estimated date of delivery should be established at the first prenatal visit so that subsequent discrepancies can be properly evaluated. There is good correlation between fundal height in centimeters measured from the symphysis pubis and gestational age in weeks beyond 20 weeks.

1. **If the uterus is smaller than expected for the estimated gestational age,** then the physician must determine if:
   a. There has been a miscalculation due to menstrual irregularity.
   b. The infant is small for gestational age, which may be caused by:
      (1) Constitutional factors
      (2) Intrauterine infection
      (3) Chromosomal abnormalities
      (4) Congenital anomalies
      (5) Uteroplacental insufficiency
   c. Oligohydramnios is present.
   d. The fetus is in a transverse lie.

2. **If the uterus is larger than expected for the estimated gestational age,** the following factors must be considered:
   a. Improper dates
   b. Uterine anomalies
   c. Polyhydramnios
   d. Multiple gestation
   e. Macrosomia
   f. Hydatidiform mole

D. **Reproductive tract abnormalities**

1. **Structural uterine anomalies**
   a. In general, the prognosis for women with **minor defects** is excellent.
   b. For women with **major defects,** the prognosis is usually fairly good; however, there is an increased risk of:
      (1) Cesarean section (when presentation is abnormal)
      (2) Perinatal loss
      (3) Low-birthweight infant
      (4) Abortion
      (5) Abruptio placentae
      (6) Preterm labor

2. **Premalignant and neoplastic lesions.** Depending on the extent of the premalignant or neoplastic lesion, management and treatment of the pregnancy and the lesion

may be quite complicated. The extent of treatment ranges from close observation to interruption of the pregnancy for more definite treatment.

3. **Leiomyomata (fibroids).** The location and size of the myomas are important in determining possible future sequelae. For example, a 5-cm myoma lying directly beneath the placenta may precipitate bleeding from a placental abruption. In general, the pregnancy has an increased risk of being complicated by:
   a. Abortion
   b. Faulty placental implantation (causing fetal growth delay)
   c. Faulty correlation of uterine size and dates
   d. Premature contractions
   e. Dysfunctional labor
   f. Postpartum hemorrhage
   g. Obstruction of labor by cervical or lower uterine segment myomas
   h. Unstable fetal lie or compound presentation
   i. Pain due to degeneration

4. **Incompetent cervix.** This is usually diagnosed by a history of a suspect second-trimester loss with minimal labor contractions with or without rupture of membranes or cervical trauma.

5. **Exposure to diethylstilbestrol (DES).** Patients exposed to DES should be closely observed throughout pregnancy because of the probability of both cervical and uterine anomalies, which could cause:
   a. Abortion or ectopic pregnancy (first trimester)
   b. Incompetent cervix (second trimester)
   c. Premature labor and rupture of membranes, leading to premature delivery (third trimester)

V. **LABORATORY DATA BASE.** Routine laboratory studies that may indicate maternal and fetal problems and thus may affect management of the pregnancy include the following.

A. **Blood type and antibody screen** are essential in all prenatal patients, most notably so that the antibody status of the woman can be determined.

1. **Rh sensitization.** Although it has very little effect on maternal health, sensitization may have profound consequences for the fetus and the management of the pregnancy. If there has been maternal sensitization to red blood cell antigens (e.g., prior transfusions), the resultant antibodies can be transferred to the fetus, which results in hemolytic disease and its intrauterine and extrauterine consequences (see Chapter 7).

2. The **antibody screen** is also essential for Rh-positive people because other blood group antigens (i.e., Kell, Kidd, and Duffy) can produce severe hemolytic disease in the fetus.

B. **Venereal Disease Research Laboratory (VDRL) test.** Syphilis involves a number of different stages, and the evaluation of each stage is important in assessing fetal risk. Pregnancy complicated by preexisting or newly acquired syphilis may result in:

1. An uninfected live infant

2. A late abortion (after the fourth month of pregnancy)

3. A stillbirth

4. A congenitally infected infant

C. **Gonorrhea culture.** Screening may be either universal or selective, depending on the prevalence of the disease in the patient population. Gonorrhea during pregnancy may be associated with:

1. Intrauterine infection, with premature rupture of membranes and preterm delivery
2. Histologic evidence of chorioamnionitis
3. Neonatal eye infection (ophthalmia neonatorum)
4. Clinical diagnosis of sepsis in the neonate
5. Associated maternal arthritis, rash, or peripartum fever

D. **Chlamydia testing.** Screening is recommended for all high-risk or symptomatic patients. Infection during pregnancy may result in:

1. Ophthalmia neonatorum
2. Neonatal pneumonia
3. Postpartum endometritis

E. **Rubella titer**

1. The **clinical course** of rubella is no more severe or complicated in the pregnant woman than it is in the nonpregnant woman of comparable age; however, active maternal infection does carry a risk for the fetus, including:
   a. First-trimester abortion
   b. Fetal infection, resulting in severe congenital anomalies
2. **Maternal infection in the first trimester** carries with it the greatest risk to the fetus.
3. **Immunization.** If a patient is diagnosed as having a rubella titer of less than 1:8, she should be immunized postpartum.
   a. The rubella vaccine is not given during pregnancy because it is a live attenuated vaccine.
   b. There have been no reported cases of congenital rubella from inadvertent administration of the vaccine to pregnant women.

F. **Complete blood count** with red blood cell indices

1. **Anemia.** If present, anemia should be evaluated further and treated. Maternal anemia may be associated with pyelonephritis, prematurity, and fetal growth retardation. **Microcytosis** without anemia may represent a thalassemia, and should also be investigated.
2. **Leukocytosis.** A mild leukocytosis is normal in pregnancy; however, a grossly abnormal value needs to be evaluated.
3. **Thrombocytopenia** may be caused by idiopathic thrombocytopenia, preeclampsia, medications, acquired immunodeficiency syndrome, sepsis, lupus, or thrombotic thrombocytopenic purpura.

G. **Urinalysis and culture.** Although the mechanism is unclear, there are specific physiologic and anatomic changes that occur during pregnancy that predispose the pregnant woman with symptomatic or asymptomatic urinary tract infections to development of pyelonephritis.

1. **Asymptomatic bacteriuria** is prevalent in 3% to 5% of pregnant women, particularly in those from lower socioeconomic groups and those at risk because of parity and age. It is important that early detection, treatment, and close follow-up be instituted.
2. **Acute systemic pyelonephritis.** Asymptomatic bacteriuria predisposes the pregnant woman to the development of acute systemic pyelonephritis, which has serious complications for the mother and fetus and has been associated with premature labor and delivery. Systemic pyelonephritis develops in approximately 20% to 40% of pregnant women with untreated asymptomatic bacteriuria.
3. **Association with pregnancy.** Few women acquire asymptomatic bacteriuria who are not bacteriuric at their first prenatal visit. Therefore, it is believed that preg-

nancy does not increase the incidence of asymptomatic bacteriuria but rather sets the stage for the development of systemic pyelonephritis in those women with preexisting bacteriuria.

H. **Pap smear.** Baseline cervical cytology should be established, and, if abnormalities are noted, proper evaluation should be instituted.

I. **Blood sugars.** Various medical centers differ on how and when to evaluate women for gestational diabetes. However, because pregnancy is a diabetogenic state and aggressive, early management can help to prevent some of the complications of diabetes, many authorities recommend that **all** pregnant women have a 1-hour 50-g glucose screen at 24 to 28 weeks' gestation.

J. **Screening for neural tube defects and trisomies** should be offered to all pregnant women and drawn at 16 to 20 weeks' gestation. This is known as the triple screen.

1. Using maternal serum **α-fetoprotein (AFP), human chorionic gonadotropin (hCG),** and **estriol,** many patients at risk for either trisomy 21 or trisomy 18 may be identified.
   a. **Trisomy 21** is associated with low AFP and estriol, and high hCG; 60% to 70% of patients may be identified.
   b. **Trisomy 18** is associated with low levels of all three markers.

2. **Elevated maternal serum AFP** is seen in 80% to 90% of pregnancies in which there is a fetal **neural tube defect** (e.g., anencephaly and spina bifida). Other disorders that elevate maternal serum AFP are:
   a. Wrong dates (i.e., the pregnancy is further along than anticipated)
   b. Multiple gestation
   c. Fetal demise
   d. Abruptio placentae
   e. Other fetal congenital defects (e.g., omphalocele, gastroschisis, and congenital nephrosis)

3. An unexplained elevated maternal serum AFP may be associated with third-trimester complications.

K. **Screening for hepatitis B** should be performed to identify fetuses at risk.

L. **HIV counseling and testing** of all pregnant women is now recommended by the CDC.

M. **A sickle cell screen** is indicated in all patients of African descent. It should also be considered for those of Indo-Pakistani, Caribbean, Mediterranean, Southeast Asian, or Latin American descent.

VI. **RISK ASSESSMENT**

A. **Preconception.** Counseling before conception affords women the opportunity to learn about fetal risks and to take appropriate action.

1. **Informational counseling sessions** are relatively inexpensive and can help prevent fetal exposure to harmful drugs, medications, infectious agents, and radiation. For example, a woman who is informed about her lack of antibodies to rubella or toxoplasmosis can take steps to avoid exposure to those infectious agents.

2. **Risk assessment is followed by health promotion.**
   a. **Preventive measures** can include rubella or hepatitis vaccination and folic acid supplements.
   b. **Education** involves measures such as informing the patient about teratogenic drugs (e.g., tretinoin and valproic acid).

    c. Encouragement of lifestyle changes is often effective only when women know about the potential fetal harm involved. Examples of changes to be encouraged include:

       (1) Cessation of smoking, alcohol use, and recreational drug use

       (2) Modification of eating habits so that blood glucose values can be closely controlled

       (3) Avoidance of situations that could result in core temperature elevation (e.g., saunas, hot tubs, and exposure to people with febrile illnesses)

       (4) Avoidance of foods harmful to the patient (e.g., avoidance of phenylalanine-containing foods by a patient with phenylketonuria)

B. **Antepartum.** Pregnancy is a dynamic state; therefore, continued assessment during the prenatal period is necessary to identify problems early and allow prompt intervention. Extensive research with high-risk patients has been conducted, and the major perinatal problems responsible for most neonatal morbidity have been identified (Table 10-4).

Table 10-4. Prenatal Assessment Objectives

Major Perinatal Problems to Be Identified Early	Associated Prenatal Problems	
	Historical Factors	**Developing Factors**
Prematurity (<37 weeks)	Mother's education Previous stillbirth Previous premature birth Previous neonatal death Multiparity (5 children or more) Uterine malformation Weight less than 100 lbs History of genitourinary infections	Moderate to severe pregnancy-induced hypertension Incompetent cervix Rh sensitization Smoking Pyelonephritis Narcotic use
Intrauterine growth retardation	Previous stillbirth Previous neonatal death Multiparity (5 children or more)	Moderate to severe pregnancy-induced hypertension
Preeclampsia/eclampsia	Chronic hypertension History of renal disease Diabetes Age younger than 17 years	Weight gain of more than 2 lbs/week Intrauterine growth retardation Positive roll-over test Multiple pregnancy
Diabetes	Age older than 35 years Previous infant over 9 lbs Family history Previous fetal anomaly	Polyhydramnios Pregnancy-induced hypertension Genitourinary infections
Congenital anomalies	Age older than 35 years Diabetes Habitual abortion Previous fetal anomaly	

Data were collected from 1417 pregnancies (1968–1972). (Reprinted with permission from Bolognese RJ, Scheider J, Schwarz R: *Perinatal Medicine: Management of the High-Risk Fetus and Neonate,* 2nd ed. Baltimore, Williams & Wilkins, 1982, p 10.)

1. **Prematurity.** Preterm labor and delivery account for much perinatal morbidity and mortality. Thus, early identification of women at risk for preterm labor and delivery allows appropriate preventive measures to be instituted (see Table 10-2).

2. **Intrauterine growth restriction (IUGR).** It is important that the progress of each pregnancy be assessed carefully, including serial weight and fundal height measurements at regular intervals. If the fundal height is noted to be lagging, ultrasonography is indicated to detect IUGR.

   a. **Definition**
      (1) Weight at birth at or below the 10th percentile for gestational age.
      (2) IUGR is differentiated from infants who are small for gestational age (SGA). IUGR is caused by a pathologic process, whereas SGA is thought to be constitutional.
      (3) IUGR may be asymmetric (head sparing) or symmetric.

   b. **Associated morbidity and mortality**
      (1) Stillbirth
      (2) Neonatal morbidity
      (3) Intrapartum asphyxia

   c. **Etiology**
      (1) Genetic/chromosomal disorders
      (2) Congenital infections
      (3) Substance abuse
      (4) Placental disease
      (5) Poor maternal weight gain
      (6) Maternal medical conditions
      (7) Multiple gestation

   d. **Management**
      (1) Improve fetal environment: bed rest, smoking cessation
      (2) Serial assessment of fetal well-being: fetal kick counts, nonstress tests, biophysical profiles
      (3) Continued assessment of fetal growth with ultrasonography
      (4) Careful monitoring of amniotic fluid status

   e. **Delivery.** Delivery should be accomplished as soon as it is thought that the extrauterine environment would be better for the fetus than the intrauterine environment.
      (1) If oligohydramnios: deliver
      (2) If poor fetal testing: deliver
      (3) If no growth on serial sonography: deliver

3. **Pregnancy-induced hypertension.** There are a number of associated historical risk factors (see Table 10-4). It is recommmended that close observation and evaluation be done for the early detection of proteinuria, edema, and hypertension.

4. **Diabetes.** It is essential that the diagnosis of diabetes be made as early as possible. The cornerstone of management is establishing an early, rigid, euglycemic metabolic control to reduce fetal and neonatal morbidity and mortality.

5. **Congenital anomalies.** It is difficult to identify the woman at risk for congenital anomalies. Some laboratory tests can be used to identify the fetus with a particular anomaly (e.g., triple screen). Routine ultrasound at 16 to 20 weeks' gestation detects many major anomalies, but has not been proven to improve perinatal outcome.

C. **Intrapartum.** Assessment of the pregnant woman must continue into the intrapartum period. Certain prenatal factors are associated with subsequent intrapartum risk and outcome. It is important to identify events associated with poor outcome so that appropriate interventions may be taken to reduce fetal and neonatal morbidity and mortality. Table 10-5 represents a prospective analysis that identifies three major perinatal problems (i.e., abnormal labor, low Apgar scores, and respiratory distress) and their related prenatal, neonatal, and intrapartum complications.

Table 10-5. Intrapartum Assessment Objectives

Major Problems to Be Prevented	Associated Problems	
	Prenatal	**Neonatal or Intrapartum**
Abnormal labor		
Prolonged latent phase of labor	Maternal age older than 35 years	None
Primary dysfunctional labor	Habitual abortion	Fetal anomalies, low 1-minute Apgar score, meconium aspiration
Prolonged second stage (more than 2.5 hours)	None	Hyperbilirubinemia
Precipitous labor	Previous stillbirth; previous premature birth	None
Prolonged labor (more than 20 hours total)	Smoking	Resuscitation at birth Fetal anomalies
Low Apgar scores		
1-minute: less than 5	Moderate to severe preeclampsia*; maternal cardiac disease; diabetes; previous stillbirth; previous neonatal death; abnormal fetal position; multiple pregnancy	Premature infant; premature rupture of membranes; abnormal presentation; multiple pregnancy; heavy meconium; primary dysfunctional labor; abruptio placentae; fetal acidosis; breech vaginal delivery*; operative forceps; shoulder dystocia
5-minute: less than 5	Moderate to severe preeclampsia*; diabetes; previous stillbirth; Rh sensitization; abnormal fetal position	Abruptio placentae; heavy meconium; abnormal presentation; premature infant; breech delivery*; fetal acidosis; operative forceps
Respiratory distress		
Respiratory distress syndrome	Moderate to severe renal disease; diabetes; previous stillbirth; previous premature birth; previous neonatal death; multiparity; uterine malformation; Rh sensitization; moderate to severe preeclampsia; pyelonephritis	Premature labor; moderate to severe toxemia; breech presentation*; abruptio placentae; fetal acidosis; breech vaginal delivery
Other respiratory distress (transient tachypnea)	Diabetes; previous neonatal death; previous cesarean section; previous infant over 9 lbs; maternal age older than 35 years	Prematurity; premature rupture of membranes; cesarean section; heavy meconium*
Meconium aspiration	Diabetes; previous stillbirth; multiparity (5 children or more); multiple pregnancy; moderate to severe preeclampsia	Moderate to severe preeclampsia*; heavy meconium*; multiple pregnancy; primary dysfunctional labor; abruptio placentae; fetal acidosis; breech delivery; shoulder dystocia

Data were collected from 1417 pregnancies (1968–1972). (Reprinted with permission from Bolognese RJ, Scheider J, Schwartz R: *Perinatal Medicine: Management of the High-Risk Fetus and Neonate,* 2nd ed. Baltimore, Williams & Wilkins, 1982, p 18.)

* An analysis of 1977 data identified these factors as no longer associated with poor outcome.

1. **Abnormal labor**
   a. **Prenatal factors** may be related to the development of the following types of abnormal labor:
      (1) Primary dysfunctional labor
      (2) Prolonged labor (more than 20 hours total)
      (3) Prolonged latent phase of labor
      (4) Precipitous labor
      (5) Secondary arrest of cervical dilation
   b. Only three types of abnormal labor have been found to be associated with **subsequent neonatal morbidity.** These are:
      (1) Primary dysfunctional labor
      (2) Prolonged second stage (more than 2.5 hours)
      (3) Prolonged labor (more than 20 hours total)

2. **Low Apgar scores in the prenatal or intrapartum period.** Many of the factors associated with low Apgar scores at birth can be identified early in the intrapartum period, and appropriate intervention can be instituted. Umbilical cord gases rather than Apgar scores are a more accurate index of the condition of the neonate.

3. **Respiratory distress** (see Table 10-5)
   a. **Respiratory distress syndrome** is often related to preterm labor and delivery.
   b. **Transient tachypnea.** Certain prenatal or intrapartum events should be evaluated and, where possible, ameliorated or controlled so that this type of respiratory distress is avoided.
   c. **Meconium aspiration.** Aggressive management intrapartum and immediately after delivery is necessary if meconium aspiration is to be avoided. Not all meconium aspiration is preventable, regardless of the measures taken.

STUDY QUESTIONS

DIRECTIONS: Each of the numbered items or incomplete statements in this section is followed by answers or by completions of the statement. Select the ONE lettered answer or completion that is BEST in each case.

1. Maternal mortality rate is defined as the number of maternal deaths per

(A) 1000 live-births
(B) 10,000 live-births
(C) 100,000 live-births
(D) 1000 pregnancies
(E) 100,000 pregnancies

2. A pregnant woman is routinely screened for which of the following disease entities?

(A) Parvovirus
(B) Toxoplasmosis
(C) Cytomegalovirus (CMV)
(D) Syphilis
(E) Herpes simplex virus (HSV)

3. Which of the following is a common reservoir for toxoplasmosis?

(A) School-age children
(B) Bird droppings
(C) Cats
(D) Contaminated seafood
(E) Blood

DIRECTIONS: Each of the numbered items or incomplete statements in this section is negatively phrased, as indicated by a capitalized word such as NOT, LEAST, or EXCEPT. Select the ONE lettered answer or completion that is BEST in each case.

4. Which of the following factors is NOT associated with an increased risk of perinatal morbidity?

(A) Low socioeconomic status
(B) Low maternal age (less than 20 years old)
(C) Heavy cigarette smoking
(D) Alcohol abuse
(E) Exercise

5. Maternal age younger than 20 years does NOT increase the risk for which of the following conditions?

(A) Low birth weight
(B) Fetal death
(C) Uterine dysfunction
(D) A genetically abnormal conceptus
(E) Premature delivery

6. Which of the following is NOT a true statement about urinary tract infections during pregnancy?

(A) Asymptomatic bacteriuria in pregnancy needs to be treated
(B) Pregnancy increases the risk for development of asymptomatic bacteriuria
(C) Acute systemic pyelonephritis resulting from asymptomatic bacteriuria is associated with premature labor and delivery
(D) Few women contract asymptomatic bacteriuria who are not bacteriuric at their first prenatal visit
(E) The incidence of asymptomatic bacteriuria is higher in pregnant women with a low socioeconomic status and increased parity and age

7. Which of the following statements about risk factors during pregnancy is NOT correct?

(A) A woman with a prior ectopic pregnancy is at risk for another ectopic pregnancy
(B) A grand multiparous woman is at risk for postpartum hemorrhage
(C) The incidence of preterm delivery increases with each subsequent preterm delivery
(D) Once a woman has had a cesarean section, all of her subsequent deliveries must be accomplished by cesarean section

8. Which of the following historical factors is NOT helpful in identifying the couple at risk for a genetic disorder?

(A) Consanguinity
(B) Parental age
(C) Ethnicity
(D) A previous spontaneous abortion

ANSWERS AND EXPLANATIONS

1. The answer is C [II A 2]. The definition of the maternal mortality rate is the number of maternal deaths per 100,000 live-births. Over the past 50 years, there has been a significant decline in maternal mortality in the United States. As recently as 1975, the maternal mortality rate was 12.8/100,000 live-births—that is, 6.7/100,000 for whites and 19.8/100,000 for others. The dramatic difference between these rates is attributed to economic and social factors, including lack of appropriate medical personnel and delivery facilities, as well as inadequate nutrition, health education, and early prenatal care.

2. The answer is D [III C 16 a–f]. Only syphilis, hepatitis B virus (HBV), human immunodeficiency virus (HIV), and rubella are serious enough and occur frequently enough to make routine screening necessary. Many authorities also recommend screening for gonorrhea and chlamydia. If sufficient clinical suspicion exists, the patient may need to be evaluated for parvovirus, toxoplasmosis, cytomegalovirus (CMV), and herpes simplex virus (HSV), all of which play a role in increasing perinatal morbidity. Prepregnancy testing for toxoplasmosis and CMV may be useful in evaluating risk involved in a future pregnancy.

3. The answer is C [III C 16 d]. Cats serve as a reservoir for toxoplasmosis. Therefore, the physician should inquire about the presence of cats in the patient's household and alert her to the potential risks. If the patient has a cat, she should be encouraged to limit her contacts with it. She should especially be encouraged to refrain from cleaning the litter box and from engaging in any other activity that could lead to contact with a cat's waste products (e.g., gardening outdoors without gloves).

4. The answer is E [III A 1–3]. Exercise during pregnancy has not been associated with an increased risk of perinatal morbidity and mortality, as long as it is done in moderation. Alcohol abuse undermines maternal health as well as produces a pattern of abnormalities in the fetus known as the fetal alcohol syndrome; the severity of the fetal involvement is related to quantity and the time during gestation of fetal exposure. The effects of the occasional social use of alcohol on the fetus are not known, so most physicians advise their patients to avoid alcohol during pregnancy. Low socioeconomic status, low maternal age, and heavy cigarette smoking all have been shown to be closely associated with an increased risk of perinatal morbidity.

5. The answer is D [III A 2 a]. Older women (i.e., older than 35 years of age), not younger, are at risk for genetically abnormal conceptuses. Young mothers, however, have an increased risk for many complications (e.g., low birth weight, fetal death, uterine dysfunction, and premature births) for unknown reasons. Speculative reasons include poor nutrition, low socioeconomic status, and late or substandard prenatal care.

6. The answer is B [V G 1–3]. Few pregnant women have asymptomatic bacteriuria who are not bacteriuric at their first prenatal visit. It is believed that pregnancy does not increase the incidence of asymptomatic bacteriuria but rather sets the stage for the development of systemic pyelonephritis in those women with bacteriuria. Asymptomatic bacteriuria does predispose the pregnant woman to the development of acute systemic pyelonephritis, which has been associated with premature labor and delivery. In addition, asymptomatic bacteriuria is more prevalent in pregnant patients with low socioeconomic status and increased parity and age.

7. The answer is D [III B 1, 3, 7, 8]. A patient with a prior cesarean section can attempt a vaginal delivery as long as there are no medical or surgical contraindications. The main surgical contraindication is a previous classic cesarean section. Current studies reveal that more than 60% of patients who have undergone a cesarean section because of cephalopelvic disproportion may have a subsequent vaginal delivery. A woman with a prior ectopic pregnancy is at increased risk for a subsequent ectopic pregnancy and must be evaluated early in the pregnancy. A woman with greater than five previous vaginal deliveries is at increased risk for postpartum hemorrhage secondary to uterine atony. Also, the incidence of preterm delivery increases with each previous preterm delivery; however, it does seem to decrease with each birth that is not preterm.

8. The answer is D [III C 9 b]. If a woman has one spontaneous abortion, it is not necessarily considered an unusual or alarming event, and it does not provide information likely to help identify a couple at risk for genetic disorders. Consanguinity and ethnicity are helpful in identifying high-risk patients because in each case a large pool of identical genes is shared, increasing the possibility of sharing similar mutant genes. Paternal age older than 55 years may increase the risk of a de novo single gene mutation. Advanced maternal age (i.e., older than 35 years) increases the risk of chromosomal anomalies.

Chapter 11

Premature Labor
William W. Beck, Jr.

I. PREMATURITY

A. Definition. Prematurity is the state of an infant born at a **gestational age of less than 37 weeks.** It is manifested by low birth weight (500–2499 g), physical signs of immaturity, and multisystem disorders. Infants who are of low birth weight but physically mature (e.g., growth-retarded infants) and infants who are large for gestational age but physically immature (e.g., infants of diabetic mothers) are not considered premature.

B. Epidemiology. Over the last 30 years, the incidence of prematurity has remained stable, although neonatal outcome has improved. Between 1970 and 1989, the neonatal mortality rate declined from a rate of 13.8/1000 live-births to 6.1/1000 live-births in the white population and from the rate of 22.8/1000 live-births to 12.1/1000 live-births in the black population.

1. **In the United States,** 9% of all neonates are born before 37 completed weeks' gestation.

2. Six percent are born before 36 completed weeks' gestation.

3. Approximately 2% to 3% are born before 33 weeks' gestation.

4. Approximately 50% of all perinatal deaths occur among children born before 33 weeks' gestation.

5. In addition, 50% to 70% of all perinatal deaths are secondary to complications arising from a preterm birth.

II. RISK FACTORS FOR PREMATURE DELIVERY.
A patient who has previously given birth to a premature infant faces a 20% to 30% risk of recurrence in the next pregnancy; 50% of the patients who deliver prematurely have no risk factor.

A. Factors in a patient's history that predispose her to a premature delivery include the following.

1. **Low socioeconomic status,** including low income, low level of education, and poor nutrition, constitutes a risk factor.

2. **Race.** African Americans tend to give birth to infants who are 1 week younger in gestational age than those born to white Americans; the preterm delivery rate for African Americans is approximately 16.3%, in contrast to 7.7% in white Americans.

3. **Age.** Gravidas who are younger than 16 years of age and primigravidas who are older than 30 years of age are at risk.

4. **Obstetric history of previous premature birth.** One premature birth increases the risk fourfold, and two premature births increase the risk sixfold.

5. **Work and activities** that are physically demanding or that are stressful and anxiety provoking increase a woman's risk.
   a. **High-risk jobs,** in terms of stress, include clerical, sales, service, manufacturing positions, nursing, and physicians.
   b. **Intermediate-risk jobs,** in terms of stress, are those in the technical and professional sectors.

    c. **Low-risk jobs,** in terms of stress, include housekeeping and positions in agricultural and fishing industries. These jobs may, however, be physically demanding.

6. **Smoking** more than 10 cigarettes per day increases a woman's risk.

7. **Cocaine use** increases a woman's risk.

8. **Complicated medical history** can increase a woman's risk, especially if it includes the following:
   a. **Previous elective termination of pregnancy,** especially after 12 weeks' gestation, possibly creating cervical incompetence.
   b. **Exposure of the patient in utero to diethylstilbestrol (DES),** resulting in a cervical or uterine abnormality, such as a T-shaped uterine cavity.
   c. **Mid-trimester loss or history of premature cervical dilation.**

B. **Complications during pregnancy that predispose a woman to premature labor**

1. **Upper urinary tract infection**
   a. Asymptomatic bacteriuria
   b. Pyelonephritis

2. **Maternal diseases**
   a. Hypertension
   b. Preeclampsia and eclampsia
   c. Asthma
   d. Hyperthyroidism
   e. Heart disease
   f. Drug addiction
   g. Cholestasis
   h. Anemia with hemoglobin levels less than 9 g/dl

3. **Conditions that overdistend the uterus**
   a. Multiple gestations
   b. Gross fetal anomalies, leading to hydramnios
   c. Diabetes
   d. Rh isoimmunization

4. Antepartum hemorrhage

5. Placental abruption or fetal death

6. Maternal abdominal surgery or general sepsis

7. Intrauterine infection

III. FACTORS INVOLVED IN PRETERM LABOR

A. **Infectious theory**

1. **Intrauterine infection rarely causes preterm labor.**

2. Progressive labor, both term and preterm, results in inflammation of the tissues exposed by cervical dilation.

B. **Other factors**

1. Abnormalities of the cervix and fundus (e.g., incompetence, myomas, müllerian anomalies)

2. Fetal anomalies

3. Multifetal pregnancies

4. Drug abuse

5. Urinary tract infection

6. Idiopathic (still representing the largest group)

IV. MANAGEMENT OF PREGNANCIES AT RISK FOR PRETERM LABOR

A. **Early detection of premature labor** is the key to successful management. The symptoms are often so subtle that they may be ignored by the patient and the physician. Once labor is established, the use of tocolytic agents is seldom effective in delaying delivery for a significant amount of time or in improving survival. To achieve early detection, the following steps should be taken.

1. **Patient education.** The patient should be educated to recognize the early signs of premature labor, including:
   a. Menstrual-like cramping
   b. Low backache
   c. Pelvic pressure
   d. Increased vaginal discharge
   e. Increased frequency of urination
   f. Vaginal bleeding (which can result from cervical dilation or rupture of the membranes and which should lead the patient to call her physician immediately)

2. **Monitoring at-risk patients.** The physician should perform **weekly cervical examinations** in patients at risk **to detect subtle changes that may herald the onset of labor,** including:
   a. Dilation of the internal and external os
   b. Cervical effacement or softening
   c. A change in the direction of the cervix (from posterior to anterior)
   d. A change in the station of the presenting part

3. If a **cervical change or uterine irritability with cramping** is noted, then hospitalization should be considered.

4. **If preterm labor is suspected,** the patient should be evaluated according to the scheme illustrated in Figure 11-1.

B. **Cervical incompetence**

1. **Evidence.** A history of a second-trimester miscarriage preceded by the absence of perceived uterine contractions is the best evidence of cervical incompetence.

2. **Hysterosalpingography** (radiograph of the uterus) before pregnancy may show abnormal widening of the cervical canal and possibly an abnormally shaped uterine cavity, such as those seen in daughters of women who took DES.

3. When **intrauterine pressure** exceeds the strength of the cervix, the cervix will open without contractions; an incompetent cervix usually begins to open in the second trimester.

4. **Cervical change without cramping in a pregnancy of less than 24 weeks** indicates a need for cervical cerclage and bed rest. A cervical cerclage, however, is of no value as prophylaxis against premature labor and the use of tocolysis. Placement of a pessary for cervical incompetence is advocated if surgery would threaten the pregnancy (i.e., if the cervix is more than 80% effaced at 16 weeks). **Complications of cervical cerclage** include the following:
   a. **Mother**
      (1) **Anesthesia risks,** such as spinal headache or aspiration of gastric contents after general anesthesia
      (2) **Cervical bleeding** from cervical dilation or usually from placement of the suture into the cervical mucosa

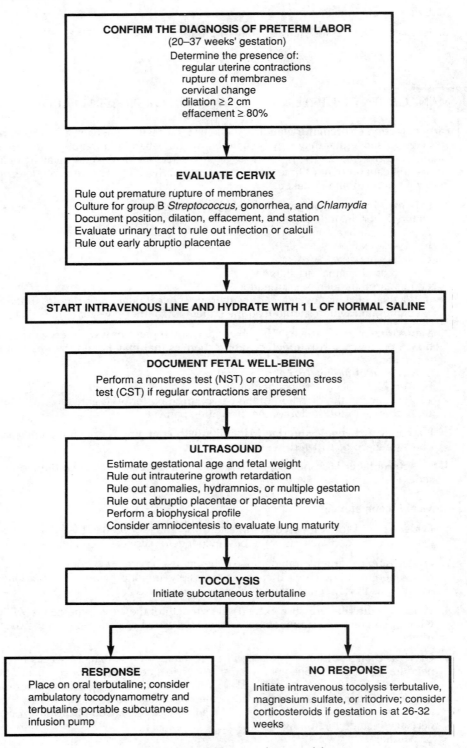

FIGURE 11-1. Management of preterm labor.

(3) Cervical deformity or autoamputation, if contractions cause the stitch to tear the cervix
(4) Chronic vaginal discharge from chronic inflammation because of a foreign body (suture)
(5) Increased incidence of amnionitis and postpartum endometritis if prolonged rupture of the membranes occurs
(6) Premature labor resulting from increased prostaglandin release because of surgical manipulation of the cervix
  b. **Fetus**
    (1) Rupture of the membranes
    (2) Chorioamnionitis, possibly resulting from overwhelming sepsis from vaginal bacteria

V. THERAPY FOR PREMATURE LABOR

A. Major tenets of therapy

1. Maintain a high-risk index of suspicion.

2. Prescribe prolonged bed rest in the left lateral position and good hydration to enhance uterine blood flow.

3. Test for asymptomatic bacteriuria, which occurs in 3% to 5% of all pregnancies.
   a. Treat with a 7-day course of antibiotics.
   b. Test for recurrent infection with a urine culture every 6 to 8 weeks.

4. Recommend cessation of cigarette smoking.

5. Suggest consultations with social workers, psychologists, and psychiatrists to reduce the psychological stress associated with preterm labor.

6. Perform therapeutic amniocentesis to remove 500 ml of fluid if hydramnios causes overdistension and contractions; may have to be repeated.

7. Recommend cessation of coitus between 20 and 36 weeks' gestation in those patients at high risk for premature delivery.

8. Consider the use of home contraction monitoring (i.e., with **ambulatory tocodynamometry**).

9. Consider home use of a **terbutaline autoinfusion pump** to inhibit uterine contractions.

B. Drug therapy

1. **Pharmacologic agents**
   a. **Inhibitors of prostaglandin synthesis,** such as ibuprofen or indomethacin, which may cause premature narrowing and closure of the fetal ductus arteriosus and, therefore, are not generally used (can be used up to 32 weeks)
   b. **Calcium ion (Ca^{2+}) channel blockers,** such as verapamil and nifedipine

2. **Intravenous tocolysis for preterm labor**
   a. **Ethanol,** which acts as a posterior pituitary inhibitor, thereby inhibiting oxytocin letdown, is rarely used today because of maternal side effects, including inebriation, vomiting, gastritis, aspiration, and lactic acidosis, and fetal depression.
   b. **Magnesium sulfate,** which competes with Ca^{2+}, has been an effective pharmacologic agent at a dose of 1 to 3 g/hr after a loading dose of 4 g. The side effects are numerous, but obstetricians are familiar with this drug, and it has a good antidote, calcium gluconate. The chief complications are shortness of breath and respiratory depression, but these can be reversed with 10 ml of a 10% solution of calcium gluconate.

c. The **family of β_2-adrenergic** agents are the most popular drugs used for arresting preterm labor.

   (1) The **mechanism of action of β_2-mimetics** is stimulation of the β_2-receptors in uterine smooth muscle, causing relaxation of the muscle and cessation of contractions.

      (a) Adenyl cyclase enhances the conversion of adenosine triphosphate to cyclic adenosine monophosphate

      (b) Increases calcium uptake by intracellular organelles

      (c) Reduces intracellular concentration of ionized calcium

      (d) Prevents activation of contractile proteins

   (2) The **most commonly used agents** are ritodrine and terbutaline. Terbutaline has the advantage of being used subcutaneously, whereas ritodrine is administered intravenously.

      (a) **Terbutaline** is given in doses of 0.25 mg subcutaneously every 30 minutes, up to a maximum of six doses, followed by oral maintenance of 5.0 mg every 4 to 6 hours.

      (b) **Intravenous administration of ritodrine,** on the other hand, should be continued for 6 to 24 hours after contractions cease, using a titration dose of a maximum of 0.35 mg/min. This may be followed by oral ritodrine, 10 mg every 2 to 6 hours.

   (3) **Maternal side effects** include tachycardia with palpitations, hypertension with widening of the pulse pressure, tremor, nausea, irritability, hyperglycemia, hypokalemia, hyperuricemia, metabolic acidosis, and pulmonary edema.

   (4) **Contraindications** to the use of β_2-adrenergic agents include maternal cardiac disease, severe eclampsia, significant hypertension, undiagnosed uterine bleeding, bleeding from placenta previa or abruptio placentae, intrauterine infection, fetal demise, severe intrauterine growth retardation, maternal hyperthyroidism, uncontrolled maternal diabetes, and any condition that mandates termination of the pregnancy.

   (5) **Maternal complications** include hyperglycemia secondary to hepatic glycogenolysis with consequent hyperinsulinemia and hypokalemia. A more significant but less common complication is pulmonary edema, which is thought to be secondary to overhydration and complicated cardiovascular, pulmonary, and renal mechanisms inherent to the gravid woman exposed to β_2 medications.

   (6) **Neonatal hypoglycemia, hypocalcemia,** and **hypotension** have been reported after use of β_2-adrenergic drugs, especially if given within 2 or 3 days of delivery. Long-term (7 years) follow-up studies of children exposed to ritodrine in utero have not reported deleterious side effects on growth or development.

3. Maternal corticosteroids have potential value in decreasing the incidence of respiratory distress syndrome when administered between 28 and 32 weeks' gestation and 24 hours before delivery, in patients with intact membranes.

a. Increase surfactant level

b. Benefit limited; must repeat corticosteroids weekly

STUDY QUESTIONS

DIRECTIONS: Each of the numbered items or incomplete statements in this section is followed by answers or by completions of the statement. Select the ONE lettered answer or completion that is BEST in each case.

1. The percentage of patients with a history of prematurity who will have another premature infant is

(A) 0% to 10%
(B) 20% to 30%
(C) 40% to 50%
(D) 60% to 70%
(E) 80% to 90%

2. A 16-year-old primigravida reports that she is experiencing regular menstrual cramping every 2 minutes. She is 28 weeks pregnant. After taking a history, the first thing that the physician should do is

(A) send her to the labor floor immediately
(B) confirm the frequency of contractions by abdominal palpation
(C) evaluate fetal well-being with a fetal monitor
(D) evaluate the cervix by speculum examination

3. The most common cause of vaginal bleeding complicating premature labor is

(A) a vaginal laceration
(B) an endocervical polyp
(C) cervical dilation
(D) placenta previa
(E) placental abruption

4. Inhibitors of prostaglandin synthesis are not generally used for tocolysis because they

(A) are ineffective
(B) produce marked hypertension
(C) may cause premature closure of the fetal ductus arteriosus
(D) are too expensive
(E) are associated with lactic acidosis

5. A 39-year-old former Olympic athlete (gravida 5, para 0311) comes for her first prenatal visit at 8 weeks' gestation. After undergoing a prenatal genetic counseling session, she asks her physician about current recommendations concerning her risk of having a premature infant. The physician should explain that

(A) she is at no risk for premature delivery
(B) she can continue her plans for running a marathon in 1 month
(C) her age has no bearing on this pregnancy
(D) he would like to see her more often to perform cervical examinations
(E) he would like to see her more often only if any symptoms of premature labor develop

6. Which of the following is a sign of late premature labor?

(A) Increased vaginal discharge
(B) Increased uterine contractions
(C) Low back pain
(D) Cervical dilation to 4 cm
(E) Worsening pelvic pressure

DIRECTIONS: Each of the numbered items or incomplete statements in this section is negatively phrased, as indicated by a capitalized word such as NOT, LEAST, or EXCEPT. Select the ONE lettered answer or completion that is BEST in each case.

7. Which of the following is NOT a predisposing factor for premature labor?

(A) Maternal age older than 30 years
(B) Smoking more than 10 cigarettes per day
(C) Exposure to diethylstilbestrol (DES) in utero with a documented uterine structural abnormality
(D) Multiparity with more than four previous deliveries
(E) Twin gestation

8. Which of the following drugs is NOT used to inhibit premature labor?

(A) Ethanol
(B) Magnesium sulfate
(C) Phenobarbital
(D) Ritodrine
(E) Terbutaline

ANSWERS AND EXPLANATIONS

1. The answer is B [II]. Unfortunately, a premature birth in one pregnancy increases the risk of a premature birth in the next pregnancy by approximately 20% to 30%. This is three times the rate of prematurity in the general population (9.0%), which has remained constant for the past 10 years. Even without apparent risk factors, it is necessary to warn patients who have had a premature birth that they are at a significant risk of having the same problem in future pregnancies.

2. The answer is B [IV A 1–4; Figure 11-1]. The regular menstrual cramping experienced by this patient is an early sign of premature labor. Other, more subtle signs of premature labor include low back pain, increase in vaginal discharge, pelvic pressure, and frequent urination. Before premature labor can be diagnosed, however, other causes of the contractions need to be considered. First, the uterus should be palpated to see if it is irritable (a condition likely to cause it to contract on palpation). Next, the fetal heart rate should be auscultated to assess fetal well-being. Evaluating the cervix with a speculum allows the physician to check for premature rupture of the membranes, to evaluate cervical dilation, and to obtain a cervical culture for gonorrhea, chlamydia, and group B streptococcus. If no rupture of the membranes has occurred, a digital pelvic examination may be performed. After this, a urine specimen should be obtained to rule out asymptomatic bacteriuria, which occurs in 3% to 5% of pregnant women and which can cause cramping.

3. The answer is C [IV A 1 f]. During premature labor, when the cervix begins to dilate and efface, the separation of the placenta and membranes may produce vaginal bleeding. The diagnosis of placenta previa should be excluded before the pelvic examination is performed. A placental abruption often causes preterm labor that cannot be inhibited with tocolytic agents. Vaginal lacerations from vaginal trauma (i.e., intercourse) usually produce vaginal bleeding without uterine contractions.

4. The answer is C [V B 1 a]. The inhibitors of prostaglandin synthesis, the most common

being indomethacin, act by blocking the endogenous production of prostaglandins. Although prostaglandin inhibitors have been used to prevent spontaneous labor, there is significant concern that this class of drugs may produce premature closure of the fetal ductus arteriosus and eventually lead to fetal death. Other potential serious side effects include thrombocytopenia, ulceration of the gastrointestinal tract, and allergic reactions. Because of these side effects, some clinicians use this drug only before 28 weeks' gestation, when the fetal ductus is more resistant to closure. Other investigators have found that indomethacin may be used safely before 32 weeks. However, it may cause decreased fetal renal perfusion, resulting in oligohydramnios.

5. The answer is D [II A 1–5; IV A]. The woman described in the question has a number of risk factors for premature labor. The four-digit code describing her parity—which translates digit by digit to number of term pregnancies (multiple gestations are counted as one pregnancy), number of preterm pregnancies, number of abortions (spontaneous or elective), and number of living children—reveals that she has had three previous premature deliveries. In addition, her maternal age is greater than 30 years, and she is at possible risk for increased physical stress. The key to preventing a premature delivery is to counsel this patient about her risk factors, recommend increased rest periods, and perform frequent cervical examinations. To await signs of premature labor before more frequent examinations would be risking premature labor that is unresponsive to therapeutic measures. Should the cervix reveal signs of dilation or effacement, tocolytic measures must be taken.

6. The answer is D [IV A 1 a–f]. One of the late signs of premature labor is cervical dilation past 2 cm. Pharmacologic inhibition of premature labor is less effective when cervical effacement is advanced beyond 80% or dilation has progressed beyond 3 or 4 cm. The early determination of premature labor, therefore, improves the chance that labor can be halted and that the pregnancy will continue until it reaches a stage that is safe for delivery of the fetus.

7. The answer is D [II A 1–8]. Multiparity with more than four previous deliveries is not a predisposing factor for prematurity. There are multiple predisposing factors for prematurity, including advanced maternal age, cigarette smoking, conditions that overextend the uterus such as a twin gestation, and exposure of the mother to diethylstilbestrol (DES) in utero. Usually more than one factor is operating at the same time. Unfortunately, over 50% of patients who deliver prematurely have no apparent risk factors.

8. The answer is C [V B 2 a–c]. Phenobarbital is an antiseizure medication and has never been shown to be an effective tocolytic agent.

Ethanol, administered by intravenous infusion, was once one of the most popular methods for the treatment of premature labor. Although it is an effective inhibitor of premature labor, it is rarely used today because of its many untoward side effects, including inebriation, nausea, vomiting, headache, lactic acidosis, respiratory depression, and aspiration. There are no significant fetal side effects, except sedation.

Ritodrine is the only β_2-mimetic agent to be approved by the Food and Drug Administration (FDA) in the United States for the inhibition of premature labor. Its mechanism of action is stimulation of β_2-adrenergic receptors, producing relaxation of the uterus and bronchi, vasodilation, and muscle glycogenolysis. Because of cross-reactivity with β_2-receptors throughout the body, there are significant cardiovascular side effects.

Magnesium sulfate is a neuromuscular blocking agent that inhibits myometrial contractions by competing with Ca^{2+}. It is the drug of choice for stopping premature labor in women with medical problems, such as diabetes mellitus.

Terbutaline is a selective β_2-agonist that is used as a bronchodilator when given orally; however, it has been used successfully to inhibit premature labor. Side effects, such as headache, tremor, hypotension, nausea, vomiting, and maternal and fetal tachycardia, are common with β_2-agonists.

Chapter 12

Prenatal Diagnosis and Obstetric Ultrasound

Jane Fang

I. INTRODUCTION

A. **Genetic counseling** assesses the risks of having a child with a genetic or congenital birth defect, interprets the risk, and assists the parents in making a decision regarding contraception, sterilization, adoption, artificial insemination, carrier detection, referrals to agencies concerned with handicapped children, prenatal diagnosis, and options regarding pregnancy termination.

B. **Prenatal diagnosis.** The diagnostic procedures currently available include ultrasound, amniocentesis, chorionic villus sampling (CVS), percutaneous umbilical blood sampling (PUBS), and fetoscopy. There is a 2% to 3% incidence of congenital malformations for low-risk couples. Prenatal diagnosis is indicated when the risks of having an affected offspring exceed this risk.

II. INDICATIONS FOR PRENATAL DIAGNOSIS

A. **Chromosomal abnormalities**

1. Advanced maternal age (i.e., at least 35 years at the time of delivery) [Table 12-1].

2. A previously affected child

3. Either parent has a chromosomal translocation or inversion

4. A history of three or more spontaneous abortions

5. Paternal aneuploidy

B. **Congenital malformations. Neural tube defects** are one of the most common congenital malformations, and occur in 1 to 2/1000 live births. They have a multifactorial inheritance pattern.

C. **Mendelian abnormalities**

1. **Inborn errors of metabolism**
   a. Mucopolysaccharidoses
   b. Mucolipidoses
   c. Lipidoses
   d. Amino acid disorders
   e. Miscellaneous biochemical disorders

2. **Abnormalities in DNA structure** (Table 12-2)

D. **Abnormal ultrasound findings**

E. **Abnormal maternal serum α-fetoprotein (MSAFP) or triple screen**

F. **Fragile X syndrome** is the most common cause of hereditary mental retardation.

1. It has an **X-linked recessive** inheritance pattern.

2. The mother who is a suspected carrier can be screened with evaluation of her chromosomes.

Table 12-1. Risk Factors for Trisomy 21

Risk Factor	Incidence/Live Births
Maternal Age*	
29	1/935
30–34[†]	1/600
35	1/365
35–39	1/300–1/100
40–44	1/60–1/50
45+	1/40

* Of children with trisomy 21, 50% are born to mothers older than 35 years of age.
[†] Risks for offspring with trisomy 21 if a previous child has trisomy 21 and maternal age is younger than 30 years is 1%–2%.

Table 12-2. Inherited Errors of Metabolism Diagnosed Prenatally

Disorder	Deficient Enzyme or Metabolic Defect
Acid phosphatase deficiency	Acid phosphatase
Adrenogenital syndrome	C-21 hydroxylase
Argininosuccinic aciduria	Argininosuccinase
Aspartylglycosaminuria	Aspartylglucosaminidase (AADG)
Ataxia, intermittent	Pyruvate decarboxylase
Cholesteryl ester storage disease	Cholesteryl ester hydrolase
Citrullinemia	Argininosuccinic acid synthetase
Combined immunodeficiency	Adenosine deaminase
Cystinosis	Cystine accumulation
Ehlers-Danlos type IV	Type III collagen
Ehlers-Danlos type VI	Collagen lysyl hydroxylase
Ehlers-Danlos type VII	Procollagen peptidase
Fabry's disease (X-linked)	Ceramide trihexosidase
Farber's disease	Ceramidase
Fucosidosis	α-Fucosidase
Galactokinase deficiency	Galactokinase
Galactosemia	D-Galactose-1-phosphate uridyl transferase
Gangliosidosis GM_1, type I	β-Galactosidase A, B, C
Gangliosidosis GM_2, type II	β-Galactosidase B, C
Gangliosidosis GM_2, type I (Tay-Sachs)	Hexosaminidase A
Gangliosidosis GM_2, type II (Sandhoff's)	Hexosaminidase A, B
Gaucher's disease	β-Glucocerebrosidase
Glucose-6-phosphate dehydrogenase deficiency (X-linked)	Glucose-6-phosphate dehydrogenase
Glycogen storage disease type II (Pompe's)	α-4-Glucosidase
Glycogen storage disease type III	Amylo-1, 6-glucosidase
Glycogen storage disease type IV	Amylo-1,4 to 1,6-transglucosidase

Table 12-2. *(continued)*

Disorder	Deficient Enzyme or Metabolic Defect
Homocystinuria	Cystathionine synthase
Hyperlipoproteinemia type II	Impaired regulation of 3-hydroxy-3-methylglutaryl CoA reductase
Hyperlysinemia	Lysine-ketoglutarate reductase
Hypophosphatasia	Alkaline phosphatase
Isovaleric acidemia	Isovaleric acid CoA dehydrogenase
Krabbe's disease	Galactocerebroside β-galactosidase
Lactosyl ceramidosis	Lactosyl ceramidase
Lesch-Nyhan disease (X-linked)	Hypoxanthine-guanine phosphoribosyl transferase
Mannosidosis	α-Mannosidase
Maple syrup urine disease	Keto acid decarboxylase
Menke's syndrome	Abnormal copper uptake
Metachromatic leukodystrophy	Arylsulfatase A
Methylmalonic aciduria I	Methylmalonic CoA mutase
Mucolipidosis type II (I-cell disease)	Lysosomal enzyme leakage
Mucolipidosis type III (pseudo-Hurler's polydystrophy)	Lysosomal enzyme leakage
Mucopolysaccharidosis I (Hurler's and Scheie's)	α-L-Iduronidase
Mucopolysaccharidosis II (Hunter's, X-linked)	Sulfo-iuronide sulfatase
Mucopolysaccharidosis III (Sanfilippo A)	Heparan sulfate sulfatase
Mucopolysaccharidosis III (Sanfilippo B)	N-Acetyl-D-glucosaminidase
Mucopolysaccharidosis IV (Morquio's)	N-Acetylhexosamine-6-sulfate sulfatase
Mucopolysaccharidosis VI (Maroteaux-Lamy)	Arylsulfatase
Mucopolysaccharidosis VII	β-Glucuronidase
Niemann-Pick disease	Sphingomyelinase
Ornithinemia	Ornithine keto acid amino transferase
Oroticaciduria I	Orotidylic pyrophosphorylase and orotidylic decarboxylase
Oroticaciduria II	Orotidylic decarboxylase
Osteogenesis imperfecta congenita	Type I collagen
Phosphohexose isomerase deficiency	Phosphohexose isomerase
Porphyria, congenital erythropoietic	Uroporphyrinogen III cosynthetase
Porphyria, acute intermittent	Porphobilinogen deaminase
Propionic acidemia	Propionyl CoA carboxylase
Refsum's disease	Phytanic acid oxidase
Testicular feminization syndrome (X-linked)	Androgen binding protein
Valinemia	Valine transaminase
Wolman's disease	Acid lipase
Xeroderma pigmentosum	Ultraviolet-specific endonuclease

Reprinted with permission from Siggers DC: *Prenatal Diagnosis of Genetic Disease.* Oxford, Blackwell Scientific, 1978, p 20.

III. GENETIC SCREENING.
In the United States, the most commonly screened genetic disorders are Tay-Sachs disease, sickle cell anemia, and the thalassemias.

A. Hemoglobinopathies

1. There are approximately 2 to 2.5 million people in the United States with inherited abnormalities of hemoglobin.

2. **Normal hemoglobin** is composed of three types of hemoglobin.
   a. **Hemoglobin A** has two α- and two β-chains, and makes up 95% of adult hemoglobin.
   b. **Hemoglobin A$_2$** has two α- and two δ-chains, and makes up 2% to 3.5% of adult hemoglobin.
   c. **Hemoglobin F** has two α- and two γ-chains, and makes up the remainder of adult hemoglobin.

3. **Sickle cell screening.** All people of African descent should undergo sickle cell screening initially with the Sickle-Dex. If this is positive for either parent, both should undergo hemoglobin electrophoresis.
   a. Sickle cell disease has an **autosomal recessive** inheritance pattern.
   b. **Sickle hemoglobin (Hb S)** results from a substitution of glutamic acid for valine in the β-globin chain.
   c. Hb S functions normally in the oxygenated state. In the deoxygenated state, hydrophobic bonds are formed, which cause red blood cell distortion, or sickling. This leads to tissue infarction and vasoocclusion.

4. **Thalassemias.** For all people at risk, screening should begin with the **mean corpuscular volume (MCV).** If the MCV is 80 fl or less, the patient should undergo hemoglobin electrophoresis.
   a. In α-**thalassemia,** there is decreased production of the α-globin chains.
   b. In β-**thalassemia,** there is decreased production of the ß-globin chains.

B. **Tay-Sachs disease** is the congenital absence of the enzyme **hexosaminidase A,** which results in an overaccumulation of sphingolipids.

1. It has an **autosomal recessive** inheritance pattern.

2. The carrier risk is 1 in 27 in Ashkenazi Jews.

3. **Preconception screening** is recommended for suspected carriers because detection is not accurate during pregnancy.

C. **Cystic fibrosis** is the most common inherited disorder in whites.

1. The carrier risk is 1 in 25 whites of northern European ancestry.

2. Seventy-five percent of carriers have the Δ-F508 gene, which can be detected with DNA studies.

3. Amniotic fluid assays for **alkaline phosphatase** can be measured in suspected pregnancies.

D. **Maternal serum** can be evaluated for neural tube defect and Down's syndrome screening.

1. **The MSAFP screen** can be performed from 15 to 19 weeks' gestation.
   a. A **low value** is indicative of a greater risk for Down's syndrome.
   b. An **elevated value** is indicative of a greater risk for a neural tube defect, and other disorders (Table 12-3).

2. **The triple screen** is offered at the same time as the MSAFP. The AFP value is integrated as one third of this screen. The other two components are human chorionic gonadotropin and estriol. All three values are evaluated together to enhance the diagnostic risk assessment for Down's syndrome.

Table 12-3. Conditions Characterized by Elevated α-Fetoprotein

Missed abortion	Cystic hygroma
Congenital nephrosis	Trisomy 30
Multiple pregnancy	Fetal bowel obstruction
Sacrococcygeal teratoma	Incorrectly dated pregnancy
Turner's syndrome	Intrauterine growth retardation
Omphalocele	

IV. TECHNIQUES OF PRENATAL DIAGNOSIS

A. **Ultrasound** is the most commonly used method of pregnancy assessment, and is a valuable tool in the prenatal diagnosis of congenital anomalies.

1. Ultrasound is **high-frequency sound waves.** Transabdominal ultrasounds performed for prenatal diagnosis operate at frequencies between 3.5 to 5 MHz.

2. **Safety**
   a. Epidemiologic studies in pregnant women have failed to reveal any association of ultrasound with congenital anomalies or adverse pregnancy outcome.
   b. Most instruments used for diagnosis produce energies far lower than what is considered a safe level of ultrasound exposure to tissues.

3. **Indications for ultrasound during pregnancy**
   a. Evaluation of gestational age
   b. Evaluation and follow-up of fetal growth and size
   c. Undiagnosed vaginal bleeding to evaluate:
      (1) Placenta previa
      (2) Placental abruption
   d. Determination of fetal presentation
   e. Confirmation of fetal life
   f. Evaluation for fetal anomalies, especially in the presence of an abnormal MSAFP or triple screen
   g. Guidance during procedures: amniocentesis, CVS, version, PUBS
   h. Evaluation of multiple gestations
   i. Assessment of fetal well-being (i.e., biophysical profile)
   j. Evaluation for ectopic gestation, missed abortion, and molar pregnancy

4. **Types of ultrasound examinations**
   a. A **basic** ultrasound examination should include:
      (1) Assessment of fetal number and presentation
      (2) Confirmation of fetal cardiac activity
      (3) Localization of the placenta
      (4) Determination of amniotic fluid adequacy
      (5) Gross evaluation for fetal anomalies
      (6) Establishment of gestational age
      (7) Evaluation for pelvic masses
   b. A **limited** ultrasound is targeted to look for specific clinical information, including:
      (1) Amniotic fluid volume
      (2) Biophysical profile
      (3) Ultrasound-guided procedures (i.e., amniocentesis, CVS, version)
      (4) To confirm fetal viability
      (5) To check placental localization
      (6) To check fetal presentation
   c. A **comprehensive** ultrasound is used to evaluate a fetus with a suspected or known anomaly.
      (1) Comprehensive ultrasound includes a careful examination of the fetal anatomy.

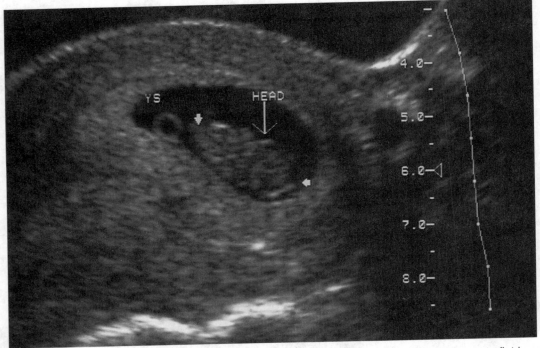

FIGURE 12-1. An ultrasound of the fetal crown–rump length. The fetus is surrounded by amniotic fluid (*dark shadow*). *Thick arrows* = ends of crown–rump length; *YS* = yolk sac.

    (2) Adequate fetal assessment may be limited by maternal obesity, fetal position, and the presence of oligohydramnios.

  5. First-trimester ultrasound is usually approached transvaginally, and is used to:
    a. Evaluate whether the pregnancy is intrauterine or ectopic. An intrauterine sac is visible transvaginally at 5 weeks' gestation.
    b. Confirm fetal viability as opposed to a missed abortion or a molar pregnancy. Fetal cardiac activity can be detected transvaginally at 6 weeks' gestation.
    c. Evaluate gestational age and number. Measurement of the fetal crown–rump length between 8 to 13 weeks' gestation can estimate fetal age within ±5 days (Figure 12-1).
    d. Evaluate pelvic masses.

  6. Second-trimester ultrasound is usually performed transabdominally with the maternal bladder full. These are routinely performed between 16 to 20 weeks' gestation for evaluation of fetal gestational age and anatomy, and for evaluation of placental location.
    a. The **biparietal diameter** is measured at the level of the thalamus and the cavum septum pellucidum. Of all the second-trimester measurements possible, the biparietal diameter reflects gestational age most closely. The correlation of the biparietal diameter measurement with gestational age decreases as the pregnancy advances (after 26 weeks) because the biologic variability of fetal head size increases dramatically (Figure 12-2).
    b. The **head circumference** is measured at the same level as the biparietal diameter.
    c. The **abdominal circumference** is measured at the level of the umbilical vein entering the liver.
    d. The **femur length** is measured.
    e. **Fetal weight** may be calculated by using the biparietal diameter, head circumference, femur length, and the abdominal circumference using a standardized regression equation; it is accurate to within 10%.

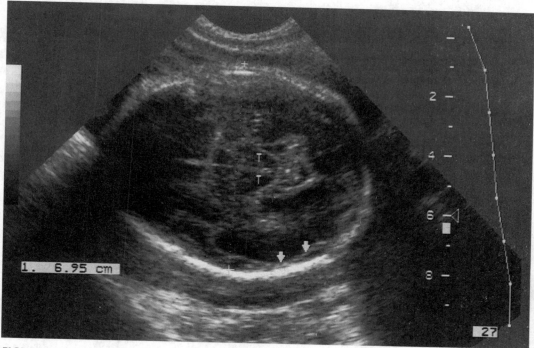

FIGURE 12-2. An ultrasound of a biparietal diameter (6.95 cm) measured between the calipers. *T* = thalamus (which always points posteriorly); *thick arrows* = edge of sylvian fissure.

   f. Placental localization is evaluated. A low-lying placenta diagnosed in the second trimester should be reevaluated in the third trimester, as the lower segment of the uterus expands.

   g. Amniotic fluid volume can be quantified by adding together the measurements of the vertical depths of amniotic fluid in the four quadrants of the uterus, the **amniotic fluid index.** Measurement of the largest single pocket of fluid indicates:

     (1) Oligohydramnios if a pocket is less than 2 cm vertically (anteriorly to posteriorly)

     (2) Adequate fluid if a pocket measures 2 to 8 cm vertically

     (3) Polyhydramnios if a pocket measures over 8 cm vertically. Polyhydramnios is associated with a higher incidence of congenital abnormalities (Table 12-4).

     (4) Normal values are about 6 to 24 cm.

Table 12-4. Fetal Malformations Commonly Associated with Polyhydramnios

Central nervous system	Respiratory tract
Anencephaly	Pulmonary hypoplasia
Hydrocephaly	Chylothorax
Encephalocele	
Gastrointestinal system	
Gastroschisis	
Omphalocele	
Tracheoesophageal fistula	
Duodenal atresia	

Reprinted with permission from Phelan JP, Martin GI: Polyhydramnios: fetal and neonatal implications. *Clin Perinatol* 16:987, 1989.

7. **Third-trimester ultrasound** is approached transabdominally. It is useful to:
   a. Follow a fetus affected with an anomaly
   b. Estimate fetal weight (see IV A 6 e). The accuracy of ultrasonographically estimated fetal weight is not as good in the very–low-birthweight or macrosomic
   fetus.
   c. Follow fetal growth
   d. Evaluate the fetus for intrauterine growth retardation. The fetal head:abdominal
   circumference ratio is maximal at 12 weeks' gestation, and falls to 1.0 at approximately 36 weeks. The fetus affected with asymmetric growth restriction has an increased ratio in the third trimester.
   e. Evaluate placental location

8. A **complete survey of the fetal anatomy** should include:
   a. Examination of the ventricles
   b. Examination of the thoracic cage and visualization of the four heart chambers
   c. Longitudinal and coronal views of the spine
   d. Visualization of the kidneys and bladder
   e. Examination of the umbilical cord and insertion site. Two small arteries and a
   large umbilical vein are seen in cross section. A two-vessel cord (single umbilical
   artery and vein) may be associated with congenital anomalies of the cardiovascular or genitourinary system, maternal diabetes mellitus, twin gestation, and increased neonatal mortality.
   f. Determination of amniotic fluid volume

9. **Biophysical profile**
   a. The biophysical profile is a method of fetal assessment that includes the following:
   (1) Amniotic fluid volume
   (2) Fetal tone
   (3) Fetal movement
   (4) Fetal breathing
   (5) Nonstress test
   b. A score of 2 (normal) or 0 (abnormal) is assigned to each component. There are
   specific guidelines in managing the abnormal biophysical profile.

10. **Placental development**
    a. **Placenta previa.** The diagnosis of placenta previa is made by ultrasound unless
    the posterior placenta is in the shadow of a fetus whose head is low. Many sec-
    ond-trimester placentas are visualized near the cervix, but this usually resolves in
    the third trimester.
    b. **Placental abruption** can sometimes be diagnosed by ultrasound. Associated find-
    ings include:
    (1) **Increased echogenicity** of one placental lobe due to fresh bleeding
    (2) **Elevation of the chorioamniotic membrane** from retroplacental blood
    (3) **Clotted blood** adjacent to the placenta
    c. **Placental thickness** increases until 32 weeks' gestation; its maximal thickness is
    usually no greater than 4 cm. There are certain conditions associated with in-
    creased placental thickness:
    (1) Maternal diabetes
    (2) Syphilis
    (3) Erythroblastosis fetalis
    (4) Some congenital anomalies

B. **Amniocentesis** is a transabdominal, fine-needle aspiration of amniotic fluid. The amniotic fluid contains fetal cells, which can be cultured and evaluated for chromosomal abnormalities. Amniocentesis can be performed from 15 to 17 weeks' gestation, at which
time ample fluid is present, diagnostic tests can be performed, and elective termination,
if desired by the patient, is still possible.

1. The **risk of fetal loss** from the procedure is **0.5%.**

2. The procedure must be performed under ultrasound guidance.

3. Rh-negative women who are not sensitized should receive Rho (D) immune globulin after the procedure.

4. Amniocentesis is used for management of the Rh-sensitized pregnancy.

5. Amniocentesis is performed in the third trimester for evaluation of fetal lung maturity with the lecithin to sphingomyelin ratio and with the presence of phosphatidyl glycerol.

6. Amniotic fluid can be assessed for acetylcholinesterase levels in the evaluation of neural tube defects.

C. **Chorionic villus sampling** can be performed at 9 to 12 weeks' gestation. Cells can be obtained either by a transabdominal or transcervical approach. The major benefit is earlier prenatal diagnosis.

1. The **risk of fetal loss** from procedure is **between 1% to 3%.**

2. The accuracy is comparable to that of amniocentesis.

3. Neural tube defect screening cannot be performed with this method.

4. Limb reduction defects have been associated with this procedure only when performed before 9 weeks' gestation.

5. Rh-negative women must receive Rho (D) immune globulin.

D. **Other techniques**

1. **Percutaneous umbilical blood sampling** is used to sample fetal blood for direct intravascular transfusion of blood into the fetus. Ultrasound is used to select the aspiration site. Bleeding from the sampling site is the main risk.

2. **Fetoscopy** is direct visualization of the fetus and intrauterine environment. Diagnostic benefit must outweigh potential fetal and maternal risks. **Pregnancy wastage can be as high as 5% to 6% from this procedure.**

3. **Fetal skin sampling** can be performed to obtain fetal cells.

E. **Molecular genetics.** With restriction enzyme techniques, DNA can be divided into fragments to which gene probes can be hybridized.

1. If a specific disorder has a known molecular basis (e.g., absence of a DNA sequence in α-thalassemia), the **DNA of the fetus can be tested** by CVS or amniocentesis for the disorder.

2. **In disorders with an unknown molecular basis,** prenatal diagnosis is still possible. In a given family with a specific inherited disorder, **restriction fragment length polymorphisms** can be traced for a mutant gene. Probes are available for Huntington's chorea, adult polycystic kidneys, Duchenne muscular dystrophy, hemophilia A or B, phenylketonuria, cystic fibrosis, and ß-thalassemia.

STUDY QUESTIONS

DIRECTIONS: Each of the numbered items or incomplete statements in this section is followed by answers or by completions of the statement. Select the ONE lettered answer or completion that is BEST in each case.

1. Which of the following procedures allows the earliest retrieval of DNA for prenatal diagnosis in pregnancy?

(A) Fetoscopy
(B) Amniocentesis
(C) Chorionic villus sampling
(D) Percutaneous umbilical blood sampling
(E) Fetal biopsy

2. Which of the following can be diagnosed from a basic ultrasound?

(A) Reverse blood flow in the umbilical artery
(B) Polyhydramnios
(C) Nuchal skin thickness
(D) Polydactyly
(E) Placenta accreta

3. A 32-year-old woman, gravida 1, para 1, comes to see you for genetic counseling. Her first child was born with sickle cell disease. She has since remarried, and is requesting prenatal testing. Which of the following is appropriate to offer the patient first?

(A) Percutaneous umbilical blood sampling at the appropriate gestational age
(B) Fetal chromosome analysis
(C) Maternal hemoglobin electrophoresis
(D) Paternal hemoglobin electrophoresis
(E) DNA linkage studies

DIRECTIONS: Each of the numbered items or incomplete statements in this section is negatively phrased, as indicated by a capitalized word such as NOT, LEAST, or EXCEPT. Select the ONE lettered answer or completion that is BEST in each case.

4. Which of the following procedures requires the LEAST technical skill and poses the lowest risk for fetal loss?

(A) Fetoscopy
(B) Chorionic villus sampling
(C) Percutaneous umbilical blood sampling
(D) Fetal biopsy
(E) Amniocentesis

5. Which of the following disorders CANNOT be diagnosed prenatally with DNA technology?

(A) Phenylketonuria
(B) Cystic fibrosis
(C) Duchenne muscular dystrophy
(D) Neural tube defects
(E) β-Thalassemia

ANSWERS AND EXPLANATIONS

1. The answer is C [IV C]. Chorionic villus sampling can be performed as early as the ninth week of pregnancy. It can be performed transcervically or transabdominally with ultrasound guidance. Chromosomal and biochemical abnormalities can be detected with DNA technology.

2. The answer is B [IV A 4 a]. Amniotic fluid volume assessment is an integral part of a basic ultrasound. Nuchal skin thickness is measured during comprehensive ultrasound. Polydactyly usually cannot be diagnosed ultrasonographically. Placenta accreta is usually diagnosed postpartum. Blood flow in the uterine artery must be examined with Doppler ultrasound techniques.

3. The answer is D [III A 3]. Because this patient has already had an affected child and is asymptomatic, she must be a heterozygous carrier. Her previous husband must also be a carrier. Because the father in this case is different, he should undergo hemoglobin electrophoresis to evaluate his carrier status. Fetal chromosome analysis will not detect an affected fetus for sickle cell disease. DNA linkage studies are not indicated unless the new father is a carrier.

4. The answer is E [IV B]. Amniocentesis is usually performed starting at 15 weeks' gestation. Although easier to perform than other prenatal diagnostic procedures, it is best done with ultrasound guidance and is not without complications. The risk of fetal loss from amniocentesis is 0.5%. All of the other methods of prenatal diagnosis listed carry a greater fetal risk.

5. The answer is D [IV E]. Neural tube defects are inherited in a multifactorial pattern. They do not have a known genetic basis. They can be diagnosed prenatally with the maternal serum α-fetoprotein test, or by ultrasound. Amniotic fluid obtained from amniocentesis can be evaluated for acetylcholinesterase, which is more specific for a neural defect than α-fetoprotein, which can be elevated from other conditions.

Chapter 13

Antepartum Bleeding

Jane Fang

I. PLACENTA PREVIA

A. **Definition.** In placenta previa, the placenta is implanted in the lower segment of the uterus instead of up in the fundus, its location over or very near the internal os of the cervix (Figure 13-1). There are three types of placenta previa.

   1. **Total placenta previa.** The placenta completely covers the internal os.

   2. **Partial placenta previa.** The placenta partially covers the internal os.

   3. **Marginal placenta previa.** The edge of the placenta comes to the margin of the internal os.

B. **Incidence.** Placenta previa is an infrequent complication of pregnancy, occurring in **1 of 250 live births.**

C. **Etiology**

   1. **Maternal factors.** Although little is known about the cause of placenta previa, the following factors are thought to play a role:
      a. **Multiparity.** About 80% of all cases of placenta previa occur in multiparas.
      b. **Age older than 35 years.** Women older than 35 years, regardless of parity, are more likely to have placenta previa than women younger than 25 years of age.
      c. **No prior history.** A previous history of placenta previa is rare.

   2. **Factors related to abnormal placentation.** Placenta previa is fundamentally an abnormality in the implantation of the placenta. Several factors that contribute to this abnormal placentation are associated with advanced maternal age and parity.
      a. **Defective vascularization of the decidua** due to atrophic changes or inflammation
      b. **Scarring of the endometrium** due to repeated pregnancies
      c. **Vessel changes at the placental site** that decrease the blood supply to the endometrium and require a greater surface area for placental attachment to provide adequate maternal blood flow
      d. **Increased surface area of placental implantation** in multiple pregnancies (e.g., twins), which causes the lower portion of the placenta to approach the region of the internal os
      e. **Erythroblastosis fetalis,** which is often accompanied by a large placenta
      f. **Altered blood supply to the endometrium** and changes in the quality of the endometrium due to a previous incision in the lower uterine segment (e.g., myomectomy, cesarean section, or hysterotomy)

D. **Clinical presentation**

   1. **Painless vaginal bleeding** in the third trimester is the most characteristic sign of placenta previa.
      a. This bleeding can occur:
         (1) During rest or activity
         (2) Suddenly and without warning
         (3) After trauma, coitus, or a pelvic examination
      b. Bleeding usually occurs for the first time early in the third trimester when the lower uterine segment begins to change, causing the cervix to efface and dilate. Bleeding is caused by the tearing of the placental attachments at or near the internal os as the cervix changes. The bleeding continues because the stretched fibers

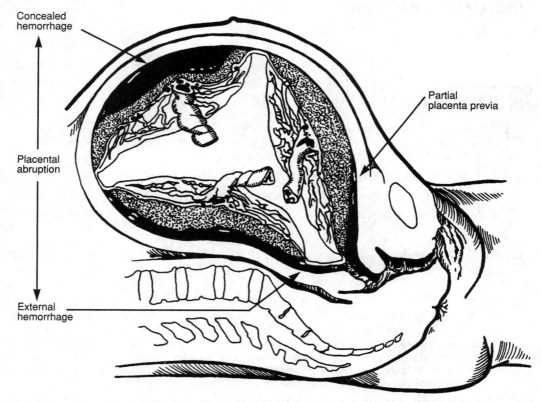

FIGURE 13-1. Hemorrhage from premature placental separation. Extensive placental abruption but with the periphery of the placenta and the membranes still adherent, resulting in completely concealed hemorrhage (*upper left*). Placental abruption with the placenta detached peripherally and with the membranes between the placenta and the cervical canal stripped from underlying decidua, allowing external hemorrhage (*lower*). Partial placenta previa with placental separation and external hemorrhage (*right*). (Reprinted with permission from Cunningham FG, MacDonald PC, Gant NF: *Williams Obstetrics,* 18th ed. East Norwalk, Connecticut, Appleton & Lange, 1989, p 702.)

of the lower uterine segment are unable to contract and compress the torn vessels.

2. **Maternal blood loss** and **fetal morbidity** are problems encountered with placenta previa.
   a. Pelvic examination can increase maternal bleeding if the diagnosis of placenta previa is not suspected. Maternal shock can result from acute blood loss.
   b. Maternal blood loss can result in fetal morbidity and mortality.
   c. **Preterm delivery** may be necessary because of maternal bleeding. In this case, the infant may experience the complications of prematurity.

E. **Diagnosis.** Placenta previa always should be suspected in the presence of vaginal bleeding in the third trimester. Women suspected of having placenta previa should undergo ultrasound examination for placental location.

1. **Suggestive findings.** The index of suspicion is heightened if any of the following clinical findings accompany vaginal bleeding:
   a. Malposition of the fetus (breech or transverse lie)
   b. Multiple gestation
   c. Multiparity or advanced maternal age

2. Placenta previa may be diagnosed at any time by **ultrasound scanning,** which is 95% accurate

3. **Definitive diagnosis of a marginal placenta previa** is made by passing a finger through the cervix and palpating the placenta or the edge of the placenta. This procedure can precipitate hemorrhage and therefore should not be undertaken unless:
   a. Delivery is contemplated at the time of the examination.
   b. The examination is performed in the delivery room with the patient prepared for a cesarean section, meaning that blood is crossmatched and anesthesia is available (i.e., the double set-up examination).
   c. The pregnancy is at or near term without ongoing bleeding.

F. Management

1. **Expectant management.** Watchful waiting is justifiable if the fetus is remote from term (i.e., before 37 weeks) and can benefit from further intrauterine development. However, an expectant attitude is appropriate only if labor has not begun, the fetus is stable, and the bleeding is not severe. Expectant therapy should proceed in the following steps:
   a. Hospitalization
   b. Careful speculum examination to rule out local lesions of the cervix and vagina
   c. Careful evaluation of the fetal monitoring strip
   d. Placental localization and determination of the type of placenta previa
   e. Close observation either in the hospital or at home; in the latter case, with careful instructions to restrict activity, to refrain from sexual intercourse, and to return to the hospital if bleeding recurs

2. **Delivery.** Decisions concerning delivery are based on the gestational age of the fetus and the amount of maternal bleeding. Delivery is accomplished by **cesarean section** with the following guidelines.
   a. **Elective.** The delivery is performed electively when the fetus weighs more than 2500 g or the gestational age is at least 37 weeks as determined by ultrasound, or the amniotic fluid lecithin to sphingomyelin ratio demonstrates fetal lung maturity, or the presence of phosphatidylglycerol.
   b. **Acute.** The delivery is performed acutely when the amount of bleeding presents a threat to the mother, regardless of fetal size or gestational age.

G. Maternal complications

1. **Severe postpartum hemorrhage** can occur because the site of placental implantation is in the lower uterine segment, which has diminished muscle content; thus, muscle contraction to control bleeding may be less effective.

2. **Placenta accreta** (the growth of placental tissue into the myometrium) may appear in patients with placenta previa because the endometrium is thinner in the lower uterine segment and cannot control the invasive properties of the trophoblast.

3. **Renal damage (acute tubular necrosis)** or **pituitary necrosis (Sheehan's syndrome)** may result from excessive blood loss and prolonged hypotension.

II. **ABRUPTIO PLACENTAE**

A. **Definition.** In abruptio placentae, or **placental abruption,** the normally implanted placenta (not a placenta previa) prematurely separates from the uterus before the delivery of the fetus (see Figure 13-1). The hemorrhage involved in placental abruption includes:

1. **Vaginal hemorrhage**

2. **Concealed hemorrhage.** Less frequently, bleeding occurs between the placenta and the uterus, with the periphery of the placenta and the membranes still adherent to the uterus. The blood is trapped behind the placenta and does not escape. This is diagnosed ultrasonographically.

B. **Incidence.** Placental abruption occurs in approximately **1 of 120 births.**

C. **Etiology.** The pathophysiology of abruptio placenta involves the spontaneous rupture of blood vessels at the placental bed, the inability of the uterus to contract and thus close off torn vessels, and the formation of a retroplacental clot.

1. **Maternal hypertension** has been associated with many cases of placental abruption. These include pregnancy-induced hypertension and chronic hypertension.

2. **Cocaine use** is associated with vasoconstriction of the placental vasculature and abruption.

3. **Less frequent associated conditions** include:
   a. Maternal abdominal **trauma**
   b. **Sudden decompression of the uterus,** with either rupture of membranes in the scenario of polyhydramnios, or the delivery of the first infant in a twin gestation, which leads to a shearing effect on the placenta as the uterus contracts
   c. **Cigarette smoking**
   d. **Uterine leiomyomata,** especially when the placenta is implanted above the fibroid
   e. **Previous history of abruption**

D. **Clinical presentation.** The clinical signs of placental abruption vary with the type and degree of placental detachment. **Peripheral detachment** and bleeding are usually less severe than **central detachment** with concealed bleeding. The designation of mild, moderate, or severe depends on both maternal and fetal conditions.

E. **Diagnosis**

1. Placental abruption is basically a clinical diagnosis that depends on **signs and symptoms** and a **high index of suspicion.**

2. **Fetal monitoring** may reveal a loss of variability or late decelerations. The **contraction monitor** may show coupled contractions with no return of uterine relaxation to baseline resting tone, and an increased frequency of contractions.

3. **Premature uterine contractions that cannot be controlled with tocolytic agents** may suggest a small or chronic abruption.

4. The demonstration of a **retroplacental clot** by ultrasound scan may help in making the diagnosis of placental abruption.

5. **Clotting studies** may reveal thrombocytopenia, hypofibrinogenemia, and elevated fibrin split products.

F. **Management.** The course of action depends on the condition of the mother and fetus and on the estimated degree of placental abruption. No matter what clinical course is followed, either **hypovolemia** or **disseminated intravascular coagulation (DIC) secondary to blood loss** can develop quickly. The patient requires adequate replacement of intravenous fluids, blood, and blood products.

1. **Immediate delivery is not necessary if the fetal monitor tracing is reassuring,** as in the case of mild placental abruption. However, the fetus requires continuous monitoring. Cesarean section is indicated whenever the monitoring is nonreassuring, or when maternal hemorrhage becomes a factor.

2. **Rapid delivery is necessary if the fetal monitor tracing is nonreassuring;** delivery by cesarean section is necessary unless vaginal delivery is imminent.

3. **Vaginal delivery is the preferred method if the fetus is dead** unless the hemorrhage is so brisk that it cannot be controlled by blood replacement. Amniotomy and oxytocin are helpful in hastening the vaginal delivery of a dead fetus.

G. **Complications**

1. **Hemorrhagic shock** from blood loss can occur with either concealed or external bleeding.

2. **Consumption coagulopathy (i.e., DIC)**
   a. **Diagnosis.** This bleeding diathesis occurs in 30% of cases of severe placental abruption with fetal demise. Abnormal laboratory values include thrombocytopenia, hypofibrinogenemia, abnormal clot formation, and elevated fibrin split products.
   b. **Treatment.** Consumption coagulopathy is treated with:
      (1) Intravenous fluid support
      (2) Replacement of blood loss
      (3) Fibrinogen and factor replacement when hypofibrinogenemia is severe and surgery is contemplated
      (4) Prompt termination of the pregnancy
      (5) Avoidance of the use of heparin

3. **Renal failure** in the form of acute tubular necrosis and cortical necrosis is rare. Renal failure in severe abruption is caused by intrarenal vasospasm as the consequence of massive hemorrhage and hypovolemia.

4. **Couvelaire uterus** is caused by widespread extravasation of blood into the uterine musculature and beneath the serosa of the uterus. These myometrial hematomas seldom interfere with uterine contractions and respond well to intravenous oxytocin. A Couvelaire uterus is not an indication for a hysterectomy.

III. OTHER CAUSES OF THIRD-TRIMESTER BLEEDING

A. Obstetric

1. **Bloody show** usually has an admixture of mucus and is associated with labor.

2. **Ruptured vasa previa** is a very rare but serious cause because the fetus can bleed to death; this condition should be considered when fetal distress accompanies **painless vaginal bleeding (no uterine contractions).**
   a. **Cause.** Ruptured vasa previa is caused by the rupture of a placental vessel, which allows the fetus to lose blood.
   b. **Diagnosis.** Fetal (nucleated) red blood cells can be identified by obtaining a glass slide smear of the blood and staining it with Wright's stain (Apt test).

3. **Ruptured uterus** must be considered when the mother has a history of previous uterine surgery (i.e., cesarean section or myomectomy) or if fetal parts are palpable abdominally.

B. Nonobstetric. Local factors in the vagina and on the cervix can cause bleeding. Visual inspection can often preclude an unnecessary cesarean section. These local causes of bleeding include:

1. **Vaginal lacerations**

2. **Erosions, polyps, or malignant lesions of the cervix**

3. **Genital condyloma**

■STUDY QUESTIONS

DIRECTIONS: Each of the numbered items or incomplete statements in this section is followed by answers or by completions of the statement. Select the ONE lettered answer or completion that is BEST in each case.

1. A woman has just delivered with a complete placenta previa by cesarean section. She is taken to the recovery room, where she is noted to have significant postpartum bleeding. Which of the following conditions best explains this bleeding?

(A) Retained placental fragments
(B) Cervical laceration
(C) Lack of response to oxytocin
(D) Consumption coagulopathy
(E) Implantation in the lower uterine segment

2. A 24-year-old hypertensive patient, who is 37 weeks pregnant, arrives on the labor floor complaining of continuous abdominal pain. The monitoring strip reveals coupled contractions and decreased fetal heart rate variability. Initial management in this situation is

(A) cesarean section delivery
(B) intravenous heparin
(C) coagulation profile
(D) induction of labor
(E) subcutaneous terbutaline

3. A woman presents with painless vaginal bleeding at 37 weeks' gestation. The fetal heart rate is stable in the 150s. Which of the following is indicated?

(A) Nonstress test
(B) Induction of labor
(C) Ultrasound examination
(D) Rupture of membranes
(E) Digital examination of the cervix

4. At what point is a digital examination of the cervix indicated in suspected placenta previa?

(A) At 27 weeks' gestation at the time of hospital admission
(B) After the patient is admitted to the hospital and the bleeding has stopped
(C) In the third trimester when there is no vaginal bleeding, and the decision for delivery has been made
(D) Before localization of the placenta by ultrasound
(E) At 40 weeks' gestation when the patient presents in labor

5. A patient who is 36 weeks pregnant reports to labor and delivery complaining of vaginal bleeding, contractions, and a very tender abdomen. In this situation, which would be atypical?

(A) Maternal hypertension
(B) Uterine hyperstimulation
(C) Fetal heart rate decelerations
(D) Placenta accreta
(E) A history of abdominal trauma

ANSWERS AND EXPLANATIONS

1. The answer is E [I G 1]. A potential problem after delivery of a placenta previa is the reduced contraction capability of the lower uterine segment because muscle content has diminished. The implantation site is in that lower uterine segment, and the muscle contraction to control the bleeding can be less effective. There should be no retained placental fragments at a cesarean section with the open uterus routinely inspected. The cervix should not be lacerated in cesarean section delivery. The uterus can respond to oxytocin and still have this type of bleeding because the fundal portion of the uterus contracts well, whereas the lower segment does not because of its reduced muscle content. Consumption coagulopathy is associated with placental abruption, not placenta previa.

2. The answer is C [II C 1, G 2; Figure 13-1]. This hypertensive woman is at risk for placental abruption. Pain, contractions, and decreased fetal heart rate variability suggest a mild abruption. Because the worst complication of an abruption is a consumption coagulopathy, a coagulation profile soon after admission would help define the urgency of the situation. Because the patient is having contractions, she does not have to be induced. Immediate delivery with cesarean section is necessary only in the face of fetal compromise. Heparin is contraindicated with any abruption. Terbutaline, a tocolytic, should not be used with a suspected abruption at term.

3. The answer is C [I D, E]. The most important aspect of painless vaginal bleeding is its cause, which may be placenta previa; therefore, an ultrasound is immediately indicated

to evaluate placental location. Digital examination, rupture of the membranes, and induction of labor are contraindicated with the diagnosis of placenta previa, and can lead to excessive bleeding. The nonstress test is used as a measure of fetal well-being, and is not necessary when continuous fetal monitoring has been initiated.

4. The answer is C [I E 3 b]. Digital examination of the cervix in a suspected marginal placenta previa is done only when delivery of the infant is necessary or indicated. This examination is contraindicated remote from term (i.e., before 37 weeks' gestation). A digital examination could precipitate massive bleeding and the need for instant delivery. The digital examination is performed in an operating room set up for a cesarean section. If the digital examination precipitates vaginal bleeding or the placenta is palpated at the cervix, cesarean section is performed. If no bleeding occurs, or if the placenta is not palpable, the patient may undergo a trial for vaginal delivery.

5. The answer is D [II A, C]. The patient is most likely experiencing a placental abruption; the diagnosis of placental abruption is essentially a clinical one. A uterine hyperstimulation pattern is common with placental abruption. A maternal history of hypertension or abdominal trauma are risk factors for abruption. Because this condition results in uteroplacental insufficiency, signs of fetal distress are expected (i.e., fetal heart rate late decelerations). A placenta accreta usually is a complication of a placenta previa, and is usually not diagnosed until after delivery.

Chapter 14

Teratology

Matthew F. Rhoa

I. **INTRODUCTION.** Teratology is the study of **abnormal fetal development.** Major birth defects are found in approximately 3% of all deliveries. A teratogenic agent can be identified in less than 50% of the cases. A teratogenic agent is any chemical (drug), infection, physical condition, or deficiency that, on fetal exposure, can alter fetal morphology or subsequent function (Table 14-1). Teratogenicity appears to be related to genetic predisposition (both maternal and embryonic), the developmental stage of the fetus at the time of exposure, and the route and length of administration of the teratogen. Because any woman in her reproductive years may be pregnant, women should be warned of any teratogenic potential a drug may have.

A. **Genetic susceptibility.** Species differences in response to teratogens have been demonstrated. Human newborns exposed to the tranquilizer thalidomide in utero demonstrated major malformation of the arms (phocomelia), whereas laboratory animals (rats) showed no effect at similar doses. Animal studies, although helpful, do not always reliably predict the response in humans.

B. **Developmental stage at time of exposure** (Figure 14-1). Susceptibility of the conceptus to teratogenic agents depends on the developmental stage at the time of exposure.

  1. Resistant period. From day 0 to day 11 of gestation (postovulation), the fetus exhibits the "all or none" phenomenon with regard to major anomalies—that is, it will either be killed by the insult or will survive unaffected. This is the period of predifferentiation when the aggregate of totipotential cells can recover from an injury and continue to multiply.

  2. Maximum susceptibility (embryonic period). From days 11 to 57 of gestation, the fetus is undergoing organ differentiation and, at this time, is most susceptible to the adverse effects of teratogens. The particular malformation depends on the time of exposure. After a certain time in organogenesis, it is thought that abnormal embryogenesis can no longer occur. For example, because the neural tube closes between days 22 and 28 postconception (5 weeks after the last menstrual period), a teratogen must be active before or during this period to initiate development of a neural tube defect (e.g., spina bifida or anencephaly).

  3. Lowered susceptibility (fetal period). After 57 days (8 weeks) of gestation, the organs have formed and are increasing in size. A teratogen at this stage may cause a reduction in cell size and number, which is manifested by:
    a. Growth retardation
    b. Reduction of organ size
    c. Functional derangements of organ systems

C. **The route and length of administration of a teratogen** alter the type and severity of the malformation produced. Abnormal developments increase in frequency and degree as the dosage increases. Agents may be less teratogenic if systemic blood levels are reduced by the route of administration (e.g., poor gastrointestinal antibiotic absorption may account for lower blood levels in pregnancy).

D. **Teratogenicity** of an agent or factor is defined by the following criteria:

  1. Presence of the agent during the critical period of development when the anomaly was likely to appear. Malformations are caused by intrinsic problems within the developing tissues at a specific time in organogenesis. Table 14-2 covers the timing and developmental pathology of certain common malformations.

Table 14-1. Causes of Congenital Anomalies

Cause	Percent of Total
Multifactorial or unknown	65%–75%
Genetic	20%–25%
Environmental	
Intrauterine infections	3%
Maternal metabolic disorders	4%
Environmental chemicals	4%
Drugs and medications	<1%
Ionizing radiation	1%–2%

2. **Production of the anomaly in experimental animals when the agent administered during a stage of organogenesis similar to that of humans.** Teratogenicity may not become apparent for several years; for example, in utero exposure to diethylstilbestrol is known to cause genital tract abnormalities, such as adenosis and carcinoma, but these abnormalities may not become apparent until the reproductive years.

3. **The ability of the agent to act on the embryo or fetus either directly or indirectly through the placenta.** For example, heparin is not teratogenic because, unlike warfarin, it cannot cross the placenta because of its large molecular weight.

E. **Structural defects** have been categorized into three groups, as shown in Figure 14-2.

1. **Malformations** are morphologic defects of an organ or other part of the body resulting from an abnormality in the process of development in the first trimester. This results

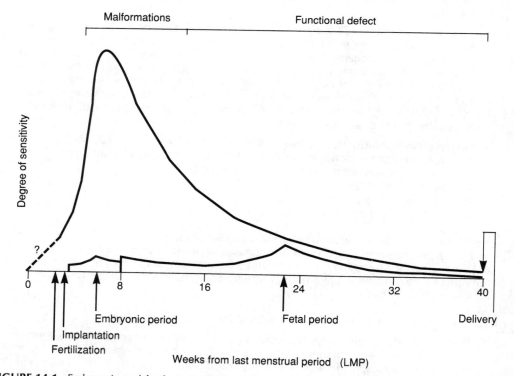

FIGURE 14-1. Embryonic and fetal sensitivity to environmental influences as a function of developmental stage. (Reprinted with permission from Creasy RK, Resnik R: *Maternal–Fetal Medicine: Principles and Practice.* Philadelphia, WB Saunders, 1984, p 95.)

Table 14-2. Relative Timing and Developmental Pathology of Certain Malformations

Tissue	Malformation	Defect	Timing of Cause	Additional Information
Central nervous system	Holoprosencephaly	Prechordal mesoderm	23 days	Associated facial defects
	Anencephaly	Closure of anterior neural tube	26 days	Subsequent degeneration of forebrain
	Meningomyelocele	Closure in portion of posterior neural tube	28 days	80% lumbosacral
Face	Cleft lip	Closure of lip	36 days	42% associated with cleft palate
	Branchial sinus or cyst	Resolution of branchial cleft	8 weeks	Preauricular and along line anterior to sternocleidomastoid
	Robin sequence	Early mandibular hypoplasia	9 weeks	U-shaped posterior cleft palate
	Cleft maxillary palate	Fusion of maxillary palatal shelves	10 weeks	
Neck	Esophageal atresia and tracheoesophageal fistula	Lateral septation of foregut into trachea and foregut	30 days	
	Posterior nuchal cystic hygroma	Lymphaticovenous communication	40 days	Common in XO Turner's syndrome
Abdomen	Rectal atresia with fistula	Lateral septation of cloaca into rectum and urogenital sinus	6 weeks	
	Diaphragmatic hernia	Closure of pleuroperitoneal canal	6 weeks	
	Duodenal atresia	Recanalization of duodenum	7–8 weeks	
	Malrotation of gut	Rotation of intestinal loop so that cecum lies to right	10 weeks	Associated incomplete or aberrant mesenteric attachments
	Omphalocele	Return of midgut from yolk sac to abdomen	10 weeks	
	Meckel diverticulum	Obliteration of vitelline duct	10 weeks	May contain gastric or pancreatic tissue
Genitourinary system	Extroversion of bladder	Migration of infraumbilical mesenchyme	30 days	Associated müllerian and wolffian duct defects
	Urethral obstruction sequence	Usually prostatic urethra valves	9 weeks	More common in males
	Bicornuate uterus	Fusion of lower portion of müllerian ducts	10 weeks	
	Hypospadias	Fusion of urethral folds (labia minora)	12 weeks	
	Cryptorchidism	Descent of testicle into scrotum	7–9 months	
Heart	D-transposition of great vessels	Directional development of bulbus cordis septum	34 days	
	Ventricular septal defect	Closure of ventricular septum	6 weeks	
	Patent ductus arteriosus	Closure of ductus arteriosus	9–10 months	
Limb	Aplasia of radius	Genesis of radial bone	38 days	Often accompanied by other defects of radial side of distal limb
	Severe syndactyly	Separation of digital rays	6 weeks	

Reprinted with permission from Graham JM: Clinical approach to human structural defects. *Semin Perinatol* 15(suppl):5, 1991.

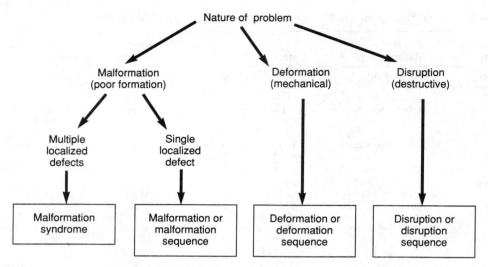

FIGURE 14-2. Categories of structural defects. (Adapted from Graham JM, Jr: *Smith's Recognizable Patterns of Human Deformation.* Philadelphia, WB Saunders, 1988, p 4.)

in incomplete or aberrant morphogenesis. An example of this is ventricular septal defect.

2. **Deformations** are abnormal forms, shapes, or positions of a body part caused by constraint within the uterus, usually occurring in the second or third trimester. An example is club feet from oligohydramnios.

3. **Disruptions** are defects from interference with a normally developing organ system, usually occurring later in gestation (i.e., in the second or third trimester, after organogenesis). An example is amniotic band syndrome.

II. TERATOGENIC AGENTS

A. **Ionizing radiation**

1. **Acute high dose (over 250 rads).** The dose of radiation as well as the gestational age during exposure are predictive of the adverse neonatal effects: microcephaly, mental retardation, and growth retardation. For example, the in utero victims of the atomic explosions in Hiroshima and Nagasaki have suffered from both birth defects and leukemia. However, follow-up studies have shown that the largest number of children with these adverse effects were those exposed before 15 weeks' gestation, during the period of organogenesis, whereas most of the children exposed during the third trimester had growth retardation but normal intelligence.

   a. **Time of exposure.** Fetal effects depend on the gestational age (postovulation) at the time of exposure.

   (1) At 2 to 4 weeks, either the fetus is normal or a spontaneous abortion occurs.

   (2) At 4 to 12 weeks, the fetus may have microcephaly, mental retardation, cataracts, growth retardation, or microphthalmia.

   (3) At 12 to 16 weeks, there is mental retardation or growth retardation.

   (4) After 20 weeks, the effects are the same as with postnatal exposure:

   (a) Hair loss

   (b) Skin lesions

   (c) Bone marrow suppression

Table 14-3. Dose to the Uterus and Embryo for Common Radiologic Procedures

Study	View	Dose*/View (mrad)	Films/Study†	Dose/Study (mrad)
Skull‡	AP, PA	<0.01		
	Lat	<0.01	4.1	<0.05
Chest	AP, PA‡	0.01–0.05		
	Lat‖	0.01–0.03	1.5	0.02–0.07
Mammogram‖	CC	0.1–0.5		
	Lat	3–5	4.0	7–20
Lumbar spine	AP§ (7″ × 17″)	30–58		
	(14″ × 17″)	33–65		
	Lat‖	11–32	2.9	51–126
Lumbrosacral spine	AP‡	92–187		
	PA‖	40–97		
	Lat‖	12–33	3.4	168–359
Abdomen	AP‡	80–163		
	PA‖	23–55		
	Lat‖	29–82	1.7	122–245
Intravenous pyelogram†	AP	130–264		
	PA	43–104		
	Lat	13–37	5.5	686–1398
Retrograde pyelogram	AP§	109–220	1.0	
Hip† (single)	AP	72–140		
	Lat	18–51	2.0	103–213

AP = anterior–posterior; *CC* = cranial–caudal; *Lat* = lateral; *PA* = posterior–anterior. Reprinted with permission from Twickler DM, Clarke G, Cunningham FG: Diagnostic imaging in pregnancy. *Williams Obstetrics,* 18th ed, suppl 18, June/July 1992, p 2. Edited by Cunningham FG, MacDonald PC, Gant NF. Norwalk, CT, Appleton & Lange, 1989.

* Calculated for x-ray beams with half-value layers ranging from 2 to 4 mm Al equivalent. Calculated using the methodology of Rosenstein M: Handbook of selected tissue doses for projections common in diagnostic radiology. Rockville, MD, Department of Health and Human Services, Food and Drug Administration. DHHS pub no (FDA) 89-8031, 1988.

† Based on data and methods reported by Laws PW, Rosenstein M: A somatic index for diagnostic radiology. *Health Phys* 35: 629, 1978.

‡ Entrance exposure data from Conway BJ: Nationwide evaluation of x-ray trends: Tabulation and graphical summary of surveys 1984 through 1987. Frankfort, KY, Conference of Radiation Control Program Directors, Inc. 1989.

§ Based on Nationwide Evaluation of X-ray Trends (NEXT) data reported in National Council on Radiation Protection and Measurements: Exposure of the US population from diagnostic medical radiation. Bethesda, MD, National Council on Radiation Protection, report no 100, p 26, 1989.

‖ Authors' estimates based on compilation of above data.

b. Dose effect

   (1) After exposure to less than 5 rads, and probably less than 10 rads, an adverse fetal outcome is unlikely to result.

   (2) After exposure to 10 to 25 rads, there may be some adverse fetal effects.

   (3) After exposure to over 25 rads, classic fetal effects, including growth retardation, structural malformations, and fetal resorption, may be detected. At this level of exposure, elective abortion should be offered as an option.

2. Chronic low dose

   a. In diagnostic radiation, the dose to the conceptus should be calculated by the hospital's radiation biologist (Table 14-3). Such a dose rarely adds up to significant exposure, even if several x-ray studies are performed. Interpretation of the fetal effects should be based on the criteria stated in II A 1 b (1)–(3).

   b. Risks of teratogenicity

   (1) The mutagenic effects of radiation, if present, have proven to be very small. The estimated risk of leukemia for children exposed in utero to radiation during maternal x-ray pelvimetry increases from 1 in 3000 among unexposed children to 1 in 2000.

       (2) The results of several studies provide no conclusive evidence linking preconception low-dose radiation exposure with an increased risk of delivering an infant with a chromosomal abnormality.

  3. Radioactive iodine. Radiation exposure from radioisotopes administered internally for organ visualization is roughly equal to that of x-ray procedures; however, after the tenth week of gestation, fetal thyroid development can be retarded in addition to any adverse effects of radiation. Iodine-containing cough preparations, antiseptic solutions, or x-ray adjuncts should be avoided throughout pregnancy.

B. **Drugs and medications.** In the United States, surveys show that 45% to 95% of pregnant women ingest either over-the-counter or prescription drugs other than iron and vitamins during their pregnancy. Many are taken before a woman realizes that she is pregnant, or without the advice of a physician. The issue of whether a medication is harmful to the fetus is raised in most pregnancies.

  1. Congenital malformation. Roughly 3% to 5% of newborns have congenital malformations caused by a host of environmental and genetic factors, most of which are unable to be identified. Drugs and medications comprise less than 1% of these factors (see Table 14-1).

  2. Access to the fetoplacental unit is critical in the causation of developmental anomalies. Factors affecting access of the drug or medication to the fetus include:
    a. Maternal absorption
    b. Drug metabolism
    c. Protein binding and storage
    d. Molecular size (molecules with a molecular weight over 1000 do not cross the placenta easily)
    e. Electrical charge
    f. Lipid solubility

  3. Animal research is helpful in identifying teratogenic potential, but results may be misleading because of species variation. The most striking example is the thalidomide debacle, in which exposure failed to produce limb defects in the animals tested (mice and rats) but caused severe limb reduction defects in humans, monkeys, and rabbits. Of the 1600 drugs that have been tested in animals, about one half cause congenital anomalies; however, there are only 30 documented human teratogens.

  4. Risk factors for adverse fetal effects have been assigned to all drugs based on the teratogenic risk that the drug poses to the fetus. The Food and Drug Administration has proposed the following outline, which is generally accepted by manufacturers and authors.
    a. Category A. Controlled studies fail to demonstrate a risk to the fetus (e.g., prenatal vitamins).
    b. Category B. Animal studies have not demonstrated a fetal risk, but there are no controlled studies in pregnant women. Also, in this category, there are drugs that may have shown an adverse effect in animals that was not reproduced in human subjects (e.g., penicillins, digoxin, epinephrine, and terbutaline).
    c. Category C. Animal studies have shown either teratogenic or embryocidal effects on the fetus, but there have been no human studies. These drugs should be administered only when their benefit outweighs the potential fetal harm (e.g., furosemide, quinidine, verapamil, and β-blockers).
    d. Category D. There is evidence of fetal risk in humans. The benefit may outweigh the fetal risk in certain extenuating circumstances (e.g., phenytoin).
    e. Category X. Studies in animals or humans have demonstrated clear fetal risk. The drugs in this category are contraindicated in women who are or may become pregnant (e.g., isotretinoin).

  5. Known teratogenic drugs. There is a surprisingly short list of proven teratogens. Certain commonly used agents should be avoided even while a patient is trying to conceive. These include the vitamin A isomer isotretinoin or doses of vitamin A over 8000 IU daily, alcohol, caffeine, and some of the sex steroids. The live-virus vaccines, such as rubella, should never be prescribed if a patient is possibly pregnant or planning to conceive within 3 months. However, if the aforementioned drugs are inadvertently given, the outcome is still usually favorable. The most common drugs and environmental chemicals known to cause congenital anomalies are listed in Table 14-4.

6. **A dose threshold** is a theoretic dose for each teratogen below which no adverse effects have been noted.

7. **"Recreational" drugs.** Because most recreational drugs are taken with other agents, such as alcohol or tranquilizers, the precise effect is difficult to ascertain. Listed below are commonly used drugs and their potential effects.
   a. **Alcohol.** Consumption of alcohol in pregnancy is the most common known teratogenic cause of mental retardation. Both abortion and stillbirth are increased in heavy drinkers. The **fetal alcohol syndrome,** which manifests as mental retardation, growth retardation, abnormal facies, ocular and joint anomalies, and cardiac defects, has been associated with the ingestion of 1 oz or more of absolute alcohol per day.
      (1) **The threshold dose of alcohol** at which point congenital anomalies are induced is unknown, so alcohol consumption in pregnancy can never be regarded as "safe."
      (2) **Early exposure.** The critical period for facial dysmorphology has been found to be around the time of conception.
      (3) **Late exposure.** Exposure late in gestation or in small quantities may result in isolated effects, such as learning or behavioral disorders.
      (4) **Heavy alcohol consumption** (over 3 oz of absolute alcohol or six drinks daily) is associated with some of the features of the fetal alcohol syndrome or the full-blown syndrome, consisting of:
         (a) **Prenatal or postnatal growth retardation.** Growth retardation is usually prenatal in onset, but postnatal catch-up generally does not occur. It is manifested by decreased birth weight, length, and head circumference.
         (b) **Central nervous system (CNS) involvement** includes small brain size and brain malformations. Functional deficits, such as moderate mental retardation, delayed motor development, poor coordination, tremulousness, hyperactivity, and poor attention spans, have been noted.
         (c) **Characteristic facial dysmorphology** includes a shortened palpebral fissure (observed in over 90% of affected children), short, upturned nose, hypoplastic maxilla, and a thinned upper lip. One study linked craniofacial abnormalities with prenatal alcohol exposure in a dose–response manner.
      (5) **Risk of the fetal alcohol syndrome.** A large number of children whose mothers drank moderately or heavily during pregnancy may exhibit features of prenatal alcohol exposure, such as developmental delay, but not the full-blown syndrome.
         (a) About 30% of children born to chronic alcoholic women will have the fetal alcohol syndrome.
         (b) The risk of major or minor congenital anomalies in infants of mothers who ingest excessive amounts of alcohol but do not meet the criteria for chronic alcoholism is around 32%.
         (c) Intrauterine fetal growth retardation is increased 2.7 times in pregnant women who drink excessively.
   b. **Marijuana.** There is no evidence that smoking marijuana is teratogenic, although the adverse effects of smoking in pregnancy should not be overlooked. Maternal smoking level correlates with:
      (1) Increased perinatal mortality
      (2) Preterm delivery
      (3) Premature rupture of the membranes
      (4) Bleeding during pregnancy
   c. **Heroin** has not been shown to cause birth defects, but the drugs that are often taken with heroin are associated with congenital anomalies. The principal adverse fetal effect in heroin addicts is **severe neonatal withdrawal,** causing death in 3%

Table 14-4. Drugs and Environmental Chemicals that Cause Congenital Defects

Substances	Defects
Alcohol	The principal features of the fetal alcohol syndrome, including prenatal-onset growth deficiency, developmental delay, short palpebral fissures, a long philtrum with a thin upper lip, multiple joint anomalies, and cardiac defects
Androgenic hormones	
Testosterone	Masculinization of the female fetus
Progestins	Masculinization of the female fetus (clitorimegaly), genital deformities of male (hypospadias) and female (fusion of the labia majora) fetuses, and cardiac defects
Cancer chemotherapeutic agents	
Aminopterin and methyl aminopterin (folate antagonists)	Small stature; abnormal cranial ossification, leading to a malformed head, hypoplastic orbital ridges, ocular hypertelorism, small, low-set ears, and micrognathia; cleft or arched palate; hydrocephaly; and myelomeningoceles
Busulfan (alkylating agents)	Cleft palate and eye defects, hydronephrosis, growth retardation, and unilateral renal agenesis (one case)
Chlorambucil	Unilateral renal and ureteral agenesis (one case)
Cyclophosphamide	Absence of toes and flattening of nasal bridge
Diethylstilbestrol	Both anatomic and functional defects in females, including cervical hood, T-shaped uterus, hypoplastic uterus, ovulatory disorders, infertility, premature labor, and cervical incompetence
Diphenylhydantoin	The fetal hydantoin syndrome, including growth and mental retardation, microcephaly, ridged metopic suture, inner epicanthal folds, eyelid ptosis, depressed nasal bridge, nail hypoplasia, and hernia (occurs only in some cases); minor craniofacial abnormalities and digital anomalies, not the full-blown syndrome, in 30% of infants exposed to phenytoin in utero; and oral clefts and congenital heart defects in many infants exposed to anticonvulsants in utero
Isotretinoin	Central nervous system (CNS) defects, facial palsy, deafness, and congenital heart defects
Lead	Abortion from embryotoxicity, growth retardation, increased perinatal mortality, and developmental delay
Lithium	Cardiac defects, including Ebstein's anomaly and malformations of the great vessels
Organic mercury	Fetal neurologic damage including seizures, psychomotor retardation, cerebral palsy, blindness, and deafness
Polybrominated biphenyls	In rats, not teratogenic unless the dosage is high enough to cause maternal death (no good human studies)
Polychlorinated biphenyls	Intrauterine growth retardation, dark brown skin pigmentation, exophthalmos, gingival hyperplasia, skull calcification, low IQ, and neurobehavioral abnormalities
Streptomycin	Fetal ototoxicity due to eighth nerve damage
Tetracycline	Deciduous teeth that are yellow, abnormally susceptible to decay, and have enamel hypoplasia from exposure after fourth month (permanent teeth are unaffected)
Thalidomide	Limb reduction, ear and nasal anomalies, cardiac and lung defects, pyloric or duodenal stenosis, and gastrointestinal atresia
Thiourea compounds	Inhibited thyroid function
Trimethadione	The features of a fetal trimethadione syndrome, including prenatal onset growth delay; mental deficiency; cardiac septal defects; and typical facies, consisting of a short, upturned nose with a broad and low nasal bridge, prominent forehead, upslanted eyebrows, and a poorly developed overlapping helix of the external ear
Warfarin	A syndrome resembling the genetic disorder Conradi's syndrome, including a stippling of the uncalcified epiphyseal regions (chondrodysplasia punctata)—primarily the axial skeleton, proximal femurs, and calcane—and severe nasal hypoplasia from first-trimester exposure (between the sixth and ninth weeks) and probably CNS problems, including mental deficiency, seizures, microcephaly, and optic atrophy, from exposure in the middle and last trimesters
Valproic acid	Neural tube defects (primary risk, in 1%–2%), cleft lip, cardiovascular, urogenital, craniofacial, and skeletal defects

to 5% of neonates. Methadone is used to replace heroin, and, although it is not teratogenic, it is also associated with severe neonatal withdrawal, which is treated with paregoric, diazepam, or phenobarbital in the neonatal period.

 d. Phencyclidine (PCP), or "angel dust," is a hallucinogenic agent associated with facial abnormalities in a small percentage of exposed infants.

 e. Cocaine is rapidly becoming the most abused drug in pregnancy, second only to alcohol. One study showed an increased risk of congenital malformations, stillbirths, and low-birthweight infants in cocaine users. There is a clear causal relationship between cocaine use and placental abruption because of the drug's vasoconstrictive properties (see also Chapter 15).

8. Cancer chemotherapy. Although there is a high incidence of fetal loss, including spontaneous abortion and stillbirth, the incidence of congenital malformations, with the exception of those agents listed in Table 14-4, is surprisingly low.

 a. When cancer chemotherapy is administered during the first trimester of pregnancy, there are varied and unpredictable effects, ranging from severe deformity to no abnormality.

 b. After the period of organogenesis, there is no teratogenic risk from chemotherapy in pregnancy.

C. **Hyperthermia.** Studies suggest that sustained maternal hyperthermia [body temperature above 38.9°C (~102°F) between 4 and 14 weeks' gestation], rather than spiking fevers, is teratogenic. Malformations noted in infants of mothers who were febrile from infectious agents or who frequented saunas in the first trimester include the following:

1. Growth retardation

2. CNS defects, such as:
 a. Mental deficiency
 b. Microcephaly
 c. Hypotonia

3. Facial anomalies, including midfacial hypoplasia, cleft lip and palate, microphthalmia, micrognathia, and external ear anomalies

4. Minor limb anomalies, such as syndactyly

D. **Maternal medical disorders.** Women with medical disorders should be counseled about the teratogenic risks from the condition being treated as well as from the treatment. In some cases, the untreated medical disorder poses greater risks to the fetus than the teratogenic potential of the specific drug therapy.

1. Diabetes mellitus. Infants of insulin-dependent diabetic mothers have up to a 22% incidence of cardiac, renal, gastrointestinal, CNS, and skeletal malformations. Most of the malformations occur between the third and sixth week postconception and are increased if there is hyperglycemia during that stage of gestation.

 a. The **level of risk** may be estimated by obtaining a glycosylated hemoglobin (hemoglobin A1c) in the first trimester. **Levels greater than 8%** (depending on the laboratory) have been associated with a significantly increased risk.

 b. Two particular **malformations** found in infants of diabetic mothers are:
  (1) Caudal regression sequence with hypoplasia of the caudal spine and lower extremities
  (2) Congenital heart disease, most commonly ventricular septal defects

 c. Testing. Because neural tube defects occur 20 times more often in infants of diabetic mothers, maternal serum α-fetoprotein screening at 16 weeks' gestation should be done. An extensive anatomic survey by ultrasound at 18 to 22 weeks' gestation should identify most of the major anomalies (i.e., cardiac and spinal defects) in an affected fetus.

2. Phenylketonuria (PKU). This is a genetic disorder characterized by a deficiency of **phenylalanine hydroxylase,** a liver enzyme that catalyzes the conversion of phenylalanine to tyrosine. The resulting high levels of phenylalanine in maternal serum result in high levels in the fetus. A special diet low in phenylalanine beginning before concep-

tion can prevent the adverse effects (mental retardation) of this disorder. Children born to mothers with PKU who have neglected their special diets have the following risks:
  a. A 92% incidence of mental retardation
  b. A 73% incidence of microcephaly
  c. A 12% incidence of congenital heart disease
  d. A 40% incidence of low birth weight

3. **Virilizing tumors (arrhenoblastoma)** can have masculinizing effects on the mother and produce pseudohermaphroditic changes in the female fetus, including fusion of the labia and clitorimegaly.

4. **Epilepsy** is a classic example of a disease process and its treatment contributing to an increase in birth defects.
  a. Epileptics who take anticonvulsants throughout the pregnancy have a two- to three-fold increased rate of giving birth to malformed infants.
  b. Untreated epileptics are also at an increased risk of delivering infants with birth defects, perhaps because of hypoxia from seizures or from an unknown factor.

E. **Infections.** Exposure to viral infections during gestation has been recognized as a significant cause of birth defects. Most infants, if infected during the first trimester, suffer from a syndrome of congenital malformations and are small for gestational age.

1. **Rubella virus (German measles).** When rubella infections occur in the first month of pregnancy, there is a 50% chance of anomalous development. This chance falls to 22% in the second month and to 6% to 10% in the third to fourth month. The timing of infection is important. If infection occurs during week 6, than cataracts may form. Deafness occurs when infection takes place between weeks 7 and 8. If a mother is infected at the time of delivery, the newborn may contract pneumonitis or encephalitis. The congenital rubella syndrome includes the following:
  a. Neuropathologic changes
    (1) Microcephaly
    (2) Mental and motor retardation
    (3) Meningoencephalitis
  b. Cardiovascular lesions
    (1) Persistent patent ductus arteriosus
    (2) Pulmonary artery stenosis
    (3) Atrioventricular septal defects
  c. Ocular defects
    (1) Cataracts
    (2) Microphthalmia
    (3) Retinal changes
    (4) Blindness
  d. Inner ear problems, resulting in sensorineural deafness
  e. Symmetric intrauterine growth retardation

2. **Cytomegalovirus (CMV)** is a ubiquitous virus that infects 1% to 2% of all infants in utero. Between 1 in 5000 to 20,000 infants suffer severe problems that are recognizable at birth.
  a. The **risk of severe complications** is much higher for infants of mothers who had a primary infection in pregnancy compared to those who had a recurrent infection.
    (1) Seronegative mothers infected with primary CMV transmit the infection to the fetus in 30% to 40% of cases. Of those infected, 2% to 4% are severely symptomatic at birth.
    (2) Seropositive mothers who have a recurrent infection transmit the infection to the fetus in only 1% of cases, and 99% of these infants appear normal at birth. Later in life, these affected infants may suffer from delayed speech development and learning difficulties due to sensorineural hearing loss. A small group has chorioretinitis.
  b. A specific relation between time of exposure and subsequent deficit has not been demonstrated, although the most damage seems to occur early in pregnancy. Gestational age at the time of exposure does not appear to influence the rate of fetal infection. The neonatal effects of a fetal CMV infection include the following:

    (1) Microcephaly and hydrocephaly
    (2) Chorioretinitis
    (3) Hepatosplenomegaly
    (4) Cerebral calcification
    (5) Mental retardation
    (6) Heart block
    (7) Petechiae

3. **Herpes simplex virus hominis type 2 (HSV-2).** Although mucocutaneous herpetic infection is quite common, less than 1 in 7500 infants suffer from perinatal transmission of HSV-2. Fetal transmission occurs by hematogenous spread during a maternal viremia or by direct contact during passage through an infected birth canal, but congenital infection, causing fetal malformations, is rare. It is thought that fetal infection during the first trimester results in miscarriage. In a few cases, a syndrome was described that resembled other infants with viral infections during the first trimester, including the following fetal anomalies:
    a. Growth retardation
    b. Microcephaly
    c. Chorioretinitis
    d. Cerebral calcification
    e. Microphthalmia encephalitis

4. **Toxoplasmosis** is caused by a protozoan, *Toxoplasma gondii,* and may be transmitted from mother to fetus antepartum. Although infection is most common outside the United States (e.g., in Sweden), the incidence of congenital infection in the United States ranges from 1 to 6 cases per 1000 live births. About 30% of infected women transmit the disease to their unborn children. In a French population of 550 women who acquired toxoplasmosis during pregnancy, 61% of the neonates had evidence of congenital infection; of these neonates, 6% died, 5% had severe clinical illness, 9% had mild disease, and 41% had subclinical disease.
    a. **Fetal infection early in pregnancy** increases the severity of infection.
        (1) The pregnancy may result in:
            (a) Spontaneous abortion
            (b) Perinatal death
            (c) Severe congenital anomalies
            (d) Abnormal growth
            (e) Residual handicap
        (2) In severe disease, the characteristic triad of anomalies includes:
            (a) Chorioretinitis
            (b) Hydrocephaly or microcephaly
            (c) Cerebral calcification, resulting in psychomotor retardation
    b. **Transmission** to the fetus is **more likely later in pregnancy,** although the neonatal handicap is much more benign and, in fact, is often subclinical.

5. **Syphilis** (*Treponema pallidum*). The incidence of syphilis in pregnant women is increasing. The rise in congenital syphilis has paralleled the increase in primary and secondary syphilis in the adult. There are several hundred cases of congenital syphilis diagnosed each year; half of these infants are born to women with no prenatal care. *T. pallidum* appears to be able to cross the placenta at any time during pregnancy. Because of an immature immune system, the fetus is rarely infected before 16 to 18 weeks' gestation. Before this time, antibiotic therapy is highly successful.
    a. The incidence of congenital infection is inversely proportional to the duration of maternal infection and the degree of spirochetemia.
        (1) Recent or secondary infection in the mother confers the greatest risk of fetal infection. All infants born to women with primary and secondary infection are infected, but 50% are asymptomatic.
        (2) Only 40% of infants born to women with early latent disease are infected, and the incidence drops to 5% to 15% for late latent infection.
    b. In utero infection may result in:
        (1) Preterm delivery or miscarriage
        (2) Stillbirth

(3) Neonatal death in up to 50% of affected infants
(4) Congenital infection (asymptomatic or symptomatic), which, when symptomatic, can manifest as:
(a) Hepatosplenomegaly
(b) Joint swelling
(c) Skin rash
(d) Anemia
(e) Jaundice
(f) Snuffles
(g) Metaphyseal dystrophy
(h) Periostitis
(i) Cerebrospinal fluid changes
c. **Adequate antibiotic therapy** for the pregnant woman is generally thought to provide adequate therapy for the unborn child. However, several case reports have described congenitally infected infants born to mothers treated with **benzathene penicillin G.** The risk of treatment failure appears to be greater for women who are treated for secondary syphilis or who are in the last trimester of pregnancy.

6. **Varicella zoster virus (VZV),** which can take the form of chickenpox and, later, herpes zoster, is an uncommon virus, occurring in 1 to 7 of 10,000 pregnancies. The infection is much more severe in adults than in children, and pregnancy does not seem to alter this risk. Transplacental transmission of VZV is now well documented and occurs in about 24% of cases after maternal varicella in the last month of pregnancy and in 0% of cases of maternal zoster (see II E 6 c). The frequency of fetal infection in the first trimester is less than 5%.

a. Inconclusive reports have described an increased risk of leukemia in infants born with gestational varicella. There is also a description of chromosome breaks in the leukocytes of a child whose mother had varicella in pregnancy.
b. There are multiple cases of congenital malformations in the offspring of women who have chickenpox during the first 20 weeks of pregnancy. These include abnormalities of several organ systems.
(1) **Cutaneous**
(a) Cicatricial skin scarring with denuded skin and limb hypoplasia
(b) Vesicular rash (hemorrhagic rash) if infection occurs in the last 3 weeks of pregnancy
(2) **Musculoskeletal**
(a) Limb hypoplasia (unilateral), involving the arm, mandible, or hemithorax
(b) Rudimentary digits
(c) Club foot
(3) **Neurologic**
(a) Microcephaly
(b) Cortical and cerebellar atrophy
(c) Seizures
(d) Psychomotor retardation
(e) Focal brain calcifications
(f) Autonomic dysfunction, such as loss of bowel and bladder control, dysphagia, and Horner's syndrome
(g) Ocular abnormalities, such as microphthalmia, optic atrophy, cataracts, and chorioretinitis
(4) **Other**
(a) Symmetric intrauterine growth retardation
(b) Fever, vesicular rash, pneumonia, and widespread necrotic lesions of the viscera, leading to death, if infection occurs in the last 3 weeks of pregnancy
c. **Herpes zoster.** There is no good evidence proving that herpes zoster causes congenital anomalies. A few case reports have described microcephaly, microphthalmia, cataracts, and talipes equinovarus in infants born to mothers suffering from zoster during pregnancy, but these cases may represent chance occurrences.

7. **Mumps.** Mumps infection is not strictly teratogenic, but, after maternal exposure, neonates have been born with:
   a. Endocardial fibroelastosis
   b. Ear and eye malformations
   c. Urogenital abnormalities

8. **Enteroviruses (coxsackie B).** Serious or fatal illness (40%) in the fetus results from maternal exposure to coxsackie B virus. Surviving infants may exhibit the following:
   a. Cardiac malformations
   b. Hepatitis, pneumonitis, or pancreatitis
   c. Adrenal necrosis

■ STUDY QUESTIONS

DIRECTIONS: The numbered item or incomplete statement in this section is negatively phrased, as indicated by a capitalized word such as NOT, LEAST, or EXCEPT. Select the ONE lettered answer or completion that is BEST.

1. Which of the following is NOT a result of insults during the course of fetal development?

(A) Death
(B) Malformation
(C) Growth retardation
(D) Dizygotic twinning

DIRECTIONS: The set of matching questions in this section consists of a list of lettered options (some of which may be in figures) followed by several numbered items. For each numbered item, select the ONE lettered option that is most closely associated with it. To avoid spending too much time on matching sets with large numbers of options, it is generally advisable to begin each set by reading the list of options. Then, for each item in the set, try to generate the correct answer and locate it in the option list, rather than evaluating each option individually. Each lettered option may be selected once, more than once, or not at all.

Questions 2–5

Match each description listed below with the viral syndrome that is most appropriately described by it.

(A) Cytomegalovirus (CMV)
(B) Toxoplasmosis
(C) Varicella zoster virus (VZV)
(D) Syphilis
(E) Rubella virus

2. Causes birth defects when a mother is infected with primary infection versus recurrent infection

3. Only very rarely leads to congenital infection before 16 weeks' gestation

4. Has a 24% incidence of congenital infection when maternal infection occurs in the last month of pregnancy

5. Infects all infants born to women with recent infection

ANSWERS AND EXPLANATIONS

1. The answer is D [I A–D]. Dizygotic twins result from the mother's propensity for multiple ovulation, not from an insult. In utero exposure to a suspected teratogen can result in a wide range of effects. Depending on the stage of gestation, the effect of the teratogen may be minimal (no perceptible effect) or so serious as to result in death in utero. The fetus exposed before the 11th day of gestation, or the 25th day from the last menstrual period, may be either unaffected or killed by the insult. This is the period of predifferentiation. Malformations are most likely to occur during the embryonic period (11–57 days postconception), when the organ systems are forming and differentiating. For instance, congenital malformations found in infants of diabetic mothers can be pinpointed to the time of gestation in which they occurred. Caudal regression syndrome, a syndrome seen only in infants of diabetic mothers that consists of severe congenital malformations, including agenesis of the sacrum and lumbar spine and hypoplasia of the lower extremities, occurs in the third week postconception. Anencephaly and other defects of neural tube closure occur before the fourth week postconception. In the fifth and sixth weeks, the common cardiac defects—transposition of the great vessels and ventricular and atrial septal defects—commonly develop. In the second and third trimesters, after the organ systems have differentiated but are continuing to develop, exposure to a specific chemical or toxic environmental agent may produce growth retardation.

2–5. The answers are: 2-A [II E 2, 3], **3-D** [II E 5], **4-C** [II E 6], **5-D** [II E 5 a (1)]. Both cytomegalovirus (CMV) and *Herpesvirus hominis* are DNA viruses of the herpesvirus group, which may reinfect the same person. CMV is now recognized as the most common cause of intrauterine infection. It causes birth defects when a mother is infected with a primary infection versus a recurrent infection. Children born to women with acute infection have neurologic sequelae in a small percentage of cases, and these cases usually involve seronegative mothers who convert to seropositive during pregnancy rather than mothers who are seropositive before pregnancy and have a reactivation of the virus. The incidence of congenital syphilis has paralleled the increase in primary and secondary syphilis in the adult population. *Treponema pallidum,* the causative agent, appears to be able to cross the placenta at any time during pregnancy, but, because of its immature immune system, the fetus is rarely infected before 16 weeks' gestation. Recent or secondary infection confers the greatest risk of fetal infection. All infants born to women with primary and secondary infections are infected, although 50% are asymptomatic. Varicella zoster virus (VZV) [chickenpox] is an uncommon virus in pregnant women, occurring in 1 to 7 of 10,000 pregnancies. Transplacental transmission of VZV is now well documented, occurring in 24% of cases after infection in the last month of pregnancy. Congenital infection is very rare before 16 weeks' gestation (5%–10%, at most).

Chapter 15

Substance Abuse in Pregnancy
William W. Beck, Jr.

I. **INTRODUCTION.** Use of illicit substances in the general population has become so prevalent that the obstetrician and neonatologist are faced daily with the effects of these drugs on their patients. The incidence of reported drug use in pregnancy ranges from 0.4% to 27%, and this level of use is consistent regardless of race. Alcohol and cocaine have become the leading abused substances, with alcohol being the most common potentially teratogenic substance used in pregnancy. Although other substances are abused in pregnancy, these two substances are paradigmatic of how a significant social problem can affect obstetric practice.

II. **DEFINITION.** Drug consumption is divided into three stages of behavior: use, abuse, and dependence.

A. **Use** involves taking low, infrequent doses of illicit substances for experimentation or social reasons. Damaging consequences are rare or minor.

B. **Substance abuse** is the persistent or repeated use of a psychoactive substance for more than 1 month, despite the persistence or recurrence of adverse social, occupational, psychological, or physical effects.

C. **A dependence syndrome,** according to the *Diagnostic and Statistical Manual of Mental Disorders* (Third Edition—Revised) is present if **three or more of the following criteria** are met continuously for 1 month or repeatedly in a given year.

1. Abandonment of social, occupational, or recreational activities

2. Continued substance use despite knowledge of social, psychological, or physical problems exacerbated by drug use

3. Substance taken to relieve or avoid withdrawal symptoms

4. Withdrawal symptoms

5. Persistent desire or one or more unsuccessful attempts to control substance use

6. Substance taken in larger amounts or over a longer period than intended

7. Frequent intoxication or withdrawal symptoms when expected to fulfill obligations at work, school, or home, or when abuse is physically hazardous

8. A great deal of time spent in getting, taking, or recovering from the substance

III. **CLASSIFICATION OF PSYCHOACTIVE SUBSTANCES**

A. **Opiates**

1. **Examples** include heroin, morphine, methadone, and codeine.

2. **Effects** include euphoria, relaxation, mood elevation, drowsiness, and respiratory depression.

B. **Depressants and alcohol**

  1. Examples include barbiturates, methaqualone, and diazepam.

  2. Effects include euphoria, relaxation, mood elevation, drowsiness, mood volatility, respiratory depression, and impaired coordination.

C. **Stimulants**

  1. Examples include cocaine and amphetamine.

  2. Effects include euphoria, alertness, sense of well-being, suppression of fatigue and hunger, increased sexual arousal, increased pulse and blood pressure, tremor, insomnia, paranoia, psychosis, cardiac arrest, placental abruption, and fetal growth retardation.

D. **Hallucinogens**

  1. Examples include lysergic acid diethylamide (LSD), mescaline, and psilocybin.

  2. Effects include altered perception, detachment, increased blood pressure, tremor, impaired judgment, and panic.

E. **Phencyclidine (PCP) and related compounds**

  1. One **example** is ketamine hydrochloride. Street names include angel dust and crystal.

  2. Effects include detachment, mental numbness, distorted perception, anxiety, and impaired coordination.

F. **Cannabinoids**

  1. Examples include marijuana and hashish.

  2. Effects include euphoria, relaxation, altered perception, sexual arousal, increased appetite, disorientation, impaired judgment, incoordination, and paranoia.

IV. ALCOHOL USE IN PREGNANCY

A. Alcohol use is the leading cause of teratogenesis by drugs or environmental agents.

B. Women who drink during pregnancy are older, have higher rates of other illicit drug use, less education, and lower social status.

C. **Fetal alcohol syndrome**

  1. Prenatal and postnatal growth deficiency

  2. Mental retardation

  3. Behavioral disturbances

  4. Atypical facial appearance—short palpebral fissure, epicanthal folds, flat midface, hypoplastic philtrum

  5. Congenital heart defects

D. **Threshold of alcohol abuse**

  1. Fetal alcohol syndrome is seen in women who drink more than 3 ounces of alcohol per day (one drink, beer, or glass of wine contains a half ounce of alcohol).

  2. Moderate growth retardation, mild mental defects, and **behavioral abnormalities** have been associated with women who drink 1 to 2 ounces of alcohol per day.

V. **COCAINE USE IN PREGNANCY.** The rise in the use of cocaine among the general population has spawned a rise in use among pregnant women, thus making the maternal and fetal complications associated with cocaine use more common.

A. **Use in general population.** Cocaine use has increased among the general population because of the availability of inexpensive **"crack"** cocaine, a highly purified form of cocaine that is named for the cracking or popping sound made when the crystals are heated in a test tube. Cocaine can be smoked as crack, taken intranasally, or injected intravenously.

B. **Pharmacologic effects**

1. Cocaine produces **complex cardiovascular effects** that depend on an intact sympathetic nervous system and direct stimulation of the myocardium and vasculature.

2. Cocaine **interferes with dopamine and norepinephrine reuptake at the postsynaptic junction,** thereby increasing central nervous system (CNS) irritability.

3. This leads to **maternal and fetal vasoconstriction and tachycardia,** as well as **stimulation of uterine contractions.**

C. **Maternal complications**

1. **Neurologic**
   a. Seizures
   b. Rupture of intracranial aneurysm
   c. Postpartum intracerebral hemorrhage

2. **Cardiovascular**
   a. Myocardial infarction
   b. Hypertension
   c. Arrhythmias
   d. Rupture of the ascending aorta
   e. Sudden death

3. **Infectious**
   a. **Intravenous use** predisposes the patient to bacterial endocarditis, hepatitis, and human immunodeficiency virus exposure.
   b. **Sexually transmitted diseases,** such as gonorrhea, chlamydia, human papillomavirus, and syphilis, are common, frequently because of the exchange of sex for drugs or for the money to buy drugs.

4. **Obstetric**
   a. Possible increase in spontaneous abortions
   b. Increased incidence of preterm labor and delivery
   c. Intrauterine growth retardation
   d. Placental abruption
   e. Possible increased risk of intrauterine fetal demise
   f. Increased risk of fetal distress
   g. Congenital anomalies
      (1) Fetal microcephaly
      (2) Nonduodenal intestinal atresia–infarction
      (3) Limb reduction defects
      (4) Urinary tract anomalies
      (5) Perinatal cerebral infarctions
   h. Neonatal and infant behavioral disturbances

D. **Management**

1. **Detection**
   a. Consider drug abuse as a differential diagnosis in, and discuss it with, all patients.
   b. Educate patients about drug use and its effects on the mother and developing infant.

   c. Ask each patient directly about types of psychoactive substances used.
   d. Examine each patient for inflammation of nasal alae and intravenous injection sites—especially patients who are failing to keep prenatal appointments or who are showing signs of anemia, fetal growth retardation, or preterm labor.
   e. Consider **urine toxicology screening.** Although this should be used as a method of monitoring and instructing a pregnant woman about drug use, some states require that these results be reported to government authorities. Although many people advocate obtaining drug screens without a patient's consent, a patient–physician alliance can be best fostered through directly confronting the patient with the suspicion of drug abuse. At that point, the physician can impress on the patient the need to treat this problem in the interest of both herself and the developing infant. Urine screening can then be obtained by way of reasoned persuasion rather than through deception.

2. **Treatment**
   a. **Refer the patient to a chemical dependency treatment center.** Ideally, treatment center options should include individual and group counseling, intensive day treatment, and residential treatment. Optimally, residential treatment should include obstetric facilities.
   b. **Marshal the assistance of social services** to coordinate a plan of management, because a patient's hostile home and social environment (e.g., pervasive poverty, easy access to drugs, and positive opinion of the drug culture) can lead to conditions that compound complications caused by cocaine use (e.g., lack of prenatal care and poor nutrition). Dealing effectively with the patient's environment may determine the success or failure of any medical intervention.
   c. **Prevent and treat premature labor and intrauterine growth retardation** through education, nutritional counseling, ultrasound examinations, and biophysical testing. Choose magnesium sulfate rather than β-mimetics to treat preterm labor because magnesium sulfate does not have stimulating effects on the heart muscle.
   d. **Begin biophysical testing** no later than 32 weeks' gestation.
   e. With symptoms of **abdominal pain,** differentiate between placental abruption and bowel ischemia. Laboratory evaluations and fetal monitoring clarify the diagnosis and point to the best treatment option. Drug screening is essential.
   f. With **cocaine overdose,** control seizures, hyperthermia, and hypertension by reducing CNS irritability and sympathetic nervous system overactivity; also evaluate the cardiovascular system.
      (1) Obtain a urine toxicology screen, a complete blood count, and coagulation studies and measure cardiac and liver enzymes, electrolytes, and arterial blood gas.
      (2) Administer oxygen and consider intubation for intractable seizures.
      (3) Monitor urine output, vital signs, and fetal heart rate.
      (4) Use ice baths or cooling blankets to treat hyperthermia.
      (5) Treat seizures with magnesium sulfate or diazepam.
      (6) Administer propranolol (1 mg intravenously), sodium nitroprusside, or phentolamine to control hypertension and tachycardia.
   g. **Consider hospitalization for detoxification,** treatment of psychological disorders, and coordination of further therapy.
   h. Once **abstinence** has been achieved, perform periodic urine screens to monitor continued abstinence.

 VI. OTHER SUBSTANCES ABUSED IN PREGNANCY

   A. Marijuana

   1. Marijuana is the most commonly used illicit substance among pregnant women.

   2. There is no evidence that marijuana is associated with congenital anomalies in humans.

3. Maternal smoking level correlates with increased perinatal mortality, preterm delivery, premature rupture of membranes, and infants of lower birth weight.

B. Heroin

1. Heroin causes no increase in congenital anomalies.
2. Intrauterine growth retardation and perinatal death are increased.
3. Behavioral disturbances and mild developmental delay have been reported.
4. The poor nutritional status of many heroin addicts may be as important as the heroin use.

C. Methadone

1. Methadone causes no increase in congenital anomalies.
2. Methadone use is associated with low-birthweight infants.

STUDY QUESTIONS

DIRECTIONS: Each of the numbered items or incomplete statements in this section is followed by answers or by completions of the statement. Select the ONE lettered answer or completion that is BEST in each case.

1. Cocaine can be best described as which of the following types of drugs?

(A) A depressant causing euphoria, mood volatility, and impaired coordination
(B) A stimulant that increases the reuptake of dopamine and norepinephrine at the postsynaptic junction, thereby increasing central nervous system (CNS) irritability
(C) A narcotic leading to suppression of endogenous endorphins, resulting in mood elevation and euphoria
(D) A hallucinogen leading to altered perception, detachment, and increased blood pressure

2. A woman at 16 weeks' gestation presents to the labor and delivery suite with the progressive onset of dyspnea, fever of 104°F, and abdominal pain. On examination, you notice evidence of intravenous drug use. Evaluation of which of the following organ systems should be undertaken first?

(A) Urinary tract
(B) Musculoskeletal system
(C) Hematologic system
(D) Cardiovascular system
(E) Neurologic system

3. An obstetric patient at 30 weeks' gestation informs her physician that she has used cocaine regularly during the pregnancy. She goes on to state that she has stopped using this drug for a number of weeks. The physician should first

(A) obtain a urine toxicology screen and begin biophysical testing
(B) advise her of the risks of congenital anomalies and of the possible risks of preterm labor and placental abruption with continued use
(C) reassure the patient that because no harm has occurred, no further evaluation or treatment is necessary, provided that no drug use occurs during the remainder of her pregnancy
(D) inform the patient that you are obligated to report her actions to the state health agency
(E) inform the patient that the effects of cocaine on her developing fetus are now permanent, and that those effects will be recognized when the child is evaluated through the first few years of life

4. A patient admitted at 32 weeks' gestation with abdominal pain and uterine contractions should be evaluated for cocaine use to determine whether she is at risk for which of the following?

(A) Fetal distress
(B) Congenital anomalies
(C) Seizure activity
(D) Intrauterine fetal demise
(E) Adverse reaction to β-mimetics

5. Which of the following is the most teratogenic?

(A) Cocaine
(B) Alcohol
(C) Methadone
(D) Marijuana
(E) Heroin

DIRECTIONS: Each of the numbered items or incomplete statements in this section is negatively phrased, as indicated by a capitalized word such as NOT, LEAST, or EXCEPT. Select the ONE lettered answer or completion that is BEST in each case.

6. Which of the following criteria CANNOT be used to determine whether a patient manifests a substance dependence syndrome?

(A) Withdrawal symptoms
(B) Increasing the amount of psychoactive substances taken
(C) Frequent intoxication
(D) Social use of a psychoactive substance
(E) Withdrawal from social activities

7. Which of the following is NOT an opiate?

(A) Heroin
(B) Morphine
(C) Mescaline
(D) Methadone
(E) Codeine

8. Which of the following obstetric complications does NOT result directly from cocaine use?

(A) Respiratory distress syndrome
(B) Intrauterine growth retardation
(C) Intrauterine fetal demise
(D) Congenital anomalies
(E) Premature labor

ANSWERS AND EXPLANATIONS

1. The answer is B [III C 1, 2; V B 2]. Cocaine is a stimulant that blocks the reuptake of dopamine and norepinephrine at the postsynaptic junction. The increase in the concentration of neurotransmitters causes central nervous system (CNS) irritability and is also responsible for the vasoconstrictive effects of cocaine that have maternal and fetal consequences.

2. The answer is D [V D 2 f]. Although a patient such as this must be evaluated by a thorough examination of each organ system, an examination of her heart may reveal signs of valvular incompetence that point to the diagnosis of bacterial endocarditis. With physical examination revealing intravenous drug abuse, a febrile patient must always have this diagnosis considered and explored through physical examination, blood studies, blood cultures, and cardiologic evaluative procedures. Hospitalization with specific intravenous antibiotic treatment is essential to treating this patient.

3. The answer is B [V C–D]. A physician should inform the patient of the risks to her and the baby from continued cocaine use. Congenital anomalies have been noted, and a patient should be apprised of this. Along with this advice, an evaluative and therapeutic plan must be orchestrated by the obstetrician. A urine toxicology screen may be used during future visits to assess compliance with abstinence. During the visit at which the patient has revealed her cocaine use to the physician, urine toxicology screening is unnecessary. Reporting the patient to a state health agency is not the physician's first obligation, although this may be necessary, depending on regulations in the state in which the physician practices. Finally, there is much controversy as to the effects of cocaine on neurologic and behavioral development because of confounding sociologic and economic variables. Consequently, effects on later life are uncertain and their permanence questionable.

4. The answer is E [V D 2 c]. A physician faced with a patient in premature labor should always consider cocaine use if only to determine the proper tocolytic medication to use in the treatment of the preterm uterine contractions. Because the effects of β-mimetics would compound the cardiovascular effects of cocaine, magnesium sulfate should be used in patients suspected of having used cocaine recently (i.e., within the past 12–24 hours). This consideration completely justifies the use of urine toxicology screening on an emergency basis in a patient with preterm labor and suspected of using cocaine, because the proper treatment for premature labor depends on whether cocaine has been used.

5. The answer is B [IV A]. Alcohol is the leading cause of teratogenesis by drugs or environmental agents. Cocaine is associated with congenital anomalies, but not to the extent that alcohol is. Marijuana, heroin, and methadone have not been shown to have an increased congenital anomaly rate.

6. The answer is D [II A, C]. Many symptoms of increasing dependence on a substance to the detriment of other life activities are listed in the criteria of the *Diagnostic and Statistical Manual of Mental Disorders,* third edition, revised (DSM-III-R) for dependence syndrome. However, using an illicit substance socially without adverse consequences can simply be classified as drug use. Although this may lead to abuse and dependence, it is very likely that no adverse consequences will occur.

7. The answer is C [III A, D]. Mescaline is a hallucinogen, not an opiate. The major effects of opiates are euphoria, relaxation, and mood elevation, whereas hallucinogens cause altered perception and detachment.

8. The answer is A [V C 4 a–h]. Respiratory distress syndrome is not directly caused by cocaine use during pregnancy. Although prematurity is directly related to the incidence of respiratory distress syndrome, the pulmonary problem is a function of prematurity and not cocaine use. Cocaine use does not delay pulmonary maturation.

Chapter 16

Operative Obstetrics
Michelle Battistini

I. **CESAREAN BIRTH.** Cesarean section is delivery of a viable fetus through an abdominal incision (laparotomy) and uterine incision (hysterotomy). Cesarean section is the most important surgical procedure in obstetrics. It can be traced back to 700 B.C.E. Rome, when the procedure was first used to remove infants from women who died late in pregnancy; in 1610, the first cesarean section was performed on a living patient. The maternal mortality rate was high up to the end of the nineteenth century, most often because of hemorrhage and infection. However, advances in surgical and anesthetic techniques, safe blood transfusions, and the discovery of effective antibiotics have led to a dramatic decline in the mortality rate.

A. **Incidence.** The incidence of cesarean sections in the United States has continued to increase over the past 30 years. Cesarean section is now the most common operative procedure performed in many hospitals throughout the country.

1. In the United States, **approximately 24% of infants are delivered by cesarean birth,** compared to 5% in 1960 and 15% in 1970. Cesarean section incidence rates in most European countries are lower than in the United States, ranging from 5% to 7%. There are several reasons contributing to the dramatic increase in cesarean births during this time period.
   a. As procedure-related morbidity and mortality rates decreased with advances in anesthetic and operative techniques, the rate of primary cesarean sections increased in the following situations.
      (1) The **widespread use of electronic fetal monitoring** has led to an increased rate of cesarean section for fetal distress.
      (2) The **growing trend of delaying childbirth,** in this country, affects the population of women in labor in two ways. There is a higher proportion of nulliparous women giving birth; and nulliparity is associated with complications that increase cesarean section rates, such as dystocia and preeclampsia. The average maternal age is increased compared to 20 years ago; cesarean section rates increase with advancing age.
      (3) There is a more liberal use of **dystocia** as an indication, with a corresponding decline in the rate of forceps deliveries.
      (4) There is a steep and marked **decrease in the number of vaginal breech deliveries.**
   b. As the number of primary sections increased, previous cesarean section increased as an indication for a repeat cesarean section. Thirty-three percent of cesarean sections performed in the United States are repeat cesarean sections.

2. **Perinatal mortality.** There is little documentation that the increase in cesarean delivery rates is associated with a decline in perinatal mortality and morbidity. Although there was an initial decrease in perinatal mortality with increasing cesarean delivery rates, the perinatal mortality rate is not higher in European countries with lower cesarean birth rates. The major causes of perinatal morbidity and mortality continue to be low birth weight and congenital anomalies.

B. **Indications.** Compared to vaginal delivery, a properly performed cesarean section carries no increased risk for the fetus; however, the risk of maternal morbidity and mortality is higher. Cesarean birth is preferred when the benefits for the mother, fetus, or both outweigh the risk of the procedure for the mother. Cesarean delivery is performed when labor is contraindicated; labor cannot be successfully induced when delivery is indicated; dystocia or fetal characteristics contraindicate a vaginal delivery; or emergent circumstances arise and vaginal delivery is not imminent.

1. **Contraindications to labor**
   a. Placenta previa
   b. Vasa previa
   c. Previous classic cesarean section
   d. Previous myomectomy with entrance into the uterine cavity
   e. Previous uterine reconstruction
   f. Certain treatable fetal malformations (e.g., hydrocephalus, meningomyelocele)
   g. Malpresentations of the fetus
   h. Active genital herpes infection
   i. Previous cesarean section and patient refuses trial of labor

2. **Failed induction for maternal or fetal indications.** Disorders include but are not limited to the following examples.
   a. Preeclampsia, eclampsia, hypertensive disorders
   b. Intrauterine growth retardation
   c. Nonreassuring antenatal testing
   d. Diabetes mellitus
   e. Isoimmunization

3. **Dystocia**
   a. Cephalopelvic disproportion, failure to descend, arrest of descent or dilation
   b. Failure to progress in normal-size infant, usually due to fetal malposition or posture
   c. Failed forceps or vacuum extractor delivery

4. **Emergent conditions that warrant immediate delivery**
   a. Placental abruption with antepartum or intrapartum hemorrhage
   b. Umbilical cord prolapse
   c. Nonreassuring intrapartum fetal heart rate tracing
   d. Intrapartum fetal acidemia, intrapartum scalp pH less than 7.20
   e. Uterine rupture
   f. Impending maternal death

C. **Types of cesarean operations.** Cesarean operations are classified according to the **orientation (transverse or vertical)** and the **site of placement (lower segment or upper segment)** of the uterine incision.

1. **Low transverse (Kerr).** The low transverse uterine incision is the preferred incision and the one most frequently used today.
   a. The incision is made in the **noncontractile portion of the uterus,** minimizing chances of rupture or separation in subsequent pregnancies.
   b. The incision requires creation of a bladder flap and lies behind the peritoneal bladder reflection, allowing reperitonealization.
   c. Uterine closure is more easily accomplished because of the thin muscle wall of the lower segment.
   d. Potential blood loss is lowest with this type of incision.
   e. The disadvantage of this incision is potential extension into the uterine vessels laterally, and into the cervix and vagina inferiorly.

2. **Low vertical (Sellheim or Kronig).** The vertical incision begins in the noncontractile lower segment but almost always extends into the contractile upper segment.
   a. The risk of uterine rupture in subsequent pregnancies is increased when the upper segment of the uterus is entered.
   b. This incision also requires creation of a bladder flap and allows reperitonealization.
   c. Uterine closure is more difficult and blood loss is greater if the upper segment is involved.
   d. This incision is used when a transverse incision is not feasible.
      (1) The lower uterine segment may not be developed if labor has not occurred; the transverse incision may not provide enough room for delivery of the infant.

(2) Malpresentations of the term or premature infant may necessitate a vertical incision to allow more room for delivery of the infant.

(3) This incision is sometimes used when an anterior placenta previa is noted to facilitate delivery without cutting through the body of the placenta.

3. Classic incision (Sanger). The classic incision is a longitudinal incision in the anterior fundus. It is infrequently used today because of the significant risk of uterine rupture in subsequent pregnancies and higher complication rate.

a. The risk of uterine rupture is higher in subsequent pregnancies and can occur before labor.

b. Uterine closure is more difficult because of the thick muscular upper segment, and the potential for blood loss is greater.

c. This incision does not require bladder dissection, and reperitonealization is not performed; the potential for intraperitoneal adhesion formation is greater.

d. This incision is indicated in cases of invasive carcinoma of the cervix; when lesions occupy the lower segment of the uterus (myomas) and prohibit adequate uterine closure; and in most cases of transverse lie with the back down. It is the **simplest and quickest incision** to perform.

D. **Complications.** The reported incidence of morbidity varies but is significantly higher after cesarean birth compared to vaginal delivery. Common postoperative complications are as follows.

1. Endomyometritis. Postoperative infection is the most common complication after cesarean section.

a. The average incidence of endomyometritis is 34% to 40%, with a range of 5% to 85%.

b. Risk factors include lower socioeconomic status, prolonged labor, prolonged duration of ruptured membranes, and the number of vaginal examinations.

c. The incidence is reduced with the use of prophylactic antibiotics administered at the time of the procedure.

d. Infection is polymicrobial in nature, including the following organisms: aerobic streptococci, anaerobic gram-positive cocci, and aerobic and anaerobic gram-negative bacilli.

e. The incidence of serious complications, including sepsis, pelvic abscess, and septic thrombophlebitis, is less than 2% with the use of modern broad-spectrum antibiotics.

2. Wound infection

a. Postcesarean wound infection rates range from 2.5% to 16%.

b. Risk factors include prolonged labor, ruptured membranes, amnionitis, meconium staining, morbid obesity, anemia, and diabetes mellitus.

c. Common isolates include *Streptococcus aureus, Escherichia coli, Proteus mirabilis, Bacteroides* sp, and group B streptococci.

3. Urinary tract infection

a. Urinary tract infections are the second most common infectious complication after cesarean delivery. Incidence varies between 2% to 16%.

b. Proper patient preparation and minimizing duration of catheter use decrease risk.

4. Thromboembolic disorders

a. Deep vein thromboses occur in 0.24% of deliveries and are three to five times more common after cesarean delivery.

b. Diagnosis and treatment are the same as in the nonpregnant state.

c. Prompt diagnosis and treatment decrease the risk of complicating pulmonary embolus to 4.5%, and that of death to 0.7%.

5. Cesarean hysterectomy

a. Hysterectomy after cesarean delivery is an emergency procedure and occurs in less than 1% of cesarean sections.

b. Indications include uterine atony (43%), placenta accreta (30%), uterine rupture (13%), extension of a low transverse incision (10%), and leiomyoma preventing uterine closure.

6. Risk of uterine rupture in future pregnancies

   a. The risk of interruption of previous cesarean scar varies with location of the incision site.

     (1) A transverse scar in the lower uterine segment carries a 0.2% to 2.3% incidence of uterine rupture.

     (2) There is a 4.3% to 8.8% incidence of rupture associated with a classic scar, and a 0.5% to 6.5% incidence with a low vertical scar.

   b. Separation of the uterine scar can be categorized as a dehiscence or a rupture.

     (1) A **dehiscence** is a separation that is frequently asymptomatic and found incidentally at the time of repeat cesarean or on palpation after a vaginal birth.

     (2) **Uterine rupture** is a catastrophic event with sudden separation of the uterine scar and expulsion of the uterine contents into the abdominal cavity. Fetal distress is usually the first sign of rupture, followed by severe abdominal pain and bleeding.

E. Procedure

1. Patient preparation. The patient should be well hydrated; preoperative hematocrit is known, and blood should be readily available as indicated by the situation. The bladder should be empty. Prophylactic antibiotics are usually given in nonscheduled procedures. Antacids are also given to reduce the acidity of the stomach contents in the event that the patient aspirates material into the lungs. Informed consent should always be obtained.

2. Anesthesia most often is regional (spinal or epidural), but can be inhalational (general) as dictated by the individual situation. General anesthesia may result in depression of the infant immediately after delivery, with the degree of depression increasing with the length of time from incision to delivery. For this reason, the patient is prepared before the induction of general anesthesia.

3. Surgical techniques

   a. Abdominal incision

     (1) The abdominal incision can be midline, paramedian, or Pfannenstiel. The Pfannenstiel incision provides the most desired cosmetic effect but requires more time to perform. The infraumbilical vertical midline incision is less bloody and allows more rapid entry into the abdominal cavity.

     (2) The incision is made with the patient on the operating table with a lateral tilt of the body to the left to prevent any maternal hypotension and uteroplacental insufficiency that may result from compression of the inferior vena cava by the uterus when the patient is supine.

     (3) The uterus can be approached in one of two ways in reference to the peritoneal cavity.

       (a) Transperitoneal cesarean section is the approach used almost exclusively today. The parietal peritoneum is opened to expose the abdominal contents and uterus.

       (b) Extraperitoneal cesarean section is mentioned for historical purposes because this approach has been virtually abandoned since the advent of effective antibiotics. This technique for approaching the uterus was devised for cases of amnionitis to avoid seeding the abdominal cavity in attempts to decrease the risk of peritonitis.

   b. Uterine incision. The pregnant uterus is palpated and inspected for rotation. The type of uterine incision is selected depending on development of the lower uterine segment, presentation of the infant, and placental location.

     (1) A **bladder flap** is created to approach the lower uterine segment if this is to be the site of incision. The reflection of bladder peritoneum is incised and dissected free from the anterior uterine wall, exposing the myometrium.

     (2) **Incision of the myometrium** is made as indicated.

   c. Delivery of the infant

     (1) The infant is delivered with the hand, forceps, vacuum extraction, or breech extraction.

     (2) The placenta is delivered spontaneously or can be manually removed.

    d. Wound closure is as follows.

        (1) The uterus is often exteriorized to massage the fundus, to inspect the adnexa, and to facilitate visualization of the wound for repair.

        (2) The uterine cavity is cleaned. Oxytocics are administered as indicated to facilitate contraction of the myometrium and hemostasis.

        (3) The transverse uterine incision is closed in one or two layers; the vertical incision usually requires three layers of closure because of the myometrial thickness of the upper segment.

        (4) The **peritoneum of the bladder reflection** can be reattached with fine absorbable sutures or left to close spontaneously.

        (5) The **abdominal incision** is closed in the usual manner.

F. **Vaginal birth after cesarean section (VBAC).** Previous cesarean section is no longer a contraindication to subsequent labor and a vaginal birth. All women who are candidates should be adequately counseled and encouraged to attempt a vaginal birth.

  1. Prerequisites

    a. No maternal or fetal contraindications to labor

    b. Previous low transverse cesarean section, with documentation of the uterine scar

    c. Informed consent regarding risks and benefits of repeat cesarean and vaginal birth

    d. Personnel and facility able to perform emergency delivery

  2. Contraindications

    a. Previous classic uterine incision

    b. Maternal or fetal contraindications to labor

    c. Trial of labor declined by mother

    d. Previous low vertical scar, unless absence of upper segment extension is well documented

    e. The risk of VBAC in multiple gestations and breech presentations has not been defined.

  3. Considerations. The risks of a vaginal birth after cesarean section, when done in the proper setting, are less than the risks of a repeat cesarean section.

    a. The risk of uterine rupture is less than 1%, with no increase in maternal or fetal mortality.

    b. There is a 60% to 80% rate of successful vaginal delivery after previous cesarean. Women with "nonrecurring" causes (e.g., breech presentation, fetal distress, hemorrhage) have higher success rates than women with recurring indications (e.g., previous cephalopelvic disproportion or failure to progress). However, up to 50% of women with previous cephalopelvic disproportion have a successful vaginal birth. A previous vaginal delivery is the best prognostic indicator for success.

    c. One third of all cesarean births are repeat cesareans. An effective strategy to decrease the current cesarean section rate is to encourage vaginal births after cesarean section, when safely indicated.

II. EPISIOTOMY

A. **Definition.** An episiotomy is an incision of the perineum made to enlarge the vaginal outlet to facilitate delivery.

  1. It is made at the end of the second stage of labor just before delivery, when indicated.

  2. It increases the area of the outlet for the fetal head during delivery, particularly in assisted deliveries with forceps or the vacuum extractor.

  3. The episiotomy is used to prevent major perineal lacerations.

  4. The role of prophylactic episiotomy to prevent pelvic relaxation has not been clearly defined and is not advocated routinely.

B. **Types**

1. The **median** or **medial episiotomy** is cut vertically in the midline of the perineal body and should be one half the length of the distended perineum.
   a. The median episiotomy results in less blood loss, is easier to repair, and is more comfortable during healing than the mediolateral technique.
   b. The disadvantage is inadvertent cutting or extension into the anal sphincter and rectum. It is important to recognize and repair this complication during repair of the episiotomy so that rectovaginal fistula does not result.

2. **Mediolateral episiotomy** is incision of the perineum, at a 45° angle to the hymenal ring, extending lateral to the anus onto the inner thigh, allowing more room than a median incision.
   a. This type of incision is more difficult to repair, results in more blood loss, and causes the patient more discomfort during healing.
   b. The advantage of this episiotomy is that it allows more room with less risk of injury to the rectum and sphincter.

III. OPERATIVE VAGINAL DELIVERY: FORCEPS AND VACUUM-EXTRACTOR OPERATIONS

A. **Indications.** An operative vaginal delivery is performed to shorten the second stage of labor for maternal or fetal indications, as listed in the following.

1. **Nonreassuring fetal status** based on heart rate pattern, auscultation, lack of response to scalp stimulation, or scalp pH

2. **Prolonged second stage of labor** secondary to malposition, deflexion, or asynclitism of the fetal head. The definition of prolonged second stage is as follows:
   a. **Nulliparous patient:** more than 3 hours with a regional anesthetic or more than 2 hours without regional anesthesia
   b. **Multiparous patient:** more than 2 hours with a regional anesthetic; more than 1 hour without regional anesthesia

3. Shortening of the second stage with avoidance of voluntary maternal expulsive efforts is indicated in certain **neurologic and maternal illnesses;** assisted vaginal delivery is indicated.

4. **Poor voluntary expulsion efforts** due to exhaustion, analgesia, or neuromuscular disease may indicate the need for instrumental delivery.

B. **Contraindications**

1. Nonvertex presentation, except for Piper forceps in the breech delivery

2. Presenting part is not engaged.

3. If the head cannot be advanced with ordinary traction when using forceps or the vacuum extractor, the attempt should be abandoned.

C. **Prerequisites for instrumental delivery.** The successful results of an instrumental delivery depend largely on the skill and judgment of the obstetrician.

1. The cervix must be fully dilated.

2. The membranes must be ruptured.

3. Position and station must be known; the head must be engaged.

4. The maternal pelvis must be judged to be adequate in size for delivery.

5. The bladder should be emptied.

6. A skilled operator must be present for delivery.

7. Adequate anesthesia must be established before forceps or vacuum application.

D. **Classification of forceps deliveries.** Forceps deliveries are classified according to station and rotation.

1. **Outlet forceps.** To be categorized as an outlet forceps delivery, the following criteria need to be fulfilled.
    a. Scalp is visible at the introitus without separating the labia.
    b. Fetal skull has reached the pelvic floor.
    c. Sagittal suture is in the anteroposterior diameter or right or left occiput anterior or posterior position.
    d. Fetal head is at or on the perineum.
    e. Rotation does not exceed 45°.

2. **Low forceps.** In low forceps delivery, the leading point of the fetal skull has descended to at least +2 station but has not reached the pelvic floor.
    a. Rotation is no more than 45°.
    b. Rotation is more than 45°.

3. **Midforceps.** The station is above +2 but the presenting part is engaged.

E. **Types of forceps.** The forceps are two matched blades that articulate and lock. The design of the blades provides standard cephalic and pelvic curves (i.e., the blades conform to the shape of the fetal head and to the vaginal canal, respectively). Each matching part of the forceps has three parts: the blade, the shank, and the handle.

1. **Classic.** These forceps are used primarily for traction when there is to be little or no rotation.
    a. **Simpson**
    b. **Elliot**
    c. **Tucker-McLean**

2. **Specialized.** These forceps are designed for rotation or special indications.
    a. **Kielland** (for rotation)
    b. **Barton** (for rotation)
    c. **Piper** (for the aftercoming head in breech deliveries)

F. **Vacuum extractors**

1. **Types.** There are two types of vacuum extractors, based on the type of cup used for application to the fetal head. Each type has three parts: a cup, a rubber hose, and a vacuum pump.
    a. **The Malmstrom vacuum extractor** consists of a metal cup (40–60 mm in diameter) that is applied to the fetal scalp. The pump is then used to create a vacuum, not exceeding 0.7 to 0.8 kg/cm^2. Traction is then applied to bring the infant's head through the introitus.
    b. **The plastic cup extractor** consists of a flexible Silastic cup that is applied to the fetal scalp more easily and with less trauma than the Malmstrom extractor. The vacuum pressures attained are about the same, but can be reached more quickly and with less trauma to the fetal scalp. This extractor is the more widely used of the two in the United States.

G. **Complications**

1. **Maternal complications** are usually of minor clinical consequence (incidence 1.4%–22%) and include lacerations of the cervix, vagina, and perineum; episiotomy extensions; and associated hemorrhage. More serious complications (incidence 0.1%–0.3%) include bladder lacerations, pelvic hematoma, and coccygeal fracture.

2. **Neonatal injury**
    a. **Scalp abrasions or lacerations** are the most common injury associated with vacuum extraction.
    b. **Soft-tissue injury** is the most common injury associated with forceps delivery.
    c. **Cephalohematoma** occurs in 0.5% to 2.5% of live births with a mean incidence of 5.0% in vacuum and midforceps deliveries.
    d. **Intracranial hemorrhage** is a rare complication, occurring in 0.75% of instrumental deliveries.

IV. CERVICAL CERCLAGE

A. Cervical cerclage is used in the treatment of **cervical incompetence.** Cervical incompetence is characterized by gradual, progressive, painless dilation of the cervix, usually leading to spontaneous pregnancy loss early in the second trimester.

1. The **cause of cervical incompetence** may be acquired or congenital. Acquired causes are primarily the result of obstetric or gynecologic trauma to the cervix (e.g., rapid delivery, use of forceps, trauma, surgical dilation, conization, breech extraction, and induced labor). Diethylstilbestrol exposure associated with other reproductive tract anomalies has been linked to an increased risk of cervical incompetence.

2. The **diagnosis** is almost always made from a characteristic history of second-trimester spontaneous losses associated with painless cervical dilation or short labors. Other methods of diagnosis (e.g., dilators, catheters) lack the sensitivity and specificity to make an accurate diagnosis. The role of ultrasound as a diagnostic modality is being explored.

3. A minority (15%–20%) of second-trimester losses are associated with cervical incompetence.

B. **Techniques.** Cerclage of the cervix involves the placement of an encircling suture around the cervical os, using a heavy, nonabsorbable suture or mersilene tape. The suturing prevents protrusion of the amniotic sac and consequent rupture by correcting the abnormal dilation of the cervix. Cerclage is usually performed between the twelfth and sixteenth weeks of gestation, but can be performed as late as the twenty-fourth week. The suture is removed at the thirty-eighth week or earlier if labor begins. Fetal viability and the absence of anomalies should be documented before performing the procedure. The following are three techniques used today for cervical cerclage.

1. The **Shirodkar** technique is the most complicated of the two procedures using a vaginal approach. The suture is almost completely buried beneath the vaginal mucosa at the level of the internal os. It can be left in place for subsequent pregnancies if a cesarean section is performed. This procedure requires dissection of the bladder and is associated with an increased blood loss.

2. The **McDonald** technique is the simplest procedure, incurring less trauma to the cervix and less blood loss than the Shirodkar procedure. It is a simple purse-string suture of the cervix.

3. **Abdominal placement** of a cervical cerclage is an uncommon procedure used for those women with a short or amputated cervix or in those who have failed a vaginal procedure. Cesarean birth is necessary for delivery.

C. **Risks and morbidity**

1. Cervical lacerations occur at 1% to 13% of deliveries after a McDonald cerclage.

2. Cervical dystocia with failure to dilate, requiring a cesarean birth, occurs in 2% to 5% of cases.

3. Displacement of the suture occurs 3% to 12% of the time. A second cerclage is then attempted, which has a lower success rate.

4. Premature rupture of the membranes complicates cerclage 1% to 9% of the time.

5. Chorioamnionitis complicates 1% to 7% of cases.

6. Early, elective cerclages have a low rate (1%) of infection; cerclage placement with dilation of the cervix has a much higher risk (30%) of infection.

D. **The success rate of cerclage** has been stated to be as high as 80% to 90%. However, there have been no randomized trials to define the efficacy and benefit of cerclage; this benefit is probably overstated. Except in those with a strong history consistent with cervical incompetence, the benefit of cerclage has not been proven.

V. **ABORTION** is the termination of pregnancy before viability, usually designated as 20 weeks' gestation (i.e., before the fetus is capable of surviving outside the uterus).

A. **Spontaneous abortion** is expulsion of the products of conception without medical or mechanical intervention. Spontaneous loss occurs in 15% of clinically recognized pregnancies; the risk increases directly with maternal age, advancing paternal age, minority race, increasing gravidity, and history of previous spontaneous losses. Chromosomal abnormalities are the most common reason for first-trimester losses, occurring at a 60% frequency. Most chromosomal abnormalities are sporadic defects; in a small percentage of cases, one of the parents carries a balanced translocation. Autosomal trisomies are the most common anomaly, followed by 45X monosomy (the most common single anomaly seen in abortuses), triploidy, tetraploidy, translocations, and mosaicism. Spontaneous abortions are classified into five types.

1. **Threatened abortion** is a term traditionally used when bleeding occurs in the first half of gestation without cervical dilation or passage of tissue. Twenty-five percent of pregnant women experience spotting or bleeding early in gestation; 50% of these proceed to lose the pregnancy. An ultrasound is obtained to document viability after 6 weeks' gestation.

2. **Inevitable abortion** is diagnosed when bleeding or rupture of the membranes occurs with cramping and dilation of the cervix. Suction curettage is performed to evacuate the uterus; Rh immune globulin is administered to the Rh-negative woman.

3. **Incomplete abortion** occurs when there has been partial but incomplete expulsion of the products of conception from the uterine cavity. Therapy is evacuation of remaining tissue by suction curettage. Rh immune globulin is administered to the Rh-negative woman.

4. **Missed abortion** is death of the fetus or embryo without the onset of labor or the passage of tissue for a prolonged period of time. Suction curettage is used to evacuate the first-trimester uterus. Dilation and evacuation (D and E) or prostaglandin induction of labor are methods used to evacuate the early second-trimester uterus.

5. **Recurrent spontaneous abortion.** In the past, this condition has been called **habitual abortion** and is defined as three or more spontaneous, consecutive first-trimester losses. This affects 2% of couples. In women with previous liveborn infants who have had a loss, the risk of a subsequent abortion is 25% to 30% regardless of whether she has had one or more losses. In women with no previous liveborn infants, the recurrence risk is 40% to 45%. Evaluation is indicated after three losses, and after two losses depending on the age of those involved.

6. The **workup for spontaneous abortion** includes the following:
   a. Detailed history and physical examination
   b. Chromosomal evaluation of the couple
   c. Endometrial biopsy to exclude luteal phase defect
   d. Thyroid function test and screening for diabetes mellitus in the woman
   e. Cervical cultures for *Ureaplasma urealyticum*
   f. Hysterosalpingogram or hysteroscopy to evaluate uterine cavity
   g. Screening test for lupus anticoagulant and anti-cardiolipin antibody

B. **Induced (elective) abortion.** Abortion first became legal in 1973 and can be induced up to approximately 20 weeks' gestation, depending on state laws. Legal abortion is one of the most frequently performed surgical procedures in the United States. Therapeutic abortions are terminations of pregnancy that are done when there is maternal risk associated with continuation of the pregnancy or fetal abnormalities associated with genetic, chromosomal, or structural defects.

1. **Techniques of pregnancy termination.** Techniques used effectively to empty the uterus of the products of conception fall under the categories of surgical evacuation or induction of labor. The preferred procedure depends on gestational age and, in

some cases, operator training. Rh status is determined in each patient and Rh immune globulin is administered to Rh-negative mothers to prevent sensitization.

a. **Surgical evacuation**

(1) **Suction curettage** is the method of dilation of the cervix and vacuum aspiration of the uterine contents used for termination of pregnancy at 12 weeks' or less gestational age. Suction curettage is the most common method of pregnancy termination in this country.

(a) *Laminaria* can be used when necessary to facilitate gentle dilation of the cervix.

(b) The administration of **prophylactic antibiotics** just before or after the procedure significantly reduces the risk of infection associated with induced abortion.

(2) **D and E** is the preferred method of termination at 13 or more weeks of gestation.

(a) As the length of gestation increases, wider cervical dilation is required to accomplish the procedure successfully. Preoperative cervical *Laminaria* is used.

(b) **Vacuum aspiration** of uterine contents is usually an adequate method of evacuation from 13 to 16 weeks. After 16 weeks, uterine evacuation is accomplished with forceps extraction. Successful completion of this procedure depends largely on operator skill. Evaluation for major fetal parts is an important component of this procedure.

(c) The routine use of **prophylactic antibiotics** is recommended.

(3) **Other mechanical methods,** which are now **obsolete,** include:

(a) Sharp curettage

(b) Hysterotomy

(c) Hysterectomy (used only when there is another indication for this procedure)

(4) **Anesthesia.** Anesthesia for induced abortion is usually sedation with a local paracervical block. General anesthesia can be used but is accompanied by a higher incidence of hemorrhage, cervical injury, and perforation because general anesthetics render the uterine musculature more relaxed and, thus, easier to penetrate.

b. **Induction of labor.** Medical means of inducing abortion include extrauterine and intrauterine administration of abortifacients, such as prostaglandins, urea, hypertonic saline, and oxytocin. These methods are used for second-trimester terminations; the frequency of use of these methods increases with increasing gestational age.

(1) **Hypertonic solutions of saline** or **urea** are injected directly into the amniotic cavity. This procedure requires amniocentesis and care to avoid intravascular injection.

(2) **Prostaglandins** are most commonly administered as vaginal suppositories of prostaglandin E_2; 90% of abortions are accomplished within 24 hours. Common side effects include fever, nausea and vomiting, and diarrhea; prophylactic medications are administered before initiation to control side effects.

(3) **Complication rates** are lowest when the uterus is successfully evacuated within 13 to 24 hours. *Laminaria* to facilitate cervical dilation is useful to shorten the length of induction.

c. **Progesterone antagonists** are not available in this country for pregnancy termination but are an effective method used in Europe and other countries.

(1) **Mifepristone (RU 486),** taken orally, is highly effective in pregnancies with up to 49 days of amenorrhea.

(2) Effectiveness can be increased with the addition of prostaglandin E.

(3) **Side effects** are minimal and complication rates, including hemorrhage and retained tissue, are low.

2. **Complications.** Complications after induced abortion are categorized into immediate, delayed, and late complications. The incidence of complications is largely deter-

mined by the method of termination and gestational age; incidence varies directly with increasing gestational age.

a. Immediate complications. These complications develop during the procedure or within 3 hours after completion.

    (1) Hemorrhage. The incidence of hemorrhage is most accurately determined by the rate of transfusion. Rates vary with method of termination and are reported to be within 0.06% to 1.72%. The lowest rates are seen with suction curettage, and the highest with saline instillation.

    (2) Cervical injury. The rates of cervical injury associated with suction curettage are within the range of 0.01% to 1.6%. Factors that decrease the risk of this complication include the use of local anesthetics instead of general anesthesia, use of *Laminaria,* and an experienced operator.

    (3) Uterine perforation. Uterine perforation is a potentially serious complication of suction curettage abortions; the incidence is approximately 0.2%.

        (a) Factors that increase the risk of perforation include multiparity, advanced gestational age, and operator inexperience. The use of *Laminaria* to facilitate cervical dilation decreases the risk of uterine perforation.

        (b) The serious consequences of uterine perforation include hemorrhage and damage to intraabdominal organs. Because of the location of the uterine vessels, lateral perforations may be associated with hemorrhage. Perforation with a suction curette may be associated with bowel or other organ injury, and requires exploration.

        (c) Many perforations require only observation. Surgical exploration is indicated when there is evidence of hemorrhage or hematoma formation, or injury to abdominal organs is suspected.

    (4) Acute hematometra. This complication occurs in 0.1% to 1% of suction curettage procedures and is evidenced by decreased vaginal bleeding and an enlarged, tender uterus. Treatment is repeat curettage and administration of an oxytocic agent.

b. Delayed complications

    (1) Postabortal infection is often associated with retained tissue; the incidence of infection varies with the method of termination.

        (a) Infection complicates less than 1% of suction curettage procedures, 1.5% of D and E terminations, and 5.3% to 6.2% of induction terminations.

        (b) Factors that increase the risk of infection include the presence of cervical gonococcal or chlamydial infection, advanced gestational age, uterine instillation methods of termination, and the use of local anesthesia instead of general anesthesia.

        (c) The uterine infection is usually polymicrobial in nature, similar to other gynecologic infections, and is treated with broad-spectrum antibiotics and prompt evacuation of retained tissue.

        (d) The use of prophylactic antibiotics significantly decreases the risk of infectious complications associated with induced abortions.

    (2) Retained tissue complicates less than 1% of suction curettage abortions.

        (a) Retained tissue may be associated with infection, hemorrhage, or both.

        (b) Treatment requires repeat curettage and antibiotic administration if infection is present.

c. Late complications

    (1) Rh sensitization. The risk of sensitization increases with advanced gestational age.

        (a) The estimated risk of sensitization associated with suction curettage is 2.6% if Rh immune globulin is not appropriately administered.

        (b) The recommended dose for Rh immune globulin prophylaxis is 50 μg up to 12 weeks' gestation, and 300 μg thereafter.

    (2) Future adverse pregnancy outcomes. The incidences of infertility, spontaneous abortion, and ectopic pregnancy are not increased after uncomplicated suction curettage procedures.

    d. Maternal mortality. The case mortality rate for induced abortion is less than 0.05 per 100,000 procedures. The risk varies with gestational age and method of termination.

        (1) The leading cause of death associated with induced abortion is anesthetic complications, followed in frequency by hemorrhage, embolism, and infection.

        (2) The risk of death is lowest for suction curettage procedures and highest for instillation procedures; risk increases with advancing gestational age.

STUDY QUESTIONS

DIRECTIONS: Each of the numbered items or incomplete statements in this section is followed by answers or by completions of the statement. Select the ONE lettered answer or completion that is BEST in each case.

1. The most significant factor responsible for the increased number of cesarean sections being performed today is

(A) decreased maternal morbidity
(B) decreased maternal mortality
(C) repeat cesarean section
(D) increased use of fetal monitoring

2. When the classic uterine incision is used in cesarean section, the major concern is

(A) rupture of the scar in a subsequent pregnancy and labor
(B) postoperative adhesion formation
(C) discomfort of the patient during healing
(D) injury to the uterine vessels
(E) inability to reach the fetal head for delivery

DIRECTIONS: Each of the numbered items or incomplete statements in this section is negatively phrased, as indicated by a capitalized word such as NOT, LEAST, or EXCEPT. Select the ONE lettered answer or completion that is BEST in each case.

3. Indications for a cesarean section include all of the following EXCEPT

(A) previous classic cesarean section
(B) failed forceps delivery
(C) nonreassuring fetal heart rate tracing
(D) McDonald cervical cerclage
(E) cord prolapse

4. Prerequisites for a forceps delivery include all of the following EXCEPT

(A) a completely dilated cervix
(B) an empty bladder
(C) the vertex in the occiput anterior position
(D) ruptured membranes
(E) the known position of the vertex

5. Which of the following complications of cesarean delivery is LEAST likely when the procedure is performed with the extraperitoneal technique?

(A) Wound infection
(B) Pyelonephritis
(C) Endometritis
(D) Cystitis
(E) Peritonitis

6. Advantages of a median episiotomy include all of the following EXCEPT

(A) increased area of vaginal outlet to facilitate delivery
(B) less blood loss compared to mediolateral technique
(C) avoidance of major perineal lacerations
(D) decreased risk of injury to the anal sphincter and mucosa
(E) greater ease of repair compared to mediolateral technique

DIRECTIONS: The set of matching questions in this section consists of a list of lettered options (some of which may be in figures) followed by several numbered items. For each numbered item, select the ONE lettered option that is most closely associated with it. To avoid spending too much time on matching sets with large numbers of options, it is generally advisable to begin each set by reading the list of options. Then, for each item in the set, try to generate the correct answer and locate it in the option list, rather than evaluating each option individually. Each lettered option may be selected once, more than once, or not at all.

Questions 7–8

For each condition described below, select the most appropriate management.

(A) Forceps delivery
(B) Cesarean delivery
(C) Oxytocin administration
(D) Prostaglandin administration
(E) Vacuum extraction

7. Aftercoming head of the breech

8. Failure of the presenting part to descend in the presence of adequate labor

ANSWERS AND EXPLANATIONS

1. The answer is C [I A 1]. The dramatic increase in cesarean section rates over the past 10 years is the result of numerous factors such as fetal monitoring and a decline in vaginal breech and forceps deliveries. However, 33% of all cesarean sections are repeat cesarean sections, making this the most frequent indication. Maternal morbidity and mortality rates are higher with cesarean section than in vaginal delivery.

2. The answer is A [I D 6]. Because the classic incision is entirely in the fundus, which is the most contractile portion of the uterus, it poses the greatest risk for rupture during subsequent pregnancy and labor; thus, it carries the greatest risk of maternal and fetal mortality. Adhesions and healing discomfort are additional problems of this incision, but these are of less consequence than rupture of the scar.

3. The answer is D [I B 1; IV B]. Previous classic cesarean section, failed forceps delivery, nonreassuring heart rate tracing, and cord prolapse are among the accepted reasons for performing a cesarean section. Cervical cerclage is not an indication for cesarean section. Most cerclages for cervical incompetence performed today are the McDonald type, which is used only for the pregnancy involved. The stitch is cut before or during labor, and cesarean section is not performed unless an acceptable obstetric indication arises.

4. The answer is C [III C]. The known position of the infant's head, a completely dilated cervix, an empty bladder, and ruptured membranes are prerequisites for a forceps delivery. The vertex does not have to be in the occiput anterior position before forceps application. The vertex can be posterior or transverse and a safe forceps application is still quite possible.

5. The answer is E [I E 3 a (3) (b)]. Although not routinely performed today, the extraperitoneal technique for cesarean delivery was once popular because it avoids contaminating the peritoneal cavity with infected contents from the uterine cavity. Therefore, postoperative peritonitis would be unlikely. However, any of the usual complications of surgery could complicate this technique or the now routinely performed transperitoneal procedure.

6. The answer is D [II]. Episiotomy is not a routine practice today. It protects the perineum from extensive lacerations and provides additional room for delivering the infant. Advantages of a median episiotomy compared to a mediolateral technique include less blood loss, ease of repair, and less patient discomfort with healing. However, it is the mediolateral technique that is associated with less risk of injury to the anal sphincter and mucosa.

7–8. The answers are: 7-A [III E 2 c], **8-B** [I B 3 a]. Often trauma to the aftercoming head of the breech can be minimized by the use of forceps (Piper type). This is done only after the head has descended to the pelvic floor and has rotated to the anteroposterior position. Forceps should never be used to bring the head into the pelvis or through an incompletely dilated cervix.

In the presence of adequate labor, significant cephalopelvic disproportion is probably the cause of failure of the presenting part to descend into the pelvis. This is a contraindication to vaginal delivery. A cesarean delivery should be done.

Chapter 17

Obstetric Analgesia and Anesthesia

Matthew F. Rhoa

I. **PHYSIOLOGIC FACTORS.** The safety of the mother and the fetus must be a constant concern when considering analgesia and anesthesia for labor and delivery. The following is a brief overview of the clinically significant physiologic changes that occur in the pregnant mother.

A. **Mother**

1. **Cardiovascular and pulmonary function changes**
   a. **Cardiac changes**
      (1) There is a 33% increase in cardiac output between the twenty-fifth and thirty-sixth weeks of pregnancy. Heart rate and blood volume increase, whereas peripheral resistance decreases.
      (2) The heavy uterus may cause a reduced venous return to the heart, which may reduce blood pressure and placental perfusion.
   b. **Pulmonary changes**
      (1) There is a 42% increase in pulmonary ventilation at term.
      (2) Pregnancy requires a 10% to 15% increase in oxygen consumption because of basic metabolic changes in the pregnant woman and the fetus.
      (3) There is an 18% reduction in the functional residual capacity of the lungs at the end of expiration; however, an increase in both the inspiratory capacity of the lungs and in the rate of respiration compensates for this reduction.

2. **Hazards of anesthesia**
   a. The **onset of labor,** with its associated fear and pain, **may cause cessation of digestion;** the stomach may contain food that was eaten 12 to 18 hours previously. Stomach contents must always be considered before anesthesia is administered.
   b. When **inhalation anesthesia** is used for delivery, there is an increased risk of aspirating the stomach contents.
   c. Because inhalation anesthesia may cause a reduction in uterine tone, it is important to monitor the depth of anesthesia closely so that it does not result in uterine atony.

B. **Fetus**

1. **Uterine blood flow.** The **maternal cardiovascular and pulmonary systems must work efficiently** to provide oxygenated blood under sufficient pressure to perfuse the placenta. In addition, normal maternal acid–base balance must be maintained to prevent fetal acidosis. Reduced uterine blood flow may result from:
   a. Low maternal blood pressure
   b. Decreased maternal cardiac output
   c. A reduction in maternal pulmonary ventilation
   d. Vascular alterations due to anesthesia

2. **Gas transfer.** Because there is **greater resistance in the placental membranes than in the pulmonary alveoli (of the mother),** the transfer of gases across the placenta is less efficient than across the alveoli.

3. **Oxygen and carbon dioxide** traverse the placenta by simple diffusion.
   a. The **oxygen pressure gradient across the placenta** is 20 to 25 mm Hg, and the carbon dioxide gradient is 4 to 5 mm Hg.
   b. The **umbilical artery pH and the umbilical vein pH** are essentially the same or only slightly less (0.02 units) than the maternal pH.

4. Fetal hemoglobin, which is more efficient than adult hemoglobin, is characterized by a shift to the left of the oxygen dissociation curve. **Characteristics of fetal hemoglobin** include the following.

   a. It allows the efficient removal of oxygen from the placenta.

   b. It allows a complete and efficient unloading of oxygen in the fetal tissues.

   c. It facilitates the transfer of carbon dioxide from fetal tissues to fetal blood and then to the maternal circulation.

C. **Placenta.** The placenta is not equipped with any natural barriers to anesthetic or analgesic agents. The respiratory center of the fetus is vulnerable to sedative and anesthetic drugs, leading to respiratory depression at birth with use of these drugs.

1. The **transfer of analgesic and anesthetic agents** from the maternal circulation to the fetal circulation occurs by simple diffusion, which depends on:

   a. The concentration gradient between maternal and fetal blood

   b. The surface area and thickness of the placenta

   c. The diffusion constant of a particular drug

2. **Lipid substances,** which are nonionized, diffuse into the placenta quite readily; therefore, anesthetic and analgesic agents that are lipid soluble and of low molecular weight enter the fetal circulation within 60 seconds. Muscle relaxants, on the other hand, are highly ionized, are of low lipid solubility, and diffuse poorly through the placenta and into the fetal circulation.

3. If only a **single dose** of an analgesic or anesthetic is administered, the mother absorbs most of it in her tissues, thus protecting the infant from the narcotizing effect of the drug. If **repeated doses** of a drug are administered, the maternal tissues absorb relatively less medication.

   a. Each succeeding dose increases the gradient between the fetal and maternal circulations.

   b. The increased gradient allows the drug to accumulate in the fetal tissues and brain, producing a greater effect on the respiratory center of the newborn.

II. **ANALGESIA AND SEDATION DURING LABOR.** Uterine contractions and cervical dilation cause pain during labor. Medication for pain relief is often indicated to allow the mother to rest between contractions and to experience only moderate discomfort at the peak of the uterine contraction.

A. **Meperidine and promethazine.** A combination of a narcotic analgesic drug, such as meperidine, and a tranquilizing drug, such as promethazine, effectively relieves pain during labor.

1. **Meperidine (50–100 mg) with promethazine (25 mg)** can be administered **intramuscularly** every 3 to 4 hours, as needed. Intramuscular administration has a maximal analgesic effect in about 45 minutes.

2. **When meperidine is administered intravenously,** the dose is usually no more than 50 mg because analgesia occurs more rapidly by this route (in about 5 minutes) and the depressant effect on the fetus is more predictable (it lasts about 90 minutes).

3. There is little evidence to suggest that meperidine affects the progress of labor, but it can cause a decrease in the beat-to-beat variability on the fetal monitor.

B. **Butorphanol and nalbuphine** are synthetic narcotic agonist–antagonist analgesics given intravenously; they cause less neonatal depression than meperidine.

C. **Morphine.** This powerful narcotic is most often used for analgesia in early labor. In doses of 10 to 15 mg intramuscularly, it is a particularly valuable analgesic for patients who are having a prolonged latent phase with frequent painful contractions.

D. **Narcotic antagonists.** When narcotic agents are given close to delivery, the infant may be significantly depressed at birth. **Naloxone** is a narcotic antagonist that is capable of reversing the respiratory depression by displacing the narcotic from specific receptors in the central nervous system (CNS).

III. CONDUCTION ANESTHESIA

A. **Neuropathways of obstetric pain.** The complete relief of pain in obstetrics can be accomplished by blocking the sympathetic pathways of the **eleventh and twelfth thoracic nerves and the parasympathetic and sensory fibers of the sacral nerves.**

1. **Uterine contractions.** The pain of the uterine contractions is transmitted from the uterus to the sympathetic nerves of the **hypogastric plexus.** The impulses are then transmitted by the paravertebral sympathetic chain and enter the gray rami of the eleventh and twelfth thoracic nerves.

2. **Cervical dilation.** The pain sensations of a dilating cervix are transmitted through the eleventh and twelfth thoracic nerves with overlap through the tenth thoracic and first lumbar nerves.

3. **Parturition.** The pain stimuli of parturition are transmitted to the cord by the pudendal nerve through the sensory fibers of the second, third, fourth, and fifth sacral nerves.

B. **Paracervical block** has been abandoned by most physicians, and is used only rarely to provide pain relief during labor.

1. **Route of administration.** By injecting local anesthetic (i.e., lidocaine) paracervically at the 3 and 9 o'clock positions or uterosacrally at 4 and 8 o'clock positions, the visceral afferent pain fibers are blocked. Pain relief for 1 to 2 hours is provided by 5 to 10 ml of 1% lidocaine injected on each side of the cervix.

2. **Complications.** Fetal bradycardia, a complication 10% to 25% of the time, is not a sign of fetal asphyxia but is secondary to the transplacental transfer of the anesthetic agent or its metabolite, which has a depressant effect on the fetal heart. The bradycardia usually lasts from 6 to 10 minutes.

C. **Pudendal block,** which is basic to obstetric anesthesia, provides perineal anesthesia by anesthetizing the pudendal nerve. It works well for a spontaneous delivery and an episiotomy repair, but it is not likely to provide adequate anesthesia for a forceps delivery.

1. **Route of administration.** The main trunk of the pudendal nerve lies on the posterior surface of the sacrospinous ligament, just medial to the ischial spine. A 1% lidocaine solution (10 ml) is injected on each side transvaginally around the tip of the ischial spine and through the sacrospinous ligament.

2. **Complications.** The intravascular injection of the local anesthetic can cause systemic toxicity in the mother, characterized by stimulation of the cerebral cortex, leading to convulsions, and depression of the medulla, leading to respiratory depression.

D. **Spinal anesthesia** is a satisfactory method of alleviating the discomfort of uterine contractions and delivery because injecting the anesthetic up to the level of the tenth thoracic nerve anesthetizes the sympathetic fibers of the eleventh and twelfth thoracic nerves and the parasympathetic and sensory fibers of the sacral plexus. Spinal anesthesia is satisfactory for both vaginal and cesarean deliveries. The main advantage is that it has a rapid onset and is easier to administer than an epidural block.

1. **Route of administration.** Spinal anesthesia is administered by injecting a local anesthetic into the subarachnoid space. Pregnant patients need smaller amounts of anesthetic agents than nonpregnant patients because the subarachnoid space is smaller in

a pregnant patient as a result of the engorgement of the internal vertebral venous plexus—a consequence of compression by the pregnant uterus on the inferior vena cava. Thus, a normal dose of an anesthetic agent could produce a much higher spinal blockade in a pregnant patient than in a nonpregnant patient. The level of the anesthesia is influenced by the:

a. Specific gravity of the agent

b. Site of the injection

c. Position of the patient

d. Concentration of the anesthetic solution

2. **Complications of spinal anesthesia** include:

   a. Hypotension. This is the most common complication; it results from the vasodilation caused by the sympathetic blockade and is compounded by obstructed venous return because of compression by the uterus on the inferior vena cava. It is treated by:

   (1) Uterine displacement to the left

   (2) Acute hydration with a saline solution

   (3) Intravenous ephedrine (10–15 mg)

   b. High spinal blockade with respiratory paralysis. This is a very dangerous complication because hypotension and apnea quickly develop and may progress to cardiac arrest. Ventilation with an endotracheal tube is indicated until the anesthesia wears off.

   c. Spinal headache. This is caused by leakage of cerebrospinal fluid from the puncture site. The headache may persist for 3 to 5 days.

   (1) When the woman stands, the diminished volume of cerebrospinal fluid allows traction on pain-sensitive CNS structures, such as the pia-arachnoid.

   (2) Bed rest, analgesics, hydration, intravenous caffeine, and the use of an abdominal binder are helpful.

   d. Meningitis. Because of sterile techniques and disposable equipment, contamination and infection of the meninges are now rare.

E. **Epidural anesthesia. Caudal anesthesia and lumbar epidural anesthesia** are accomplished by injecting suitable local anesthetic agents into the epidural or peridural space—a potential space that immediately surrounds the dura and extends from the foramen magnum to the sacral hiatus.

1. **Route of administration**

   a. Caudal anesthesia is produced by injecting a local anesthetic, such as **bupivacaine** (0.25% or 0.5%), through the sacral hiatus into the caudal space. This method is rarely used in modern obstetrics.

   (1) The **sacral hiatus** is a foramen at the lower end of the sacrum, which results from the nonclosure of the last sacral vertebra.

   (2) This foramen leads to the **caudal space**—the lowest extent of the peridural space.

   (3) A rich network of sacral nerves runs through the caudal space; an anesthetic agent injected into this space abolishes the sensation of pain carried by the sacral nerves, producing anesthesia suitable for delivery.

   b. Lumbar epidural anesthesia is injected into the same anatomic space as caudal anesthesia, but the anesthetic agent is injected into the **lumbar area** of the space rather than through the sacral hiatus.

   (1) Anesthesia for the pain of labor and vaginal delivery depends on a block from the tenth thoracic nerve to the fifth sacral nerve. For an abdominal delivery, an anesthetic level from the fourth thoracic nerve to the eighth thoracic nerve must be achieved.

   (2) **The spread of lumbar anesthesia** depends on the:

   (a) Location of the catheter tip in the peridural space

   (b) Dose of the anesthetic agent

   (c) Head-down, horizontal, or head-up position of the patient

   (3) **If the meninges are perforated** with the needle and the usual amount of anesthetic agent is injected, the anesthesia will be subarachnoid and may rapidly produce a total spinal blockade.

2. Epidural analgesics
  a. Epidural morphine can provide satisfactory analgesia during the first stage of labor.
  b. Fentanyl and its derivatives, in combination with local anesthetics, are used as a continuous epidural infusion for first-stage analgesia.
  c. Postcesarean section epidural morphine is more effective for pain relief than the same dose of intramuscular morphine.
    (1) A single dose provides pain relief for 12 to 24 hours.
    (2) Side effects can include pruritus, nausea, vomiting, urine retention, and delayed respiratory depression.

3. Complications of epidural anesthesia
  a. Inadvertent spinal anesthesia may occur with puncture of the dura and injection of the anesthetic agent. The complications of a high spinal block may follow (see III D 2 b).
  b. Intravenous injection of the anesthetic agent can result in **CNS toxicity,** with slurred speech, tinnitus, convulsions, or even cardiac arrest.
  c. Ineffective anesthesia
    (1) Anesthesia may be ineffective in a rapidly progressive labor because of the time it takes for peridural anesthesia to become effective.
    (2) Perineal anesthesia for delivery may be difficult to obtain with the lumbar epidural anesthesia because the block may not include the sacral nerves.
  d. Hypotension and decreased placental perfusion occur because of the blockade of the sympathetic tracts and pooling of blood below the pregnant uterus.
  e. An epidural block induced before well established labor may be followed by **desultory** labor, which is characterized by ineffective contractions. In addition, the patient's expulsive efforts may be hampered, leading to an increased incidence of operative delivery.

IV. GENERAL ANESTHESIA. Because the placenta is not a barrier to general anesthesia, all anesthetic agents that depress the CNS of the mother cross the placenta and depress the CNS of the fetus. General anesthesia is used in obstetric emergencies when the fetus must be delivered quickly or if conduction anesthesia (epidural or spinal) is contraindicated because of back problems or coagulation disorders.

A. Types

1. Gas anesthetics. Nitrous oxide is not commonly used to provide pain relief during labor. This method continues to be used, however, in developing countries.
  a. Nitrous oxide does not prolong labor or interfere with uterine contractions.
  b. Satisfactory analgesia can be obtained with a concentration of 50% nitrous oxide and 50% oxygen, with the patient breathing the mixture intermittently while pushing during the second stage of labor.

2. Volatile anesthetics
  a. Halothane produces significant uterine relaxation and should be restricted to situations that require a relaxed uterus, such as internal podalic version, breech extraction, and repositioning of the acutely inverted uterus. Prompt discontinuation of the anesthetic is necessary to prevent hemorrhage from an atonic uterus.
  b. Isoflurane is the most commonly used agent for general anesthesia.

B. Aspiration during general anesthesia. Pneumonitis from inhalation of gastric contents is the most common cause of anesthetic death in obstetrics.

1. Prophylaxis. Important factors in preventing aspiration include the following.
  a. The **patient should fast** for as long as possible before the induction of general anesthesia.
  b. After labor has begun, only **clear liquids** should be permitted.

    c. Before the induction of anesthesia, gastric acidity should be neutralized with ant-acids, such as sodium citrate.

    d. With **intubation,** cricoid pressure is administered to compress the esophagus just as the patient is being induced with sodium pentothal.

2. **Pathology.** When the pH of aspirated gastric fluid is below 2.5, a severe **chemical pneumonitis** develops.

    a. Aspiration of particles without acidic fluid leads to:

        (1) Patchy atelectasis

        (2) Bronchopneumonia

    b. Aspiration of acidic fluid leads to:

        (1) Tachypnea

        (2) Bronchospasm

        (3) Rhonchi

        (4) Rales

        (5) Atelectasis

        (6) Cyanosis

        (7) Hypotension

    c. Exudate into the lung interstitium and alveoli causes:

        (1) Decreased pulmonary compliance

        (2) Shunting of blood

        (3) Severe hypoxemia

3. **Treatment**

    a. Suction. As much inhaled material as possible must be removed immediately from the mouth, pharynx, and trachea.

    b. Bronchoscopy. This procedure is indicated if large particulate matter is causing airway obstruction.

    c. Corticosteroids. Large doses of intravenous corticosteroids should be adminis-tered every 8 hours for 24 hours in an attempt to maintain cell integrity in the presence of strong acid.

    d. Oxygen and ventilation. Endotracheal intubation with intermittent positive pres-sure may be necessary to maintain the arterial P_{O_2} at 60 mm Hg. Frequent suc-tion is necessary to remove secretions and edema fluid.

    e. Antibiotics. Infection after aspiration is most frequently caused by **anaerobes.** Therefore, antibiotic coverage with clindamycin or metronidazole is indicated.

STUDY QUESTIONS

DIRECTIONS: Each of the numbered items or incomplete statements in this section is followed by answers or by completions of the statement. Select the ONE lettered answer or completion that is BEST in each case.

1. The laboring patient has progressed through labor without any analgesia. She pushes effectively and brings the vertex to the perineum. Effective anesthesia will be needed for an episiotomy and repair. Where should the needle be placed?

(A) Through the perineum
(B) Into the hypogastric plexus
(C) Into the uterosacral ligament
(D) Through the sacrospinous ligament
(E) Into the tip of the sacrum

2. The patient has just delivered her fifth child, and she used no analgesia. The physician is anxious to remove the placenta and pulls on the umbilical cord. As the placenta delivers, the physician notices that the uterus has inverted and is protruding through the vagina. Which of the following agents would be appropriate anesthesia for repositioning the uterus?

(A) Halothane
(B) Cyclopropane
(C) Bupivacaine
(D) Nitrous oxide

DIRECTIONS: Each of the numbered items or incomplete statements in this section is negatively phrased, as indicated by a capitalized word such as NOT, LEAST, or EXCEPT. Select the ONE lettered answer or completion that is BEST in each case.

3. The physician is called to see a patient the morning after her delivery. She states that her headache is so bad that she cannot raise her head off the pillow. It is noted that she had an epidural for pain relief during labor. Which of the following is NOT a possible explanation for her headache?

(A) Leakage of cerebrospinal fluid at the puncture site
(B) Traction on the pia-arachnoid
(C) Diminished cerebrospinal fluid volume
(D) Collapse of the maternal vertebral venous plexus
(E) Diminished intravascular volume

4. The patient had a crash induction with general anesthesia for an emergency cesarean section because of fetal distress. After the surgery, the anesthesiologist notes a tachypnea and absent breath sounds in both lower lobes of the lungs. All of the following would be appropriate actions in this case EXCEPT

(A) antibiotic administration
(B) corticosteroid administration
(C) ventilation
(D) antacid administration
(E) suction

5. Which of the following statements concerning maternal physiology during pregnancy is NOT correct?

(A) Cardiac output is increased
(B) Pulmonary ventilation is increased
(C) Oxygen consumption is increased
(D) Functional residual capacity of the lungs is increased
(E) Inspiratory capacity of the lungs is increased

6. Which of the following is NOT a result of epidural anesthesia in a pregnant woman?

(A) Hypotension
(B) Decreased placental perfusion
(C) Decreased venous return
(D) Increased venous pooling
(E) Increased cardiac output

7. Which of the following statements concerning placental transfer of analgesic agents is NOT correct?

(A) It occurs by simple diffusion
(B) It is rapid with ionized substances
(C) It depends on the concentration gradient between maternal and fetal blood
(D) Analgesic agents enter the fetal circulation quickly
(E) It is a function of placental surface area and thickness

DIRECTIONS: The set of matching questions in this section consists of a list of lettered options (some of which may be in figures) followed by several numbered items. For each numbered item, select the ONE lettered option that is most closely associated with it. To avoid spending too much time on matching sets with large numbers of options, it is generally advisable to begin each set by reading the list of options. Then, for each item in the set, try to generate the correct answer and locate it in the option list, rather than evaluating each option individually. Each lettered option may be selected once, more than once, or not at all.

Questions 8–10

For each of the following obstetric presentations, select the analgesic or anesthetic modality that would be most appropriate.

(A) Pudendal block
(B) Spinal anesthesia
(C) Intramuscular morphine
(D) Epidural anesthesia
(E) Intravenous meperidine

8. A woman presents with painful uterine contractions that occur every 2 to 3 minutes. On examination, she is dilated 2 cm and 60% effaced. Three hours later, she is even more uncomfortable, with the same contraction pattern, but her cervix is still only 2-cm dilated.

9. A woman is in active labor having contractions every 2 to 3 minutes. She is 3-cm dilated with the vertex at the −1 station. Two hours later, she is 5- to 6-cm dilated with the vertex at the +1 station; she requests pain relief.

10. A woman is in the delivery room ready for delivery. She has had no analgesia or anesthesia up to this point. The vertex is on the perineum; the infant's head is visible at the perineum with each push.

ANSWERS AND EXPLANATIONS

1. The answer is D [III B 1, C 1]. At this stage, delivery is imminent, and perineal anesthesia is needed. A pudendal block gives the most effective local perineal anesthesia. The needle goes through the vagina to the tip of the ischial spine (not the sacrum) and through the sacrospinous (not the uterosacral) ligament. The paracervical block is injected into the uterosacral ligament. Local infiltration of the perineum could be used, but this is not as effective anesthesia as the pudendal block.

2. The answer is A [IV A]. The postpartum inverted uterus is one of the true obstetric emergencies; death can occur quickly because of both blood loss and neurogenic shock. Epidural and spinal anesthesia take too much time to administer and become effective. The patient needs to be anesthetized with a general anesthetic that also relaxes the uterus so that it can be repositioned. Neither nitrous oxide nor cyclopropane is a good myometrial relaxant; however, halothane produces significant uterine relaxation.

3. The answer is E [III D 2 c (1)]. The patient had an epidural, at which time the dura was punctured, resulting in a spinal headache. Spinal headaches are caused by leakage of cerebrospinal fluid from the puncture site through the dura. With delivery, some of the pressure from the now nonpregnant uterus on the inferior vena cava lessens, and the engorgement of the vertebral venous plexus diminishes. This, combined with the loss of cerebrospinal fluid volume (through leakage), results in traction on the pain-sensitive structures of the central nervous system (CNS), such as the pia-arachnoid, with the resultant headache. The headache is accentuated when the patient tries to raise her head. Decreased intravascular volume is not an immediate factor in the usual postspinal headache.

4. The answer is D [IV B 1–3]. This patient aspirated gastric contents during crash intubation before her surgery. Aspiration is always a potential problem with the obstetric patient because she often will have a full stomach going into labor. The chief concern in this situation is the development of a chemical pneu-

monitis, which can be fatal. The patient already has partial atelectasis and tachypnea. Immediate therapy would be endotracheal intubation with suction, ventilation, and oxygen. In addition, the patient would be placed on antibiotics and corticosteroids. Antacids are given before, not after, the induction of the general anesthesia in an attempt to neutralize the gastric acidity.

5. The answer is D [I A 1]. Because of an increased fluid volume and changes in the basic metabolic rate in pregnant women, cardiac output, pulmonary ventilation, oxygen consumption, and the inspiratory capacity of the lungs are increased. However, because of the enlarging uterus, which pushes the intraabdominal contents under the diaphragm, there is an actual decrease in the functional residual capacity of the lungs at the end of expiration.

6. The answer is E [I A 1 a; III E 3 d]. Because of the blockade of the sympathetic tracts with epidural anesthesia in a pregnant woman, there is pooling in the lower extremities below the large uterus with a decreased venous return. This can result in hypotension and decreased placental perfusion, which in turn can cause fetal distress. There would not be an increased cardiac output because the anesthesia would cause a decrease in the venous return to the heart, resulting in a decreased maternal cardiac output.

7. The answer is B [I C 1, 2]. The placental transfer of analgesic agents occurs by simple diffusion, which, in turn, is influenced by concentration gradients and surface area. Most anesthetic agents are lipid soluble, of low molecular weight, and nonionized—features that permit rapid transfer across the placenta and entry into the fetal circulation within 60 seconds. Ionized agents traverse the placenta slowly.

8–10. The answers are: 8-C [III C], **9-D** [III E], **10-A** [III C]. The woman who is still only 2-cm dilated after 3 hours of labor is experiencing a nonprogressive, painful type of labor; she is having regular contractions but showing no cervical change. Her labor is hypertonic and dysfunctional. Potent sedation with morphine is indicated at this point to give the patient a much-needed rest. Often the labor will become progressive when the morphine wears off.

The woman who is 5- to 6-cm dilated is in active, progressive labor. The vertex is well within the pelvis. A vaginal delivery can be anticipated in such a patient. Because she needs pain relief, an epidural is appropriate because she needs an anesthetic that will last for an indefinite period of time and that will provide anesthesia for the delivery. Neither a spinal nor a pudendal block will accomplish both purposes: a spinal lasts for a finite period of time, and a pudendal block will not block the pain of labor.

The woman who is in the delivery room needs a quick, simple anesthesia for the perineum. A spinal and an epidural would take too long to take effect and involve much more anesthesia than is needed. An analgesic like meperidine would have a depressant effect on the infant and would do nothing for the perineal pain. The pudendal block is a quick, easy method for last-minute anesthesia of the perineum for episiotomy.

Chapter 18

Gestational Trophoblastic Disease

Jane Fang

I. INTRODUCTION. Gestational trophoblastic disease (GTD) is the general term for a spectrum of proliferative trophoblastic abnormalities originating from the placenta.

A. Clinical classification (Table 18-1)

1. **Hydatidiform mole** is characterized by proliferation of the trophoblast, which suggests an advanced normal pregnancy when it fills the uterine cavity. Hydatidiform moles may be **complete (classic)** or **incomplete (partial).**

2. **Gestational trophoblastic neoplasia (GTN)** is malignant GTD, which arises from the trophoblastic elements of the developing blastocyst, retains the invasive tendencies of the normal placenta, and remains able to secrete the polypeptide hormone, **human chorionic gonadotropin (hCG).** GTN can be either **metastatic** or **nonmetastatic.** These include invasive moles, placental site trophoblastic tumors, and choriocarcinoma.

B. Incidence

1. **Benign GTD** (hydatidiform mole) occurs in 1 of 1200 pregnancies in the United States and up to 1 of 120 pregnancies in other parts of the world (e.g., East Asia).
   a. **Socioeconomics.** Incidence is highest among women with low socioeconomic status and women in underdeveloped areas, such as Southeast Asia.
   b. **Age.** Moles tend to occur in older women.
   c. **Remission.** Spontaneous remission is common in 80% to 85% of patients after dilation and evacuation.

2. **Malignant GTD,** which develops in 20% of moles, occurs in 1 of 20,000 pregnancies in the United States and may follow:
   a. Hydatidiform mole (25%)
   b. Normal pregnancy (50%)
   c. Spontaneous abortion or ectopic pregnancy (25%)

II. HYDATIDIFORM MOLE

A. Characteristics (microscopic features)

1. **Complete, or classic, mole**
   a. Marked edema and **enlargement of the villi**
   b. Disappearance of the villous blood vessels
   c. Proliferation of the trophoblastic lining of the villi
   d. Absence of fetus, cord, or amniotic membrane
   e. Normal karyotype (usually 46,XX, rarely 46,XY); all the chromosomes are paternally derived
   f. Uterine size usually larger than expected
   g. A higher incidence of postmolar complications (i.e. GTD, hyperemesis, theca-lutein cysts, hyperthyroidism)

2. **Incomplete, or partial, mole**
   a. Marked swelling of the villi with **atrophic trophoblastic cells**
   b. Presence of normal villi
   c. **Presence of fetus,** cord, and amniotic membrane

TABLE 18-1. Clinical Classification of Gestational Trophoblastic Disease (GTD)

Hydatidiform mole (molar pregnancy)
    Complete, or classic
    Incomplete, or partial
Gestational trophoblastic neoplasia (GTN)
    Nonmetastatic
    Metastatic
        Low risk (good prognosis)
        High risk (poor prognosis)

---

    d. Abnormal karyotype, usually triploidy or trisomy (69,XXX, or 69,XXY); the chromosomes are derived from a duplicated paternal set and a haploid ovum
    e. Uterine size usually smaller than expected
    f. Postmolar GTD less common

B. **Symptoms**

    1. **Bleeding** usually occurs in the first trimester.

    2. **The uterus is often larger than expected** in terms of the last menstrual period.

    3. **Nausea and vomiting** occur in about one-third of patients.

    4. **Preeclampsia** in the early second trimester should raise high suspicion of a molar pregnancy.

    5. **Clinical hyperthyroidism** occurs occasionally. It is hypothesized to be caused by binding of the hCG molecule (with elevated levels of hCG) to the thyroid-stimulating hormone receptor site and by hyperfunction of the thyroid gland.

    6. **Abdominal pain** secondary to theca-lutein cysts is found in 15% of patients because the molar pregnancy produces excessive hCG, which stimulates excessive growth of the ovaries.

C. **Diagnosis**

    1. The first evidence of a molar pregnancy may be bleeding or the **passage of vesicular tissue.**

    2. A **quantitative hCG** titer of greater than 100,000 mIU/ml with an enlarged uterus and bleeding is highly suggestive of a mole.

    3. **Ultrasonography** has replaced other diagnostic methods.

D. **Management**

    1. **Diagnostic studies** should include complete blood count with platelets, quantitative β-hCG level, chest radiograph, coagulation studies, type and screen, and baseline renal function studies.

    2. **Suction curettage** is the primary tool for evacuating a mole even when the uterus has enlarged beyond the size expected for a 20-week pregnancy.
        a. Suction curettage has almost eliminated the need for hysterotomy, which was commonly used before suction was available.
        b. Suction curettage is used in conjunction with **intravenous oxytocin.**

    3. **Primary hysterectomy** may be the selected method of evacuation if the patient does not want future pregnancies.
        a. If **theca-lutein cysts** are encountered, the ovaries are left untouched because the cysts will regress as the hCG level falls to normal.

b. Despite the hysterectomy, the follow-up is the same as for suction evacuation in molar pregnancy.

4. Prophylactic chemotherapy. Because 80% of patients with molar pregnancies have spontaneous remission and do not require any therapy, and because serial hCG determinations can identify the 20% of patients in whom malignancies will develop, it is not appropriate to treat all patients. The toxicity from prophylactic chemotherapy can be severe, even leading to death.

E. **Follow-up.** The average time to expect complete elimination of hCG is 73 days; however, this time period depends on the initial level of hCG, the amount of viable trophoblastic tissue remaining after evacuation, and the half-life of hCG. Follow-up of a molar pregnancy should include:

1. Determinations of hCG at 48 hours postevacuation, then every 1 to 2 weeks until the results are negative twice, then every 1 to 2 months for 1 year; patients must be advised to use contraception for 1 year. Oral contraceptives prevent pregnancy and suppress luteinizing hormone production.

2. Physical examination, including a pelvic examination at regular intervals during the first year until remission to ensure adequate involution of pelvic organs

3. A repeat **chest radiograph** to rule out pulmonary metastases if the hCG titer plateaus or rises

4. Chemotherapy started immediately if the hCG titer rises or plateaus during follow-up or if metastases are detected at any time

III. **GESTATIONAL TROPHOBLASTIC NEOPLASIA** (Table 18-2)

A. **Characteristics**

1. Abnormal uterine bleeding due to GTN can appear within a relatively short time or years after a pregnancy.

2. Bleeding from lesions in the lower genital tract can occur at any time.

3. Metastatic disease can be found in the gastrointestinal tract, the genitourinary system, the liver, the lung, and the brain; it is often associated with hemorrhage because of the propensity of trophoblastic tissue to invade vessels.

TABLE 18-2. Classification of Gestational Trophoblastic Neoplasia (GTN)

Nonmetastatic—disease confined to the uterus
Metastic—disease spread outside the uterus
   Good prognosis (low risk)
      Short duration—disease present less than 4 months
      Pretreatment hCG titer less than 40,000 mIU/ml
      No prior chemotherapy
   Poor prognosis (high risk)
      Long duration—disease present more than 4 months
      Pretreatment hCG titer greater than 40,000 mIU/ml
      Brain or liver metastases
      Failure of prior chemotherapy
      Disease after term pregnancy

hCG = human chorionic gonadotropin.

B. **Diagnosis**

1. With a high index of suspicion, a **quantitative hCG** is diagnostic.
2. **Workup of the patient with GTN** should include the following:
   a. Chest film and intravenous pyelogram
   b. Liver and computed tomography scans
   c. Hematologic survey and serum chemistries
   d. Determination of the pretreatment hCG titer
   e. Ultrasound of the pelvis

C. **Nonmetastatic GTN** is the most common form of this disease, which is confined to the uterus.

1. **Treatment** of nonmetastatic GTN has been almost 100% successful.
   a. **Patients** with nonmetastatic disease can be **treated with single-agent chemotherapy** (e.g., methotrexate, actinomycin D, and high-dose methotrexate with folinic acid rescue) until negative hCG titers are obtained for consecutive weeks or unless one of the following toxic reactions occurs:
      (1) Thrombocytopenia
      (2) Leukopenia
      (3) Oral or gastrointestinal ulceration
      (4) Febrile course
      (5) Abnormal blood urea nitrogen, or serum transaminases
   b. In **patients who fail single-agent chemotherapy,** secondary hysterectomy can be performed. In **patients who want no further pregnancies,** primary hysterectomy is recommended during the first course of chemotherapy. Hysterectomy shortens the duration of chemotherapy necessary to obtain remission.
   c. Patients who fail one single-agent therapy may be changed to another single agent. Patients who fail this should be switched to multiagent chemotherapy.
   d. Almost 50% of **those who want pregnancy after treatment for nonmetastatic GTN** have been successful, with normal infants in 80% to 85% of cases.

2. **Follow-up**
   a. Titers of hCG every 2 weeks for 3 months, then monthly for 3 months, then every 6 months
   b. Frequent pelvic examinations
   c. Chest radiograph at regular intervals
   d. Contraception (usually birth control pills) for a minimum of 1 year

D. **Metastatic GTN** is disease outside the uterus. Patients have various symptoms, such as **hemoptysis (pulmonary metastases)** or **neurologic signs (brain metastases).**

1. **Good-prognosis metastatic GTN**
   a. The following factors are **associated with a good prognosis:**
      (1) Short duration (less than 4 months)
      (2) Low pretreatment hCG titer (less than 40,000 mIU/ml)
      (3) No metastatic spread to the brain or liver
      (4) No prior chemotherapy
   b. **Single-agent chemotherapy** can be used to treat good-prognosis metastatic GTN. However, a greater number of courses of chemotherapy are usually required, and alternative therapy is more frequently necessary.
   c. **Primary and secondary hysterectomy** are used as for nonmetastatic GTN.
   d. **Follow-up** is similar to that for nonmetastatic GTN (see III C 2).

2. **Poor-prognosis metastatic GTN**
   a. The following factors are **associated with a poor prognosis:**
      (1) Long duration (symptoms more than 4 months)
      (2) High pretreatment hCG titer (greater than 40,000 mIU/ml)
      (3) Liver or brain metastases
      (4) Failure of prior chemotherapy
      (5) Disease after a term pregnancy

   b. Treatment. A significant problem in treating patients with a poor prognosis occurs because many have been treated previously with chemotherapy and are thus resistant to therapy.

      (1) These patients are treated with multiagent chemotherapy and a multiple modality approach (i.e., chemotherapy, surgery, radiation).

      (2) They should be treated in centers that have special interest and expertise in this disease, especially when life-threatening toxicity from therapy is a factor.

      (3) The survival rate is between 60% to 84%.

      (4) Hysterectomy usually does not improve the outcome.

   c. Follow-up

      (1) Three additional courses of chemotherapy after three consecutive normal weekly hCG assays

      (2) Monitoring of hCG levels (similar to that for nonmetastatic GTN)

      (3) Chest radiograph at regular intervals

      (4) Contraception for at least 1 year after negative levels of hCG

E. **Recurrence rates**

1. Nonmetastatic GTN: 2%

2. Good-prognosis metastatic GTN: 5%

3. Poor-prognosis metastatic GTN: up to 20%

STUDY QUESTIONS

DIRECTIONS: Each of the numbered items or incomplete statements in this section is followed by answers or by completions of the statement. Select the ONE lettered answer or completion that is BEST in each case.

1. Which of the following is consistent with a partial mole?

(A) 46 chromosomes
(B) Villous edema
(C) Theca-lutein cysts
(D) A uterus that is large for dates
(E) The presence of a fetus

2. A 25-year-old nulligravid woman presents with a molar gestation at 12 weeks from her last menstrual period. Which of the following is the most appropriate management for this patient?

(A) Single-agent chemotherapy
(B) Obtain a quantitative β-hCG titer
(C) Hysterotomy
(D) Total abdominal hysterectomy with preservation of the ovaries
(E) Thyroid function studies

3. Which of the following factors is a poor prognostic indicator for metastatic gestational trophoblastic neoplasia?

(A) Lung metastases
(B) Patient age of 35 years
(C) Diagnosis of disease at 6 weeks post-partum
(D) Presence of a fetus
(E) Hysterectomy as treatment

ANSWERS AND EXPLANATIONS

1. The answer is E [II A 2]. Partial moles are differentiated from complete moles by the presence of a fetus, umbilical cord, or amniotic membranes. Their karyotypes have 69 chromosomes rather than the diploid makeup of complete moles. The villi of partial moles tend to be small and atrophic, rather than edematous, which is why the uterine size is not larger than expected.

2. The answer is B [II D 1]. Once the diagnosis of molar gestation has been established, a preoperative β-hCG level is necessary so that this value can be followed after surgery. Once uterine evacuation is performed, β-hCG levels must be evaluated 48 hours later, then at least every other week until the level falls to zero. If the level plateaus or rises, a chest radiograph is indicated to rule out metastases to the lung, and chemotherapy must be initiated.

3. The answer is C [III D 2; Table 18-2]. The poor prognostic indicators for metastatic gestational trophoblastic neoplasia are listed in Table 18-2. When a molar pregnancy is diagnosed after a term pregnancy, this confers a high risk for failure of treatment. Lung metastases do not confer a poorer prognosis for treatment. Age has not been shown to influence the prognosis.

Chapter 19

Pediatric and Adolescent Gynecology

Matthew F. Rhoa

I. **INTRODUCTION.** An awareness of the problems that are unique to pediatric and adolescent gynecology is basic for proper management of the young patient. Particular care is essential in performing a pelvic examination because both physical and emotional trauma may be inadvertently inflicted. Often, a complete physical examination before the pelvic examination can help to establish rapport and reassurance in a patient unaccustomed to pelvic examinations. The adolescent patient should have a pelvic examination at menarche or at least by high school age, then regularly when she becomes sexually active.

A. **Pelvic examination of a pediatric patient** may reveal the following:

1. A mucoid vaginal discharge and even vaginal bleeding in an infant for up to 2 weeks after birth as a result of maternal estrogens

2. An introitus that is located more anteriorly than normal and a clitoris that is more prominent than normal (1–2 cm)

3. A redundant hymen that may protrude on straining and that remains essentially the same size until age 10 years

4. A vaginal epithelium that is uncornified and erythematous with an alkaline pH

5. A small uterus (2.5–3 cm in length), with the cervix comprising two thirds of the organ—the reverse of adult proportions

6. A cervical os that normally appears as an ectropion

B. **Visualization of the vagina.** Instruments for visualizing the vagina include the vaginoscope, the urethroscope, and the pediatric speculum. Stirrups are usually not necessary for the preadolescent; a simple "frog-leg" position is usually sufficient. In an occasional patient, intravenous sedation may be necessary to accomplish a thorough genital examination. To determine the presence or absence of internal genitalia, ultrasound and magnetic resonance imaging are helpful when indicated.

C. **Rectal examination** is often more informative because the short posterior vaginal fornix cannot be distended and a cul-de-sac does not exist.

II. **VULVOVAGINAL LESIONS**

A. **Lichen sclerosus et atrophicus**

1. **Clinical picture.** A white, papular lesion resembling leukoplakia may cover the vulva and perianal regions.

2. **Etiology** is unknown.

3. **Diagnosis.** Biopsy, which shows superficial hyperkeratosis with basal atrophic and sclerotic changes, should be performed to clarify the diagnosis.

4. **Therapy.** This condition is benign and can be self-limiting. Improved hygiene is the first line of therapy. Cortisone may be used temporarily for itching. Some may require progesterone cream. Testosterone, used in the treatment of adults with this condition, should be avoided. The condition may resolve at puberty, but usually is a chronic condition.

B. **Trauma**

1. **Clinical picture**

   a. **Tears, abrasions, ecchymoses, and hematomas** are common in preadolescent girls. The incidence is highest in children aged 4 to 12 years. The most common mechanisms of injury are sexual abuse, straddle injuries, accidental penetration, sudden abduction of the extremities, and pelvic fractures. Most genital trauma results from straddle injuries such as a child landing on the center bar of a boy's bicycle. The injury may appear as a small ecchymotic area or a large vulvar hematoma. The clinician must always suspect sexual abuse when a child presents with genital trauma.

   b. **Sexual abuse** necessitates immediate medical attention, including a complete physical examination, cervical and rectal smears, serologic tests, and psychological evaluation and follow-up. Genital findings, when present, should be recorded very carefully because of their importance in supporting allegations of abuse in court proceedings. The colposcope is used to document specific normal and abnormal findings. However, in cases of sexual abuse, 96% of patient abnormalities are detected with the unaided eye.

2. **Therapy**

   a. **Conservative therapy** for most trauma consists of rest, ice, and analgesics. When vaginal bleeding occurs as a result of pelvic trauma, a complete and thorough examination is mandatory. This includes evaluation of the urinary system and rectum. A vaginoscope is used to visualize the vagina to locate sources of bleeding. If a large vaginal laceration exists, a laparotomy may be necessary to ensure that an expanding hematoma is not present in the retroperitoneal space. Superficial abrasions and lacerations of the vulva, if not actively bleeding, may be cleaned and left alone.

   b. In sexual abuse, **antibiotic therapy** is advised as prophylaxis against some sexually transmitted diseases (STDs).

C. **Labial agglutination**

1. **Clinical picture.** Adhesion of the labia minora in the midline, usually the result of inflammation or skin disease, is the usual presentation. A line extends vertically downward and distinguishes labial agglutination from imperforate hymen or vaginal atresia. The agglutination encourages retention of urine and vaginal secretions. These patients frequently present with vulvovaginitis or a urinary tract infection.

2. **Therapy**

   a. If asymptomatic, **improved hygiene** may be all that is necessary. Treatment is indicated if there is a chronic vulvovaginitis or difficulty urinating.

   b. **Topical estrogen,** applied twice daily, induces cornification of the epithelium and promotes spontaneous separation. The use of estrogen in the prepubertal female, if prolonged, may stimulate breast growth and vaginal bleeding. Therapy must be limited to 2 weeks.

   c. **Surgical separation** is rarely necessary.

D. **Imperforate hymen**

1. **Clinical picture.** The usual presentation is a bulging introitus, which is usually an isolated anomaly.

2. **Therapy**

   a. Most are asymptomatic and will resolve at puberty.

   b. **Surgical correction** at puberty may be necessary if there is no spontaneous resolution.

   c. A **cruciate incision** is made in the hymen and excess tissue is removed. This creates enough space for the flow of menses as well as sexual activity.

E. **Prolapsed urethra**

1. **Clinical picture.** A small, hemorrhagic, friable mass surrounding the urethra is the most common presentation. The average age at diagnosis is 5 years. The bleeding is usually painless. The prolapse is thought to result from increased intraabdominal pressure. The lesion can easily be confused with condyloma. Acetic acid applied to con-

dyloma turns that tissue white. A prolapsed urethra will remain pink and fleshy in appearance.

2. Therapy

a. If voiding is uninhibited, local therapy may be all that is needed. Topical estrogen and sitz baths are the mainstays of therapy. The prolapse usually resolves after 4 weeks of therapy.

b. If urinary retention or necrosis is present, surgical removal and catheterization are necessary.

F. **Vaginal discharge**

1. Clinical picture

a. A **mucoid discharge** is common in infants for up to 2 weeks after birth as a result of maternal estrogen. It is also a common finding in prepubertal and postpubertal girls, as a result of increased estrogen production by maturing ovaries.

b. **Discharge** may also result from any of the following conditions:

(1) **Infections with organisms,** such as *Escherichia coli, Proteus, Pseudomonas,* yeast, *Gardnerella, Neisseria gonorrhoeae, Chlamydia,* and *Trichomonas*

(2) **Hemolytic streptococcal vaginitis,** which results in a bloody or serosanguineous discharge, usually after a streptococcal infection elsewhere (e.g., skin or throat)

(3) **Monilial vaginitis,** which is common in diabetic children or after antibiotic therapy

(4) **A foreign body,** which can cause persistent vaginal discharge, sometimes with pain and bleeding

(5) **Nonspecific vaginitis** from local irritation, scratching, manipulation, or poor hygiene

2. Therapy. Conservative management is advisable, as follows:

a. **Culture** to identify causative organisms. Preliminary search for *Monilia,* nonspecific bacteria, and *Trichomonas* can be accomplished with saline and sodium hydroxide (20%) preparations added to laboratory slides.

b. **Urinalysis** to rule out cystitis

c. **Review proper hygiene.** Instruct the child's mother to avoid tight clothing, perfume soaps, bubble bath, and powders. The child should avoid prolonged periods in moist clothing.

d. **Perianal examination** with transparent tape to test for pinworms

III. CONGENITAL ANOMALIES

A. **Vaginal atresia**

1. Clinical picture. Vaginal atresia represents a failure of caudal müllerian duct or sinovaginal bulb development of the urogenital sinus. Ovarian development is normal, but the uterus is functional in less than 10% of cases.

2. Therapy. Surgical correction should be deferred until the structures are well developed unless a functional uterus is present.

B. **Ectopic ureter with vaginal terminus**

1. Clinical picture

a. Ectopic ureter, the most common cause of vaginal cysts in infants, presents as a **ureterocele,** which appears as a cystic mass protruding from the vagina. If the ureter is patent, constant irritation and vaginitis may be presenting signs.

b. The ectopic ureter is usually one of a pair to a single kidney, and it almost always drains the rudimentary upper renal pole of the kidney.

c. **Hydroureter** and **hydronephrosis** may also develop.

2. Diagnosis is made through **intravenous pyelography,** which allows visualization of the entire urinary tract.

3. **Therapy.** Resecting the lowest portion of the ureter, then implanting it into the bladder is preferable to removing the ureter and the associated portion of the kidney.

C. **Vaginal ectopic anus**

1. **Clinical picture.** Vaginal ectopic anus is an imperforate anus associated with rectovaginal communication. Only a skin dimple is found at the normal anal site.

2. **Therapy.** Surgical correction is indicated.

IV. NEOPLASMS

A. **Tumors of the vagina,** although uncommon, are most often malignant. **Sarcoma botryoides** is the most common malignant vaginal tumor.

1. **Clinical picture**
   a. Sarcoma botryoides is a tumor that arises from mesenchymal tissue of the cervix or vagina, usually on the anterior wall of the upper vagina.
   b. It grows rapidly, fills the vagina, then protrudes through the introitus.
   c. It appears as an edematous, grape-like mass that bleeds readily on touch.
   d. It is usually multicentric, and extension is usually local, with rare instances of distant metastases.

2. **Therapy.** A combination of surgery and chemotherapy is most commonly used.

B. **Ovarian tumors**

1. **Clinical picture.** Although uncommon in children, these tumors can present as torsion (twisting) of the ovaries. Among ovarian neoplasms, 40% are of non–germ-cell origin (coelomic epithelium), and 60% are of germ-cell origin. Most ovarian neoplasms in adolescents are endocrine secreting, regardless of whether they are of germ-cell origin.
   a. **Non–germ-cell origin**
      (1) Lipoid cell tumors (feminizing)
      (2) Granulosa-theca cell tumors (feminizing), of which approximately 20% are malignant
   b. **Germ-cell origin**
      (1) Benign cystic teratomas
      (2) Benign cysts
      (3) Arrhenoblastomas (virilizing)
      (4) Germinomas and gonadoblastomas (tumors of dysgenetic gonads)
      (5) Endodermal sinus tumors
      (6) Embryonal carcinomas (gonadotropin secreting)
      (7) Immature teratomas, which account for 20% of malignant germ-cell tumors

2. **Therapy** is surgical, alone or in combination with radiation and chemotherapy, depending on the tumor.

V. DEVELOPMENTAL DEFECTS OF THE GENITALIA. Early diagnosis is important so that proper assignment of sex can take place during the neonatal period, and the management plan established at that point can minimize psychological problems and help establish the gender role.

A. **Congenital adrenal hyperplasia** results when enzymatic regulation of the biosynthesis of cortisol and aldosterone is impaired at various steps in the pathway. Adrenocorticotropic hormone secretion by the pituitary is increased as a result of low levels of blood cortisol. Both the precursors immediately preceding the impaired step and the by-products have biologic activity that can lead to the clinical and biochemical features observed. The 21-hydroxylase defect is the most common cause of distinct virilization of the female newborn. Its incidence is 1/5000 births, and it accounts for 95% of all cases of congenital adrenal hyperplasia, which is inherited as an autosomal recessive trait.

1. **Clinical picture.** The chromosomes, gonads, and internal genitalia are female, and the degree of closure of the urogenital orifice varies. Clitoral enlargement and accentuation of labial folds are characteristic. The disorder is progressive if untreated.

2. **Diagnosis.** Urinary levels of pregnanetriol and 17-ketosteroids and plasma levels of 17-hydroxyprogesterone are elevated.

3. **Therapy.** Hydrocortisone is administered indefinitely to all patients.

B. **Adrenal tumors,** which may cause virilization of the external genitalia after infancy, should be suspected in children with very high levels of urinary 17-ketosteroid excretion.

C. **Maternal ingestion of synthetic progestins** can result in **masculinization of the female fetus.**

1. **Clinical picture.** Masculinization is limited to the external genitalia. The clitoris is enlarged, and the labia may be fused, but the vagina, tubes, and uterus are normal. Growth and development are normal, and progressive virilization does not occur.

2. **Diagnosis** can be made from a positive history and by exclusion.

3. **Therapy.** Clitoral reduction and surgical correction of fused labia may be necessary.

D. **Androgen ingestion** by children is usually through preparations that have androgenic activity.

1. **Clinical manifestations** are the same as those resulting from maternal ingestion of synthetic progestins (i.e., masculinization; see V C 1).

2. **Therapy** involves clitoral reduction and surgical correction of fused labia, if necessary.

E. **Androgen insensitivity syndrome (testicular feminization)**

1. **Clinical picture.** Androgen insensitivity is characterized by a 46,XY genotype and a female phenotype. The vagina ends as a blind pouch, and testicles are present in the labia. These patients, who are often reared as girls, have a deficiency of androgen receptors. The external genitalia can appear virilized in the incomplete form (Reifenstein's syndrome).

2. **Therapy.** The testicles should be removed after puberty and maturation because of an increased risk of malignancy (3%–4% before age 25 years).

F. **True hermaphroditism**

1. **Clinical picture.** The genotype of most true hermaphrodites is 46,XX. The external genitalia may appear male, female, or ambiguous. Both male and female internal genitalia may be present. Sex assignment and rearing should be consistent with the dominant appearance of the external genitalia and with surgical correctability.

2. **Therapy.** The genitalia that are inconsistent with sex assignment should be surgically removed or modified.

G. **Maternal virilizing tumor during pregnancy** (luteoma of pregnancy) can result in masculinization of the female fetus. The clinical picture and the therapy are similar to those for the maternal ingestion of synthetic progestins (see V C).

VI. SPECIAL PROBLEMS OF THE ADOLESCENT

A. Dysmenorrhea

1. **Clinical picture**
   a. Dysmenorrhea may be secondary to obstructions and other anatomic causes.
   b. Nausea, vomiting, and diarrhea are common accompaniments.

2. **Etiology.** Frequently, no organic cause is found.

3. **Therapy** includes antiemetics and prostaglandin inhibitors.

B. Dysfunctional uterine bleeding (DUB) is defined as excessive, prolonged, or irregular bleeding that is not associated with an anatomic lesion. Most adolescent girls have anovulatory menstrual periods for the first 2 to 3 years after menarche. Approximately 2% of adolescents ovulate regularly in the first 6 months after menarche, and 18% by the end of the first year, making DUB secondary to anovulation very common in this age-group.

1. **Etiology.** The cause of DUB in 75% of cases is an **immature hypothalamic–pituitary axis,** which results in anovulation. Other causes include psychogenic factors, juvenile hypothyroidism, and coagulation disorders (von Willebrand's disease).

2. **Clinical picture**
   a. **Menometrorrhagia** is the most characteristic symptom.
   b. The condition is usually self-limited, but if symptoms persist for more than 4 years, the chance of future DUB is 50%.

3. **Therapy** is cyclic hormonal manipulation with estrogens and progestins.

C. Amenorrhea. Primary amenorrhea categorizes menarche that has not yet occurred, and secondary amenorrhea categorizes menstruation that ceases for more than 6 months. Late menarche or oligomenorrhea are common before age 16 years. Evaluation is indicated if menarche is delayed beyond 16 years of age. Chromosomal abnormalities account for approximately 30% to 40% of all cases of primary amenorrhea. Other causes of amenorrhea include malnutrition; delayed puberty; systemic illness; central nervous system (CNS) lesions; tumors; and psychogenic (anorexia nervosa), anatomic, hypothalamic, and metabolic disorders.

1. **Müllerian anomalies and vaginal atresia** represent the cause in 20% of cases of amenorrhea. Of these patients, 45% have associated urinary tract abnormalities.
   a. **Mayer-Rokitansky-Küster-Hauser syndrome** involves vaginal agenesis with or without uterine agenesis. Adolescents may present with cyclic abdominal pain and amenorrhea when a partial endometrial cavity is present.
   b. An **imperforate hyman** is easily diagnosed. A bulging introitus with cyclic abdominal pain is a classic presentation. Secondary sexual characteristics are abnormal.

2. **Hypogonadotropic hypogonadism,** which is characterized by a deficiency of pituitary or hypothalamic hormone secretion (particularly gonadotropin), accounts for 40% to 50% of all cases of amenorrhea. **Kallmann's syndrome** is an autosomal dominant disorder that involves a deficiency of gonadotropin-releasing hormone (GnRH). Hypopituitarism with obesity (adiposogenital dystrophy) manifests as adiposity of breasts, mons pubis, and pelvic girdle, accompanied by atrophy of the genitalia. The etiology is unknown.

3. **Systemic illnesses,** including infections; hepatic, thyroid, and adrenal diseases; diabetes mellitus; cystic fibrosis; and hemoglobinopathies (e.g., sickle cell anemia and thalassemia) may be responsible for amenorrhea.

4. **CNS lesions,** including space-occupying lesions (e.g., craniopharyngioma, pinealomas, adenomas), **trauma,** and **vascular lesions** may play a role in amenorrhea and delayed adolescent development.

5. **Anorexia nervosa,** characterized by extreme weight loss with no known organic cause, can affect adolescent development and cause amenorrhea. Psychiatric symptoms can be present, and, occasionally, the outcome is fatal.

6. **Gonadal dysgenesis** (hypergonadotropic hypogonadism) is characterized by absence of secondary sex characteristics, infantile but normal genitalia, and streak-like gonads that are devoid of germ cells and appear as fibrous white streaks. The presence of a Y chromosome dictates early removal of the gonads because of their propensity to malignancy (25% of cases by age 15 years). The different forms of gonadal dysgenesis are as follows:

   a. **Turner's syndrome (45,X)** is characterized at birth by low weight, short stature, edema of the hands and feet, and loose skin folds on the neck. Adolescent patients have short stature, lack of sexual maturation, low posterior hairline, prominent ears, broad chest, and epicanthal folds.

   b. **Swyer's syndrome (46,XY)** is characterized by a female phenotype with amenorrhea and a lack of secondary sex characteristics. Growth is usually normal, and some virilization may occur after puberty, especially when gonadal tumors are present. This clinical picture without virilization and tumor propensity can also occur in 46,XX individuals, whose condition is termed **pure gonadal dysgenesis.** Swyer's syndrome is inherited as an X-linked recessive trait. Pure gonadal dysgenesis is compatible with autosomal recessive inheritance.

   c. **Mixed gonadal dysgenesis (45,X/46,XY mosaicism)** is characterized by sexual ambiguity in the newborn. Internal structures include müllerian and wolffian derivatives. Asymmetric development of the gonads is expressed as a testis or gonadal tumor on one side, with a rudimentary gonad, a streak, or no gonad on the other side.

   d. **Abnormalities of the X chromosome** (mosaicism, isochromosome, short arm X deletion, long arm X deletion, and translocation) result in amenorrhea and varying degrees of Turner's syndrome features.

D. **Delayed puberty.** Although most adolescents with delayed puberty prove to have no underlying physiologic or anatomic (constitutional) abnormality, evaluation is indicated if no secondary sex characteristics appear by 13 years of age.

1. **Etiology.** The causes of amenorrhea mentioned previously apply to delayed puberty as well. Disorders that are only associated with delayed puberty include Hand-Schüller-Christian disease, developmental defects of the midbrain, dwarfism, Prader-Willi syndrome, and Laurence-Moon-Biedl syndrome.

2. **Diagnosis** is based on neurologic, physical, and pelvic examinations; measurement of gonadotropin levels; karyotype; and endocrine profiles.

3. **Therapy** is simply gonadal steroid replacement (estrogen with progesterone).

E. **Precocious puberty** is characterized by early sexual maturation with menarche before 9 years of age.

1. **Types of precocious puberty**

   a. **Heterosexual precocious puberty** is the development of secondary sex characteristics that are inconsistent with genetic sex. The causes may include tumors (arrhenoblastomas), congenital adrenal hyperplasia, and chronic ingestion of androgenic preparations.

   b. **Isosexual precocious puberty** is the development of secondary sex characteristics consistent with genetic sex. Precocious puberty can be divided into **true sexual precocity,** in which the hormones are secreted by maturing gonads, and **precocious pseudopuberty,** in which maturing normal gonads are not the source of the sex steroids.

   (1) **Clinical picture.** It has been found that 80% to 90% of cases of isosexual precocious puberty have no obvious underlying etiology (i.e., they are idiopathic). A family history can sometimes be elicited. The clinical course is usually benign. Patients are larger than normal for chronologic age (height, weight, and bone age). Somatic and genital development are consistent with bone age. Early closure of the epiphyses causes the final height to be less than normal. Intellectual capacity is not accelerated or reduced, although abnormalities have been noted on the electroencephalogram for most of these

patients. Psychological development and mental capacity are consistent with chronologic age. Sexual activity is usually not premature. Reproductive potential is not adversely affected, and the patient can become pregnant.

(2) **Therapy.** Progestational agents have been used in the past but are associated with significant side effects. GnRH agonists are effective and represent the most significant advance in the management of precocious puberty. The agents are potent and long-acting. They can be given intranasally and subcutaneously. When treatment is stopped, pubertal development resumes. Menses occur by 6 to 12 months after treatment. Predictions of height outcome improve with agonist therapy. Because height is always compromised in children with precocious puberty, any therapy should be evaluated by its effect on height improvement.

2. **Causes of precocious puberty**
   a. **CNS disorders**
      (1) Trauma to the hypothalamus
      (2) Postinflammatory reactions (e.g., toxoplasmosis, congenital syphilis, tuberculosis, encephalitis, and meningitis)
   b. **Congenital anomalies**
      (1) McCune-Albright syndrome, a polyostotic fibrous dysplasia characterized by café au lait spots distributed unilaterally over the osseous lesions, with fractures and deformities of the long bones
      (2) Hemangioma of the hypothalamus
      (3) Tuberous sclerosis
      (4) Hydrocephalus
      (5) Neurofibromatosis
      (6) Intracranial neoplasms that occupy the floor of the third ventricle
   c. **Chronic ingestion of estrogens,** usually oral contraceptives or tonics, lotions, or creams containing estrogen
   d. **Adrenal estrogen-secreting tumor** (rare)
   e. **Estrogen-producing ovarian neoplasm or cyst,** such as granulosa-theca cell tumor

3. **Diagnosis** of precocious puberty is based on physical, ophthalmologic, and radiologic signs; endocrine profile; and, possibly, laparoscopy or laparotomy to diagnose occult tumors.

4. **Therapy** is aimed at slowing down the accelerated growth, reducing pituitary, ovarian, or adrenal function, and inducing regression of secondary sex characteristics. In cases of known or organic etiology, therapy is with surgery, chemotherapy, or radiation, as indicated.

F. **Contraception.** Most sexually active adolescents do not use contraception, especially at the time of the first sexual act. In addition, the young patient will probably not mention contraception; therefore, a discussion about using contraceptives and preventing the transmission of STDs should follow a physical examination, regardless of whether the patient is sexually active.

G. **Sexual abuse** is defined as sexual touch by someone at least 5 years older than the adolescent. It incorporates a wide range of behavior, from coerced seduction to violent assault. Rape is a form of sexual abuse.

1. **Incidence.** Seven percent of American men and women at ages 18 to 22 years have experienced at least one episode of nonvoluntary sexual intercourse.

2. **Diagnosis.** Lack of findings on examination does not mean that abuse did not occur. A thorough history, assessment of family and environment, and laboratory studies should accompany the findings on examination to establish the diagnosis.

3. **Follow-up studies** suggest that many people, particularly adolescents, may remain disabled long after the abuse has ended.

STUDY QUESTIONS

DIRECTIONS: Each of the numbered items or incomplete statements in this section is followed by answers or by completions of the statement. Select the ONE lettered answer or completion that is BEST in each case.

1. Sexual ambiguity may be seen in which of the following conditions?

(A) Androgen insensitivity syndrome
(B) Pure gonadal dysgenesis
(C) Swyer's syndrome
(D) Mixed gonadal dysgenesis
(E) Structural abnormalities of the X chromosome

2. In idiopathic precocious puberty, the parents should be warned that

(A) final height will be less than that of peers
(B) premature heterosexual activity is common
(C) future reproductive potential is adversely affected
(D) mental capacity is also advanced
(E) there is no satisfactory therapy

3. Which of the following conditions is commonly encountered in the female newborn and usually requires no therapy?

(A) Enlarged clitoris
(B) Labial fusion
(C) Mucoid vaginal discharge
(D) Prolapsed urethra
(E) Ectopic anus

4. The most common characteristic of ovarian neoplasms in adolescents is

(A) endocrine secreting, germ-cell origin
(B) endocrine secreting, coelomic epithelial origin
(C) nonendocrine secreting, germ-cell origin
(D) non–germ-cell origin
(E) coelomic epithelial origin

5. Persistent vaginal discharge in a pediatric patient should prompt a search for which of the following?

(A) Foreign body
(B) Pinworms
(C) Illicit drug use
(D) Vaginal lacerations
(E) Ectopic ureter

DIRECTIONS: The numbered item or incomplete statement in this section is negatively phrased, as indicated by a capitalized word such as NOT, LEAST, or EXCEPT. Select the ONE lettered answer or completion that is BEST.

6. Which of the following statements concerning congenital adrenal hyperplasia is NOT correct?

(A) The incidence is 1/5000 births
(B) It is self-limiting and rarely requires therapy
(C) The internal genitalia are normal
(D) It is the most common cause of virilization in the newborn female
(E) The most common defect is of 21-hydroxylase

DIRECTIONS: The set of matching questions in this section consists of a list of lettered options (some of which may be in figures) followed by several numbered items. For each numbered item, select the ONE lettered option that is most closely associated with it. To avoid spending too much time on matching sets with large numbers of options, it is generally advisable to begin each set by reading the list of options. Then, for each item in the set, try to generate the correct answer and locate it in the option list, rather than evaluating each option individually. Each lettered option may be selected once, more than once, or not at all.

Questions 7–9

For each diagnosis listed below, select the underlying etiology.

(A) Immature hypothalamic–pituitary axis
(B) Sarcoma botryoides
(C) 21-Hydroxylase defect

7. Dysfunctional uterine bleeding (DUB) in an adolescent girl

8. Heterosexual precocious puberty

9. Congenital adrenal hyperplasia

■ANSWERS AND EXPLANATIONS

1. The answer is D [V E; VI C 6 b–d]. Most patients with mixed gonadal dysgenesis have the genotype XO/XY or some form of mosaicism. The Y chromosome results in a unilateral testis and, therefore, ambiguous genitalia at puberty. Patients with testicular feminization and other types of gonadal dysgenesis have female external genitalia.

2. The answer is A [VI E 1 b (1)]. In idiopathic precocious puberty, early tall stature is followed by short adult height secondary to early closure of the epiphyses—a factor that may cause emotional problems. Children who have idiopathic precocious puberty do not exhibit accelerated intellectual and psychological development. Ongoing studies have shown that gonadotropin-releasing hormone (GnRH) analogues are the most effective therapy.

3. The answer is C [I A 1]. A thin and mucoid vaginal discharge is often seen in newborns and is secondary to the high levels of maternal estrogens present in pregnancy. The discharge resolves without intervention as the maternal estrogen levels in the infant decline.

4. The answer is A [IV B 1 a, b]. Most ovarian neoplasms in adolescents are endocrine secreting regardless of whether the neoplasms are of germ-cell origin. The germ-cell variety is the most common.

5. The answer is A [II F 1 b (4)]. Persistent vaginal discharge, which is often associated with pain (regardless of the cause of the discharge) should raise suspicion for the presence of a foreign body in the vagina. General anesthesia may be necessary to perform a thorough examination of the vagina.

6. The answer is B [V A 1–3]. Elevation of androgenic steroids preceding the block in the biosynthetic pathway leads to persistent virilization of the external genitalia (internal genitalia are normal) and heterosexual precocity if therapy is not instituted. The steroids secreted do not affect the negative feedback on adrenocorticotropic hormone production, which is also increased. Hydrocortisone is administered indefinitely to all patients; the disorder is progressive if untreated.

7–9. The answers are: 7-A [VI B 1], **8-C** [VI E 1 a], **9-C** [V A]. Irregular bleeding in adolescent girls in the absence of organic pathology is known as dysfunctional uterine bleeding (DUB). The usual cause is an immature hypothalamic–pituitary axis. Sarcoma botryoides is a malignant tumor of the vagina. Heterosexual precocious puberty is the development of secondary sex characteristics that are inconsistent with genetic sex. The etiology may include tumors (arrhenoblastomas), congenital adrenal hyperplasia, or chronic ingestion of androgenic preparations. Congenital adrenal hyperplasia results when enzymatic regulation of the biosynthesis of cortisol and aldosterone is impaired. The 21-hydroxylase defect is the most common cause of distinct virilization of the female newborn.

Chapter 20

The Menstrual Cycle

William W. Beck, Jr.

I. **INTRODUCTION.** The menstrual cycle is characterized by the regular occurrence of ovulation throughout the reproductive life of a woman. The cycle is divided into two phases: the follicular (or proliferative) phase and the luteal (or secretory) phase.

A. **Length of the cycle**

1. The **mean duration** of the cycle is **28 days,** plus or minus 7 days.
   a. **Polymenorrhea** is defined as menstrual cycles that occur at short intervals (less than 21 days).
   b. **Oligomenorrhea** is defined as menstrual cycles that occur at long intervals (more than 35 days).

2. Menstrual cycles are the most irregular during the 2 years after menarche (i.e., the first menses) and during the 3 years before menopause. At both times, **anovulation** (i.e., absent ovulation) is most common.

B. **Follicular or proliferative phase.** This phase lasts from the first day of menses until ovulation, during which time the **endometrial glands** proliferate under the influence of **estrogen,** primarily **estradiol.** The follicular phase is characterized by:

1. Variable length
2. Low basal body temperature
3. Development of ovarian follicles
4. Vascular growth of the endometrium
5. Secretion of estrogen from the ovary

C. **Luteal or secretory phase.** The second part of the cycle extends from ovulation until the onset of menses. Under the influence of progesterone, the endometrial glands develop the secretory status necessary for implantation of the embryo. The luteal phase is characterized by:

1. A fairly constant duration of 12 to 16 days
2. An elevated basal body temperature (over 98° F)
3. The formation of the **corpus luteum** in the ovary, with the secretion of progesterone and estrogen
4. An endometrium that reveals gland tortuosity and secretion, stromal edema, and a decidual reaction

D. **Cycle integration.** The integration of the menstrual cycle involves the interaction among **gonadotropin-releasing hormone** (GnRH), the **gonadotropins** [i.e., follicle-stimulating hormone (FSH) and luteinizing hormone (LH)], and the **sex steroids** (i.e., androstenedione, estradiol, estrone, and progesterone).

II. **GnRH** is the hypothalamic hormone that controls gonadotropin release.

A. **Characteristics**

1. GnRH is a decapeptide with 10 amino acids.
2. It is produced by hypothalamic neurons, principally from the arcuate nucleus, and is

transported along axons that terminate in the median eminence around capillaries of the primary portal plexus.

3. It is secreted into the portal circulation, which carries it to the anterior lobe of the pituitary gland.

B. **Secretion**

1. GnRH is secreted in a **pulsatile manner;** the amplitude and frequency of the secretions vary throughout the cycle.
   a. One pulse every hour is typical of the follicular phase.
   b. One pulse every 2 to 3 hours is typical of the luteal phase.

2. The **amplitude and frequency** are regulated by:
   a. Feedback of estrogen and progesterone
   b. Neurotransmitters within the brain, mainly the catecholamines dopamine (inhibitory) and norepinephrine (facilatory)

C. **Action of GnRH on gonadotropin production**

1. Synthesis and storage (the reserve pool) of gonadotropins

2. Activation and movement of gonadotropins from the reserve pool to a pool ready for secretion

3. Immediate release of gonadotropins

4. Stimulates the synthesis and release of both FSH and LH from the same cell

5. When GnRH binds to specific receptors on the surface membrane of target cells, it:
   a. Activates a second messenger, **adenyl cyclase**
   b. Changes the concentration of cyclic adenosine monophosphate (**cAMP**)

6. High, prolonged GnRH exposure saturates the GnRH receptors and inhibits FSH and LH secretion. This is desensitization or downregulation.

III. **GONADOTROPINS: FSH AND LH**

A. **FSH receptors** exist primarily on the **granulosa cell membrane.**

1. FSH acts primarily on the granulosa cells, where it stimulates follicular growth.

2. It stimulates formation of LH receptors.

3. It activates the aromatase and 3-hydroxysteroid dehydrogenase enzymes.

4. It stimulates follicular growth by increasing both FSH and LH receptors in granulosa cells; the estradiol being produced by the granulosa cells enhances this action.

B. **LH receptors** exist on **theca cells** at all stages of the cycle and on **granulosa cells** after the follicle matures under the influence of FSH and estradiol.

1. LH stimulates **androgen synthesis** by the theca cells.

2. With a sufficient number of LH receptors on the granulosa cells, LH acts directly on the granulosa cells to cause **luteinization** (i.e., the formation of the corpus luteum) and the production of progesterone.

C. **Two-cell hypothesis of estrogen production** (Figure 20-1)

1. LH acts on the theca cells to produce androgens (i.e., androstenedione and testosterone).

2. Androgens are transported from the theca cells to the granulosa cells.

3. Androgens are aromatized to estrogens (i.e., estradiol and estrone) by the action of FSH on the enzyme aromatase in the granulosa cells.

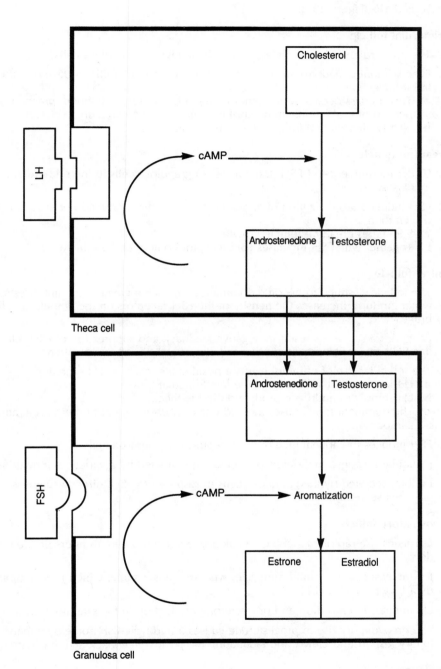

FIGURE 20-1. Two-cell hypothesis of estrogen production. *cAMP* = cyclic adenosine monophosphate; *FSH* = follicle-stimulating hormone; *LH* = luteinizing hormone. (Reprinted with permission from Speroff L, Glass RH, Kase NG: Regulation of the menstrual cycle. In *Clinical Gynecologic Endocrinology and Infertility*. Baltimore, Williams & Wilkins, 1989, p 94.)

IV. OOGENESIS (Figure 20-2)

A. Primordial follicle

1. The primordial follicle is covered by a single layer of granulosa cells.

2. Even without gonadotropin stimulation, some primordial follicles develop into preantral follicles.
   a. This process occurs during times of anovulation (i.e., childhood, pregnancy, and periods of oral contraceptive use) as well as during ovulatory cycles.
   b. Nearly all preantral follicles become atretic.

B. Preantral follicle

1. Under the influence of FSH, the number of granulosa cells in the primordial follicle increases.

2. FSH-induced aromatization of androgen results in the production of estrogen. The **estrogen** then:
   a. Stimulates preantral follicle growth
   b. Together with FSH increases FSH receptor content of the follicle

C. Antral follicle

1. The follicle destined to become dominant secretes the greatest amount of estradiol, which, in turn, increases the density of the FSH receptors on the granulosa cell membrane.

2. Rising estradiol levels result in negative feedback and suppression of FSH release; this halts the development of other follicles, which then become atretic.

3. The follicular rise of estradiol exerts a positive feedback on LH secretion.
   a. LH levels rise steadily during the late follicular phase.
   b. LH stimulates androgen production in the theca.
   c. The dominant follicle uses the androgen as substrate and further accelerates estrogen output.

4. FSH induces the appearance of LH receptors on granulosa cells.

5. Follicular response to the gonadotropins is modulated by a variety of growth factors.

6. Inhibin, secreted by the granulosa cells in response to FSH, directly suppresses pituitary FSH secretion.

D. Preovulatory follicle

1. Estrogens rise rapidly, reaching a peak approximately 24 to 36 hours before ovulation.

2. LH increases steadily until midcycle, when there is a surge, which is accompanied by a lesser surge of FSH.

3. LH initiates luteinization and progesterone production in the granulosa layer.

4. The preovulatory rise in progesterone causes a midcycle FSH surge by enhancing pituitary response to GnRH and facilitating the positive feedback action of estrogen.

E. Ovulation

1. Ovulation occurs approximately 10 to 12 hours after the LH peak and 24 to 36 hours after the estradiol peak; the **onset** of the LH surge, which occurs 34 to 36 hours before ovulation, is the most reliable indicator of the timing of ovulation.

2. The LH surge stimulates the following:
   a. Completion of reduction division in the oocyte
   b. Luteinization of the granulosa cells
   c. Synthesis of progesterone and prostaglandins within the follicle

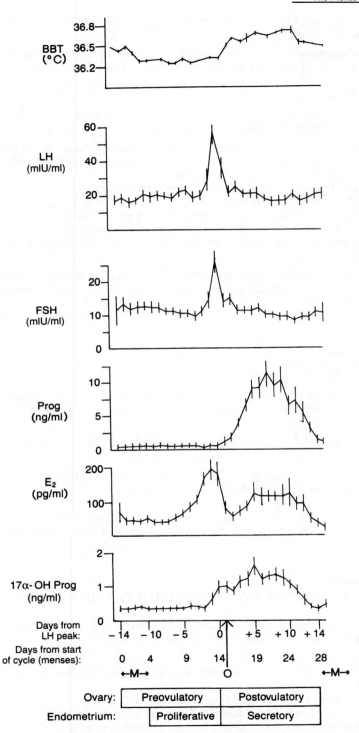

FIGURE 20-2. Hormonal (ovarian and pituitary), uterine (endometrial), and basal body temperature (*BBT*), correlates of the normal menstrual cycle. Mean plasma concentrations (±SEM) of luteinizing hormone (*LH*), follicle-stimulating hormone (*FSH*), progesterone (*Prog*), estradiol (*E₂*) [day +1] and 17 α-hydroxyprogesterone (17 α-OH Prog) are shown as a function of time. Ovulation occurs on day 15 (day +1) after the LH surge, which occurs at midcycle on day 14 (day 0). *M* = menses; *O* = ovulation. (Adapted from Thorneycroft IA, et al: The relation of serum 17-hydroxyprogesterone and estradiol 17-β levels during the human menstrual cycle. *Am J Obstet Gynecol* 111:947–951, 1971.)

3. Prostaglandins and proteolytic enzymes are responsible for the digestion and rupture of the follicle wall.

4. The progesterone-dependent midcycle rise in FSH frees the oocyte from follicular attachments and ensures sufficient LH receptors for an adequate luteal phase.

F. Corpus luteum

1. Peak levels of progesterone are attained 8 to 9 days after ovulation, which approximates the time of implantation of the embryo.

2. Normal luteal function requires optimal preovulatory follicular development.
   a. Suppression of FSH during the follicular phase is associated with:
      (1) Low preovulatory estradiol levels
      (2) Depressed midluteal progesterone production
      (3) Small luteal cell mass
   b. The accumulation of LH receptors during the follicular phase sets the stage for the extent of luteinization and the functional capacity of the corpus luteum.
   c. A defective luteal phase can contribute to both infertility and early pregnancy wastage.

3. In early pregnancy, human chorionic gonadotropin maintains luteal function, with secretion of progesterone, until placental steroidogenesis (production of progesterone) is established.

V. MENSTRUATION

A. In the absence of a pregnancy, decreasing steroid levels lead to increased coiling and constriction of the spiral arteries, which supply the upper two thirds of the functional endometrium.

1. The decreased blood flow to the functional portion of the endometrium causes **ischemia** and degradation of endometrial tissue.

2. The bleeding, or **menses,** is the result of the degraded endometrial tissue, which is desquamated, or shed, into the uterine cavity.

B. Within 2 days of the onset of menses, the surface epithelium begins to regenerate under the influence of estrogen and continues this process while the endometrium is shedding.

VI. CLINICAL PROBLEMS ASSOCIATED WITH THE MENSTRUAL CYCLE

A. **Dysmenorrhea.** Painful menses usually begin with ovulatory menstrual periods and are the most common medical problem in young women.

1. **Clinical aspects**
   a. Dysmenorrhea begins just before or with the onset of menses and lasts 24 to 48 hours.
   b. The pain is suprapubic, sharp, and colicky.
   c. Nausea, diarrhea, and headache may accompany the pain.
   d. Dysmenorrhea does not occur in anovulatory cycles.

2. **Physiology**
   a. Menstrual cramps are the result of **uterine contractions.**
   b. **Prostaglandins** are potent **stimulators** of uterine contractions.
   c. Endometrial prostaglandins are produced during the luteal phase. If ovulation does not occur, there is no luteal increase in prostaglandins.

  d. In the first-day menstrual endometrium, the prostaglandin level increases until it is several times higher than its concentration in the luteal phase.

3. Management
  a. Prostaglandin synthetase inhibitors (e.g., nonsteroidal antiinflammatory drugs) have the following properties; they:
   (1) Decrease levels of endometrial prostaglandin
   (2) Lessen uterine contractions
   (3) Relieve dysmenorrhea
  b. Combination (estrogen plus progestin) **oral contraceptive agents** eliminate ovulation.
   (1) Estrogen followed by progesterone (in ovulatory cycles) is necessary to produce high menstrual levels of prostaglandin in the endometrium.
   (2) Combination oral contraceptives prevent dysmenorrhea by eliminating the natural estrogen–progesterone progression found only in ovulatory cycles.
   (3) In the absence of ovulation, there is little or no dysmenorrhea.

B. **Premenstrual syndrome (PMS).** This set of symptoms (or molimina) occurs with the approach of menses and usually ends abruptly with the onset of bleeding.

1. Clinical aspects
  a. Over 100 symptoms have been attributed to PMS. The most common are:
   (1) Abdominal bloating
   (2) Anxiety
   (3) Breast tenderness
   (4) Crying spells
   (5) Depression
   (6) Fatigue
   (7) Irritability
   (8) Weight gain
  b. Premenstrual symptoms can exist in women with stable or unstable personalities.

2. Etiology. The etiology of PMS is elusive and has been associated with excesses or deficiencies of progesterone, estrogen, prolactin, aldosterone, pyridoxine, opioids, unrecognized mineralocorticoids, and monoamine oxidase activity.

3. Management. Both the physiologic and the psychosocial aspects of PMS must be considered when designing a therapeutic program. Basic measures include:
  a. Regular exercise and a balanced diet
  b. Vitamin B_6, 200 mg/day, on a daily basis
  c. Luteal-phase progesterone or estrogen, depending on perceived need
  d. Diuretics
  e. Oral contraceptives and elimination of the ovulatory sequence
  f. Therapy with psychoactive drugs such as alprozolam (Xanax) and fluoxetine hydrochloride (Prozac), in relatively small doses given during the luteal phase, has been helpful in relieving PMS symptoms

STUDY QUESTIONS

DIRECTIONS: Each of the numbered items or incomplete statements in this section is followed by answers or by completions of the statement. Select the ONE lettered answer or completion that is BEST in each case.

1. The average length of the menstrual cycle is

(A) 22 days
(B) 25 days
(C) 28 days
(D) 35 days
(E) 38 days

2. The establishment and maintenance of the menstrual cycle depend on

(A) prolactin release by the anterior pituitary
(B) pulsatile secretion of gonadotropin-releasing hormone (GnRH)
(C) a follicular phase of variable length
(D) progesterone synthesis by the corpus luteum
(E) estrogen secretion by the ovary

3. Gonadotropin-releasing hormone (GnRH) controls the synthesis and secretion of which of the following substances?

(A) Follicle-stimulating hormone (FSH) and luteinizing hormone (LH)
(B) Dopamine
(C) Prolactin
(D) Norepinephrine
(E) Thyrotropin-releasing hormone (TRH)

4. The best predictor of ovulation is

(A) estrogen peak
(B) follicle-stimulating hormone (FSH) surge
(C) onset of the luteinizing hormone (LH) surge
(D) preovulatory rise in progesterone
(E) the LH peak

5. Which of the following is fundamental in the etiology of dysmenorrhea?

(A) Prostaglandin release
(B) Drop in progesterone
(C) Ovulation
(D) Secretory endometrium
(E) Corpus luteum

6. Dysmenorrhea would be most likely to occur in which of the following women?

(A) A young teenager
(B) A woman on birth-control pills
(C) A 48-year-old woman with irregular cycles
(D) A marathon runner with one menses per year
(E) A 35-year-old woman with regular cycles

DIRECTIONS: Each of the numbered items or incomplete statements in this section is negatively phrased, as indicated by a capitalized word such as NOT, LEAST, or EXCEPT. Select the ONE lettered answer or completion that is BEST in each case.

7. Which of the following changes in the endometrium do NOT occur during the menstrual cycle?

(A) Proliferation of glandular cells
(B) Plasma cell infiltration
(C) Vascular growth
(D) Stromal edema
(E) Decidual reaction

8. Which of the following statements about the two-cell hypothesis of estrogen production is NOT correct?

(A) Theca cells produce androstenedione
(B) Luteinizing hormone (LH) stimulates theca cells
(C) Aromatization of androgens takes place in the granulosa cells
(D) Follicle-stimulating hormone (FSH) activates the enzyme aromatase
(E) Estradiol is transported to the theca cells

9. Which of the following is NOT characteristic of the follicular phase of the menstrual cycle?

(A) Variable length
(B) Growth and development of the ovarian follicles
(C) Basal body temperature over 98° F
(D) Vascular growth of the endometrium
(E) Secretion of estrogen from the ovary

10. Which of the following is NOT a physiologic characteristic of menstruation?

(A) Constriction of spiral arteries
(B) Desquamation of endometrial tissue
(C) Ischemia of endometrial tissue
(D) Estrogen secretion
(E) Decline in prostaglandin

DIRECTIONS: The set of matching questions in this section consists of a list of four to twenty-six lettered options (some of which may be in figures) followed by several numbered items. For each numbered item, select the ONE lettered option that is most closely associated with it. To avoid spending too much time on matching sets with large numbers of options, it is generally advisable to begin each set by reading the list of options. Then, for each item in the set, try to generate the correct answer and locate it in the option list, rather than evaluating each option individually. Each lettered option may be selected once, more than once, or not at all.

Questions 11–14

For each activity listed, select the hormone that is most likely to be responsible for it.

(A) Follicle-stimulating hormone (FSH)
(B) Luteinizing hormone (LH)
(C) Both
(D) Neither

11. Stimulates androgen secretion

12. Stimulates aromatase activity

13. Stimulates prolactin release

14. Stimulates target cells in the ovary

ANSWERS AND EXPLANATIONS

1. The answer is C [I A 1]. The length of the normal menstrual cycle varies between 21 and 35 days, the average length being about 28 to 30 days. The preovulatory phase of a normal cycle often varies in length, from 8 to 21 days, whereas the postovulatory phase (about 2 weeks) usually is fairly constant in length.

2. The answer is B [II B, C 1]. Hourly pulses of gonadotropin-releasing hormone (GnRH) given intravenously lead to the onset and establishment of menses in prepubertal monkeys. Discontinuation of the GnRH infusion results in amenorrhea. Thus, this pulsatile activity is a prerequisite for the establishment and maintenance of the menstrual cycle; what follows this activity are the components of a normal menstrual cycle: estrogen secretion from the ovary, a follicular phase of variable length, ovulation, the establishment of the corpus luteum, and the secretion of progesterone from the corpus luteum.

3. The answer is A [II B 2, C 1]. Gonadotropin-releasing hormone (GnRH) controls the synthesis and secretion of the gonadotropins follicle-stimulating hormone (FSH) and luteinizing hormone (LH). The catecholamines dopamine and norepinephrine are neurotransmitters that influence the release of GnRH. Thyrotropin-releasing hormone (TRH) stimulates prolactin and thyroid-stimulating hormone (TSH) secretion. However, GnRH has no effect on prolactin.

4. The answer is C [IV D 1, 2, E 1]. The onset of the luteinizing hormone (LH) surge, which occurs 28 to 32 hours before ovulation, is the most reliable indicator of the timing of ovulation. The estrogen peak occurs about 24 to 36 hours before ovulation, the LH peak is about 10 to 12 hours before ovulation, and a small follicle-stimulating hormone (FSH) rise occurs along with the LH surge. However, none of these events is as predictive of ovulation as the onset of the LH surge. The preovulatory rise in progesterone is important in stimulating the midcycle rise in FSH, but it is not a predictor of ovulation.

5. The answer is C [VI A 1 d, 3 b (3)]. In the absence of ovulation, dysmenorrhea does not occur. All the other factors are involved, but they are the consequences of ovulation. With ovulation comes the formation of a corpus luteum, which establishes a secretory endometrium under the influence of progesterone. The drop in progesterone that occurs at the end of a cycle may relate to the release of prostaglandin. However, all of this activity depends on ovulation. Dysmenorrhea does not occur in anovulatory cycles.

6. The answer is E [I A 2; VI A 1 d, 3]. Among the five women, the 35-year-old woman with regular cycles is the most likely to have dysmenorrhea. She is having regular cycles, which can be assumed to be ovulatory in nature. Dysmenorrhea does not occur in the absence of ovulation. The young teenager is postmenarchal and characteristically has had anovulatory cycles for 1 to 2 years. At the other end of the spectrum is the 48-year-old perimenopausal woman, who usually has irregular, anovulatory cycles. The woman on the birth-control pills does not ovulate, and the marathon runner has irregular (anovulatory) cycles or even amenorrhea because of the intensity of her training and her low body fat content.

7. The answer is B [I B 4, C 4]. The presence of plasma cells has nothing to do with the phase of the menstrual cycle. Plasma cells indicate the existence of a chronic infection of the endometrium. However, under the influence of estrogen, the endometrium proliferates, with replication of both glandular and stromal cells and vascular growth. During the postovulatory phase, progesterone influences an increase in the tortuosity and secretory activity of the glands plus stromal edema. A decidual reaction appears toward the end of the cycle.

8. The answer is E [III A 3, B 1, C]. In the two-cell hypothesis of estrogen production, luteinizing hormone (LH) acts on the theca cells by stimulating their production of the androgens androstenedione and testosterone, which are transported to the granulosa cells. Follicle-stimulating hormone (FSH) activates both the aromatase and 3-hydroxysteroid dehydrogenase enzymes; the androgens are aromatized in the granulosa cells to form the estrogens estradiol and estrone. Once the estradiol is produced in the granulosa cells, it is secreted into the circulation, not transported to the theca cells.

9. The answer is C [I B, C 2]. The follicular, or proliferative, phase of the menstrual cycle extends from day 1 of menstrual bleeding to ovulation. Basal body temperature is usually low rather than above 98° F. Other characteristics of this phase are variable length, growth and development of the ovarian follicles, vascular growth of the endometrium, and secretion of estrogen from the ovary. The postovulatory, or luteal phase, of the cycle is marked by the secretion of progesterone, which has a slight thermogenic effect on the body; in the luteal phase, the basal body temperature is over 98° F.

10. The answer is E [V; VI A 2 d]. When pregnancy does not occur in a cycle, steroid production (progesterone) from the corpus lu-teum declines, leading to increased coiling and constriction of the spiral arteries in the endometrium. At the same time, prostaglandin increases in the endometrium. The decreased blood flow leads to ischemia and degradation of the endometrial tissue, with subsequent desquamation, or shedding, of that tissue, which results in bleeding. Soon after the menses begin, regeneration of the surface epithelium under the influence of estrogen occurs just as the endometrium is shedding.

11–14. The answers are: 11-B, 12-A, 13-D, 14-C [III A, B 1, C]. Luteinizing hormone (LH) stimulates the theca cells to produce androgens, which are important precursors in the synthesis of estrogens. Follicle-stimulating hormone (FSH) stimulates the granulosa cells, follicular growth and maturation, and aromatase activity, which is necessary for the synthesis of estradiol. The two-cell hypothesis of estrogen production involves the aromatization of theca cell androgen to estradiol in the granulosa cells. Both FSH and LH stimulate target cells in the ovary; FSH stimulates granulosa cells, and LH stimulates theca cells. Neither is responsible for prolactin release.

Chapter 21

Family Planning: Contraception and Complications
William W. Beck, Jr.

I. **NATURAL FAMILY PLANNING** entails planning or avoiding pregnancies by abstaining from sexual intercourse during the fertile phase of the menstrual cycle. Drugs, devices, and surgical procedures are not used. In Western countries, the **pregnancy rate** among women using natural family planning is 10 to 15/100 woman-years of exposure.

A. **Fertility cycle.** The fertile and infertile phases of the menstrual cycle bring bodily signs and symptoms that result from the changing concentrations of estrogen and progesterone over the cycle. Estrogen and progesterone have their most marked effects on the cervical mucus and the basal body temperature. The fertility cycle has three phases.

1. **Phase 1, the relatively infertile phase,** extends from menstruation to the beginning of development of the egg follicle.
   a. The length of this phase of the menstrual cycle depends on how rapidly the follicles respond to the pituitary hormones.
   b. This phase can be a problem in terms of fertility assessment because of the potential variation from cycle to cycle.

2. **Phase 2, the fertile phase,** extends from the beginning of follicular development until 48 hours after ovulation.
   a. The 48 hours allow 24 hours for the fertilizable life span of the ovum and 24 hours for the clinical imprecision of detecting ovulation.
   b. Spermatozoa retain the capacity to fertilize the ovum for up to 5 days in the cervical mucus, which is produced abundantly during this phase of the cycle.
   c. This combined fertile phase, therefore, lasts approximately 6 to 8 days per cycle.

3. **Phase 3, the absolutely infertile phase,** extends from 48 hours after ovulation until the onset of menstruation. This phase lasts approximately 10 to 16 days and is much more consistent than phase 1.

B. **Cervix.** Changing concentrations of estrogen and progesterone affect the quantity and quality of cervical mucus.

1. **Phase 1.** Just after menstruation, little, if any, mucus is produced.
   a. If mucus is found at the vulva, it is thick, tacky, and opaque.
   b. When held between the thumb and forefinger and stretched, mucus of this type breaks quickly.
   c. When mucus is present, women note stickiness at the entrance to the vagina.
   d. When mucus is not present, women have a sensation of dryness in the vulva.

2. **Phase 2.** As the follicles produce increasing amounts of estrogen, the cervix responds with increased mucus production.
   a. The mucus becomes more abundant, increasingly thin, stretchy, clear, and watery.
   b. If held between the thumb and forefinger, mucus of this type stretches for several inches before it breaks.
   c. Women have a sensation of wetness and slipperiness in the vulva at this time.
   d. Peak cervical mucus occurs at the height of estrogen secretion, no more than 3 days before ovulation; peak cervical mucus can be identified only in retrospect (i.e., after the mucus again changes and becomes thick, sticky, and opaque).
   e. If a 24-hour period is allowed for ovum fertilization, then the fourth day after the peak marks the end of the fertile phase.

3. **Phase 3.** With ovulation and the production of progesterone comes a rapid change in the amount and characteristics of the mucus.
   a. The quantity of mucus drops sharply and sometimes disappears altogether.

    b. Mucus, if present, becomes thick, sticky, and opaque as in the infertile-type mucus in the first stage of the cycle.

C. **Basal body temperature** is the temperature of the body at complete rest after a period of sleep and before normal activity, including eating.

    1. The basal body temperature **increases** 0.4° F to 1.0° F **during the postovulatory phase** of the cycle because the secretion of progesterone has a thermogenic effect.

    2. As an **indicator of fertility,** the basal body temperature can detect only the end of the fertile phase because the temperature remains elevated for 3 days after the shift.

    3. To avoid pregnancy using the basal body temperature method alone, a couple must restrict sexual intercourse to the period from the third day of temperature elevation until the end of the cycle.

II. BARRIER METHODS OF CONTRACEPTION—diaphragms, condoms, sponges, and spermicides—protect users against sexually transmitted diseases (STDs) and, thus, indirectly against carcinoma of the cervix; these contraceptives are also thought to be relatively free from side effects.

A. **Condoms** are one of the oldest surviving forms of birth control. They are effective, safe, and relatively inexpensive; moreover, their effects are reversible. Condoms are highly effective, but only when couples use them with every act of coitus.

    1. **Pregnancy rate** is 5 to 10/100 woman-years of use; **effectiveness** depends on the following features:
        a. Age of the couple (primarily because of the lower fertility level in older couples)
        b. Family income
        c. Interest in spacing or preventing pregnancies
        d. Education level of the couple

    2. **STDs.** Because latex condoms are airtight, watertight, and impermeable to microorganisms, they can prevent the spread of STDs. Transmission of the following organisms is prevented by the use of latex—but not lambskin—condoms:
        a. Herpes simplex virus (HSV)
        b. *Neisseria gonorrhoeae*
        c. *Chlamydia trachomatis*
        d. *Ureaplasma urealyticum*
        e. Human papillomavirus
        f. *Mycoplasma hominis*
        g. *Trichomonas vaginalis*
        h. *Treponema pallidum*
        i. Human immunodeficiency virus

    3. **Carcinoma of the cervix.** Barrier contraception is thought to protect the cervix from sexually transmitted agents that promote cervical neoplasia, such as HSV, papillomavirus, and *C. trachomatis*. Another speculation is that the use of condoms may help to reverse the progression of cervical dysplasias.

B. **Spermicides**—including creams, jellies, aerosol foams, and nonfoaming and foaming suppositories—are commonly used with other forms of contraception, such as diaphragms, sponges, and condoms. Only about 3% of women use spermicides alone.

    1. Mode of action
        a. The barrier substances are important for the following reasons:
            (1) Their speed in releasing the active ingredient
            (2) Their ability to spread over the cervix and vagina
            (3) Their ability to act as physical barriers at the cervix to prevent sperm penetration

    b. The **active agents** work by killing the sperm, decreasing sperm motility, or inactivating the enzymes needed for the sperm to penetrate the ova. **Surface-active agents** (e.g., nonoxynol 9 and octoxynol 9) are spermicidal agents that disrupt the outer lipoprotein surface layer of spermatozoa.

2. Pregnancy rate is 5 to 25/100 woman-years of use and reflects a wide range of factors. **Effectiveness** depends on the couple's motivation to use this form of contraceptive correctly for *every* act of coitus.

3. Safety. No serious side effects have been reported with the currently available spermicides. Concerns about a higher spontaneous abortion rate and a higher incidence of congenital abnormalities among users of spermicides compared with nonusers have not been substantiated by epidemiologic analysis.

C. **Vaginal sponges.** The most widely used sponge is made of polyurethane impregnated with 1 g of nonoxynol 9.

1. Mode of action. Vaginal sponges release spermicide during coitus, absorb ejaculate, and block the entrance to the cervical canal. They may be used for 24 hours regardless of the frequency of coitus.

2. Pregnancy rate is reported to be 10 to 15/100 woman-years of use.

3. Safety. There is no risk of toxic shock syndrome (TSS), as originally feared.
    a. TSS is a serious illness characterized by sudden onset of high fever, vomiting, diarrhea, and body rash; the cause is toxins produced by *Staphylococcus aureus*.
    b. Nonoxynol 9 retards staphylococcal replication and toxin production.

D. **Diaphragms.** All diaphragms are dome-shaped, 50 to 105 mm in diameter, and made of latex rubber. The base of the dome is a rubber-covered metal spring, which is either a flat spring, a coil spring, or an arcing spring. Diaphragms rest between the posterior aspect of the symphysis pubis and the posterior fornix of the vagina; they cover the anterior vaginal wall and the cervix.

1. Mode of action. Diaphragms act as physical barriers to sperm and are effective vehicles for carrying spermicidal creams or jellies. They prevent the cervical mucus from neutralizing the vaginal acidity so the vagina remains hostile to sperm.

2. Pregnancy rate is reported to be 5 to 10/100 woman-years of use. **Effectiveness** depends on leaving the diaphragm in place for 6 hours after intercourse and introducing more spermicide if intercourse occurs again.

3. Safety. Few side effects are associated with use of the diaphragm. A reported increase in the frequency of urinary tract infections possibly results from urethral compression. The diaphragm may protect against pelvic inflammatory disease.

E. **Cervical cap**

1. The cervical cap is about as effective as the diaphragm, but harder to fit.

2. It can be left in place for longer than a diaphragm (up to 36 hours), and it need not be used with a spermicide.

3. There is no evidence that it causes TSS.

4. Like the diaphragm, it must be left in place for at least 6 hours after intercourse to ensure that no motile sperm are left in the vagina.

III. **INTRAUTERINE DEVICES (IUDs)**

A. **Advantages** include:

1. A high level of effectiveness

2. A lack of associated systemic metabolic effects

3. A single act of motivation (the IUD insertion) required for long-term use

B. **Mode of action**

1. **Nonmedicated IUD.** Contraception involves a local, sterile inflammatory reaction caused by the presence of a foreign body in the uterus.
   a. Tissue breakdown products from the increased number of endometrial leukocytes produce an intrauterine environment that is spermicidal.
   b. The addition of copper increases the inflammatory reaction.
   c. With removal of both copper-bearing and non–copper-bearing IUDs, the inflammatory reaction rapidly disappears and resumption of fertility follows.

2. **Medicated IUD.** The **medicated (progesterone) IUD** exerts its contraceptive effect locally on the endometrium and the cervix.
   a. The influence of progesterone renders the endometrium incapable of sustaining an implantation.
   b. Changes in the cervical mucus make the passage of sperm difficult.

C. **Types.** The types of IUDs that were in general use are listed next. Because of medicolegal costs, only the progesterone-releasing device and the copper-containing device are still being produced.

1. **The barium-impregnated plastic devices** may be left in situ indefinitely.

2. **The copper-bearing devices** must be replaced every 6 years because of the constant dissolution of copper.

3. **The progesterone-releasing T-shaped device** must be replaced each year; the reservoir of progesterone becomes depleted after 18 months of use.

D. **Adverse effects**

1. **Uterine bleeding.** Heavy or prolonged menses and intermenstrual bleeding are the major reasons for discontinuing use of the IUD.
   a. **Vascular erosions** may occur in areas of the endometrium in direct contact with the IUD, and evidence of increased vascular permeability has appeared in areas not in direct contact with the IUD.
   b. **Excessive bleeding** in the first few months after IUD insertion should be treated with reassurance and supplemental oral iron; the bleeding frequently diminishes as the uterus adjusts to the presence of the foreign body. If bleeding continues, the IUD should be removed.

2. **Perforation of the uterine fundus** is one of the potentially serious complications associated with IUD use.
   a. Perforation initially occurs at insertion in about 1/1000 insertions.
   b. Perforation should be suspected if a patient reports that she cannot feel the attached string and did not notice that the IUD was expelled.
   c. Rotation of the device can occur, with the string being drawn into the cavity.
      (1) **X-ray film or ultrasound** can be used to locate the device.
      (2) **Contrast media** in the uterine cavity with a radiograph help to locate the IUD within or outside the uterus.
   d. If an IUD is found outside the uterus, it should be removed because complications, such as adhesions and bowel obstruction, have been reported.

3. **Infection.** In the first 24 hours after insertion of an IUD, the normally sterile cavity is infected with bacteria; the natural defenses destroy these bacteria in most cases.
   a. **Pelvic infection rates** are highest in the first 2 weeks after insertion and then steadily diminish. The **risk for development of pelvic infection** is greatest in women who have:
      (1) A prior history of pelvic infection
      (2) No children (women who are nulliparous) and who are younger than 25 years of age
      (3) Multiple sexual partners
   b. The **incidence of salpingitis** is about three times greater in IUD users than in diaphragm or oral contraceptive users, with the highest incidence in nulliparous women younger than age 25 years.

c. It is prudent not to insert the IUD in a nulliparous woman because of the risk of impairing her future fertility.

d. **Treatment**

   (1) Salpingitis can usually be treated effectively with removal of the IUD and antibiotics.

   (2) The unilateral tuboovarian abscess occasionally found in IUD users may be removed without a pelvic cleanout. This abscess is unique to IUD users.

E. **Complications related to pregnancy**

1. **Spontaneous abortion.** The rate of spontaneous abortion is about 50% if an IUD is left in situ. If the IUD is removed in early pregnancy, the subsequent abortion rate is about 20% to 30%. The possibility of serious infection associated with an IUD pregnancy mandates an attempt at IUD removal.

2. **Ectopic pregnancy.** If pregnancy occurs while an IUD is in place, the chance of an ectopic pregnancy is greater than if no IUD were used, possibly because of IUD effectiveness in preventing a uterine pregnancy. Chances of having an ectopic pregnancy while an IUD is in place range from 3% to 7% compared to 1% to 2% in non–IUD-using women.

3. **Prematurity.** The chance of prematurity is 12% to 15% in pregnancies producing live births while an IUD is in situ. This prematurity may be caused by IUD irritation of the myometrium during the third trimester.

F. **Pregnancy rate** among IUD users is 2 to 3/100 woman-years of use.

IV. ORAL CONTRACEPTIVES

A. **Composition.** The oral contraceptive agents contain either an estrogen/progestin combination or a progestin alone.

1. **The combination pills** contain various amounts of estrogen (ethinyl estradiol or mestranol) and one of a variety of progestins. The current preparations contain low doses of estrogen (usually 20–50 μg per pill). They are taken for 21 days, with 1 week between pill packs. Most are either monophasic or triphasic combinations.

2. **The progestin-only pills** are taken continuously without a break.

B. **Mode of action**

1. **Suppression of ovulation** is the primary mechanism of action. Either the estrogen or the progestin can suppress gonadotropins and inhibit ovulation.

2. The cervical mucus changes to a thick, rather viscous material, which is hostile to sperm migration through the endocervix.

3. The endometrium, under the influence of the progestins, becomes flat and inactive and is thus unprepared for implantation of the embryo.

C. **Side effects.** The frequency of side effects appears to relate to estrogen dosage. These side effects include the following:

1. Troublesome breakthrough bleeding or amenorrhea, either one often seen when very low-dose preparations are used

2. Nausea, headaches, weight gain, and breast tenderness, which usually disappear or lessen in severity after two or three cycles of pill use

D. **Complications**

1. **Thromboembolism.** Estrogen causes an increase in plasma levels of a number of clotting factors, especially factor VII, presumably by acting on the liver. Antithrombin III

levels fall within 10 days of starting oral contraceptives. Incidences of both superficial and deep vein thromboses are increased in oral contraceptive users.

2. **Cardiovascular disease.** The relative risk of dying from cardiovascular or cerebrovascular diseases for women currently taking oral contraceptives is increased fourfold.
   a. Most deaths result from **myocardial infarction;** there is no relationship between the incidence of death due to cardiovascular disease and the length of oral contraceptive use.
   b. **Cardiovascular disease morbidity and mortality,** which are **related to the estrogen content** of the oral contraceptives, are significantly reduced by use of preparations containing 50 μg or less.
   c. **Age and cigarette smoking** have an important influence on the risk of death from myocardial infarction among oral contraceptive users; women who smoke and are 35 years of age or older are at greatest risk.

3. **Hypertension**
   a. Renin substrate, plasma renin activity, and angiotensin levels are elevated in oral contraceptive users. There is an increase in aldosterone secretion and renal retention of sodium.
   b. The resulting hypertension in a small number of oral contraceptive users may represent the failed suppression of renin substrate and plasma renin activity that occurs with elevated levels of angiotensin.
   c. The length of oral contraceptive use seems to relate to the development of hypertension; hypertension develops in about 5% of users after 5 years of use.
   d. Almost all women in whom hypertension develops while taking oral contraceptives return to normotensive levels when they discontinue the medication.

4. **Postpill amenorrhea.** The occurrence of amenorrhea after ceasing oral contraceptive use ranges between 0.2% and 3.1%; this condition is not associated with length of use of the pill.
   a. Studies indicate that **preexisting menstrual irregularities** were present in 35% to 56% of women who had amenorrhea after discontinuing oral contraceptives.
   b. The possibility of a **pituitary adenoma** with any amenorrhea must be explored even when the amenorrhea seems to result from oral contraceptive use; a check of serum prolactin level is indicated with postpill amenorrhea.

5. **Liver tumor.** An association between the use of oral contraceptives and the subsequent development of a rare liver tumor, the **hepatocellular adenoma,** has been reported; the risk for development of this tumor increases when oral contraceptives have been used for 5 years or more. It occurs at a rate of 3/100,000 woman-years of use.

E. **Continual use**

1. **Break.** The impression that oral contraceptive use should be discontinued every 2 to 3 years has no scientific basis.
   a. The incidence of complications does not decrease with such a break.
   b. A high incidence of unwanted pregnancies occurs during such "rest" periods.

2. **Elective surgery.** Oral contraceptives should be discontinued when elective surgery is scheduled. Any estrogen-containing formulation should be stopped 1 month before planned surgery to lessen the incidence of postoperative thrombophlebitis.

3. **Age.** Oral contraceptives can be used safely by women between 35 and 45 years of age if they are in good health and do not smoke.
   a. Low-dose formulations should be used.
   b. Obesity, hyperlipidemia, diabetes, and cardiovascular disease are additional risk factors that contraindicate oral contraceptive use by women older than age 35 years.

F. **Neoplasia.** At present, no statistically valid data support a cause-and-effect relationship between use of oral contraceptives and neoplasia in the breast, cervix, endometrium, or ovary.

1. **Breast**
    a. Progestins antagonize the stimulating effect of estrogen on breast tissue.
    b. There is a decreased incidence of benign breast disease in oral contraceptive users.
    c. The incidence of breast cancer has remained fairly constant during the past 15 to 20 years despite widespread use of the birth control pill.

2. **Cervix**
    a. Cervical hypertrophy and eversion are seen in pill users.
    b. The pill does not induce carcinoma of the cervix, but neither does it protect against it. Its nonbarrier mode of action does not prevent exposure to potential carcinogenic agents, such as the papillomavirus or HSV.

3. **Endometrium**
    a. Progestins compete with estrogen for binding sites in the endometrial cells.
    b. Progestins reduce the stimulating effect of estrogen and prevent the normal proliferative endometrium from progressing to hyperplasia.
    c. The regressive effect of the pill on the endometrium has led to its use as a therapeutic agent in treating adenomatous hyperplasia in some cases.

4. **Ovary**
    a. Functional cysts are fewer in oral contraceptive users than in nonusers.
    b. Oral contraceptive use suppresses ovarian activity and inhibits ovulation.
    c. One hypothesis is that the interruption of a significant number of ovulatory cycles in oral contraceptive users may lead to a decreased incidence of ovarian cancer.

G. **Effectiveness.** The combination oral contraceptives are the most effective reversible method of birth control. When properly used, these preparations are virtually 100% effective.

V. OTHER HORMONAL CONTRACEPTION

A. **Injectable medroxyprogesterone**

1. Medroxyprogesterone, a progestin, acts on the hypothalamic–pituitary–ovarian axis to inhibit ovulation. As a result, it also affects the endometrium and the cervical mucus.

2. The usual dose is 150 mg intramuscularly every 2 to 3 months. At this dosage schedule, the drug is a very effective contraceptive, with reported failure rates of zero.

3. The main reason for discontinuing this drug, or any other progestin-only contraception, is menstrual disturbances, ranging from frequent, irregular, sometimes heavy menses to amenorrhea.

4. An initial delay in the return of fertility follows medroxyprogesterone use because it takes time to eliminate the drug completely and resume ovulation. The median time to conception is 9 months, which is double the median time for conception after stopping other forms of birth control.

B. **Gonadotropin-releasing hormone (GnRH) analogues**

1. **Agonistic analogues** of GnRH were originally developed to facilitate treatment of hypogonadism. Paradoxically, chronic GnRH agonist treatment resulted in desensitization, or downregulation, of the pituitary processes responsible for gonadotropin synthesis and release.

2. **The superagonist, buserelin,** a GnRH analogue, can be absorbed when given intranasally—a fact that has stimulated further clinical trials of this new approach to birth control.
    a. One study revealed that women given daily doses of 400 or 600 μg of buserelin

intranasally over 3 to 6 months obtained a safe and effective method of birth control that works by interfering with normal ovulation; no pregnancies occurred.

    b. The bleeding pattern during the chronic superagonist treatment varied from fairly regular menstrual-like bleeding to oligomenorrhea or amenorrhea; dysfunctional uterine bleeding did not occur.

    c. No side effects occurred, except bleeding disturbances caused by the induced anovulation.

  3. The main mechanism of action of chronic GnRH agonist treatment seems to be pituitary desensitization of the processes responsible for gonadotropin secretion. The reserve capacity for gonadotropin secretion is rapidly reduced during repeated administration of GnRH agonists.

C. **Postcoital contraception**

  1. The **"morning after pill"** can be used after unprotected coitus around the time of ovulation.

    a. It must be taken within 72 hours of coitus; however, use within 24 hours is preferable.

    b. The high doses of steroids just after ovulation may disrupt the endometrium enough so that implantation of the embryo does not take place.

  2. One of the first regimens was diethylstilbestrol 25 mg twice a day for 5 days; this regimen can cause severe nausea and vomiting and thus should include an antiemetic.

  3. Four tablets that are a combination of ethinyl estradiol (0.03 mg) and norgestrel (0.3 mg), given as two tablets twice over 12 hours, is the most common approach.

  4. Ethinyl estradiol alone at 5 mg/day for 5 days is another alternative.

  5. Because of the potential teratogenic effects of the steroids, a therapeutic abortion must be recommended if the postcoital contraception fails and a pregnancy occurs.

D. **The levonorgestrel implant** is a long-acting, reversible, and effective birth control device.

  1. Administration

    a. Six flexible silicone rubber implants containing levonorgestrel are placed under the skin of the woman's arm.

    b. Small amounts of the levonorgestrel are released at a relatively constant rate for 5 years.

  2. Mode of action

    a. Ovulation is suppressed in many, but not all, users.

    b. Low levels of levonorgestrel cause the cervical mucus to become thick and scanty, preventing migration of the sperm.

    c. Development and growth of the endometrium are suppressed.

  3. Side effects most commonly involve a change in a woman's bleeding pattern, with more frequent and irregular bleeding episodes, spotting between periods, or amenorrhea. Many of the bleeding irregularities diminish after several months.

E. **Mifepristone** (RU-486) is an antiprogesterone steroid.

  1. Mifepristone has been studied as both an abortifacient and a contraceptive agent.

  2. It binds the progesterone receptor and prevents or interrupts progestational action.

  3. A single dose given in the midluteal phase induces menses in about 72 hours and, thus, has potential as a once-a-month form of fertility control.

  4. When given with prostaglandin, it is very effective in inducing abortion in early pregnancy.

STUDY QUESTIONS

DIRECTIONS: Each of the numbered items or incomplete statements in this section is followed by answers or by completions of the statement. Select the ONE lettered answer or completion that is BEST in each case.

1. Increased thromboembolic activity with the birth control pill may result from an increase in which of the following?

(A) Levels of factor VII
(B) Plasma renin activity
(C) Levels of antithrombin III
(D) Platelet counts
(E) Angiotensin

2. Which of the following methods of contraception suppresses ovulation as its primary mechanism of action?

(A) Medicated intrauterine device (IUD)
(B) Postcoital norgestrel and ethinyl estradiol
(C) Levonorgestrel
(D) Mifepristone
(E) Gonadotropin-releasing hormone (GnRH) agonists

DIRECTIONS: Each of the numbered items or incomplete statements in this section is negatively phrased, as indicated by a capitalized word such as NOT, LEAST, or EXCEPT. Select the ONE lettered answer or completion that is BEST in each case.

3. Which of the following is NOT a characteristic of the fertile phase of the menstrual cycle?

(A) Peak levels of estrogen
(B) Clear, abundant cervical mucus
(C) Ovulation
(D) Production of progesterone
(E) Sensation of vulvar slipperiness

4. Which of the following is NOT a contraceptive action of the spermicides?

(A) Killing the sperm
(B) Decreasing sperm motility
(C) Inactivating acrosomal enzymes
(D) Disrupting the outer lipoprotein surface layer
(E) Neutralizing vaginal acidity

5. Which of the following is NOT a physiologic change effected by oral contraceptives?

(A) Suppression of ovulation
(B) Hostile cervical mucus
(C) A hypoestrogenic state
(D) Inactive endometrium
(E) Reduction of gonadotropins

6. Which of the following is NOT associated with hypertension from oral contraceptive use?

(A) Increased plasma renin activity
(B) Increased aldosterone secretion
(C) Elevated levels of angiotensin
(D) Increased renal excretion of sodium

7. Which of the following advantages is NOT associated with barrier methods of contraception?

(A) They protect the user against sexually transmitted diseases (STDs)
(B) Regular office visits are not required
(C) They are relatively free from side effects
(D) They prevent cervical cancer
(E) They are effective, safe, and immediately reversible

DIRECTIONS: The set of matching questions in this section consists of a list of four to twenty-six lettered options (some of which may be in figures) followed by several numbered items. For each numbered item, select the ONE lettered option that is most closely associated with it. To avoid spending too much time on matching sets with large numbers of options, it is generally advisable to begin each set by reading the list of options. Then, for each item in the set, try to generate the correct answer and locate it in the option list, rather than evaluating each option individually. Each lettered option may be selected once, more than once, or not at all.

Questions 8–9

Match the description of the phase of the menstrual cycle with the appropriate phase.

(A) Relatively fertile phase (phase 1)
(B) Fertile phase (phase 2)
(C) Absolutely infertile phase (phase 3)
(D) Menstrual phase (phase 4)
(E) Postmenstrual phase (phase 5)

8. This phase of the cycle is characterized by peak estrogen secretion with abundant, clear cervical mucus and a sensation of vulvar wetness.

9. This phase of the cycle is characterized by a rise in the basal body temperature, thick, scant cervical mucus, and the presence of progesterone.

■ ANSWERS AND EXPLANATIONS

1. The answer is A [IV D 1, 3]. The incidence of superficial and deep vein thromboses is increased in oral contraceptive users, perhaps because of an increase in clotting factors, such as factor VII, and a decrease in antithrombin III. Platelet counts do not increase in pill users. An increase in renin substrate, plasma renin activity, and angiotensin in pill users occurs in association with the pathophysiology of hypertension, not with thromboembolic disease.

2. The answer is E [III B; V B 1, 2, C 1 b, D 2, E 2]. Gonadotropin-releasing hormone (GnRH) agonists primarily suppress ovulation and offer contraception. The medicated intrauterine device (IUD) with its progesterone prevents the endometrium from sustaining implantation and creates a cervical mucus that is hostile to sperm migration. The postcoital norgestrel and ethinyl estradiol disrupt the endometrium enough to prevent implantation of the embryo. Levonorgestrel can suppress ovulation, but it also influences the endometrium and the cervical mucus in much the same manner as the medicated IUD. Mifepristone (RU-486) does not prevent ovulation but binds the progesterone receptor and interrupts progestational action through lysis of the corpus luteum.

3. The answer is D [I A 2, B 2, 3]. Progesterone production occurs after ovulation and characterizes the infertile phase of the menstrual cycle. The fertile phase of the menstrual cycle is characterized by ovulation. Estrogen levels rise to a peak just before ovulation, and this peak triggers ovulation. With the rise of estrogen, the cervix is stimulated to produce clear, abundant mucus, which gives the vulva a feeling of slipperiness.

4. The answer is E [II B 1 b]. If spermicides neutralized vaginal acidity, they would decrease their effectiveness because sperm are naturally inactivated in an acidic vagina. Spermicides have two basic components—the active agent and the carrier substance. The active agent works by disrupting the outer lipoprotein surface layer of the spermatozoon, which kills it. In addition, the spermicides de-

crease sperm motility and inactivate the enzymes that the sperm need to penetrate the ovum.

5. The answer is C [IV B]. Patients on oral contraceptives are not hypoestrogenic. Either mestranol or ethinyl estradiol is a pill component, and both maintain normal estrogen levels. The oral contraceptives are effective for several reasons. They reduce the gonadotropins and thus inhibit ovulation. Because of the dominant progestin effect, they also cause the cervical mucus to be scant and viscous and the endometrium to be inactive; both of these features contribute to contraception.

6. The answer is D [IV D 3]. Aldosterone secretion and renal retention, not excretion, of sodium lead to increased hypertension from oral contraceptive use. Renin substrate, plasma renin activity, and angiotensin are elevated in oral contraceptive users. The resulting hypertension, which is usually seen in users of at least 5 years, may represent the failed suppression of renin substrate and plasma renin activity with elevated levels of angiotensin.

7. The answer is D [II]. The barrier forms of contraception (condoms, sponges, diaphragms, spermicides, and cervical caps) do not prevent cervical cancer. However, because they protect the cervix from sexually transmitted diseases (STDs) such as human papillomavirus and herpes simplex virus (HSV), which promote cervical neoplasia, they may indirectly decrease the incidence of cervical cancer. They all are good forms of birth control when used faithfully.

8–9. The answers are 9-B [I A 2, B 2], **10-C** [I A 3, B 3]. Phase 2 of the cycle is the fertile phase, the time when a woman can get pregnant. It is characterized by high levels of estrogen, which stimulate the cervix to secrete clear, abundant cervical mucus. When the estrogen level peaks, ovulation occurs. Because spermatozoa can live in the cervical mucus for several days, birth control is necessary when a woman notices vulvar wetness or mucus that stretches out to several inches when held between two fingers. For a woman who does not want pregnancy or for whom pregnancy is contraindicated, birth control should be used with every act of intercourse, no matter what phase of her cycle she is in, for optimal efficacy. Phase 3 of the cycle is the absolutely infertile phase, the time when a woman cannot get pregnant. Ovulation has occurred, and the corpus luteum secretes progesterone. The progesterone causes the basal body temperature to rise 0.4° F to 1.0° F and causes the cervical mucus to become thick and hostile to sperm penetration and migration. There is no such thing as a post-menstrual phase (phase 5). Once phase 4 is completed, phase 1 begins.

Chapter 22

Pelvic Pain

William W. Beck, Jr.

I. **INTRODUCTION. Pelvic pain and abdominal pain** are the most common complaints in a gynecologic practice, and their evaluation is often difficult. Not only do innumerable pathologic entities and functional disorders cloud the diagnostic picture, but also individual responses to pain and pain thresholds make localization of pain a taxing diagnostic dilemma.

II. **NEUROPHYSIOLOGY.** Nerve endings extend into all internal pelvic organs but are few in number. Because there is no great concentration of sensory nerve ganglia in the pelvis, the central nervous system (CNS) has difficulty differentiating the pain that arises from the deep pelvic viscera. Moreover, pelvic pain is characterized as secondary because it is poorly localized and slowly conducted; it also persists after a stimulus is removed.

A. **Sources of pelvic pain.** Pelvic pain is **visceral** and thus does not respond to thermal, chemical, or tactile sensations. Visceral pain is **referred** or **splanchnic.**

1. **Referred pain** occurs when autonomic impulses arise from a diseased visceral organ and elicit an irritable response within the spinal cord, exciting cells receiving somatic impulses. Pain is then sensed by the corresponding CNS site as originating in the skin. Referred pain most likely occurs because a common pathway is shared by visceral and somatic fibers.

2. **Splanchnic pain** occurs when an irritable stimulus is appreciated in the specific organ secondary to:
    a. **Tension**
        (1) Distention and subsequent contraction of a hollow viscus
        (2) Traction as a result of fibrosis or a fibrotic process
        (3) Stretching of the capsule of a solid organ
    b. **Peritoneal irritation or inflammation**
        (1) Inflammation from an adjacent viscus: tends to be well localized and well defined
        (2) Generalized peritonitis: may result from spillage of an irritant (e.g., pus, blood, intestinal contents)
        (3) Chemical irritation
        (4) Tissue ischemia

B. The **autonomic nervous system** innervates the pelvic organs. Visceral abdominal pain tends to be poorly localized because sensory impulses from several viscera overlap within the same segment of the spinal cord. Three pathways transmit sensations from the pelvic organs, as follows:

1. The **parasympathetic nerves (S2, S3, and S4)** transmit sensations to the spinal cord via the hypogastric plexus from the:
    a. Upper third of the vagina
    b. Cervix
    c. Lower uterine segment
    d. Posterior urethra
    e. Trigone of the bladder
    f. Lower ureters
    g. Uterosacral ligaments

      h. Cardinal ligaments

      i. Rectosigmoid

      j. Dorsal external genitalia

  2. The **thoracolumbar sympathetic nerves (T11, T12, and L1)** transmit impulses to the spinal cord via the hypogastric and inferior mesenteric plexus from the:

      a. Uterine fundus

      b. Proximal third of the fallopian tube

      c. Broad ligaments

      d. Upper bladder

      e. Appendix

      f. Cecum

      g. Terminal large bowel

  3. The **superior mesenteric plexus (T5–T11)** transmits impulses to the spinal cord from the:

      a. Ovaries

      b. Lateral two thirds of the fallopian tubes

      c. Upper ureters

III. **HISTORY.** Because pelvic pain is often difficult to describe, a meticulous history should be taken. Important considerations are the onset (acute or chronic), location, quality, duration (constant or cyclic), and severity of the pain episode as well as any associated complaints, such as fever, chills, anorexia, nausea, vomiting, or bleeding. The physician must also determine whether the pain is related to the menstrual cycle, is life threatening, necessitates resuscitative efforts, or is related to reproductive processes.

A. **Onset**

  1. **Sudden onset** suggests an acute intraperitoneal event, such as perforation, hemorrhage, rupture, or torsion. Acute colic of the urinary or gastrointestinal tract may present similarly.

  2. **Gradual onset** suggests inflammation, obstruction, or a slowly evolving problem.

B. **Location**

  1. **Abdominal pain** that is generalized suggests extensive peritoneal irritation.

  2. **Epigastric pain** suggests problems in structures innervated by T6–T8.

      a. Stomach

      b. Duodenum

      c. Pancreas

      d. Liver

      e. Gallbladder

  3. **Periumbilical pain** suggests problems in structures innervated by T9 and T10.

      a. Small intestine

      b. Appendix

      c. Upper ureters

      d. Ovaries

  4. **Hypogastric or suprapubic pain** suggests problems in structures innervated by T11 and T12.

      a. Colon

      b. Bladder

      c. Lower ureters

      d. Uterus

  5. **Pelvic pain** suggests problems in structures innervated by S2, S3, and S4 (e.g., cervix) or T10–T12 (e.g., ovaries, fallopian tubes).

6. Shoulder pain may indicate referred pain from diaphragmatic irritation.

C. **Quality**

1. **Cramping, rhythmic pain** suggests:
   a. Muscular contractions of a hollow viscus
   b. Intraluminal pressure in a hollow viscus

2. **Constant pain** suggests:
   a. An inflammatory process
   b. Overdistention of a solid organ
   c. Compromise of blood supply

3. **Intermittent pain** suggests an adnexal mass with partial torsion.

4. **Positional pain** suggests a mobile pelvic mass that is symptomatic in certain positions.

5. **Sharp pain** suggests obstruction or an acute peritoneal event.

6. **Dull pain** suggests an inflammatory process.

D. **Duration and recurrence** of pain episodes help to establish whether the problem is acute or chronic. If the patient has had similar pain in the past or similar pain for a prolonged period, an acute problem is unlikely. Acute attacks of pain over long periods, which last less than 48 hours and are recurrent, may be secondary to a chronic problem (e.g., ovulatory pain).

E. **Severity.** The appearance of the patient must be evaluated for the presence or absence of pallor and diaphoresis.

F. **Associated symptoms**

1. **Vaginal bleeding** associated with pelvic pain usually indicates reproductive tract pathology.

2. **Fever and chills** often indicate a pelvic infection that has spread systemically.

3. **Anorexia, nausea, and vomiting,** although nonspecific, often indicate intestinal tract pathology, pelvic malignancy, or acute pelvic accident.

4. **Syncope, vascular collapse, and shock** usually indicate intraperitoneal hemorrhage and instability secondary to hypovolemia.

5. **Frequency, dysuria, flank pain, or hematuria** usually indicate urinary tract pathology, such as pyelonephritis or kidney stone.

6. **Shoulder pain** indicates irritation of the undersurface of the diaphragm by blood, such as a ruptured ectopic pregnancy or a bleeding ovarian cyst.

7. **Dyspareunia** must be investigated because it can have many causes.

8. **Other.** A history of ectopic pregnancy, pelvic inflammatory disease (PID), appendectomy, tubal repair, and endometriosis should also be investigated.

IV. **PHYSICAL SIGNS**

A. **General examination**

1. **Vital signs:** blood pressure, pulse, respiratory rate, temperature

2. **General appearance:** relaxed, anxious, agitated, septic, rigid, level of consciousness

3. **Heart and lungs.** Abdominal pain may be referred from pulmonary and cardiac disease.

4. **Activity level**

B. **Abdominal examination**

1. The physician should **inspect** visually to evaluate distention and contour and to determine the location of the pain.

2. **Auscultation** must be performed gently to evaluate hypoactive or hyperactive bowel sounds, concomitantly evaluating for guarding, rebound tenderness, and abdominal rigidity. Initially, the area of maximum pain should be avoided.

3. **Percussion** localizes the area of tenderness and aids in evaluating ascites, distention, masses, and organ size.

4. **Palpation** should be gentle to evaluate tenderness or masses.

C. **Pelvic examination.** Tenderness or masses, when identified, need further evaluation. Careful evaluation of the cervix, uterus, and adnexa is imperative. The clinician should:

1. **Inspect the external genitalia and cervix** for evidence of trauma, infection, hemorrhage, or asymmetry

2. Without placing the hand on the abdomen, **palpate the vaginal wall** for tenderness, and **palpate the cervix** for cervical motion tenderness, localizing the side of tenderness

3. **Palpate the adnexa,** starting with the side of least tenderness as elicited by the cervical motion test

4. Use the hand on the abdomen to **evaluate masses or tenderness**

V. **LABORATORY TESTS.** The evaluation of pelvic pain presents the clinician with a diagnostic challenge. Valuable diagnostic information can be gleaned from the following tests.

A. **Complete blood count with a differential smear.** An increased white blood cell count, especially with a shift to the left, may indicate systemic infection. Decreased hemoglobin levels may indicate blood loss.

B. **Urinalysis with microscopic examination and culture and sensitivity testing.** The presence of bacteria, white blood cells, or red blood cells suggests that the urinary tract is the site of disease.

C. **Blood type and antibody screen.** If intraabdominal bleeding is suspected or diagnosed, then blood should be sent to the blood bank for typing and should be crossmatched.

D. **Pregnancy test,** with serial human chorionic gonadotropin β-subunit measurements if indicated. This test is important in the evaluation of the patient who may be pregnant. A negative serum pregnancy test essentially excludes this possibility. A positive serum pregnancy test needs to be followed with serial β-subunit measurements if the exact location of the pregnancy is in doubt. Anything other than the 2- to 3-day doubling time needs to be viewed with suspicion and evaluated with care.

E. **Cervical cultures** for gonorrhea and chlamydia are indicated if a pelvic infection is suspected. If sexually transmitted disease is suspected, testing for human immunodeficiency virus should be included.

F. **Culdocentesis** may be helpful in evaluating the posterior cul-de-sac for intraperitoneal blood or free fluid.

G. **Radiographs.** Abdominal radiographs, including upright, supine, and lateral decubitus films, may reveal evidence of:

1. Intestinal obstruction
2. Free air under the diaphragm, suggesting perforation of an air-filled viscus
3. Free fluid, suggesting bleeding or a ruptured cyst
4. Calcifications, suggesting renal stones, gallstones, calcified myomas, and dermoid cysts

H. **Ultrasound** is particularly useful in evaluating the pelvis for diagnosis of the following:

1. An early intrauterine pregnancy or ectopic pregnancy
2. An adnexal mass

I. **Laparoscopy** is quite useful in the assessment of pelvic pain because it is a well-controlled procedure, it allows visualization of the pelvic structures, it allows time for reflection about the optimal mode of management, and it is an opportunity to diagnose and treat a problem without extensive surgery. This procedure is contraindicated, however, in patients with hypovolemic shock or gastrointestinal obstruction. Despite the usefulness of laparoscopy, it will not lead to a better understanding of the reason for pelvic pain because approximately 30% of patients will have a normal pelvis.

VI. DIFFERENTIAL DIAGNOSIS

A. **Acute pelvic pain**
1. **Related to pregnancy**
   a. **Abortion** is characterized by vaginal bleeding and abdominal pain that is suprapubic, involves cramps, and varies in intensity. It is classified as:
      (1) **Spontaneous.** The categories of spontaneous abortion are:
         (a) In **threatened abortion,** blood exits from the cervical os even though it is closed.
         (b) **Inevitable abortion** is manifested by prolonged, profuse bleeding with an open cervical os.
         (c) **Incomplete abortion** is characterized by a partial passage of tissue through the cervical os.
         (d) **Complete abortion** is characterized by a complete passage of tissue, resulting in resolution of symptoms.
         (e) **Missed abortion** is the death of the embryo or fetus without the onset of labor or passage of tissue and often without any bleeding.
      (2) **Induced.** Subsequent to an induced abortion, pelvic pain can occur secondary to:
         (a) **Incomplete evacuation**
         (b) **Septic abortion,** which is characterized by abortion symptoms along with fever and sepsis secondary to infection of the uterine contents. **Treatment** consists of obtaining appropriate cultures, performing dilation and evacuation, and instituting intravenous broad-spectrum antibiotics.
   b. **Ectopic pregnancy**
      (1) **Location.** Ninety-five percent of all ectopic pregnancies occur in the fallopian tubes. A pregnancy may exist in any portion of the tube, including the cornua, interstitium, isthmus, ampulla, or infundibulum, each of which is associated with particular complications and surgical considerations. Ectopic pregnancies may also occur in the abdomen, cervix, or ovary, although these locations are uncommon.
      (2) The **mechanism of pain** may involve distention of the tube due to the growing pregnancy. The presenting symptoms may be so vague that the physician must always suspect ectopic pregnancy when a patient presents with pelvic pain. The low abdominal pain is usually unilateral; however, it may be bilat-

eral or generalized. The pain may be either crampy due to tubal distention by the enlarging pregnancy or sudden and sharp due to acute rupture with intra-abdominal bleeding.

(3) **At-risk patients.** A patient who has a history of an ectopic pregnancy or a pelvic infection or who uses an intrauterine device is at increased risk for a future ectopic pregnancy.

(4) **Associated symptoms** include:

(a) Vaginal bleeding or spotting

(b) Delayed or missed menses

(c) Syncope

(d) Orthostatic changes

(e) Rectal pressure and the urge to defecate as a result of blood in the posterior cul-de-sac

(f) Nonspecific symptoms of pregnancy, including nausea, vomiting, and breast enlargement

2. **Unrelated to pregnancy**

a. **Mittelschmerz** is pain in the lower abdomen noticed around ovulation and believed to be secondary to chemical irritation of the peritoneum from ovarian follicular cyst fluid. The pain usually lasts only a few hours, but usually no longer than 2 days.

b. **Ovarian accidents.** Bleeding, rupture, and torsion may be associated with inflammatory cysts, endometriomas, benign or malignant cysts or solid tumors, or variations in the normal ovarian cycle. The mechanisms of pain involve acute distention, peritoneal irritation by blood or cyst fluids, or ischemia.

(1) **Bleeding** may cause pain by irritation of the peritoneal cavity by extruded blood or acute distention of the ovary.

(2) **Rupture of a cyst** releases cyst fluid, which is quite irritating to the peritoneum.

(3) **Torsion** (i.e., rotation of a tumor around its pedicle) leads to ischemia and tissue necrosis; the clinical presentation depends on the extent of interference with the ovarian blood supply. Torsion can also involve the fallopian tube. The more complete the vascular occlusion, the more extensive the ischemia, and then the more severe the pain. The pain is usually paroxysmal and unilateral but becomes more constant if infarction occurs. In pregnancy, torsion is more likely to occur during the period of rapid uterine growth (8–16 weeks) or involution postpartum.

(a) **Associated symptoms** may include nausea, vomiting, syncope, shock, and shoulder pain.

(b) **Therapy** involves laparoscopy or laparotomy with isolation and clamping of the infundibulopelvic ligament before untwisting of torsive adnexae and subsequent excision.

c. **Ovarian hyperstimulation syndrome** may occur in patients who have a history of infertility that is currently being treated with fertility hormones (e.g., clomiphene, human menopausal gonadotropins). The ovaries are enlarged with multiple follicular cysts, a large cystic corpus luteum, and stromal edema. Associated symptoms include:

(1) **Mild cases**

(a) Weight gain

(b) Abdominal distention

(c) Abdominal pain

(2) **Severe cases** may also include:

(a) Ascites

(b) Pleural effusion

(c) Hypovolemia

(d) Oliguria

(e) Electrolyte disturbances

(f) Dyspnea

(3) **Therapy** involves:

        (a) Hospitalization
        (b) Observation
        (c) Bed rest
        (d) Fluid and electrolyte replacement

    d. PID is an infection of the pelvic organs by pathogenic microorganisms, usually *Neisseria gonorrhoeae, Chlamydia trachomatis,* and *Mycoplasma hominis.*

    e. Appendicitis. The pain is not well localized and is referred initially as a result of distention of the lumen of the appendix by inflammatory exudate. The pain is colicky with a gradual onset. It localizes to the right lower quadrant (i.e., to the site of the appendix) once the overlying parietal peritoneum becomes locally involved in the inflammatory process. In pregnancy, the appendix is usually displaced upward by the enlarging uterus, and symptoms tend to localize at the site where the appendix would be for that stage of pregnancy. **Associated symptoms** include:

        (1) Anorexia
        (2) Nausea
        (3) Vomiting

B. | Chronic pelvic pain

  1. Cyclic

    a. Mittelschmerz (see VI A 2 a)

    b. Dysmenorrhea is defined as pain accompanying menstruation. It is further categorized as primary or secondary.

      (1) Primary dysmenorrhea is defined as painful menstruation in the absence of organic pelvic lesions. Primary dysmenorrhea usually accompanies ovulatory cycles. The pain is spasmodic and throbbing. Originally located in the lower abdomen, it often radiates to the lower back and the front of the thighs. Its onset is concurrent with the menses, and it lasts for 1 to 3 days. Associated symptoms include backache, nausea, vomiting, diarrhea, headache, and fatigue.

        (a) Although primary dysmenorrhea may have a psychological component, it is generally thought that decreasing progesterone levels at the end of the menstrual cycle cause a release of phospholipase A_2 from the endometrial cells. This enzyme acts on the lipid cell membrane to produce arachidonic acid and, through the action of prostaglandin synthetase, forms prostaglandins E_2 and F_{2a}. These prostaglandins cause uterine contractions, resulting in areas of ischemia, which ultimately causes pain.

        (b) Therapy entails the following:

          (i) Discussions regarding the nature of the pain
          (ii) Suppression of ovulatory cycles with oral contraceptives to decrease prostaglandin levels in menstrual fluid
          (iii) Use of prostaglandin synthetase inhibitors, such as ibuprofen, naproxen, and mefenamic acid. These should be administered 48 hours before onset of menses and for 1 to 3 days of menstrual flow.
          (iv) Laparoscopy if the medications discussed previously are not effective

      (2) Secondary dysmenorrhea is defined as painful menstruation in the presence of organic disease, occurring more than 2 years after menarche. Numerous conditions may precipitate this complaint, including the following:

        (a) Endometriosis is characterized by the proliferation of foci of normal endometrium outside the uterine cavity. The usual affected areas include the ovaries, uterosacral ligaments, and posterior cul-de-sac; however, the intestinal tract and urinary tract may also be involved. Endometriosis can cause local destruction, distortion, obstruction, adhesions, and scar formation.

        (b) Adhesive disease occurs secondary to chronic PID, endometriosis, or postsurgical formation. Therapy consists of surgical lysis of adhesions.

        (c) Uterine pathology

          (i) Adenomyosis is uterine pathology characterized by the presence of ectopic foci of endometrial glands and stroma in the myometrium.

This condition is associated with heavy menstrual bleeding secondary to swelling of the ectopic endometrial islands in the myometrial wall. Antiprostaglandin medications may decrease both dysmenorrhea and heavy menstrual flow. Hysterectomy should be considered in refractory cases.

   (ii) **Leiomyomas** (i.e., fibroids or myomas) are benign uterine tumors composed of muscle and fibrous connective tissue in various locations: intramural, subserosal, or submucosal. Chronically, they may cause a crampy secondary dysmenorrhea associated with vaginal bleeding, which may progressively worsen. Therapy involves hysteroscopic resection of submucosal myomas, abdominal myomectomy, or hysterectomy.

   (d) **Congenital anomalies** may cause an obstruction to the menstrual flow with resultant **hematometra** (i.e., accumulation of menstrual blood in the uterus secondary to cervical obstruction) or **hematocolpos** (i.e., accumulation of menstrual blood in the vagina secondary to introital obstruction). Imperforate hymen and noncommunicating horn of the uterus are examples. These conditions must be repaired surgically.

   (e) **Cervical stenosis** occurs secondary to previous surgery. Treatment involves dilation or laser-directed opening of the cervical os.

   c. **Ovarian remnant syndrome** results from residual ovarian tissue after bilateral oophorectomy. Patients present with symptoms of a pelvic mass, pelvic pain, or flank pain from associated ureteral obstruction. This diagnosis should be considered in any woman with cyclic pain after extirpative surgery.

2. **Acyclic pelvic pain** is prolonged, intractable pelvic pain that is unrelated to menstruation. The goal in treating this type of pain is to localize the organic problem and separate it from any psychogenic influence.
   a. **Organic etiologies**
      (1) **Endometriosis**
      (2) **Pelvic adhesions**
      (3) **Ovarian remnant syndrome**
      (4) **Pelvic congestion syndrome.** The existence of this syndrome as a true pathologic entity is controversial, although many claim that it is secondary to dilated pelvic varicosities.
      (5) **Urinary tract.** Although the kidney is located at a distance from the urinary tract, it can, along with the more distal ureters and the bladder, refer pain to the lower abdomen. As a result, any pathologic process in the urinary tract, such as **cystitis** or **ureteral colic secondary to renal calculi,** may be responsible for chronic pelvic pain.
      (6) **Intestinal tract.** Gastrointestinal disease should be regarded as one explanation for the etiology of pelvic (lower abdominal) pain and thus appropriately evaluated. These diseases include **diverticulitis** and **colitis.**
      (7) **Orthopedic conditions.** A number of disease processes, congenital deformities, or inflammatory processes may cause pain with an abdominal reference. These include:
         (a) Spina bifida
         (b) Scoliosis
         (c) Osteoarthritis
         (d) Fibromyositis
         (e) Herniated intervertebral disc
   b. **Abdominal and soft tissue pain.** Recently, a number of researchers have broadened the diagnostic differential in chronic pelvic pain. They have found that many patients have sensitive trigger points that elicit pain reflexes when irritated.
      (1) **Location.** The trigger points may be located in:
         (a) The abdominal wall
         (b) The skeletal muscle or muscle fascia
         (c) The pelvic soft tissue (e.g., the vestibule, levator muscles, and paracervical tissues)

(2) **Diagnosis** is assisted by selective infiltration of suspected areas with local anesthetic agents to determine pain relief.

(3) The **cause** is unclear but may involve systemic illness, immunologic dysfunction, or an infectious agent.

c. **Psychogenic causes.** When organic disease has been eliminated as the source of pelvic pain, patients should be evaluated for evidence of borderline personality, hypochondriasis, depression, and hysteria. In addition, studies have shown that these patients may have difficulty with interpersonal relationships, a history of sexual abuse as a child, and emotional instability during adolescence.

(1) Results of the **Minnesota Multiphasic Personality Index** show that patients with chronic pelvic pain have a fourfold increase in the manifestation of somatization, depression, and borderline personality.

(2) **Management** should revolve around a team approach, including a social worker or psychiatrist, to evaluate psychosocial difficulties that may be in part responsible for the pain. It is important, however, to rule out all other possible causes before deciding that the root cause of the pain is psychogenic.

STUDY QUESTIONS

DIRECTIONS: Each of the numbered items or incomplete statements in this section is followed by answers or by completions of the statement. Select the ONE lettered answer or completion that is BEST in each case.

1. A 29-year-old woman comes to see the physician with the complaint of chronic pelvic pain. The pain is dull and continuous. She has a history of oligomenorrhea as well as several hospitalizations for suicidal ideation. She is taking numerous medications for arthritic complaints, asthma, peptic ulcer disease, and depression. The most likely etiology for her chronic pain is

(A) endometriosis
(B) uterine fibroids
(C) mittelschmerz
(D) pelvic adhesions
(E) psychogenic cause

2. An 18-year-old woman complains of a long history of extremely painful menses, which last 5 to 7 days. She states that her last menstrual period was 5 weeks ago and was very heavy. Examination reveals a fairly normal pelvis. The first step that the physician should take in treating this patient is

(A) performing a dilation and curettage
(B) ruling out pregnancy
(C) ruling out thyroid dysfunction
(D) administering oral contraceptives and antiprostaglandins
(E) administering a progestational agent

3. A woman has seen her physician for many years with complaints of pelvic pain. During her early evaluation, her condition had been diagnosed as endometriosis. Over the years, after numerous operations, she decides to have a total abdominal hysterectomy and bilateral salpingo-oophorectomy. The operation is performed uneventfully. Eight months later she returns, complaining of pelvic and flank pain. This examination shows a right pelvic mass. Which of the following should be one of the leading diagnoses?

(A) Pelvic adhesions
(B) Cecum
(C) Urinoma
(D) Pelvic kidney
(E) Ovarian remnant

DIRECTIONS: Each of the numbered items or incomplete statements in this section is negatively phrased, as indicated by a capitalized word such as NOT, LEAST, or EXCEPT. Select the ONE lettered answer or completion that is BEST in each case.

4. Which of the following statements concerning pain episodes is NOT true?

(A) The sudden onset of pain usually suggests an acute episode
(B) Generalized abdominal pain suggests extensive peritoneal irritation
(C) Crampy, rhythmic pain usually suggests muscular contractions or increased intraluminal pressure of a hollow viscus
(D) Primary dysmenorrhea is usually unilateral and associated with a specific structural or organic abnormality
(E) Vaginal bleeding in association with pelvic pain usually indicates reproductive tract pathology

5. Which of the following symptoms is NOT associated with ectopic pregnancy in the fallopian tube?

(A) Unilateral lower abdominal pain
(B) Vaginal bleeding or spotting
(C) Missed menstrual period
(D) Rectal bleeding
(E) Shoulder pain

ANSWERS AND EXPLANATIONS

1. The answer is E [VI B 2 c]. Although the etiology of this woman's pelvic pain is psychogenic, this type of patient is one of the most difficult for a gynecologist to manage. The physician must not only be alert to the real possibility of organic pain but also be aware of numerous medical problems—real or imagined. Given the history of somatization and depression, chronic pelvic pain is most apt to be another manifestation of deep-rooted psychological difficulties. A team approach, using a gynecologist, internist, psychiatrist, and social worker, would most benefit this patient.

2. The answer is B [VI B 1 b (1)]. The young woman described complains of primary dysmenorrhea. Because her menses were 5 weeks ago, a physician is obligated to rule out pregnancy. This assessment can be determined by measuring the human chorionic gonadotropin β-subunit levels. However, irregular menses within several years of menarche are not unusual. After her next menses, this young woman should begin oral contraceptives and antiprostaglandins to limit the prostaglandin effects on the uterus, which are responsible for her symptoms. However, pregnancy must be ruled out before contraceptives or antiprostaglandins are begun.

3. The answer is E [VI B 1 c]. This clinical situation is typical of ovarian remnant syndrome, which results from fragments of ovarian tissue left after surgery. This tissue responds to central stimulation as ovarian tissue would. If a corpus luteum forms, then a cyst may form from hemorrhage into that area. The diagnosis can be confirmed by ultrasound. Surgery is the only effective way of managing the syndrome.

4. The answer is D [VI B 1 b (1), (2)]. Primary dysmenorrhea is usually symmetric with no associated pelvic disease, and often improves with pregnancy. On the other hand, secondary dysmenorrhea is usually associated with a structural or organic abnormality and more frequently is unilateral. Sudden onset of pain usually suggests an acute episode, whereas a gradual onset suggests inflammation, obstruction, or a more slowly evolving entity. Extensive peritoneal irritation is usually associated with generalized abdominal pain, whereas peritoneal inflammation associated with specific structures is usually more localized. Crampy, rhythmic pain is usually associated with muscular contractions, whereas steady, persistent pain suggests an inflammatory process. Vaginal bleeding in association with pelvic pain usually indicates reproductive tract pathology.

5. The answer is D [VI A 1 b]. The presenting symptoms of an ectopic pregnancy may be so vague that the physician should always consider that possibility in the differential diagnosis of pelvic pain. Rectal bleeding is not a symptom associated with ectopic pregnancy in the fallopian tube, although rectal symptoms do include rectal pressure and the urge to defecate as a result of blood in the posterior cul-de-sac. The lower abdominal pain is usually unilateral; however, it may be bilateral or generalized. The patient may also present with vaginal bleeding or spotting and a delayed or missed menstrual period. Nonspecific symptoms of pregnancy may also exist. Shoulder pain may point to peritoneal irritation by means of referred pain.

Chapter 23

Pelvic Inflammatory Disease

Kavita Nanda

I. **INTRODUCTION. Pelvic inflammatory disease (PID)** comprises a spectrum of inflammatory diseases of the upper genital tract of women. PID can involve infection of the endometrium **(endometritis)**, the oviducts **(salpingitis)**, the ovary **(oophoritis)**, the uterine wall **(myometritis)**, or portions of the parietal peritoneum **(peritonitis)**.

A. **Acute PID** mostly involves the tubes and the sequelae of tubal infection, such as destruction of tubal architecture and function and pelvic adhesions.

B. **Chronic PID** is a misnomer because the chronic problems associated with PID—hydrosalpinx, infertility, adhesions, and pain—no longer have direct bacteriologic association. True chronic PID, such as pelvic tuberculosis (TB) and actinomycosis, is rare.

II. **EPIDEMIOLOGY OF PID**

A. **Costs.** PID is usually the result of a sexually transmitted disease (STD), which has become a major health concern, although PID can also have iatrogenic causes.

1. Approximately 1 million cases of acute PID occur each year in the United States.

2. Direct and indirect costs of PID and its sequelae have been greater than $4 billion annually in the 1990s.

3. In the United States, these costs involve 267,000 inpatient hospital admissions and 119,000 operations annually.

B. **Incidence**

1. PID is a disease of the young woman. The **peak incidence** occurs in women in their late teens and early twenties.

2. Acute PID occurs in 1% to 2% of young, sexually active women annually and is the most common serious infection in women 16 to 25 years of age. Initiation of intercourse at age 15 years results in a one in eight chance of PID. Fifty percent of these adolescents have four or more sexual partners that first year.

3. **Medical sequelae** develop in one in four women with acute PID.
   a. **Ectopic pregnancy rate** increases sixfold to tenfold in women with PID. Approximately 50% of all ectopic pregnancies are thought to result from the tubal damage caused by PID.
   b. **Chronic pelvic pain** develops in 20% of women with acute PID. Both chronic pelvic pain and dyspareunia (90,000 new cases each year) are related to PID.
   c. **Infertility** results after acute PID in 6% to 60% of cases, causing more than 100,000 women per year to become infertile. The risk of **tubal obstruction** depends on the severity and the number of episodes of infection:
      (1) After one episode of PID: 11.4%
      (2) After two episodes of PID: 23.1%
      (3) After three episodes of PID: 54.3%
   d. **Mortality,** although rare, does occur, particularly in neglected cases in which a **ruptured tuboovarian abscess** can lead to septic shock and death.

C. **Contraceptive use.** Women who are not sexually active and use no contraception do not contract PID. Conversely, women who are sexually active but use no contraception contract 3.42 cases of PID per 100 woman-years.

1. **Condoms,** when used consistently and correctly, are very effective in preventing PID, as well as other STDs.

2. **Oral contraceptives** appear to protect the user against PID: only 0.91 case of PID per 100 woman-years has been reported among women using the pill. This relationship between the pill and PID may be the result of:
   a. Decreased menstrual flow
   b. Decreased ability of pathogenic bacteria to attach to endometrial cells
   c. Progestin-induced changes in the cervical mucus that retard the entrance of bacteria

2. **Other barrier methods of contraception** (e.g., the diaphragm, sponge, and contraceptive foam) also protect against PID. Spermicides may also be bactericidal. Any barrier to spermatozoa also acts as a barrier to pathogenic bacteria.

3. **Intrauterine devices (IUDs)** have been linked to an increased risk of PID (5.21 cases per 100 woman-years). The risk is confounded by epidemiologic factors such as history of STD and sexual promiscuity, and is lower in monogamous, healthy women. Possible mechanisms for the increased risk include:
   a. Creation of a sanctuary for bacteria from the body's defenses
   b. Establishment of a chronic anaerobic endometritis within the uterine cavity

III. **BACTERIOLOGY.** Acute PID is usually a **polymicrobial infection** caused by organisms that are considered normal flora of the cervix and vagina.

A. **Organisms cultured from the fallopian tube**

1. *Neisseria gonorrhoeae,* a gram-negative diplococcus

2. *Chlamydia trachomatis,* an obligate intracellular organism due to its inability to produce adenosine triphosphate

3. Endogenous aerobic bacteria, such as *Escherichia coli* and *Proteus, Klebsiella,* and *Streptococcus* sp

4. Endogenous anaerobic bacteria, such as *Bacteroides, Peptostreptococcus,* and *Peptococcus* sp

5. *Mycoplasma hominis*

6. *Actinomyces israelii,* which is found in 15% of IUD-associated cases of PID, particularly in unilateral abscesses. It is rarely found in women who do not use an IUD.

B. **Organism prevalence**

1. *N. gonorrhoeae* is the only organism recovered by direct tubal or cul-de-sac culture in one third of women with acute PID.

2. One third have a positive culture for *Neisseria* plus a mixture of endogenous aerobic and anaerobic flora.

3. One third have only aerobic and anaerobic organisms.

4. *C. trachomatis* alone is found in tubal cultures of approximately 20% of all women with salpingitis.

5. *N. gonorrhoeae* and *C. trachomatis* coexist in the same individual 25% to 40% of the time.

IV. **PATHOPHYSIOLOGY.** There is a multifactorial microbiologic etiology. Salpingo-oophoritis is usually preceded by vaginal and cervical colonization of pathologic bacteria, a state that may exist for months or years. An inciting event occurs that allows bacteria to ascend the uterus to the tubal lumen, usually bilaterally.

A. **Inciting events**

1. **Menstrual periods.** Degenerating endometrium is a good culture medium. Two thirds of acute PID cases begin just after menses.

2. **Sexual intercourse.** Bacteria-laden fluids may be pushed into the uterus, and uterine contractions may assist their ascent.

3. **Iatrogenic events**
   a. Elective abortion
   b. Dilation and curettage or endometrial biopsy
   c. IUD insertion or use
   d. Hysterosalpingography
   e. Chromopertubation at laparoscopy
   f. Radium insertion into the endometrial cavity

B. **Chronology of salpingo-oophoritis.** Infection is usually bilateral, but unilateral infection is possible, especially in association with an IUD. The presence of chronic anaerobic endometritis near one tubal ostium may explain this. The **clinical course** is as follows:

1. **Endosalpingitis** develops initially with edema and ultimately proceeds to destruction of luminal cells, cilia, and mucosal folds. Bacterial toxins are most likely to be responsible.

2. Infection spreads to the tubal muscularis and serosa. It then spreads by direct extension to the abdominal cavity through the fimbriated end of the tube.

3. **Oophoritis** develops over the surface of the ovaries, and microabscesses may develop within the ovary.

4. **Peritonitis** can develop, and upper abdominal infection may result either by direct extension of infection up the abdominal gutters laterally or by lymphatic spread. Development of **perihepatitis** with adhesions and right-upper-quadrant abdominal pain is known as the **Fitz-Hugh–Curtis syndrome.**

5. **Low-grade, smoldering, or inadequately treated infections** allow less virulent bacteria to contribute to the process, resulting in mixed infections. **Anaerobes** then play a major role in the development of pelvic abscesses.

6. **Sequelae of PID** are:
   a. Pyosalpinges (tubal abscesses)
   b. Hydrosalpinges (fluid-filled, dilated, thin-walled, destroyed tubes, usually totally obstructed)
   c. Partial tubal obstruction and crypt formation, resulting in ectopic pregnancies
   d. Total tubal obstruction and infertility
   e. Tuboovarian abscesses
   f. Peritubular and ovarian adhesions
   g. Dense pelvic and abdominal adhesions
   h. Ruptured abscesses, resulting in sepsis and shock
   i. Chronic pelvic pain and dyspareunia

V. **DIAGNOSIS**

A. **Signs and symptoms of PID** are relatively nonspecific. Thus, they produce both a high false-positive rate and a high false-negative rate of diagnosis. Laparoscopic studies have revealed the inadequacy of diagnosing acute PID by means of the usual history and physical examination and laboratory studies (Tables 23-1 and 23-2).

TABLE 23-1. Laparoscopic Findings in Patients with False-Positive Clinical Diagnosis of Acute Pelvic Inflammatory Disease (PID) with Pelvic Disorders Other Than PID

Laparoscopic Finding	No.
Acute appendicitis	24
Endometriosis	16
Corpus luteum bleeding	12
Ectopic pregnancy	11
Pelvic adhesions only	7
Benign ovarian tumor	7
Chronic salpingitis	6
Miscellaneous	15
Total	98

Reprinted with permission from Jacobson LJ: Differential diagnosis of acute pelvic inflammatory disease. *Am J Obstet Gynecol* 138:1007, 1980.

1. Based on symptoms, a **high degree of suspicion** is essential in making the diagnosis.

2. Sometimes, only very mild symptoms appear in spite of serious infection. Women with *C. trachomatis* infection may present with a few symptoms but then exhibit a severe inflammatory process when examined with the laparoscope.

B. **Clinical criteria for diagnosis**

1. **Minimum criteria for diagnosis.** Empiric treatment of PID should be given if all of the following criteria are met in the absence of another established cause for pelvic inflammation:
   a. Lower abdominal tenderness
   b. Adnexal tenderness
   c. Cervical motion tenderness

TABLE 23-2. Laparoscopic and Laparotomy Diagnosis in Patients with False-Negative Clinical Diagnosis of Acute Pelvic Inflammatory Disease (PID)

Clinical Diagnosis	Visual Diagnosis: Acute PID (No.)
Ovarian tumor	20
Acute appendicitis	18
Ectopic pregnancy	16
Chronic salpingitis	10
Acute peritonitis	6
Endometriosis	5
Uterine myoma	5
Uncharacteristic pelvic pain	5
Miscellaneous	6
Total	91

Reprinted with permission from Jacobson LJ: Differential diagnosis of acute pelvic inflammatory disease. *Am J Obstet Gynecol* 138:1007, 1980.

2. **Additional criteria.** For women with severe signs, these additional criteria are used to increase the specificity of the diagnosis:
   a. Oral temperature above 38.3° C
   b. Abnormal cervical or vaginal discharge
   c. Elevated erythrocyte sedimentation rate
   d. Elevated C-reactive protein
   e. Positive test for gonorrhea or chlamydia
   f. Tuboovarian abscess seen on ultrasound
   g. Evidence of endometritis on endometrial biopsy
   h. Laparoscopic evidence of PID

C. **Differential diagnosis** for PID should include:

1. Ectopic pregnancy

2. Ruptured ovarian cyst

3. Appendicitis

4. Endometriosis

5. Inflammatory bowel disease

6. Degenerating fibroids

7. Spontaneous abortion

8. Diverticulitis

D. **Diagnostic techniques**

1. **Cervical Gram stain.** If gram-negative intracellular diplococci are present, gonorrhea is the presumed diagnosis. However, Gram stain alone misses one half of the gonorrhea cases.

2. **Serum human chorionic gonadotropin.** A sensitive pregnancy test is important in the differential diagnosis of pelvic pain to rule out the possibility of ectopic pregnancy. In the past, approximately 3% to 4% of women admitted with the diagnosis of PID had an ectopic pregnancy.

3. **Ultrasound** may help to define adnexal masses and intrauterine or ectopic pregnancies, especially when a patient has a tender abdomen and will not permit an adequate pelvic examination. Response to therapy can be measured objectively as pelvic masses and induration regress.

4. **Laparoscopy.** If the disease process is unclear, this technique is the ultimate way to establish the diagnosis.

5. **Culdocentesis.** If purulent fluid is obtained, a culture may assist in antibiotic selection. However, infections may be secondary to another primary process.

6. **Blood studies**
   a. **Leukocytosis** is not a reliable indicator of acute PID. Less than 50% of women with acute PID have a white blood cell count greater than 10,000 cells/ml.
   b. An **increased sedimentation rate** is a nonspecific finding, but the sedimentation rate is elevated in approximately 75% of women with laparoscopically confirmed PID.

VI. **THERAPY**

A. **Individualized treatment** and a **high index of suspicion for infection** are mandatory. Treatment should always include the sex partners. The physician must decide between outpatient management of the woman with close follow-up in 48 to 72 hours, or hospitalization. Many experts recommend that all patients be hospitalized. **Hospitalization of PID patients** should be especially considered if:

1. The diagnosis is uncertain
2. Surgical emergencies, such as appendicitis or ectopic pregnancy, must be excluded
3. A pelvic abscess is suspected
4. Severe illness (e.g., vomiting, dehydration, high fever, or signs of peritonitis) precludes outpatient management
5. The patient is pregnant
6. The patient is an adolescent, and may not comply with therapy
7. The patient is nulliparous
8. The patient has human immunodeficiency virus infection
9. The patient is unable to follow or tolerate an outpatient regimen
10. The patient has failed an outpatient course of management
11. Clinical follow-up within 72 hours of beginning antibiotics cannot be arranged

B. **Mild PID. Outpatient regimens** for patients with mild PID include:

1. **Ceftriaxone** 250 mg intramuscularly plus **doxycycline** 100 mg orally twice a day for 14 days
2. **Ofloxacin** 400 mg orally twice daily for 14 days and either **clindamycin** 450 mg four times a day or **metronidazole** 500 mg orally two times a day for 14 days

C. **Acute severe PID.** One of the following combination antibiotic regimens that cover the three major pathogens—N. gonorrhoeae, C. trachomatis, and anaerobes—should be used.

1. **Cefoxitin** 2 g intravenously every 6 hours or **cefotetan** 2 g intravenously every 12 hours plus **doxycycline** 100 mg intravenously or orally every 12 hours
2. **Clindamycin** 900 mg intravenously every 8 hours plus a **gentamicin** loading dose of 2.0 mg/kg intravenously, followed by gentamicin, 1.5 mg/kg intravenously every 8 hours
3. **Conservative therapy** with intense intravenous antibiotics should be tried first. Signs of clinical improvement, which include defervescence, reduction in direct or rebound abdominal tenderness, and reduction in uterine and adnexal tenderness, should occur within 72 hours of initiating therapy.
   a. If clinical improvement results, treatment should be continued for at least 48 hours after the patient demonstrates substantial clinical improvement, then followed by doxycycline 100 mg twice a day for 14 days total. Sonographic resolution of tuboovarian masses may take weeks.
   b. **Surgical intervention** must be considered if the patient shows no response to antibiotic therapy in 72 hours.
      (1) **Laparoscopy** may be considered for diagnosis, and may be followed by laparotomy. Unless a well-defined unilateral abscess allows a unilateral salpingo-oophorectomy, the treatment of choice is a total abdominal hysterectomy, bilateral salpingo-oophorectomy, and drainage of the pelvic cavity. The patient, regardless of her age, should be prepared for this possibility before surgery.
      (2) If an abscess is accessible through the cul-de-sac or radiologically, **catheter drainage** may be possible.

VII. OTHER CAUSES OF PELVIC INFECTION

A. **Granulomatous salpingitis**

1. **Tuberculous salpingitis** almost always represents systemic TB. The incidence is high in underdeveloped countries and very low in developed countries. It usually

affects women in their reproductive years, but an increased incidence has been reported among postmenopausal women. Primary genital TB is extremely rare in the United States.

    a. Physical findings are variable. Patients usually present with adnexal masses. Induration may be noted in the paracervical, paravaginal, and parametrial tissues. The typical patient is 20 to 40 years of age with known TB and a pelvic mass. Symptoms are related to a family history of TB, low-level pelvic pain, infertility, and amenorrhea.

    b. Pathology. Grossly, the uterine tube has a classic "tobacco pouch" appearance—enlarged and distended. The proximal end is closed, and the fimbria are edematous and enlarged. Microscopically, tubercles show an epithelioid reaction and giant cell formation. Inflammation and scarring are intense and irreversible.

    c. Treatment involves the standard regimens for disseminated TB, including isoniazid, rifampin, and ethambutol. Prognosis for cure is excellent, but the outlook for fertility is dismal.

2. Leprous salpingitis. The histologic picture is similar to the one for TB, and the two are often difficult to distinguish on a histologic basis. Langerhans' giant cells and epithelioid cells are present. Positive cultures are necessary for a diagnosis of TB.

3. Actinomycosis. *A. israelii,* the causative agent, is pathogenic for humans but not for other mammals. Most gynecologic involvement is infection secondary to appendiceal infection, gastrointestinal tract disorders, or IUD use. A total of 100 cases are reported annually, and the age range of prevalence is about 20 to 40 years.

    a. Physical findings. Half the lesions are bilateral and are characterized by adnexal enlargement and tenderness. Presenting symptoms may be confused with those for appendicitis.

    b. Pathology. Grossly, there is tuboovarian inflammation, and there is copious necrotic material on sections of the tube. The tubal lumen may have an adenomatous appearance. Microscopically, actinomycotic "sulfur" granules are present. Club-like filaments radiate out from the center. A monocytic infiltrate is apparent, and giant cells may be present.

    c. Treatment. Therapy is a prolonged course of penicillin.

4. Schistosomiasis occurs most commonly in the Far East and Africa.

    a. Physical findings are pelvic pain, menstrual irregularity, and primary infertility. The diagnosis is usually made by histopathologic findings.

    b. Pathology. Grossly, lesions appear as a nonspecific tuboovarian process. Microscopically, the ova or schistosome is seen surrounded by a granulomatous reaction with giant and epidermoid cells. An egg within an inflammatory milieu is a dramatic sight.

5. Sarcoidosis. Although very rare, sarcoidosis can lead to a granulomatous salpingitis.

6. Foreign-body salpingitis occurs after the use of non–water-soluble dye material for hysterosalpingography; it may also be secondary to medications placed within the vagina, such as starch, talc, and mineral oil.

B. **Nongranulomatous salpingitis** refers to any other bacterial infection, usually of the peritoneal cavity, that can secondarily cause tubal infection, including:

    1. Appendicitis

    2. Diverticulitis

    3. Crohn's disease

    4. Cholecystitis

    5. Perinephric abscess

STUDY QUESTIONS

DIRECTIONS: Each of the numbered items or incomplete statements in this section is followed by answers or by completions of the statement. Select the ONE lettered answer or completion that is BEST in each case.

1. The pathogenesis of a tuboovarian abscess initially involves which of the following?

(A) Perihepatitis
(B) Endometritis
(C) Endosalpingitis
(D) Cervicitis
(E) Myometritis

2. Which of the following procedures confirms the diagnosis of pelvic inflammatory disease (PID)?

(A) White blood cell count
(B) Cervical Gram stain
(C) Culdocentesis
(D) Laparoscopy
(E) Pelvic ultrasound

3. Which of the following bacteria has been found almost exclusively in women with pelvic inflammatory disease (PID) who use an intrauterine device (IUD)?

(A) *Actinomyces israelii*
(B) *Bacteroides fragilis*
(C) *Chlamydia trachomatis*
(D) *Mycoplasma hominis*
(E) *Neisseria gonorrhoeae*

4. Which of the following drug combinations would be most appropriate in the inpatient treatment of acute pelvic inflammatory disease (PID)?

(A) Clindamycin/norfloxacin
(B) Cefoxitin/doxycycline
(C) Ampicillin/tetracycline
(D) Ampicillin/gentamicin
(E) Cefoxitin/cefotetan

DIRECTIONS: Each of the numbered items or incomplete statements in this section is negatively phrased, as indicated by a capitalized word such as NOT, LEAST, or EXCEPT. Select the ONE lettered answer or completion that is BEST in each case.

5. Which one of the following factors is NOT associated with an increased risk of pelvic inflammatory disease (PID)?

(A) Onset of intercourse at age 15 years
(B) An elective abortion
(C) Oral contraceptive use
(D) Hysterosalpingography
(E) Use of a copper intrauterine device (IUD)

6. Which of the following procedures does NOT aid in the diagnosis of pelvic inflammatory disease (PID)?

(A) Laparoscopy
(B) Ultrasound
(C) Culdocentesis
(D) Hysterosalpingography
(E) Rectal examination

7. Which of the following diseases does NOT cause pelvic inflammatory disease (PID)?

(A) Crohn's disease
(B) Syphilis
(C) Appendicitis
(D) Sarcoidosis
(E) Schistosomiasis

8. Which of the following is NOT a known consequence of pelvic inflammatory disease (PID)?

(A) Endometriosis
(B) Ectopic pregnancy
(C) Pelvic adhesions
(D) Dyspareunia
(E) Hydrosalpinx

9. An 18-year-old woman enters the emergency room with acute lower abdominal pain, which started 1 week after a period that was 7 days late. She is sexually active and not using birth control. Her temperature is 99.4° F, and her white blood cell count is 12.4. On examination, her pain extends to the upper abdomen on the right side. The differential diagnosis should NOT include which of the following?

(A) Ectopic pregnancy
(B) Fitz-Hugh–Curtis syndrome
(C) Appendicitis
(D) Pelvic tuberculosis (TB)
(E) Acute salpingitis

DIRECTIONS: The set of matching questions in this section consists of a list of four to twenty-six lettered options (some of which may be in figures) followed by several numbered items. For each numbered item, select the ONE lettered option that is most closely associated with it. To avoid spending too much time on matching sets with large numbers of options, it is generally advisable to begin each set by reading the list of options. Then, for each item in the set, try to generate the correct answer and locate it in the option list, rather than evaluating each option individually. Each lettered option may be selected once, more than once, or not at all.

Questions 10–12

For each of the following clinical situations describing a typical picture of pelvic inflammatory disease (PID), select the organism that is most likely to be responsible for it.

(A) *Staphylococcus aureus*
(B) *Bacteroides fragilis*
(C) *Actinomyces israelii*
(D) *Neisseria gonorrhoeae*
(E) *Chlamydia trachomatis*

10. A sexually active, 15-year-old girl comes to the emergency room complaining of acute pain in the lower abdomen that makes walking difficult. She states that the pain began 2 days after her menses ended and that she has a vaginal discharge.

11. A 40-year-old woman has had several admissions to the hospital for PID. On the present admission, a tender, fluctuant pelvic mass is noted. She has a temperature of 102° F and looks septic. After 5 days of intravenous antibiotics, there is no response. Exploratory surgery reveals a tuboovarian abscess.

12. A 24-year-old woman had an intrauterine device (IUD) inserted after her first delivery 2 years ago. She comes to the emergency room with lower abdominal pain and uterine tenderness. Pelvic examination reveals bilateral adnexal fullness. The IUD is removed and sent to pathology. The patient is started on penicillin.

ANSWERS AND EXPLANATIONS

1. The answer is C [IV B 1–5]. The offending pathogen initially stimulates an endosalpingitis. The infection spreads to the tubal muscularis and the serosa and, by direct extension, to the peritoneal cavity and the ovary, where an oophoritis usually proceeds to a tuboovarian abscess. Cervicitis (inflammation of the cervix), endometritis (inflammation of the endometrium), and myometritis (inflammation of the uterine muscularis) are not necessarily part of the pathophysiology of tuboovarian abscess. A perihepatitis involves infection in the right upper quadrant with adhesions and right-upper-quadrant pain, and is known as the Fitz-Hugh–Curtis syndrome.

2. The answer is D [V D 1–6]. Laparoscopy is the gold standard in terms of diagnosing pelvic inflammatory disease (PID). Direct visualization of the pelvis, tubes, and ovaries confirms or rules out the diagnosis of PID. Most other studies are supportive but not diagnostic. For example, 50% of cases of *Neisseria gonorrhoeae* PID are missed by cervical Gram stain, and less than 50% of women with PID have a white blood cell count above 10,000 cells/ml. The purulent fluid obtained from the cul-de-sac through culdocentesis may be helpful in making the diagnosis, but that fluid could be coming from an infection elsewhere in the peritoneal cavity. Pelvic ultrasound may be helpful in defining and following adnexal masses, but it cannot confirm the diagnosis of PID.

3. The answer is A [III A, B]. *Actinomyces israelii* is found in 15% of intrauterine device (IUD)-associated cases of pelvic inflammatory disease (PID) and is rarely found in women who do not use an IUD. *Neisseria gonorrhoeae* may be responsible for as many as 40% of PID cases, and penicillinase-producing strains, should they continue to proliferate, will make it difficult to eradicate. *Chlamydia trachomatis* may be responsible for up to 40% of cases of PID, but rigid laboratory growth requirements have made it difficult to link *C. trachomatis* with PID. *Mycoplasma hominis* may be responsible for 20% of cases of PID.

4. The answer is B [VI C 1,2]. The combination of medications used to treat acute pelvic inflammatory disease (PID) must cover a variety of pathogens—aerobes, anaerobes, gonorrhea, and chlamydia. The two regimens that are recommended by the Centers for Disease Control and Prevention for inpatient treatment are cefoxitin or cefotetan plus doxycycline, or clindamycin and gentamicin.

5. The answer is C [II C 2]. Oral contraceptive use appears to protect the user against pelvic inflammatory disease (PID) because of decreased menstrual flow, which inhibits the transport of bacteria; decreased ability of bacteria to attach to endometrial cells; and the presence of progesterone. Intrauterine devices (IUDs) have been linked to an increased risk of PID as has early initiation of intercourse. Iatrogenic events that may allow bacteria to ascend the uterus to the tubal lumen include elective abortion, hysterosalpingography, dilation and curettage, and IUD insertion.

6. The answer is D [V D 1–6]. Hysterosalpingography should never be performed if pelvic inflammatory disease (PID) is suspected because it can disseminate the infection. The signs and symptoms of PID are relatively nonspecific; thus, a high degree of suspicion is essential for the diagnosis. Techniques that aid in the diagnosis include laparoscopy, culdocentesis, and ultrasound. A rectal examination should always be performed during a pelvic examination to detect pelvic masses.

7. The answer is B [VII A, B]. Although syphilis can occur in association with pelvic inflammatory disease (PID) because both are sexually transmitted, it is not a direct cause of PID. Bacterial infections that can secondarily cause tubal infection include appendicitis, which often causes pelvic adhesions and perisalpingo-oophoritis, and Crohn's disease, which can cause damage and inflammation of the oviducts. Although rare, schistosomiasis and sarcoidosis can also lead to granulomatous salpingitis.

8. The answer is A [IV B 6]. Endometriosis can cause symptoms similar to those associated with pelvic inflammatory disease (PID), but its occurrence is not related to pelvic infection. At present, 6% to 60% of female infertility is caused by the tubal obstruction from PID, and 50% of all ectopic pregnancies are thought to result from the tubal damage caused by PID. Pelvic adhesions and hydrosalpinges are consequences of the peritubal infection that occurs. Chronic pelvic pain and dyspareunia can be related to a prior history of PID.

9. The answer is D [V C; VII A 1 a]. Pelvic tuberculosis (TB) rarely causes acute abdominal pain; it is usually suspected as a causative agent when there is a history of pulmonary TB, a pelvic mass, long-standing infertility, and pelvic adhesions. Ectopic pregnancy should always be considered in a young woman who presents with abdominal pain, particularly if she is sexually active and if her period is late. The pain of an ectopic pregnancy results from tubal distention and intraabdominal blood. Acute salpingitis is the primary diagnosis in a young woman whose signs and symptoms of lower abdominal infection begin during or after a menses. The Fitz-Hugh–Curtis syndrome is a pelvic inflammatory disease (PID) that spreads to the upper abdomen; it presents as perihepatitis and right-upper-quadrant abdominal pain. Appendicitis is part of the differential diagnosis when there is lower abdominal pain and evidence of infection.

10–12. The answers are: 10-D [II B 1,2; III B], **11-B** [III A; IV B 5], **12-C** [VII A 3]. The picture of the sexually active teenager is one of acute pelvic inflammatory disease (PID). Initiation of intercourse at age 15 years results in a one in eight chance of PID, with 50% of these women having four or more sexual partners in the first year. *Neisseria gonorrhoeae* is thought to be the chief pathogen in the development of acute primary PID. It usually can be cultured from the cervix, especially when there is a discharge present, as there is in this case. The clinical picture of the 40-year-old woman is one of chronic PID with pelvic abscess formation. The pathogens in chronic PID are usually different from those of acute primary PID. There is likely to be a mixture of aerobic and anaerobic organisms. *Haemophilus, Streptococcus,* and *Escherichia coli* are the prominent aerobic organisms found with such abscesses, and *Bacteroides, Peptococcus,* and *Peptostreptococcus* are the prominent anaerobes. *Actinomyces israelii* is the organism that has been associated with intrauterine device (IUD) users in 15% of IUD-associated cases of PID. It is not usually found in non-IUD users. The adnexae may be enlarged and tender. "Sulfur" granules are seen microscopically. The therapy is penicillin.

Chapter 24

Endometriosis

Matthew F. Rhoa

I. INTRODUCTION

A. Definition. Endometriosis is the presence of functioning endometrial glands and stroma outside their usual location in the uterine cavity, often resulting in significant pelvic adhesions with or without associated inflammatory cells or hemosiderin-laden macrophages. It is primarily a pelvic disease with implants on, or adhesions of, the ovaries, fallopian tubes, uterosacral ligaments, rectosigmoid, and bladder. Less commonly, endometriosis can be found outside the pelvis, suggesting a metastatic spread. Endometriosis is in general a **benign disease** that usually affects women in their reproductive years. There have been, however, several cases in the recent literature of endometrioid carcinoma arising within endometriosis. Endometriosis is often associated with:

1. Crippling dysmenorrhea

2. Severe dyspareunia

3. Chronic pelvic pain

4. Infertility

B. Infertility. Pregnancy, with its positive effect on improving endometriosis, often is very difficult to achieve.

1. Infertility among women with endometriosis is approximately 30% to 40%.

2. Endometriosis in infertile women has been demonstrated by **laparoscopy** in 15% to 25% of cases.

II. THEORIES OF PATHOGENESIS

A. Retrograde menstrual flow. One theory postulates that the backward flow of menstrual debris through the fallopian tubes causes the endometrial cells to spread into the pelvis. These cells implant there or set up irritative foci, which stimulate coelomic metaplasia and differentiation of the peritoneal cells into endometrial-type tissue.

1. **Clinical evidence.** Endometriosis is commonly found in dependent portions of the pelvis, most frequently on the ovaries, cul-de-sac, and uterosacral ligaments. Flow of menstrual blood from the fallopian tubes has been observed during laparoscopy.

2. **Experimental evidence.** Endometrial fragments from the menstrual flow can grow both in tissue culture and after injection beneath the skin of the abdominal wall.

B. Hematogenous or lymphatic spread. Endometriosis at sites distant from the pelvis may be caused by vascular or lymphatic transport of endometrial fragments. This could explain the presence of endometriosis at distant sites such as the brain and lungs.

C. Metaplasia of coelomic epithelium. The transformation of coelomic epithelium results from some as yet unspecified stimuli. Endometriosis has been reported in a prepubertal girl, and in many adolescents who have had very few menstrual cycles.

D. **Genetic and immunologic influences.** The relative risk of endometriosis is 7% in siblings, compared to 1% in a control group. In addition, an immunologic deficiency may be involved in the pathogenesis of endometriosis. Monkeys with spontaneous endometriosis were found to have a cell-mediated response to autologous endometrial tissue that was significantly lower than that of control animals. Thus, a genetic influence could manifest itself through a deficient immunologic system.

III. DIAGNOSIS

A. **Signs and symptoms.** Endometriosis should be suspected in any woman complaining of infertility. Suspicion is heightened when she also complains of dysmenorrhea and dyspareunia.

1. **Dysmenorrhea.** Painful menses are suggestive of endometriosis if they begin after years of relatively pain-free menses. With the increased use of laparoscopy, many adolescents with primary dysmenorrhea are being diagnosed with endometriosis.

2. **Pelvic pain.** Pain can be diffuse in the pelvis, or it can be more localized, often in the area of the rectum. The degree of endometriosis often does not correlate with the amount of pain experienced. Many women who have endometriosis are asymptomatic.

3. **Dyspareunia.** Painful intercourse may be caused by:
   a. Endometrial implants of the uterosacral ligaments
   b. Endometriomas of the ovaries
   c. Fixed retroversion of the uterus secondary to the endometriosis

4. **Infertility.** When endometriosis involves the ovaries and causes adhesions, there is no question of its role in causing infertility. The association between minimal endometriosis and infertility is less well documented. Medical therapy in these cases does not improve fertility. Significant quantities of **prostaglandin,** reported to be secreted from the endometrial implants near the tubes and ovaries, may:
   a. Interfere with tubal function and mobility, ovulation, steroidogenesis, and luteal function
   b. Contribute to the **luteinized unruptured follicle syndrome,** in which the ovum is trapped within the follicle and not released with the luteinizing hormone surge

5. **Other signs of endometriosis.** Irregular menses, cyclic rectal bleeding or pain, and hematuria may be signs of endometriosis of the ovaries, rectosigmoid, and bladder, respectively.

B. **Examination.** The diagnosis of endometriosis combines the findings from the history, pelvic examination, and laparoscopy. The only way to diagnose endometriosis is by visualization at surgery and laparoscopy or by biopsy of an implant; history and physical examination are suggestive, but not diagnostic.

1. **History.** The symptoms described by the patient are correlated with the physical examination and the diagnostic procedures in arriving at a diagnosis. A history of endometriosis in the patient's mother or sisters is important.

2. **Pelvic examination.** With minimal endometriosis, the pelvic examination may provide only normal findings.
   a. **Beading, nodularity, and tenderness of the uterosacral ligaments** are characteristic of endometriosis and can be best appreciated on rectovaginal examination.
   b. **Endometriomas, or chocolate cysts of the ovaries,** are palpated as adnexal masses, often fixed to the lateral pelvic walls or posterior to the broad ligament.
   c. The **uterus** is often in a **fixed, retroverted** position.

3. The **CA-125** assay tests for a cell surface antigen found on derivatives of the coelomic epithelium, which includes the endometrium.
   a. Serum levels are elevated in patients with endometriosis.

    b. The assay correlates with the degree of disease and response to treatment.

    c. It can be used as a marker for the recurrence of endometriosis.

  4. Laparoscopy. Visual diagnosis of endometriosis with the laparoscope is essential because ovarian enlargement and nodularity of the cul-de-sac may result from metastatic ovarian carcinoma, bowel cancer, or calcified mesotheliomas.

C. **Classification of endometriosis.** Because both treatment and prognosis of endometriosis are determined, to some extent, by the severity of the disease, it would be desirable to have a uniform system of classification that takes into account both the extent and severity of the disease. Unfortunately, the diversity of the different classification systems precludes accurate comparisons, and questions regarding the most efficacious treatment of varying degrees of endometriosis go unanswered. The most commonly used classification system, developed by the American Fertility Society, is based on findings from laparoscopy or laparotomy.

IV. **MANAGEMENT.** The **age of the patient,** the **extent of the disease,** the **reproductive plans of the couple,** the **duration of the infertility,** and the **severity of the symptoms** are all important considerations.

A. **Expectant therapy.** No therapy has proven to be a logical approach to patients with minimal disease. This situation is especially relevant to the young woman with short-term infertility. In a comparison of patients with mild endometriosis, the pregnancy rate in 1 year was 72% in patients managed with an expectant approach and 76% in patients treated with conservative surgery.

B. **Medical therapy.** Ectopic endometrium responds to cyclic hormone secretion in a fashion similar to normal endometrium; thus, **hormonal suppression of a woman's menses** constitutes the basis of medical therapy.

  1. Oral contraceptives. The use of a **continuous combination estrogen with progestin pill** creates a pseudopregnancy with amenorrhea. The pseudopregnancy causes a deciduation, necrobiosis, and resorption of the ectopic endometrium. This form of treatment is **appropriate only in mild endometriosis** that does not involve much distortion of the pelvic anatomy by adhesions or endometriomas. An oral contraceptive with strong progestational properties should be taken continuously for 9 months in the following manner.

    a. Dosage. The pills are given daily on a continuous basis. Breakthrough bleeding can be controlled by adding conjugated estrogens for short periods. The therapy is continued for 6 to 12 months.

    b. The **pregnancy rate after pseudopregnancy** has generally been between 25% and 50%.

    c. Recurrence rate. The fact that pseudopregnancy does not cure endometriosis is reflected in the recurrence rate of the disease—about 17% to 18% in 1 year, and higher with extended periods of posttreatment observation.

  2. Danazol. Danazol, commonly used in the past, is being replaced by the gonadotropin-releasing hormone (GnRH) agonists. Danazol creates a high-androgen, low-estrogen environment.

    a. Dosage. The effective dose is 400 to 800 mg/day (200-mg tablets) for 6 months.

      (1) Lower doses offer mainly symptomatic relief.

      (2) Higher doses. The **pregnancy rate** when the higher doses are used is 40% to 60% after 6 months of pseudomenopause.

    b. Side effects are related both to the hypoestrogenic environment that danazol creates and to its androgenic properties.

      (1) Hypoestrogenic properties include water retention, decreased breast size, atrophic vaginitis, dyspareunia, hot flashes, muscle cramps, and emotional lability.

      (2) Androgenic properties include weight gain, acne, oily skin, deepening of the voice, and growth of facial hair.

      c. Prognosis with danazol is related to the extent of the endometriosis and the dose of the drug; with a regimen of 800 mg/day for 4 to 9 months, the pregnancy rate is approximately 60%.

      d. Recurrence rates are highest (23%) during the first year after stopping the danazol treatment.

    3. Progestogens. Long-acting, intramuscular progestogens (medroxyprogesterone acetate 100–200 mg/month) suppress hypothalamic–pituitary function, leading to amenorrhea and decidual, rather than atrophic, endometrial changes.

      a. Breakthrough bleeding is a nuisance side effect, but weight gain and depression are potential problems for the patient.

      b. Prolonged amenorrhea after treatment makes this regimen undesirable in women who want immediate fertility.

    4. GnRH agonists. With continuous administration, these agents first stimulate gonadotropin release, then suppress pituitary–ovarian function, leading to a "medical hypophysectomy."

      a. Administration. The drug is administered either daily in the form of intranasal spray or subcutaneous injection or monthly in a depot injection.

      b. Effects. Amenorrhea and atrophic endometrial changes occur.

      c. Menopausal-type symptoms (e.g., hot flashes, decreased libido, and vaginal dryness) occur because of the hypoestrogenic state.

      d. Prolonged use can result in significant bone loss leading to osteoporosis.

C. **Surgical therapy.** If there are anatomic factors such as tuboovarian adhesions or large endometriomas indicative of moderate to severe disease, the treatment of choice is surgery. Medical therapy and hormone suppression do not dissolve the adhesions or eliminate the endometriomas. The success of surgery in relieving infertility is directly related to the severity of the endometriosis.

    1. Conservative surgery involves the excision, fulguration, or laser vaporization of endometriotic tissue, the excision of ovarian endometriomas, and the resection of severely involved pelvic viscera, leaving the uterus and at least one tube and ovary intact. Additional infertility surgery measures for endometriosis include the gentle handling of tissue, lysis of adhesions, precise dissection, and meticulous hemostasis.

      a. Reconstruction of all peritoneal surfaces is essential. The raw areas in the pelvis can be covered with free peritoneal or omental grafts to prevent adhesions.

      b. Postoperative use of hormones has been the subject of great controversy because the highest pregnancy rates occur in the first year after conservative surgery; thus, most physicians are reluctant to use hormones that prevent pregnancy, even for a few months. If pregnancy does not occur within 2 years of surgery for endometriosis, the long-term prognosis is poor.

    2. Radical surgery, which involves a total abdominal hysterectomy and bilateral salpingo-oophorectomy, is used in patients whose childbearing is finished or in those whose endometriosis is so severe that it precludes any attempt at reconstruction. A less than complete pelvic cleanout in these patients guarantees reoperation at a later date. Radical surgery for endometriosis in women in their reproductive years means castration at an early age. In these women, replacement estrogen is essential to prevent problems with loss of calcium from bones, atrophic changes in the pelvis, especially the vagina, and premature aging of the cardiovascular system. Estrogen replacement therapy carries only a small risk of inciting growth of residual endometriosis.

V. **MAINTENANCE OF FERTILITY AND SYMPTOMATIC RELIEF.** Finding endometriosis (by laparoscopy) in a young woman who has pelvic pain and no immediate interest in pregnancy is a common occurrence. The goals for this type of patient are relief of the dysmenorrhea and prevention of further growth of the endometriosis.

A. **Birth control pills.** Cyclic birth control pills are appropriate treatment for mild disease because they reduce the amount of endometrial buildup and shedding, thereby preventing further growth of the endometriosis.

B. **Nonsteroidal antiinflammatory drugs (NSAIDs).** Women with endometriosis show increased concentrations of prostaglandins in the peritoneal fluid. The prostaglandin synthetase inhibitors (i.e., NSAIDs) are effective in controlling the endometriosis-related dysmenorrhea.

C. **Birth control pills and NSAIDs.** The two may be administered simultaneously if neither one individually controls the dysmenorrhea.

STUDY QUESTIONS

DIRECTIONS: Each of the numbered items or incomplete statements in this section is followed by answers or by completions of the statement. Select the ONE lettered answer or completion that is BEST in each case.

1. Oral contraceptive therapy for endometriosis is appropriate in which of the following situations?

(A) Presence of endometriomas
(B) Minimal endometriosis and mild symptoms
(C) Infertility
(D) Severe endometriosis with debilitating symptoms
(E) After radical surgical therapy

2. The diagnosis of endometriosis is made by

(A) clinical history
(B) physical examination
(C) history of infertility
(D) CA-125 blood test
(E) direct visualization and biopsy

3. The most likely site for implantation of endometriosis is

(A) small bowel serosa
(B) omentum
(C) appendix
(D) bladder
(E) peritoneum of cul-de-sac

4. The most appropriate therapy for a 35-year-old woman who just underwent radical surgery for endometriosis would be

(A) gonadotropin-releasing hormone (GnRH) agonists
(B) nonsteroidal antiinflammatory drugs (NSAIDs)
(C) danazol
(D) oral contraceptive pills
(E) estrogen replacement therapy

DIRECTIONS: Each of the numbered items or incomplete statements in this section is negatively phrased, as indicated by a capitalized word such as NOT, LEAST, or EXCEPT. Select the ONE lettered answer or completion that is BEST in each case.

5. Which of the following is NOT a theory for the pathogenesis of endometriosis?

(A) Coelomic metaplasia
(B) Endometrial hyperplasia
(C) Retrograde menstruation
(D) Immunologic deficiency
(E) Lymphatic spread of endometrial fragments

6. Which of the following is NOT a hormonal therapy for endometriosis?

(A) Gonadotropin-releasing hormone (GnRH) agonists
(B) Progesterone
(C) Oral contraceptive pills
(D) Methotrexate
(E) Danazol

DIRECTIONS: The set of matching questions in this section consists of a list of four to twenty-six lettered options (some of which may be in figures) followed by several numbered items. For each numbered item, select the ONE lettered option that is most closely associated with it. To avoid spending too much time on matching sets with large numbers of options, it is generally advisable to begin each set by reading the list of options. Then, for each item in the set, try to generate the correct answer and locate it in the option list, rather than evaluating each option individually. Each lettered option may be selected once, more than once, or not at all.

Questions 7–9

For each clinical presentation listed below, select the most appropriate therapeutic modality.

(A) Expectant management
(B) Danazol therapy
(C) Conservative endometriosis surgery
(D) Cyclic oral contraceptives
(E) Radical endometriosis surgery

7. A 26-year-old medical student presents with an established diagnosis of mild endometriosis. She states that she wants to finish a residency program before even thinking of a pregnancy.

8. A 24-year-old woman presents with a 6-month history of infertility. A laparoscopic diagnosis of mild endometriosis shows scattered cul-de-sac implants. This woman has no other infertility factors.

9. A 32-year-old lawyer presents with a 5-year history of infertility. A laparoscopic diagnosis of moderate endometriosis is made. Scattered endometrial implants in the pelvis, a 2-cm endometrioma on the left ovary, and adhesions between the tube and ovary on each side are found.

ANSWERS AND EXPLANATIONS

1. The answer is B [IV B 1 a, b, 2]. Oral contraceptive use as medical therapy for endometriosis induces a pseudopregnancy; that is, the continuous use of the estrogen with progestin medication results in amenorrhea for about 9 months. The medication causes deciduation, necrobiosis, and resorption of the endometrial implants, but it does not eliminate structural abnormalities, such as endometriomas. After radical surgery, estrogen replacement therapy would be most appropriate. The pregnancy rate after a pseudopregnancy is 25% to 50%.

2. The answer is E [III B]. The diagnosis of endometriosis can be made only by direct visualization and biopsy. History and physical examination are suggestive, but not diagnostic.

3. The answer is E [II A 1]. Endometriosis is commonly found in dependent portions of the pelvis, most frequently on the ovaries, cul-de-sac, and uterosacral ligaments.

4. The answer is E [IV C 2]. Radical endometriosis surgery means a bilateral oophorectomy. Castration in a woman in her reproductive years induces an immediate hypoestrogenic state, which has short- and long-term consequences. Hot flashes, atrophic vaginitis, and a decreased libido are symptoms that women notice days to weeks after surgery. Osteoporosis and premature aging of the cardiovascular system are long-term sequelae of early castration that does not involve estrogen replacement.

5. The answer is B [II A–D]. Endometrial hyperplasia occurs in anovulatory patients who have unopposed estrogen stimulation of the endometrium and has nothing to do with endometriosis. The classic theory of endometriosis involves the retrograde flow of menstrual debris out through the tubes, resulting in implantation in the pelvis. The fragments appear to serve as irritative foci, which then stimulate coelomic metaplasia into endometrial-type tissue. Lymphatic spread may explain endometriosis at sites distant from the pelvis. Because endometriosis is found in siblings, a genetic influence could be manifested through a deficient immunologic system.

6. The answer is D [IV B 1–4]. Methotrexate is a chemotherapeutic agent used most commonly in gestational trophoblastic neoplasia and ectopic pregnancy.

7–9. The answers are: 7-D [V A], **8-A** [IV A], **9-C** [IV C 1]. The 26-year-old woman with mild endometriosis—but not infertility—currently does not need any therapy for her endometriosis. However, because she wants to maintain her fertility, her disease should not be allowed to progress. Cyclic use of oral contraceptives helps to prevent progression of the endometriosis by reducing both the amount of endometrial shedding (compared with the endometrial proliferation and shedding of a natural cycle) and further growth of the endometriosis. The 24-year-old woman with a 6-month history of infertility has mild endometriosis without any anatomic alterations of her pelvis. There is no need for immediate medical or surgical therapy. An expectant approach in a young woman with mild endometriosis should yield a pregnancy rate of 60% to 70% within 1 year. The woman in her thirties with a 5-year history of infertility has anatomic changes in her pelvis as a result of the endometriosis. Because of this woman's age and the significant length of her infertility, medical therapy would be inappropriate because it takes 6 to 9 months and has questionable results in women with anatomic changes, such as endometriomas and pelvic adhesions. Thus, the indicated therapy is conservative surgery to resect the endometrioma, lyse the adhesions, and remove the implants.

Chapter 25

Vulvovaginitis

Michelle Battistini

I. **INTRODUCTION.** Vulvovaginitis is one of the most common gynecologic problems seen by the practicing gynecologist. Moreover, a wide spectrum of disorders can create vulvovaginal symptoms.

II. **VULVOVAGINAL ANATOMY**

A. **Vulva.** The vulva is made up of the **mons pubis, labia majora and minora, clitoris, and vestibule;** it contains the urinary meatus, vaginal orifice, Bartholin's glands (major vestibular glands), Skene's ducts, and minor vestibular glands. The vulva is subject to any conditions that may affect the skin and related structures, including psoriasis, hypersensitivity reactions, and benign and malignant neoplasms.

   1. **Anatomy**
      a. The entire vulva is covered by a keratinized squamous epithelium.
      b. Hair-bearing regions contain associated hair follicles, sebaceous glands, and apocrine and eccrine sweat glands.
      c. Regions without hair, such as the labia minora and prepuce, contain sebaceous glands, but hair follicles and eccrine and apocrine sweat glands are absent.
      d. The **labia majora** are composed of skin enclosing a variable amount of fat and smooth muscle.
         (1) They extend from the mons anteriorly to the fourchette posteriorly.
         (2) The embryologic homologue in the male is the scrotum.
      e. The **labia minora** are erectile tissue, devoid of fat and composed of skin and vascular and connective tissue.
         (1) They extend from the prepuce two thirds of the distance of the perineum.
         (2) The embryologic homologue in the male is the floor of the penile urethra.
      f. The **clitoris** is a highly vascular and innervated, erectile organ located between the bifurcating folds of the labia minora.
         (1) It consists of the glans and the body, covered by the prepuce.
         (2) The embryologic homologue in the male is the penis.
      g. The **vestibule** is the space between the labia minora extending from the clitoris to the vaginal introitus. It contains the urethral meatus and the openings of the major and minor vestibular glands as well as Skene's glands.
      h. **Bartholin's glands** are the major vestibular glands.
         (1) They lie posterior and lateral to the vaginal introitus.
         (2) The embryologic homologue in the male is Cowper's glands.
      i. **Skene's ducts** and **minor vestibular glands** are paraurethral structures.

   2. **Nerve supply.** The nerve supply to the vulva includes sensory nerves, special receptors, and autonomic nerves to vessels and glands. Symptoms of vulvovaginal disorders are frequently caused by irritation of the sensory nerves of the vulva. The major nerves supplying the vulva include those derived from the pudendal, ilioinguinal, and posterior femoral cutaneous nerves.
      a. The **pudendal nerve** gives rise to the inferior hemorrhoidal nerve, the perineal nerve, and the dorsal nerve of the clitoris.
      b. The **ilioinguinal nerve** gives rise to the anterior labial nerves.
      c. The **posterior femoral cutaneous nerve** gives rise to the labial nerves.

   3. **Vascular supply.** The major blood vessels supplying the vulva derive from the inter-

nal pudendal artery, which arises from the internal iliac artery, and the superficial and deep external pudendal arteries, which arise from the femoral artery.

4. **Lymphatic supply.** The femoral and inguinal lymph nodes receive the lymphatic drainage from the vulva. The superficial inguinal lymph nodes are the initial site of drainage. Many infections or inflammatory conditions of the vulva and distal vaginal wall are accompanied by an increase in lymphatic drainage, resulting in tender lymphadenopathy at this site.

B. **Vagina.** This structure is a hollow cylinder approximately 9 to 10 cm in length; it extends from the introitus to the uterus and lies dorsal to the bladder and ventral to the rectum.

1. **Anatomy.** The vaginal wall has three layers: the mucosa, muscularis, and adventitia.
   a. The **mucosa** is covered by a stratified, nonkeratinized, squamous epithelium.
      (1) It is a mucous membrane that is under the hormonal influence of the ovarian steroids; estrogen stimulates the proliferation and maturation of vaginal epithelial cells, whereas progesterone is inhibitory.
      (2) There are no glandular structures; lubrication is derived form endocervical secretions and transudation of fluid across the vaginal epithelium.
   b. The **muscularis** is composed of an outer longitudinal and inner circular layer.
   c. The **adventitia** is a strong sheet of connective tissue, condensed anteriorly to form the pubocervical fascia, fused to the fascial coverings of the pelvic and urogenital diaphragms.

2. **Nerve supply.** The nerve supply is derived from the lumbar plexus and the pudendal nerve. The pudendal nerve, which supplies the vagina, does not have as rich a distribution of fine sensory nerves as do the nerves supplying the vulva.

3. **Vascular supply.** The major vessels supplying the vagina include the vaginal artery, arising from the internal iliac or uterine artery; the azygous artery of the vagina, arising from the cervical branch of the uterine artery; and branches of the pudendal artery. Venous drainage forms a plexus surrounding the vagina, and major vessels follow the arterial course.

4. **Lymphatic supply.** The lymphatic drainage of the vagina includes a complex anastomotic plexus that involves drainage to the internal iliac, pelvic, sacral, inferior gluteal, anorectal femoral, and inguinal nodes.

III. **VAGINAL PHYSIOLOGY.** The vaginal ecosystem is a finely balanced environment maintained by a complex interaction among vaginal flora, microbial by-products, estrogen, and host factors. The vagina is **usually resistant to infection** for two reasons: **marked acidity** and a **thick protective epithelium.** Other host factors such as the immune system also play a role in vaginal defense mechanisms.

A. **Microbiology.** The vaginal flora play a critical role in vaginal defenses by maintaining the normally acidic pH (pH 3.8–4.2) of the vagina.

1. There are normally 5 to 15 different bacterial species (i.e., group B *Streptococcus, Escherichia coli),* both aerobic and anaerobic, that inhabit the vagina. The type and number can vary in response to normal and abnormal changes in the vagina

2. *Lactobacillus acidophilus* is the dominant bacteria in a healthy vaginal ecosystem. Lactobacilli play a critical role in maintaining the normal vaginal environment.
   a. The acidic environment of the vagina is maintained through the production of lactic acid.
   b. Lactic acid and hydrogen peroxide produced by lactobacilli are toxic to anaerobic bacteria in the vagina.

3. **Insults that affect the acidic pH** and lead to a more alkaline environment result in a decrease in lactobacilli, with an overgrowth of pathogenic organisms.

B. **Host factors**

1. **Normal estrogen levels** are necessary for a normal vaginal environment and resistance to infection.
   a. Estrogen stimulates proliferation and maturation of the vaginal epithelium, providing a physical barrier to infection.
   b. Mature vaginal epithelium provides **glycogen,** necessary for lactobacillus metabolism. If glycogen levels are decreased, lactobacillus counts decrease as well.
   c. Conditions associated with decreased estrogen levels are associated with an increase in susceptibility to vaginal infections.

2. **Cellular and humoral immunity** play a role in the normal vaginal defense mechanisms.

C. **Factors that alter the vaginal environment.** Insults that affect the vaginal microbiology, vaginal epithelium, or vaginal pH lead to an increased susceptibility to vaginal infections.

1. **Antibiotics** alter the microbiology of the vagina and can increase the risk of infection.

2. **Hormones.** Decreasing the estrogen level or increasing the progesterone level can affect the vaginal epithelium and increase the risk of infection.

3. **Intravaginal preparations.** Douching or the use of intravaginal medications can change the vaginal pH or affect the vaginal flora, changing the resistance to infection.

4. **Intercourse.** Semen has an alkaline pH, thus affecting the microenvironment of the vagina. New organisms that may be introduced into the vagina also affect the microenvironment.

5. **Sexually transmitted diseases (STDs)** affect the microbiology of the vagina, changing the resistance to infection. Other organisms may be the cause of vaginal symptomatology.

6. **Stress, poor diet, and fatigue** probably play a role by affecting microbiology, pH, and the immune system.

7. **Foreign bodies** alter the pH and microbiology of the vagina.

8. Changes in immune function associated with **human immunodeficiency virus (HIV) infection** are associated with recurrent vaginal candidiasis.

IV. **DIAGNOSIS.** A thorough history, physical examination, and judicious use of ancillary tests are critical in establishing the correct diagnosis underlying the patient's symptoms. The medical history is an essential step in evaluating the potential causes of vulvovaginal symptoms. It is especially important to characterize both the patient's symptomatology and contributing features.

A. **Symptomatology**

1. **Vulvar symptoms.** The two **most common symptoms** are:
   a. **Burning.** Vulvar irritation or burning is a symptom associated with a variety of disorders, including vulvovaginitis, vulvovestibulitis, or vulvodynia. Intensity, progression, and inciting factors are important aspects of the history.
   b. **Itching/pruritus.** Vulvar pruritus is a common symptom that can result from vulvovaginitis. Other possible causes include any skin disorder associated with pruritus, including allergic reactions.

2. **Vaginal discharge.** Description of the discharge is crucial to diagnosis and the differentiation from a normal physiologic finding. The characteristics of note are:
   a. **Consistency (thick, watery).** A thin, white discharge is often normal.

    b. Viscosity. Cervical mucus changes normally during the menstrual cycle. Follicular mucus is normally watery and abundant; postovulatory mucus can be thick and viscid. Patients may observe such changes and report them as abnormal.

    c. Color. Normal discharges are usually white to beige. Green, yellow, or brown discharges are usually associated with an infection, a foreign body, or some other abnormality.

   3. Odor. Description of the odor is useful in establishing a differential diagnosis.

    a. An odor may be present without an associated discharge noticed by the patient.

    b. Complaints of a severe, offensive odor are most often noted with retained foreign bodies, such as tampons.

B. **Contributing factors.** Certain factors can predispose to certain types of vulvovaginal infections. Inciting factors may also point to other etiologies, such as allergic reactions.

   1. Sexual activity

    a. Are there complaints of irritation?

    b. What is the relation of the onset of symptoms to intercourse or other sexual activity?

    c. Any unusual sexual practices, new partners?

   2. Recent systemic or local infection

   3. Use of antibiotics

   4. History of diabetes

   5. Previous vulvovaginal infections

   6. Vaginal hygienic practices (e.g., douching)

   7. Contraceptive methods

   8. Menstrual history

   9. Previous treatments, use of self-prescribed medications, herbal or home remedies

V. PHYSICAL EXAMINATION

A. **Pelvic examination,** which is essential in the management of vulvovaginitis, should consist of a thorough evaluation of the following:

   1. The **external genitalia** to detect gross lesions, edema (and discoloration) of the labia, ulceration, and condylomata; and to rule out pubic lice

   2. The **inguinal area,** which should be palpated for the presence or absence of lymphadenopathy, and any discoloration noted

B. **Speculum examination,** using water as the only lubricant to avoid interfering with specimen collection and culturing, should reveal:

   1. Nature of the vaginal discharge, in particular, the consistency, viscosity, color, and odor.

   2. Evidence of trauma, congenital abnormalities, or characteristic lesions of the vaginal walls (e.g., "strawberry spots" if *Trichomonas vaginalis* is suspected).

   3. Presence or absence of cervical abnormalities. A culture of the endocervix detects gonorrhea or chlamydial infection, and Papanicolaou's test (Pap smear) detects carcinoma or infection.

C. **Laboratory tests**

   1. When an infectious vaginitis is suspected, a **vaginal pH** helps to differentiate the various types of infections.

2. A specimen should be obtained for **wet mount preparation.** Microscopic inspection of the vaginal secretions in saline and a 10% potassium hydroxide solution (KOH) is pivotal in making a diagnosis of vaginitis.

3. Occasionally, **cultures** are useful in difficult cases.

VI. **VULVOVAGINAL CONDITIONS.** Vaginitis is characterized by one or more of the following symptoms: **increased volume of discharge; abnormal color (yellow or green) of discharge; vulvar itching, irritation, or burning; dyspareunia; and malodor.** Vaginitis may be caused by infectious agents, such as *Candida, Gardnerella,* and *Trichomonas,* or by atrophic changes. Other vulvovaginal conditions may present with symptoms similar to vaginitis, including vulvar dystrophies, vulvar dermatitis, and other skin conditions of the vulva. Acute herpes simplex genitalis can cause acute vulvar symptoms, necessitating prompt evaluation and treatment.

A. *Candida* **vaginitis (candidiasis or moniliasis)** is the second most common vaginal infection in the United States, accounting for 1.3 million cases a year.

1. **Etiology**
   a. The etiologic agent for this infection is a yeast (fungi) organism, usually *Candida albicans.* The organism is a common inhabitant of the bowel and perianal region. Thirty percent of women may be colonized vaginally and be without symptoms of infection.
   b. Several factors have been identified that can lead to a symptomatic infection as opposed to colonization. These include the following:
      (1) Contraceptive practices (e.g., birth control pills and vaginal spermicides, which influence the vaginal pH)
      (2) Use of systemic steroids, which influence the immune system
      (3) Use of antibiotics, which alters the microbiology of the vagina; 25% to 70% of women report yeast infections after antibiotic use. Any antibiotic can play a causative role, particularly broad-spectrum agents.
      (4) Tight clothing, panty hose, and bathing suits, because yeast thrive in a dark, warm, moist environment
      (5) Undiagnosed or uncontrolled diabetes
   c. Another reason for a refractory monilial infection can be a **compromised immune status;** with recurrent monilial vaginitis, a test for HIV infection is indicated.
   d. There has been a recent **increase in the number of infections caused by non-albicans** species. Up to 20% of infections may be caused by organisms such as *Candida tropicalis* and *Torulopsis glabrata.* These organisms may be resistant to standard treatment regimens.

2. **Clinical presentation**
   a. Characteristically, patients with monilial vaginitis present with complaints of a thick, white discharge and extreme vulvar pruritus. The vulva may be red and swollen.
   b. Symptoms may recur and be most prominent just before menses or in association with intercourse.
   c. Yeast infections may occur more frequently during pregnancy.
   d. Patients with infections due to *C. tropicalis* and *T. glabrata* may have an atypical presentation. Irritation may be paramount, with little discharge or pruritus.

3. **Diagnosis.** Diagnosis is made by history, physical examination, and microscopic examination of the vaginal discharge in saline and 10% KOH.
   a. On examination, excoriations of the vulva may be noticeable; the vulva and vagina may be erythematous, with patches of adherent "cottage cheese"-like discharge.
   b. Infection with *C. tropicalis* and *T. glabrata* may not be associated with the classic discharge; discharge may be white-gray and thin.

    c. Vaginal pH may be normal or slightly more basic (pH 4.5–4.8) than normal.
    d. Wet mount microscopic examination reveals hyphae or pseudohyphae with budding yeast in 50% to 70% of women with yeast infections.
    e. Cultures are not necessary to make the diagnosis except in some cases of recurrent infections.

4. Treatment. Many agents are available for the treatment of vulvovaginal candidiasis. These include topical agents, which can be over-the-counter (OTC) or prescription agents, and oral agents, which are available by prescription only.
    a. Antifungal intravaginal agents are administered as suppositories or creams; are available as a single-dose, 3-day or 7-day course; and include butoconazole, clotrimazole, miconazole, tioconazole, and terconazole.
        (1) OTC regimens include clotrimazole for 7 to 14 days and miconazole for 7 days.
        (2) OTC regimens should be used only by women who have been diagnosed with a yeast in the past and are experiencing identical symptoms.
    b. Oral agents include fluconazole and ketoconazole.
        (1) Fluconazole is available as a single-dose (150 mg) treatment for uncomplicated vaginal candidiasis.
        (2) Ketoconazole is used effectively for the treatment of chronic and recurrent candidiasis; a 5% incidence of hepatotoxicity limits more widespread use. The dosing schedule is 200 mg bid × 5 days, then 100 to 200 mg daily for 6 months.
    c. Boric acid capsules, 600 mg for 14 days, may be effective.

5. Chronic recurrent yeast infections. Five percent of women experience chronic relapsing yeast infections. In most women, no exacerbating factor can be found, but the following possibilities should be considered.
    a. Failure to complete a full course of therapy
    b. HIV infection. Recalcitrant candidiasis may be a presenting symptom in women with HIV infection. HIV testing should be considered and offered to the patient.
    c. Chronic antibiotic therapy
    d. Infection with a resistant organism such as *C. tropicalis* or *T. glabrata*
    e. Sexual transmission from the male partner
    f. Allergic reaction to partner's semen, or vaginal spermicide

B. *Trichomonas vaginalis* vaginitis (trichomoniasis) is the third most common vaginitis, accounting for 25% of cases.

1. Etiology. The etiologic agent is the motile protozoan *T. vaginalis.*
    a. *Trichomonas* vaginitis is a multifocal infection involving the vaginal epithelium, Skene's glands, Bartholin's glands, and the urethra.
    b. The trichomonad can be recovered from 70% to 80% of the male partners of the infected patient; *Trichomonas* vaginitis is therefore an STD.

2. Clinical presentation
    a. Unless asked directly, 25% to 50% of women may not report symptoms.
    b. Most women complain of a discharge that is described as copious, green, and frothy.
    c. The discharge may be associated with a foul odor and vulvar irritation or pruritus.

3. Diagnosis
    a. Physical examination may reveal classic evidence of trichomoniasis.
        (1) Copious, green, frothy discharge may be evident.
        (2) Punctation, described classically as the "strawberry cervix," is evident only in 25% of patients.
    b. Laboratory tests
        (1) The vaginal pH is usually greater than 4.5.
        (2) Saline wet mount of the vaginal discharge reveals numerous leukocytes and the highly motile, flagellated trichomonads in up to 75% of cases.
        (3) Cultures are not usually necessary to make the diagnosis. They should be ob-

tained when the diagnosis is suspected but cannot be confirmed by wet mount examination.

(4) Pap smears may be positive in up to 65% of cases. Positive Pap smears should be confirmed by wet mount examination because of the high false-positive rate.

4. Treatment
  a. Because of the multiple sites of infection, vaginal therapy alone is ineffective, and **systemic agents are necessary.**
  b. Because the causative agent is sexually transmitted, **both partners require therapy;** 25% of women will be reinfected if their partner is not treated.
  c. Cure rates of 90% are achieved with treatment with **metronidazole** at the following recommended doses, if the partner is treated simultaneously. Patients should be warned of a disulfiram-like reaction and told to abstain from alcohol use with treatment.
    (1) The preferred regimen is 2 g by one dose (four 500-mg tablets) because of ease of compliance; up to 10% of patients may experience vomiting on this regimen.
    (2) Alternatively, 500 mg bid for 7 days or 250 mg tid for 7 days can be given.
  d. Resistant cases may require treatment with intravenous metronidazole. Because resistance is rare, other causes should be considered, such as noncompliance of the patient or partner.
  e. Metronidazole is contraindicated for use during the first trimester of pregnancy. After this, it can be can be used to treat *Trichomonas* infections.
  f. Infected patients should be screened for other STDs.

C. **Bacterial vaginosis** is the most common vaginal infection in the United States today.

1. Etiology
  a. Bacterial vaginosis is caused by an **overgrowth of a variety of bacterial species,** particularly anaerobes, often found normally in the vagina. Organisms most often involved include *Bacteroides, Peptostreptococcus, Gardnerella vaginalis*, and *Mycoplasma hominis.*
  b. The anaerobic bacteria produce enzymes that break down peptides to amino acids and amines, resulting in compounds associated with the discharge and odor characteristic of this infection.
  c. Bacterial vaginitis has also been known as nonspecific vaginitis and *Gardnerella* vaginitis in the past.

2. Clinical presentation
  a. Fifty percent of women with bacterial vaginitis are asymptomatic.
  b. The most common presentation is a malodorous, gray discharge.

3. Diagnosis. The diagnosis is based on finding three of the following four criteria.
  a. The vaginal pH is consistently greater than 4.5.
  b. Wet mount preparations with saline reveal a "clean" background with minimal or no leukocytes, an abundance of bacteria, and the characteristic "clue" cell. The clue cell is a squamous cell in which coccobacillary bacteria have obscured the sharp borders and cytoplasm.
  c. Application of 10% KOH to the wet mount specimen produces a fishy odor, indicating a positive "whiff" test.
  d. The presence of a gray, homogenous, malodorous discharge is noted.

4. Treatment is based on the use of agents with anaerobic activity and uses both topical and systemic agents. Both appear to be 90% effective.
  a. Vaginal preparations
    (1) Intravaginal 2% **clindamycin cream** is used at bedtime for 7 days.
    (2) Intravaginal **metronidazole** is applied twice a day for 5 days.
  b. Oral regimens
    (1) Metronidazole 500 mg bid for 7 days, or 250 mg tid for 7 days, or a single 2-g dose.

(2) **Clindamycin,** 300 mg tid for 7 days, may be associated with a higher incidence of diarrhea.
c. Sexual partners should be treated in cases of repeated episodes of bacterial vaginitis. Routine treatment of the patient's partner has not been shown to improve cure rates or lower reinfection rates.
d. Treatment during pregnancy is critical because data suggest an association of adverse maternal and fetal outcomes with bacterial vaginitis.
(1) Clindamycin can be used throughout pregnancy.
(2) Metronidazole can be used after the first trimester.
e. Patients with recurrences should be screened for other STDs.

D. **Atrophic vaginitis**

1. **Etiology.** Atrophic vaginitis, associated with decreased estradiol levels, is most often seen in postmenopausal women, but also may be seen in women who are breast-feeding (lactating). Atrophic changes in the vulvovaginal tissues result from **estrogen withdrawal** because the normal protective thickness of the vaginal epithelium depends on estrogen stimulation.

2. **Clinical presentation**
   a. Without consistent and sufficient estrogen, the vaginal epithelium becomes thin; the vulvar structures may atrophy.
   b. The amount of glycogen also decreases, and the pH changes to an alkaline state.
   c. The vagina is often pale with punctate hemorrhagic spots throughout the vaginal wall. There is an absence of superficial epithelial cells and a predominance of parabasal cells.

3. **Diagnosis**
   a. Atrophic vaginitis must be suspected in the hypoestrogenic woman who presents with signs and symptoms of leukorrhea, pruritus, burning, tenderness, and dyspareunia.
   b. Physical examination of the vagina reveals atrophic, sometimes inflamed vaginal walls.
   c. Vaginal pH is usually above 4.5; a discharge may be present.
   d. No other vaginal infection is identified on wet mount preparation.

4. **Treatment.** Topical administration of vaginal cream containing estrogen reverses symptoms and tissue changes.
   a. Symptoms respond to short-term therapy but recur on discontinuation.
   b. Changes in the tissues require long-term therapy and may not be noticed until after 3 to 4 months of treatment. Proliferation and maturation of the vaginal epithelium and compliance and elasticity of the vaginal wall are restored.
   c. Treatment is with systemic or topical agents.
   (1) **Hormone replacement therapy** given in accordance with a standard regimen is acceptable treatment.
   (2) **Estrogen cream** is administered intravaginally every night for up to 2 weeks, and then continued once or twice a week to maintain results.

E. **Vulvar dystrophies**

1. **Etiology.** Vulvar dystrophies are dermatologic conditions of the vulvar skin of uncertain etiology. Most frequently seen in postmenopausal women, these conditions often accompany a history of chronic candidal vulvovaginitis. The dystrophies can be:
   a. Hyperplastic when the epithelium is markedly thickened
   b. Atrophic (lichen sclerosus et atrophicus)
   c. A mixture of both

2. **Clinical presentation**
   a. With **hyperplastic dystrophy,** the most common symptom is constant pruritus. Scratching frequently exacerbates the pruritus, creating a vicious cycle.
   b. With **lichen sclerosus,** vulvar burning, pruritus, or chronic soreness associated with "vulvar dysuria" frequently occurs.

3. **Diagnosis. Vulvar biopsy** is ultimately necessary to make the diagnosis, but a preliminary diagnosis can be made based on **physical examination.**
    a. **Hyperplastic dystrophy** presents as very thickened skin ("elephant hide") accompanied by linear excoriations from scratching. Areas of leukoplakia may also be noted.
    b. **Lichen sclerosus** presents as extremely pale, thin skin, often with subepithelial hemorrhages. In its most severe form, painful contraction of the introitus or clitoral hood is noted.

4. **Treatment**
    a. **Hyperplastic dystrophy** responds well to a 6- to 8-week trial of topical fluorinated steroid cream. Chronic therapy may be necessary on an intermittent basis.
    b. **Lichen sclerosus** responds to long-term topical testosterone preparations. If this treatment is not tolerated, a topical progesterone preparation may be helpful. Fluorinated steroid creams may also provide relief in women who cannot tolerate other preparations.

F. **Traumatic vaginitis**

1. **Etiology.** Traumatic vaginitis is usually the result of injury or chemical irritation.
    a. **In adults,** the most common cause of injury to the vagina is a "lost" tampon.
    b. **In pediatric patients,** foreign bodies placed in the vagina serve as sources of infection or trauma (e.g., wads of paper, chewing gum, paper clips).
    c. **Chemical irritation** can be secondary to douches, deodorants, lubricants, or topical intravaginal preparations.

2. **Treatment.** Vulvovaginitis resulting from foreign bodies or chemical irritants responds immediately to withdrawal of the causative agent.

G. **Neoplasia**

1. **Etiology.** Malignancies can masquerade for months as vulvar lesions; thus, they are often ignored by patients or mistreated by physicians as irritations or infections.

2. **Diagnosis.** Patients who present with a long-term history of symptoms and treatment failures of vulvar lesions should undergo biopsy before further therapeutic trials are instituted.

3. **Treatment** is as indicated for the condition described in the pathology report.

H. **Herpes simplex genitalis**

1. **Etiology**
    a. Herpes genitalis is caused by the herpes simplex virus (HSV), a member of the *Herpesviridae* family of viruses, which are capable of establishing latent status and causing recurrent disease.
    b. Seventy to 90% of cases of herpes genitalis are caused by HSV type 2 (HSV-2); HSV type 1 (HSV-1) is the etiologic agent in only 13% of cases.
    c. Sixty to 85% of women with antibodies to HSV-2 have never had a recognized genital ulcer.
    d. Transmission is through direct contact with someone who is actively shedding virus from skin or mucous membrane lesions.
    e. Incubation period is 2 to 7 days.

2. **Clinical presentation**
    a. **Primary infection**
        (1) The infection is usually acquired from sexual contact, with symptoms appearing in 3 to 7 days.
        (2) Primary infection is often associated with systemic "flu-like" symptoms of malaise, myalgias, headache, and the like.
        (3) Pain and itching may precede the development of vesicular lesions, which may appear on the labia, perineum, buttocks, urethra, vagina, cervix, and bladder. Cervical involvement is seen in 70% of women with genital involvement.

    (4) Vesicles progress to ulcer and may coalesce. Lesions are exquisitely tender.

    (5) Tender inguinal lymphadenopathy may be present.

    (6) Local symptoms consist of hyperesthesia, burning, itching, dysuria, and frequently exquisite pain and tenderness of the vulva.

    (7) Vulvar pain makes intercourse unbearable and may lead to urinary retention.

    (8) Primary lesions persist for 3 to 6 weeks and usually heal without scarring.

        (a) Primary symptoms may last from 2 days to 3 weeks. Symptoms may be milder in women with antibodies to HSV-1.

        (b) Viral shedding may persist for 12 days.

        (c) Complications include sacral radiculopathy with urinary or fecal retention.

        (d) Aseptic meningitis is a rare complication.

  b. Recurrent infection

    (1) The dormant herpesvirus resides in the neurons of the sacral ganglia, which supply the areas of cutaneous involvement.

    (2) Periodic asymptomatic viral shedding occurs, particularly during the first 6 months after infection.

    (3) Recurrences are most frequent during the first year. Frequency of recurrence varies; some patients never have another outbreak; others have frequent recurrences.

    (4) Systemic symptoms usually do not occur with recurrences.

    (5) Many women experience prodromal symptoms of itching and burning, from 30 minutes to 2 days before an outbreak.

    (6) Recurrent lesions tend to be less severe and are of shorter duration (3–7 days).

3. Diagnosis

  a. A presumptive diagnosis of herpes genitalis can be made on physical examination when typical lesions are present. HSV-2 should be suspected when superficial ulcerations of the vulvovaginal tissues are identified.

  b. Viral culture is the gold standard by which the diagnosis of HSV infection is made and requires 48 hours for completion. Sensitivity of cultures is 90% if vesicles are present, but only 30% if lesions are crusted.

  c. Cytologic studies and direct identification methods such as immunofluorescence offer confirmatory evidence of an HSV infection, but have only a 50% sensitivity.

4. Treatment

  a. Local measures used for comfort during the acute outbreak include sitz baths and topical anesthetic creams. The area should be kept clean and dry to avoid secondary infection.

  b. Catheterization may be necessary for acute urinary retention.

  c. Antiviral therapy. Acyclovir is an antiviral drug that is effective against herpesvirus. Other antiviral agents are being developed as well.

    (1) Acyclovir is a cyclic purine nucleoside analogue with in vivo and in vitro activity against HSV.

    (2) It can be applied topically or taken orally for the **primary** episode of HSV-2 infection.

    (3) Oral acyclovir decreases the time of viral shedding, duration of symptoms, and the time to healing in primary herpes outbreaks. The recommended dose is 200 mg, taken five times a day for 10 days.

    (4) If initiated at the time of initial onset of a recurrence, oral acyclovir also decreases duration of viral shedding, time to healing, and local symptoms. Recommended dose is 200 mg five times a day for 5 days.

    (5) Oral acyclovir has been shown to decrease the frequency of recurrences by up to 75%. Suppressive therapy has been approved for up to 5 years. The recommended dose is 200 mg tid or 400 mg bid. Therapy is discontinued on an annual basis and frequency of recurrences is documented. Treatment is restarted as indicated.

STUDY QUESTIONS

DIRECTIONS: Each of the numbered items or incomplete statements in this section is followed by answers or by completions of the statement. Select the ONE lettered answer or completion that is BEST in each case.

1. Infection with which organism results in vaginitis that requires treatment of both partners?

(A) *Trichomonas*
(B) *Candida*
(C) Group B *Streptococcus*
(D) Herpes simplex virus
(E) *Lactobacillus*

2. Hyperplastic vulvar dystrophy is associated with which statement?

(A) Treatment is topical testosterone ointment
(B) Marked atrophy of the vulvar structure results
(C) The etiologic agent is herpes simplex virus type 2 (HSV-2)
(D) It responds well to fluorinated steroid cream
(E) Treatment of choice is a 1% progesterone cream

DIRECTIONS: Each of the numbered items or incomplete statements in this section is negatively phrased, as indicated by a capitalized word such as NOT, LEAST, or EXCEPT. Select the ONE lettered answer or completion that is BEST in each case.

3. If a woman presents with a chronic yeast infection, the physician should elicit a history for all of the following EXCEPT

(A) diabetes
(B) pregnancy
(C) use of antibiotics
(D) use of oral contraceptives
(E) use of vinegar douches

4. All of the following statements about vulvar anatomy are true EXCEPT

(A) the nerve supply includes contributions from the perineal, genitofemoral, and ilioinguinal nerves
(B) the lymphatic drainage is to the superficial inguinal lymph node group
(C) both Skene's and Bartholin's glands drain into the vestibule of the vagina
(D) the vulva is covered exclusively by keratinized epithelium
(E) the labia minora have sebaceous glands

5. Bacterial vaginosis is associated with all of the following features EXCEPT

(A) a pH of 5.0
(B) "clue" cells
(C) marked inflammatory background in vaginal secretions
(D) positive "whiff" test
(E) response to metronidazole

ANSWERS AND EXPLANATIONS

1. The answer is A [VI B 4 b]. The sexual partners of the patient with *Trichomonas* vaginitis should be treated to prevent reinfection. Treatment of partners of patients with *Candida* vaginitis has reduced recurrent infections in women with refractory infections. Group B *Streptococcus* and *Lactobacillus* are common inhabitants of the vagina and do not cause vaginitis. Infection with herpes simplex virus does not result in vaginitis, and treatment is symptomatic only.

2. The answer is D [VI E 1–4]. Hyperplastic dystrophy of the vulva is of uncertain etiology but has been associated with chronic candidal vulvovaginitis, not herpes simplex virus (HSV). The most common symptom of hyperplastic vulvar dystrophy is incessant pruritus, which responds well to a short course of topical fluorinated steroid cream. This disorder is probably caused by chronic vulvar irritation, which produces a thickened epithelium resembling elephant skin. It is not associated with atrophy of the vulvar structures, as is lichen sclerosus. Testosterone ointment and progesterone cream are used in the chronic treatment of lichen sclerosus.

3. The answer is E [VI A 1, 2]. Various changes in the vaginal environment contribute to chronic yeast infections in some women. Antibiotics change the normal vaginal flora. Pregnancy and oral contraceptives alter the vaginal epithelium by hormone-induced changes that reflect a progesterone rather than an estrogen dominance. Douching with a vinegar solution is often used as a prophylaxis against vaginitis because of the acidic nature of the douche; it would not be a predisposing factor for a yeast infection.

4. The answer is D [II A]. The sensory nerve supply of the vulva includes contributions from the pudendal, posterior femoral cutaneous, and ilioinguinal nerves. These sensory nerves are responsible for most of the symptoms of vulvovaginitis (i.e., pruritus, burning, and soreness). Many times, superficial inguinal adenopathy can be seen in acute vulvovaginitis. The vestibule, which many physicians mistake as being part of the vagina, is a nonkeratinized mucous membrane between the inner aspect of the labia minora and the hymenal ring. The labia minora do not have hair follicles but do have sebaceous glands. The secretory glands (Skene's and Bartholin's) empty into the vestibule. The vulva is covered predominantly, but not exclusively, by keratinized epithelium.

5. The answer is C [III A; VI B 3 b, C 3, 4]. Bacterial vaginosis is characterized by a malodorous, watery vaginal discharge. Vaginal pH in the normal vagina is approximately 4.5. In bacterial vaginosis, the organism involved is *Gardnerella vaginalis,* and the vaginal pH is between 5.0 and 5.5. Wet mount preparations in bacterial vaginosis have "clue" cells and a "clean" background, unlike those in *Trichomonas* infections, which show an intense inflammatory reaction, with many white blood cells on the slide. The clue cell is diagnostic of bacterial vaginosis in that coccobacillary bacteria obscure the sharp borders and cytoplasm of this squamous cell. Application of 10% potassium hydroxide to the wet mount specimen produces a fishy odor that indicates a positive "whiff" test. Bacterial vaginosis is best treated with oral metronidazole.

Chapter 26

Dysfunctional Uterine Bleeding

Michelle Battistini

I. DEFINITIONS

A. **Dysfunctional uterine bleeding (DUB)** is abnormal uterine bleeding, usually excessive in amount, reflecting a disturbance in normal ovulatory function.

1. It results from **abnormalities of endocrine origin;** there is no demonstrable organic cause.

2. DUB is most often associated with **anovulation,** but can occur with ovulatory cycles that have shortened or inadequate follicular or luteal phases.

3. DUB is a manifestation of **abnormal hormonal stimulation of the endometrial lining.**

B. **Patterns of abnormal bleeding**

1. **Intermenstrual bleeding** is bleeding that occurs between regular menstrual periods and is variable in amount.

2. **Menorrhagia (hypermenorrhea)** is prolonged (exceeding 7 days) and excessive (greater than 80 ml) uterine bleeding that occurs at regular intervals.

3. **Metrorrhagia** is prolonged and excessive uterine bleeding that occurs at irregular intervals.

4. **Polymenorrhea** is uterine bleeding that occurs at intervals of less than 21 days.

5. **Oligomenorrhea** is infrequent uterine bleeding that occurs at intervals greater than 35 days.

II. PHYSIOLOGY OF HORMONALLY BASED ENDOMETRIAL BLEEDING

A. **Postovulatory estrogen–progesterone withdrawal bleeding.** This mechanism of bleeding occurs normally with the menstrual cycle.

1. **Estrogen** stimulates endometrial growth during the normal follicular phase; after ovulation, subsequent progesterone stimulation induces endometrial differentiation. This results in structurally stable endometrial lining throughout the uterine cavity.

2. **In the absence of fertilization,** the corpus luteum regresses and hormonal stimulation is withdrawn. The withdrawal of hormonal support is a universal endometrial event occurring at all sites simultaneously.

3. **Progesterone** withdrawal initiates rhythmic vasoconstriction of spiral arterioles leading to ischemia, necrosis, and sloughing of the endometrial lining. Vasoconstriction continues, allowing initiation of hemostatic mechanisms to control bleeding sites. Healing continues with resumption of estrogen stimulation. The events that lead to bleeding are also self-limiting.

4. **Bleeding occurs in a controlled fashion** because endometrial shedding occurs in a universal, synchronous fashion that is self-limiting and involves a structurally stable lining.

B. **Estrogen breakthrough bleeding.** This is the hormonal event associated with anovulatory DUB.

1. **In the absence of ovulation,** estrogen stimulates the lining of the endometrium unop-

posed by progesterone. This leads to excessive proliferation of endometrial glands with lack of differentiation and development of stromal support. This results in an unstable and fragile endometrial lining that exhibits superficial breakdown and bleeding.

2. **Continuous unopposed estrogen** stimulates further endometrial proliferation and healing. As one site heals, another site breaks down, resulting in continuous bleeding. Endometrial shedding occurs randomly and is not a universal event.

3. **In the absence of progesterone withdrawal,** there is a loss of the rhythmic, progressive vasoconstriction of the spiral arteries. Without this, there is a loss of the periodic, orderly shedding of the endometrial lining; bleeding is not self-limited.

4. **Bleeding occurs in an unpredictable fashion** because endometrial shedding is not universal, synchronous, or self-limiting and involves a structurally unstable lining.

C. **Estrogen withdrawal bleeding.** This hormonal mechanism accounts for midcycle bleeding that is not caused by a structural lesion; it occurs during an ovulatory cycle when estrogen levels decline just before ovulation.

1. **Estrogen stimulation** leads to a proliferative endometrium.

2. When **estrogen stimulation is removed,** the endometrium loses hormonal support and is shed.

3. **Healing** occurs when estrogen support is restored.

D. **Progesterone breakthrough bleeding.** This hormonal event is associated with prolonged corpus luteum function and methods of progestin-only contraception.

1. **Prolonged progesterone stimulation** leads to an unfavorable estrogen–progesterone ratio, with inadequate estrogen to stimulate proliferation of the endometrial lining.

2. With **inadequate estrogen stimulation,** the endometrium becomes thin and atrophic.

3. With **continued progesterone stimulation,** the endometrial surface bleeds irregularly, varying in amount and duration.

III. PATHOPHYSIOLOGY OF DUB

A. **Anovulatory cycles.** DUB most often occurs in the absence of cyclic hormonal changes that determine the menstrual cycle. About 90% of all DUB is anovulatory in nature and is an example of **estrogen breakthrough bleeding.**

1. **Bleeding patterns** correlate with the duration of unopposed estrogen exposure of the endometrial lining; the amount and duration of bleeding vary directly with the duration and level of unopposed estrogen stimulation.

2. **Prolonged exposure of the endometrial lining to unopposed estrogen stimulation** increases the risk of endometrial hyperplasia and endometrial carcinoma.

3. Anovulatory cycles are a symptom of a loss of the normal regulatory mechanisms controlling the menstrual cycle. Ovulatory cycles are the result of a complex interaction of a multitude of factors involving the hypothalamic–pituitary–ovarian axis. Abnormalities at any of these sites interfere with normal ovulation; a variety of etiologies cause a loss of normal ovulatory function.
   a. **Immaturity of the hypothalamic–pituitary axis.** Anovulation and DUB are often seen in the postpubertal adolescent shortly after menarche. The onset of the first menses may occur before full maturation of the hypothalamic control mechanisms of ovulation; gonadotropin-releasing hormone (GnRH) secretion has not yet attained the pulsatile nature characteristic of ovulatory cycles.
   b. **Dysfunction of the hypothalamic–pituitary axis.** Anything that interferes with the

normal pulsatile secretion of GnRH leads to anovulatory states; a prolonged insult leads to progressive dysfunction and amenorrhea.

(1) **Hyperprolactinemia.** An elevation of circulating prolactin can be the result of pituitary adenomas or a side effect of medications, most notably psychotropic drugs.

(2) **Stress and anxiety.** Often anovulation and menstrual irregularities are seen during times of stress and major life changes; this results from loss of pulsatile GnRH secretion.

(3) **Rapid weight loss.** Sudden and rapid weight loss after crash dieting may also interfere with normal GnRH secretion, resulting in ovulatory dysfunction and menstrual irregularities.

(4) **Borderline anorexia nervosa.** Anovulation occurs early in the course of anorexia nervosa. If the condition progresses in severity, complete loss of ovarian function results in amenorrhea and hypoestrogenism.

c. **Abnormalities of normal feedback signals. Estradiol** levels play a critical role in controlling the sequence of events during a normal ovulatory cycle. The rise and fall of estradiol at critical points in the cycle are important feedback mechanisms of cycle control. Estradiol primarily exerts a negative feedback effect on follicle-stimulating hormone (FSH) secretion and must drop appropriately before menses to allow the rise in FSH necessary for initiation of a new cycle. Sustained estradiol levels at this time prevent normal cycling and are the result of persistent secretion, abnormal clearance and metabolism, or production by extragonadal sources.

(1) The most common cause of persistent estrogen secretion is **pregnancy.** Other, less common causes are ovarian or adrenal tumors.

(2) Metabolism and clearance of estradiol can be affected by medical conditions, most commonly **hepatic disease** or **thyroid abnormalities.** Hyperthyroidism and hypothyroidism affect the clearance and peripheral conversion of estradiol, leading to abnormalities in ovulation. Laboratory tests to detect abnormalities of thyroid function should be part of the evaluation in any patient with ovulatory dysfunction.

(3) **Extragonadal production of estrogen** occurs with conditions that lead to an increase in the production or conversion of estrogen precursors. Physical or psychological stress can lead to an increase in secretion of estrogen precursors from the adrenal gland. Adipose tissue is a site for peripheral conversion of adrenal precursors; conversion increases with increasing body weight. This is one explanation for the association between obesity and anovulation and related conditions such as DUB.

4. Ovulation depends on a **midcycle luteinizing hormone (LH) surge** that is induced by a concomitant estradiol surge. If estrogen levels fail to reach a critical value, LH levels do not peak; ovulation fails to occur.

a. This condition most commonly occurs in the premenopausal woman before the cessation of menses. Failure of ovarian follicles to produce critical estradiol levels necessary for induction of the LH surge leads to anovulatory cycles common in this age-group. The postmenarchal and premenopausal periods are the most common times to see anovulatory, estrogen breakthrough bleeding, although the underlying mechanism may be different in each case.

b. **Local ovarian conditions.** Normal follicular function is highly dependent on intrinsic factors as well as external stimulation. The follicular hormonal environment is critical for normal activity; disruption of this balance results in anovulatory cycles.

c. **Follicular growth and development.** There are numerous, well-defined factors involved in normal follicular growth and development, such as inhibin, activin, and insulin-like growth factors I and II, that act in an orderly sequence. Abnormalities of these local factors or defects in the sequence of events lead to disruption of the ovulatory process.

d. **Androgens in the ovarian follicle.** A critical concentration of androgens is necessary for normal follicular function and steroidogenesis. Increasing the androgen level locally within the ovary above this level leads to defects in ovulation.

    (1) **Obesity** is commonly cited as a cause of anovulation and a risk factor for DUB and related conditions. Obesity is associated with an increase in peripheral and ovarian androgens. The androgenic environment as well as increased peripheral conversion of androgen to estrogen are responsible for the ovulatory dysfunction associated with obesity.

    (2) **Polycystic ovary** is a consequence and not a cause of chronic ovulatory dysfunction. A local ovarian environment that is androgenic contributes to the perpetuation of this condition.

B. **Ovulatory cycles.** Abnormal bleeding secondary to a hormonal etiology can also occur during ovulatory cycles, although this a less common cause of DUB. These patterns can occur at any age, but are most common with declining ovarian function characteristic of the years preceding the menopause.

    1. **Midcycle spotting** is a scanty intermenstrual discharge that is associated with a decrease in estrogen at midcycle, just before ovulation.

    2. **Frequent menses,** or polymenorrhea, is associated with a shortened follicular phase.

    3. **Luteal phase deficiency,** which may be associated with premenstrual spotting, results when the luteal phase is shortened by prematurely decreased progesterone levels.

    4. **Prolonged corpus luteum activity** is the result of persistent progesterone production in the absence of pregnancy, resulting in prolonged cycles or protracted menstrual bleeding.

IV. **EVALUATION AND DIAGNOSIS OF ABNORMAL UTERINE BLEEDING.** Abnormal uterine bleeding can be associated with a variety of conditions that are not endocrine in nature (Table 26-1). Organic conditions, such as polyps, uterine fibroids, endometritis, endometrial hyperplasia, intrauterine malignancy, pregnancy, and blood

TABLE 26-1. Abnormal Uterine Bleeding: Differential Diagnosis

Reproductive tract pathology	**Endocrine gland dysfunction**
Cervicitis	Hypothyroidism
Cervical neoplasia	Hyperthyroidism
Endometritis	Pituitary adenoma
Endometrial polyps	**Ovulatory dysfunction**
Endometrial hyperplasia	Anovulation
Uterine leiomyomas	Shortened follicular phase
Adenomyosis	Luteal phase deficiency
Uterine sarcomas	Prolonged corpus luteum function
Ovarian neoplasms (estrogen producing)	**Pregnancy-related conditions**
Medications	Threatened abortion
Estrogen administration	Spontaneous abortion
Oral contraceptives	Ectopic pregnancy
Progesterone-only contraceptives	Gestational trophoblastic neoplasm
Aspirin	**Systemic disease**
Anticoagulants	Hematologic disorders
Psychotrophic medications	von Willebrand's disease
Trauma	Thrombocytopenia
Foreign body	Hepatic disease
Lacerations	Renal disease
Intrauterine device	

dyscrasias, must be considered as possible causes. Elimination of anatomic or structural causes of abnormal bleeding is the first step in the diagnosis of DUB.

A. **Complete history.** Most often, a presumptive diagnosis of DUB can be made or ruled out based on history alone, with examination and diagnostic tests used as confirmation.

1. **Current bleeding history.** It is critical to define accurately the current pattern of bleeding and how it deviates from previous bleeding patterns.

2. **Menstrual history.** Age of menarche, cycle frequency and duration, and presence of moliminal symptoms establish the presence or absence of ovulatory cycles. A history of prolonged anovulation identifies the patient at risk for endometrial hyperplasia, requiring endometrial sampling.

3. **Contraceptive use.** Pregnancy-related causes should be considered early in the evaluation of a woman who presents with bleeding during the reproductive years. A complete sexual and contraceptive history needs to be obtained. Progesterone breakthrough bleeding can be associated with combined oral contraceptives and progesterone-only contraceptive methods, including oral contraceptives, implants, and injections. Intrauterine devices can also be associated with abnormal bleeding patterns.

4. **Medical history.** The presence of a medical condition associated with abnormal bleeding (e.g., coagulation disorders) should be considered. Thirty percent of adolescents presenting with severe blood loss have an associated coagulopathy such as von Willebrand's disease. In addition, thyroid disease and pituitary adenomas may be the underlying cause of bleeding associated with anovulatory cycles.

5. **Medication history.** Certain medications can be associated with abnormal uterine bleeding, e.g., anticoagulants. Psychotropic medications may secondarily cause DUB through an elevation of prolactin.

B. **Complete physical examination.** Physical examination detects organic causes of abnormal uterine bleeding and also signs associated with causes of anovulation and DUB.

1. **General physical examination.** The presence of thyroid enlargement, galactorrhea, ecchymosis, and purpura should be determined by physical examination.

2. **Gynecologic examination.** A complete gynecologic examination, including Pap smear, detects organic causes of abnormal uterine bleeding.

C. **Laboratory studies.** The necessity of additional laboratory studies is determined by history and physical examination. Not all tests are necessary in all patients.

1. **Pregnancy test.** Modern urine pregnancy tests are highly sensitive, inexpensive, and easy to perform; one should be obtained in all women with abnormal bleeding before the menopause except in select circumstances.

2. **Complete blood count.** In patients with heavy or prolonged bleeding, a hemoglobin/hematocrit should be obtained. A platelet count detects thrombocytopenia; a white blood cell count may be useful in the diagnosis of endometritis or rare conditions such as leukemia.

3. **Thyroid-stimulating hormone/prolactin.** These studies should be performed in all women with bleeding associated with anovulation. Treatment of these conditions restores normal ovulatory function.

4. **Coagulation profile.** Prothrombin time, partial thromboplastin time, and bleeding time are obtained when an associated coagulation disorder is suspected.

5. **Androgen profile.** Testosterone, dehydroepiandrosterone, and hydroxyprogesterone are obtained in the woman who presents with anovulatory bleeding and hirsutism.

D. **Diagnostic studies.** The need for additional diagnostic testing is determined on an individual basis.

1. **Endometrial biopsy.** A sample of the endometrial lining is obtained in all women thought to be at risk for endometrial hyperplasia or carcinoma. This includes all women older than 40 years of age and those younger than 40 years who have chronic anovulatory bleeding.

2. **Dilation and curettage (D and C).** D and C is performed in those women thought to have DUB who fail to respond to medical management with hormonal manipulation.

3. **Hysteroscopy, or direct visualization of the endometrial cavity.** Hysteroscopy is performed at the time of D and C or when an organic lesion such as a polyp or fibroid is suspected.

V. TREATMENT OF DUB. The treatment of anovulatory DUB is hormonal therapy with a progestin, estrogen, or a combination of the two. The choice of therapy is based on the duration of bleeding, age of the patient, and preference of the patient.

A. Hormonal therapy

1. **Progestins. Progesterone supplementation** is the treatment of choice because most women with DUB are anovulatory. Bleeding is estrogen breakthrough bleeding and is a manifestation of unopposed estrogen stimulation of the endometrial lining. Addition of progesterone restores the normal controlling influences to the endometrium.
   a. Progestins act as antiestrogens; they exert an antimitotic, antigrowth effect.
      (1) They enhance the conversion of estradiol to estrone, which is then displaced from the cell.
      (2) They diminish the effect of estrogen on target cells by inhibiting estrogen receptor replenishment in the cell.
   b. A progestin **supports and organizes the endometrium** so that an organized sloughing of the endometrium occurs after its withdrawal. **Medroxyprogesterone** (10 mg/day for 10 days) produces regular withdrawal bleeding in patients with adequate amounts of endogenous estrogen.
   c. Progestins may not stop the acute episode of DUB as effectively as estrogen, especially if bleeding has been prolonged. However, progestin, either alone or in combination with estrogen, is warranted for long-term control after the acute episode of DUB is controlled.
   d. The **antimitotic, antigrowth effect of progestins** supports their use in the treatment of endometrial hyperplasia.

2. **Oral contraceptive therapy.** Frequently, in the younger patient, DUB is associated with prolonged endometrial buildup and heavy bleeding. Combined estrogen–progestin therapy using oral contraceptives is used to treat the acute bleeding episode.
   a. The combined oral contraceptive converts a fragile, overgrown endometrium into a pseudodecidualized, structurally stable lining.
   b. Bleeding usually is controlled within 24 hours of initiation of therapy. If there is no response by this time, another etiology should be pursued.
   c. Any low-dose combined pill can be used. The pill is administered two or three times a day for a total of 5 to 7 days.
   d. A heavy withdrawal bleed is expected after cessation of therapy.
   e. Cyclic therapy with once-a-day administration is continued for 3 months to reduce the endometrial lining to baseline height.
   f. After 3 months of treatment, the oral contraceptive is continued if birth control is desired; progestins are administered (10 mg × 10 days/month) if spontaneous resumption of normal menses does not occur.

3. **Estrogens.** High-dose estrogen therapy rapidly stops bleeding within 12 to 24 hours and is the treatment of choice in some situations.
   a. **When bleeding has been prolonged,** the endometrium is denuded to the basalis layer and is insufficient in quantity to respond to progestin stabilization. High-

dose estrogen stimulates a rapid growth of endometrial tissue over the denuded and raw epithelial surfaces.

b. **When bleeding is hemorrhagic,** high-dose estrogen administered intravenously most rapidly halts the bleeding and initiates the healing process.

c. **When bleeding is secondary to progesterone breakthrough bleeding,** addition of estrogen adds height to the atrophic endometrium and brings a halt to the bleeding.

d. The acute mechanism of action is thought to be **initiation of clotting at the capillary level.** Proliferation of the endometrial surface is a later effect.

e. **Conjugated estrogens,** 1.25 mg, or estradiol, 2 mg, are administered daily for 7 to 10 days. If bleeding is moderately heavy, the same doses are administered every 4 hours during the first 24 hours of therapy. Treatment is continued for another 10 days with the daily dose of estrogen combined with 10 mg medroxyprogesterone. A withdrawal bleed is expected after cessation of therapy.

f. **Parenteral estrogen** is effective in treating acute profuse DUB. Estrogen, 25 mg, is administered intravenously every 4 hours until the bleeding lessens, or up to 12 hours. A progestin must be started at the same time.

g. After control of the acute episode, **chronic therapy** is initiated with the oral contraceptive or periodic progesterone for at least 3 months.

B. Medical therapy

1. **Nonsteroidal antiinflammatory agents (NSAIDs)**

   a. **Prostaglandins** have important pharmacologic actions on the endometrial vasculature and on endometrial hemostasis.

   b. The concentration of endometrial prostaglandins increases progressively during the menstrual cycle.

      (1) **Thromboxane** promotes platelet aggregation and is a potent vasoconstrictor.

      (2) **Prostacyclin** prevents platelet aggregation and is a potent vasodilator.

   c. NSAIDs inhibit prostaglandin synthesis and may work by altering the balance between thromboxane and prostacyclin.

   d. The NSAIDs are primarily effective in reducing menstrual blood loss in women who ovulate, and reduce excessive blood flow by up to 50%.

2. **GnRH agonists.** After control of the acute episode, GnRH agonist may be useful to achieve amenorrhea in the chronically ill patient. Expense and the long-term effects of hypoestrogenism limit therapy. If long-term therapy is chosen, hormone replacement therapy with estrogen and progestin is advised.

3. **Desmopressin.** A synthetic analogue of arginine vasopressin, desmopressin is used as a treatment of last resort in patients with coagulation disorders.

C. Surgical therapy

1. **D and C** with or without hysteroscopy is not the treatment of first choice in the patient thought to have DUB. It is undertaken in the patient who fails to respond to initial hormonal therapy and is used as a diagnostic rather than a therapeutic modality.

2. **Hysterectomy.** In women who have completed childbearing, persistent abnormal bleeding is often both worrisome and bothersome. Some may not tolerate or choose not to pursue continued hormonal or medical management. Hysterectomy is a realistic option in this situation to restore quality of life.

3. **Endometrial ablation.** Ablation of the endometrium is a surgical option for women who are not candidates for hysterectomy because of medical conditions or who wish to avoid hysterectomy but choose not to pursue hormonal therapy.

   a. Ablation of the endometrium is achieved using laser, electrocautery, or thermal destructive techniques.

   b. Fifty percent of women achieve amenorrhea; 90% achieve a decrease in bleeding.

   c. The long-term risk of the occurrence of undetectable endometrial carcinoma in isolated segments of endometrium has yet to be defined.

STUDY QUESTIONS

DIRECTIONS: Each of the numbered items or incomplete statements in this section is followed by answers or by completions of the statement. Select the ONE lettered answer or completion that is BEST in each case.

1. Dysfunctional uterine bleeding (DUB) is frequently associated with

(A) endometrial polyps
(B) anovulation
(C) cervicitis
(D) systemic lupus erythematosus
(E) von Willebrand's disease

2. The abnormal pattern of bleeding that appears in conjunction with a short follicular phase is called

(A) menorrhagia
(B) menometrorrhagia
(C) polymenorrhea
(D) anovulatory bleeding
(E) metrorrhagia

3. Which diagnosis might be associated with dysfunctional uterine bleeding (DUB)?

(A) Thrombocytopenia
(B) Endometrial polyps
(C) Hydatidiform mole
(D) Polycystic ovarian disease
(E) Leukemia

4. A 15-year-old girl is brought to the physician's office by her mother because she thinks that her daughter is having abnormal bleeding. The patient had her first menses 18 months before the office visit. Which of the following characterizes bleeding in young women of this age?

(A) Regular cycles with heavy menses
(B) Midcycle spotting
(C) Anovulatory bleeding
(D) Progesterone withdrawal bleeding
(E) Hypothalamic–pituitary maturity

5. Which term best describes menses with a 100-ml blood loss every 35 days?

(A) Menometrorrhagia
(B) Metrorrhagia
(C) Polymenorrhea
(D) Menorrhagia
(E) Oligomenorrhea

DIRECTIONS: The numbered item or incomplete statement in this section is negatively phrased, as indicated by a capitalized word such as NOT, LEAST, or EXCEPT. Select the ONE lettered answer or completion that is BEST.

6. Functions of progestins include all of the following EXCEPT

(A) treating endometrial hyperplasia
(B) diminishing the effect of estrogen on target cells
(C) supporting and organizing the endometrium
(D) providing antimitotic activity
(E) enhancing estrogen receptor replenishment in the cell

DIRECTIONS: The set of matching questions in this section consists of a list of four to twenty-six lettered options (some of which may be in figures) followed by several numbered items. For each numbered item, select the ONE lettered option that is most closely associated with it. To avoid spending too much time on matching sets with large numbers of options, it is generally advisable to begin each set by reading the list of options. Then, for each item in the set, try to generate the correct answer and locate it in the option list, rather than evaluating each option individually. Each lettered option may be selected once, more than once, or not at all.

Questions 7–9

For each clinical situation listed, select the most closely related laboratory finding.

(A) Platelet dysfunction
(B) Elevated progesterone level
(C) Hematocrit
(D) Positive pregnancy test or elevated human chorionic gonadotropin (hCG) levels
(E) None of the above

7. Anovulation

8. Ectopic pregnancy and hydatidiform mole

9. von Willebrand's disease

ANSWERS AND EXPLANATIONS

1. The answer is B [I A; IV]. Dysfunctional uterine bleeding (DUB) is associated with anovulation in 90% of cases. DUB is a diagnosis of exclusion, which is made after organic causes of bleeding, such as endometrial polyps, cervicitis, systemic lupus erythematosus, and von Willebrand's disease, have been ruled out. If another etiology or source can be found for the bleeding, it is not DUB.

2. The answer is C [I B; III B 2]. One type of dysfunctional bleeding associated with ovulatory cycles is polymenorrhea, which is characterized by menses that occur at regular intervals of less than 21 days. Cycle length is determined by the length of the follicular phase. Because the cycle is short, so is the follicular phase. Menorrhagia, menometrorrhagia, and metrorrhagia are characterized by heavy, prolonged, and irregular bleeding. These conditions are usually associated with anovulatory cycles.

3. The answer is D [I A; III A 1–3, 4 d (2)]. Dysfunctional uterine bleeding (DUB) is usually anovulatory in nature and is usually the result of estrogen breakthrough bleeding. Polycystic ovarian disease is the result of a chronic anovulatory condition with sustained estrogen secretion. Thrombocytopenia, polyps, hydatidiform mole, and leukemia are organic causes of uterine bleeding and, therefore, not DUB. DUB is the diagnosis after organic causes of bleeding have been excluded.

4. The answer is C [III A 3 a, B 1]. This patient is the postmenarchal adolescent who has irregular bleeding characteristic of this time period. The uterine bleeding during the first few years after the menarche is often both irregular and anovulatory because of an immaturity of the hypothalamic–pituitary–ovarian axis. The irregular bleeding that does occur is caused by the sustained estrogen secretion with breakthrough bleeding. Both midcycle spotting and progesterone withdrawal bleeding are associated with ovulatory cycles and are not, therefore, compatible with the anovulatory nature of the postmenarchal bleeding. Regular cycles with heavy bleeding also suggest an ovulatory state with menorrhagia; however, the menorrhagia in the postmenarchal years is usually associated with anovulation.

5. The answer is D [I B 2]. Menses characterized by prolonged and excessive bleeding at regular intervals is called menorrhagia. Menometrorrhagia and metrorrhagia are characterized by bleeding that occurs at irregular intervals, whereas polymenorrhea is normal uterine bleeding that occurs at frequent regular intervals. Oligomenorrhea is infrequent uterine bleeding that occurs at intervals greater than 40 days.

6. The answer is E [V A 1]. Progestins are one of the synthetic steroids. Because they have a progesterone-like quality, they are used in treating dysfunctional uterine bleeding (DUB). DUB is most frequently associated with anovulation and continuous or unopposed estrogen secretion. Thus, a progesterone-like compound is an excellent substance to use in treating DUB because such a compound is basically an antiestrogen. The progestins diminish the effect of estrogen on target cells by inhibiting, not enhancing, estrogen receptor replenishment in the cell. The progestins are antimitotic and antigrowth in nature because they oppose the effects of estrogen at the cellular level. Thus, they are effective agents in treating endometrial hyperplasia, which usually results from unopposed estrogen. The progestins support and organize the endometrium, so sloughing occurs after progestin withdrawal.

7–9. The answers are: 7-E, 8-D, 9-A [I A; II B; III A, Table 26-1]. None of the laboratory findings listed in the question would be useful in diagnosing anovulation, which can be diagnosed by an endometrial biopsy that reveals a proliferative endometrium. Human chorionic gonadotropin (hCG) is the hormone secreted by a conceptus from the trophoblastic tissue; thus, a positive pregnancy test and elevated hCG levels indicate pregnancy or a pregnancy-related complication, such as hydatidiform mole. von Willebrand's disease is associated with a factor VIII deficiency and platelet dysfunction, but not with abnormal platelet counts. An elevated progesterone level indicates ovulation and, thus, is not present in an anovulatory cycle.

Chapter 27

Sexual Abuse

William W. Beck, Jr.

I. INTRODUCTION. Sexual abuse incorporates a wide range of behavior, from coerced seduction to violent assault.

A. Rape. Sexual assault is a term used to describe manual, oral, or genital contact with the genitalia of the victim without the victim's consent. **Rape and incest** are coital forms of sexual assault. **The primary motive for rape is aggression.** Three basic components of rape are:

1. The genitalia of the offender must contact the genitalia of the victim.

2. The offender must accomplish the act **against the victim's will.**

3. The act must involve an **element of force** or threat of physical harm.
   a. **Force** often involves a weapon that may injure or kill.
   b. **Resistance to force** is no longer a requirement for proving rape.

B. Statutory rape involves sexual activity with a person who is unable to consent either because she or he is below the age of consent or because consciousness has been altered by illness, sleep, drugs, or alcohol.

II. EPIDEMIOLOGY

A. Incidence. Although rape is one of the least reported crimes, because victims fear being further victimized by the attitudes of society, reported rape is increasing by an annual rate of 9%. The number of rapes peaks in the summer, and rape is more frequent in the more highly populated southern states and in lower socioeconomic groups.

B. Profile. The offenders are typically young men between the ages of 16 and 25 years; they have a low social status and poor education.

C. Act. Rape is foremost a crime of violence.

1. In 86% of all rapes, the assailant either carries a weapon or threatens the victim with death.

2. Victims experience violence as roughness or beatings.

3. Approximately 0.5% of rapes terminate in death.

III. MEDICAL EVALUATION

A. Initial contact. The physician should try to help the victim overcome feelings of helplessness created by the experience of rape. The victim may object to being examined, especially by a male physician, for she may perceive the examination as a continuation of the violation. If she has no threatening injuries, the physician can, without hesitation, delay the examination until a family member, a friend, a member of a woman's support organization, or a female nurse has comforted the patient. The physician must remain objective while offering reassurance and emotional support.

B. **History.** Both the victim's history and the physical examination are important in evaluating the actual and potential harm and in providing information for possible future legal action.

1. A precise description of all forms of sexual activity, including the areas of the body involved, is mandatory.

2. The physician must note whether the victim has changed clothes, urinated, bathed, showered, douched, or brushed her teeth since the alleged attack.

3. The victim should report the last time she had sexual intercourse before the assault.

4. The date of the victim's last menstrual period and her birth control status are important.

C. **Physical examination.** Sketches or photographs made during the physical examination are ideal for documentation and notation of the precise location of any cuts or bruises sustained by the victim.

1. **Signs of resistance**—choke marks on the neck, bites, or scratches—should be described. Because the signs of blunt trauma—ecchymoses and hematomas—often do not appear for some time after injury, the victim should be asked to return when such marks appear.

2. **Evidence of semen.** Semen, which is high in **histone,** fluoresces when exposed to **Wood's light** in a darkened room. This characteristic is an effective means of localizing **moist** or **dried semen** during the physical examination or examination of the clothing. The presence of semen indicates only that the victim has had sexual intercourse, not necessarily with her attacker.

3. A **complete neurologic examination,** including a mental status evaluation, is mandatory.

4. **Pelvic examination.** This part of the physical examination is the most critical because of the legal implications of the findings and their documentation.
   a. The **perineum** is examined for bruising and laceration.
   b. The **presence or absence of blood and moist or dried secretions** on the mons pubis, vulva, perineum, rectum, buttocks, or thighs is noted.
   c. Pubic hair is combed for a **hair sample.**
   d. **Fingernail scrapings** are collected where appropriate.
   e. The **status of the hymen** is observed and recorded, remembering that:
      (1) Penetration by a penis through an elastic hymen may occur without lacerations.
      (2) The hymen may be ruptured by trauma other than sexual intercourse, including masturbation or introduction of foreign objects into the vagina.
   f. **Speculum examination** includes visual inspection and collection of vaginal pool samples.
      (1) The **vaginal mucosa** is carefully inspected for abrasions, lacerations, and ecchymoses.
      (2) Swabs of the cervix and vagina should be taken for a **gonococcal and chlamydial culture.**
      (3) A **wet mount** is obtained from the vaginal pool to determine the presence or absence of spermatozoa and sperm motility.
      (4) Swabs of the vaginal pool are obtained, smeared on two glass slides, and allowed to air-dry, and are then tested for the presence of **acid phosphatase** (see III D 2) and the **ABO antigen** (see III D 3).

D. **Laboratory studies**

1. **Spermatozoa.** At the time of the rape examination, a wet mount is obtained from the vaginal pool and checked for the presence or absence of spermatozoa.
   a. The **presence of motile spermatozoa** suggests sexual intercourse within the previous 24 hours.
   b. The **presence of nonmotile spermatozoa** has little significance.

    c. The **absence of spermatozoa** does not disprove recent sexual intercourse; the rapist may be azoospermic, may be severely oligospermic, or may have had a vasectomy.

  2. Acid phosphatase. Although all ejaculates contain acid phosphatase, it is not unique to semen; it is found in urine, normal vaginal fluid, and all tissues of the human body. However, **the concentration of acid phosphatase in semen is important;** a fresh ejaculate contains between **400 and 8000 King-Armstrong units/ml.** Thus, identification of significant quantities of acid phosphatase in specimens from the vagina, anus, or mouth is strong evidence of recent ejaculation in these areas.

  3. ABO antigen. Approximately 80% of men secrete ABO antigens into body fluids, including semen. Thus, ABO typing is excellent confirmatory evidence for the identity of the assailant. If no vaginal fluid is available, the vagina can be washed with sterile saline, which then can be saved for ABO antigen testing.

  4. Other studies. Blood should be drawn for a complete blood count and a serum test for syphilis, hepatitis B, and human immunodeficiency virus. Urine should be sent for urinalysis. At follow-up, appropriate repeat cultures and serologies should be obtained.

IV. PROTECTION OF THE VICTIM

A. **Venereal disease.** Prophylaxis against venereal disease should be administered to all victims at the time of the initial examination. After a pediatrician is consulted, pediatric doses should be administered to children who weigh less than 100 lbs.

  1. Antibiotic regimens include:
    a. Single-dose **ceftriaxone,** 250 mg intramuscularly (IM), plus **doxycycline,** 100 mg orally twice daily for 7 days
    b. Alternatively, **spectinomycin,** 2 g IM, followed by **doxycycline**

  2. Efficacy
    a. Gonorrhea. Because of the emergence of resistant strains of gonorrhea, all victims should be recultured in 4 weeks.
    b. Syphilis. The victim should have a repeat serum test for syphilis in 6 weeks.

B. **Pregnancy.** Human chorionic gonadotropin (hCG) determination, if initially negative, should be repeated weekly until it becomes positive or until menses occur. To be effective, pregnancy prophylaxis should begin within 72 hours of the assault.

  1. The standard dose of **diethylstilbestrol (DES)** is 25 mg twice daily for 5 days; the extreme nausea that can accompany this therapy can be helped with prochlorperazine. Because of the teratogenic effects of DES, a therapeutic abortion is recommended if the therapy fails.

  2. Another approach is to prescribe the **oral contraceptive Ovral.** The **dosage** is two tablets taken immediately and two tablets taken 12 hours later. The backup is the same as with DES.

  3. Insertion of an **intrauterine device** is also effective in preventing pregnancy, and the physician should offer this alternative to the victim.

C. **Psychological sequelae**

  1. Support groups should be recommended to victims because these organizations can provide:
    a. Immediate postevaluation counseling and an ongoing relationship with the victim
    b. Group sessions with other victims, thus providing opportunities for the patient to reenact the traumatic episode with understanding, objective people
    c. Assistance to victims as they convert feelings of rage and shame to healthy anger

2. **Reactions to rape** typically involve three phases:
   a. The **first phase,** which lasts several days or weeks, is an acute reaction period, in which the patient has difficulty talking about the assault. Anxiety usually replaces shock and dismay as time passes. Recall of the event may so affect the patient that she becomes totally unable to function in her everyday activities. The victim typically suffers from feelings of anger, immerses herself in self-recrimination, and fears the reactions of others.
   b. The **second phase** represents a pseudoadjustment period. Anxiety and anger in this stage are managed by denial, repression, and rationalization; the victim frequently withdraws from group sessions and therapeutic efforts.
   c. The **third phase** is the adjustment or reorganization phase and is long term; it is often marked by **depression.**
      (1) It may be associated with flashbacks and nightmares.
      (2) It may be associated with the development of phobias about men or the sex act.
      (3) The victim's lifestyle, including friends, job, and residence, may change.
      (4) The patient may require extensive, nonjudgmental, sensitive counseling or psychotherapy.

3. **Psychological problems in pediatric victims** may be more complex and intense than those in older victims.
   a. Acquisition of relevant information may be difficult because of the child's severe anxiety combined with the inability to communicate clearly.
   b. Parents of assaulted children frequently display considerable anxiety about the psychological and physical well-being of the child. Their irrational behavior toward medical personnel is their way of expressing their anger, guilt, and helplessness.

V. SEXUAL ABUSE OF CHILDREN.

V. **SEXUAL ABUSE OF CHILDREN.** In addition to rape, the sexual abuse of children includes fondling, oral and anal sodomy, incest, pornography, and prostitution. Often no physical evidence is present to show what has occurred or whether force was exerted, but the offender may be using other means, such as threats, bribery, or coercion, to get the child to submit to sexual acts.

A. **Incidence.** As with rape, the incidence of sexual abuse of children is an underreported problem, in part because it is perceived as a social taboo.

1. It occurs in families of every racial and ethnic background and at every educational and income level.

2. No age-group of children is spared.

3. It is estimated that 1 in 5 girls and 1 in 10 boys are sexually abused before age 18 years.

4. Most sexually abused children are victims of someone they know.

B. **Predisposing factors.** At high risk are children:

1. Who are born to single-parent families

2. Whose mothers and fathers are divorced or separated

3. Who are born into families with mental illnesses

4. Who have a history of abusive parents

5. Who live with homeless families or reside in overcrowded units

6. Whose parents work and leave them home alone

7. Who return to an empty house after school

VI. THE BATTERED WOMAN (also called **domestic violence** and **spouse abuse**)

A. **Definition:** any woman older than 16 years of age with evidence of physical abuse on at least one occasion at the hands of an intimate male partner

1. Physical abuse can vary in intensity, from verbal abuse or threats of violence to pushing, hitting, beating, threatening with a weapon, or using a weapon.

2. This violence is accompanied by mental abuse or intimidation.

B. There is a significant **relationship between spouse battering and child abuse** by men.

C. **Signs of domestic violence**

1. **Presenting complaints** in office or emergency room include headaches, insomnia, choking sensation, hyperventilation, and chest, back, or pelvic pain.

2. **Other signs or symptoms** include shyness, fright, embarrassment, passivity, evasiveness, crying, drug or alcohol abuse, and injuries.

STUDY QUESTIONS

DIRECTIONS: Each of the numbered items or incomplete statements in this section is followed by answers or by completions of the statement. Select the ONE lettered answer or completion that is BEST in each case.

1. A victim experiencing the second phase of the psychological reaction to rape typically exhibits

(A) shame and dismay
(B) denial and rationalization
(C) anger and self-recrimination
(D) acute anxiety
(E) inability to function in everyday activities

2. Motile spermatozoa found on a wet mount of vaginal secretions are indicative of intercourse within the past

(A) 6 hours
(B) 12 hours
(C) 24 hours
(D) 48 hours
(E) 72 hours

DIRECTIONS: Each of the numbered items or incomplete statements in this section is negatively phrased, as indicated by a capitalized word such as NOT, LEAST, or EXCEPT. Select the ONE lettered answer or completion that is BEST in each case.

3. Which of the following statements about rape is NOT correct?

(A) Rape is a crime of aggression
(B) Victims experience violence in most rape cases
(C) Aggression is the primary motive for sexual assault
(D) The frequency of rape is highest in northeastern cities
(E) Demonstrated resistance is not necessary to prove rape

4. Which of the following is NOT supportive evidence in a rape case?

(A) Motile spermatozoa found on a wet mount 2 hours after the assault
(B) Acid phosphatase found on a dried slide taken from the vaginal pool
(C) A lacerated hymen
(D) Positive Wood's light examination of dried vulvar secretion
(E) A positive gonococcal culture

5. Which of the following family patterns is NOT a risk factor that predisposes children to sexual abuse?

(A) Families with divorced or separated parents
(B) Families in which the mother works and the father stays home
(C) Families with mental illness
(D) Single-parent families
(E) Families below the poverty level

6. Which of the following is NOT evidence of ejaculation at the time of a rape?

(A) Positive Wood's light examination
(B) Positive acid phosphatase test
(C) Wet mount of vaginal secretions showing motile spermatozoa
(D) Presence of the B antigen in the vaginal fluid
(E) Positive human chorionic gonadotropin (hCG) test

7. Which of the following statements about sexual abuse of children is NOT correct?

(A) It is underreported
(B) It is seen in all ethnic groups
(C) It occurs among all socioeconomic groups
(D) Most sexually victimized children do not know their abuser
(E) No age-group among children is spared

ANSWERS AND EXPLANATIONS

1. The answer is B [IV C 2 a–c]. Shame, dismay, anxiety, anger, self-recrimination, and the inability to function in everyday activities are characteristic of the first phase of the reaction to rape. The second phase is a pseudoadjustment period, which is marked by denial, repression, and rationalization.

2. The answer is C [III D 1 a]. Motile spermatozoa found on a wet mount of vaginal secretions indicate that the spermatozoa have been deposited there within the previous 24 hours. Spermatozoa cannot live longer than 24 hours because of the vaginal acidity, which irreversibly inactivates them.

3. The answer is D [I A; II A, C]. Rape is a crime of violence, the major motive being aggression; however, although beatings occur with great frequency, occurrence is less than 50% of reported cases. It is no longer necessary to show resistance to force to prove rape. The occurrence of rape peaks during the summer months and is more frequent in the highly populated southern states.

4. The answer is E [III C 2, 4 a, D 1 a, 2]. In an alleged rape, anything that suggests intromission and ejaculation is positive evidence. A lacerated hymen can indicate forceful intromission. A positive Wood's light examination and the finding of acid phosphatase suggest the presence of semen. Motile spermatozoa indicate intercourse within 24 hours. A positive gonococcal culture is not evidence of rape because the gonococci could have been acquired before the rape from a different source.

5. The answer is B [V B]. A number of factors predispose children to sexual abuse. Chil-dren who are left alone while parents work or who return home to an empty house after school are at risk. Children from broken homes, families with mental illness, single-parent families, families with histories of abuse, families below the poverty level, and homeless families are also at risk. However, no evidence suggests that children of families in which the mother works and the father stays home are at risk.

6. The answer is E [III C 2, 4 f (3), D 1–3; IV B]. Motile spermatozoa found on a wet mount preparation indicate that those spermatozoa were deposited within the previous 24 hours. Wood's light fluoresces in the presence of histone, which is found in semen. Acid phosphatase is suggestive of semen, especially if found in large concentrations. Because 80% of men secrete ABO antigens into body fluids, including semen, the finding of a B antigen in the vaginal fluid, especially if the victim is blood type A or O, would be evidence that an ejaculation had occurred. A human chorionic gonadotropin (hCG) test is for pregnancy. The only thing that a positive hCG test would indicate in a rape victim is that she was already pregnant at the time she was raped.

7. The answer is D [V A 1–4]. Like rape, sexual abuse of children is underreported, often because the abuser is a family member or member of the community; in most cases, sexually abused children are victims of someone they know. Children of all ages, including infants and toddlers, are abused. There is no racial, ethnic, educational, or economic barrier to sexual abuse of children; it occurs without regard to social status.

Chapter 28

Ectopic Pregnancy

William W. Beck, Jr.

I. INTRODUCTION

A. **Definition.** An ectopic pregnancy is any gestation occurring outside the uterine cavity. The most common site for an ectopic pregnancy is the fallopian tube (98%), but other sites are the ovary, cervix, and abdominal cavity (Figure 28-1).

B. **Incidence.** The frequency of ectopic pregnancy is about 1 in 200 pregnancies. In urban medical centers, which serve high indigent populations, the frequency of ectopic pregnancy is 1 in 80 pregnancies.

C. **Mortality.** A substantial maternal mortality rate still occurs with ectopic pregnancy because hemorrhage and shock occur rapidly and the prerupture diagnosis is elusive, with a consequent delay in surgical treatment.

   1. Serum human chorionic gonadotropin (hCG) testing, ultrasonography, and laparoscopy allow prerupture intervention in 80% of cases.

   2. Fatality rate has decreased in 10 years from 35.5 to 3.8 per 10,000 ectopic pregnancies, a decrease of 90%.

II. ETIOLOGY OF ECTOPIC PREGNANCY

A. **Pelvic infection.** Chronic salpingitis is a common pathologic finding (30%–50%) in a fallopian tube with an ectopic pregnancy. The high incidence of ectopic pregnancy in indigent populations, where pelvic inflammatory disease (PID) is endemic, supports this observation.

   1. **Infection of the tube** leads to fibrosis and scarring of intraluminal structures, which may result in transport dysfunction because of constriction of the tube, false passage formation, altered cilia, and abnormal tubal muscular action. All of these features retard the progress of the fertilized ovum on its way through the tube to the uterus, fostering implantation in the tube.

   2. **Chronic PID** usually involves both tubes. The 10% to 15% recurrent ectopic pregnancy rate in the contralateral tube confirms the relation between PID and ectopic pregnancy.

B. **Narrowing of the tube.** Conditions causing a significant narrowing of the passageway for the fertilized ovum and, thus, an increased incidence of ectopic pregnancy include:

   1. Congenital defects of the tube, such as diverticula and sacculations

   2. Benign tubal tumors and cysts

   3. Uterine fibroids at the uterotubal junction

   4. Endometriosis of the tube, which has the capacity to undergo early decidua-like changes

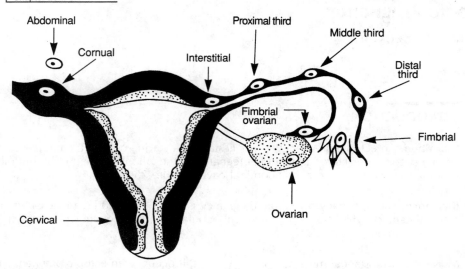

FIGURE 28-1. Anatomic site of ectopic pregnancy. (Reprinted with permission from Breen JL: A 21-year survey of 654 ectopic gestations. *Am J Obstet Gynecol* 106:1004, 1970.)

    5. Peritubal adhesions secondary to appendicitis or pelvic or abdominal surgery

    6. Surgical repair of the tube. Ectopic pregnancy is seen with increased frequency in patients who undergo repair of the tube after previous PID or tubal anastomosis after a previous tubal ligation.

C. **Intrauterine device (IUD) usage.** About 3% to 4% of pregnancies conceived with the IUD in place are ectopic. This occurrence is probably caused by the relative efficiency of the device in preventing intrauterine pregnancies rather than a specific relationship between the IUD and ectopic pregnancy.

D. **Use of assisted reproductive technology**

    1. Incidence of heterotopic pregnancies (both intrauterine and ectopic) is 1 in 100 pregnancies

    2. Seen with in vitro fertilization, gamete intrafallopian transfer, and superovulation

III. SIGNS AND SYMPTOMS OF ECTOPIC PREGNANCY

A. **Bleeding.** The most common symptom is abnormal uterine bleeding or spotting, which usually begins 7 to 14 days after the missed menstrual period.

    1. Abnormal bleeding may occur at the time of the expected menses and be interpreted by the patient as a menses.

    2. Major hemorrhage is uncommon, but menstrual-type bleeding occurs in 25% of ectopic pregnancies, and the patient or physician may consider it delayed menses.

    3. The amount, timing, and character of the bleeding should not obviate the possibility that ectopic pregnancy could be the diagnosis.

B. **Pain.** Unilateral pelvic pain, which may be knife-like and stabbing or dull and less well defined, is the next most common symptom. With intra-abdominal hemorrhage and blood under the diaphragm, shoulder pain is a common symptom.

C. **Clinical picture.** Few patients actually present with the classic picture of ectopic pregnancy, which entails amenorrhea and signs of early pregnancy followed by abnormal bleeding, abdominal pain, and fainting (due to hypotension from intraperitoneal bleeding).

1. Ectopic pregnancy can occur with an acute, subacute, or chronic presentation.

2. The mass of the unruptured ectopic pregnancy may be small and not palpable.

3. The uterus is usually enlarged to a 6-week size and is soft. The palpable, only slightly tender, tubal ectopic pregnancy may be confused with an ovary that contains a corpus luteum of pregnancy.

4. The bleeding and pain may be interpreted as a threatened abortion.

IV. DIAGNOSIS OF ECTOPIC PREGNANCY

A. **Index of suspicion.** Ectopic pregnancy must be suspected when pregnant patients present with abnormal bleeding and pelvic pain or give a history of PID or pelvic surgery, because this history places them at increased risk.

B. **Differential diagnosis.** The diagnosis of ectopic pregnancy may be straightforward in a patient with amenorrhea, symptoms of pregnancy, pelvic pain, and bleeding. However, other clinical conditions are likely also and should be ruled out.

1. **Adnexal torsion or acute appendicitis.** Although these conditions are suggested by unilateral pelvic pain, they do not produce amenorrhea, syncope, anemia, and early shock.

2. **Aborting intrauterine pregnancy.** In an aborting intrauterine pregnancy, the external bleeding is much more severe than the pain, whereas the reverse is true with an ectopic pregnancy.

3. **Bleeding corpus luteum of a normal intrauterine pregnancy.** The bleeding corpus luteum usually does not produce the severity of pain or shock typical of ectopic pregnancy. In addition, uterine bleeding is usually absent. When heavy internal bleeding is accompanied by shock, the physician has no other option but to observe the process directly by laparoscopy or laparotomy.

C. **Tests for diagnosing ectopic pregnancy**

1. **Serial testing of hCG.** Serum hCG tests are positive in 100% of ectopic pregnancies.
   a. The **rate of rise of serum hCG** can help to differentiate normal from abnormal pregnancies (i.e., ectopic and blighted ovum pregnancies); in a normal pregnancy, the serum hCG level doubles every 2 days.
   b. **At threshold levels of 6000 mIU/ml and 1500 mIU/ml of hCG,** an intrauterine pregnancy should be detected by abdominal ultrasound and vaginal ultrasound, respectively. Failure to detect fetal echoes within the uterus suggests an ectopic pregnancy.

2. **Pelvic ultrasound.** Ultrasound is only helpful in ruling out ectopic pregnancy by identifying a clearly defined intrauterine sac at 7 weeks from the last menstrual period; this finding correlates with an hCG level of 5000 to 6000 mIU/ml. An enlarged uterus and an adnexal mass observed by ultrasound are not helpful because these findings may simply represent an early intrauterine pregnancy and a corpus luteum.

3. **Vaginal ultrasound.** Ultrasound performed through the vagina with a vaginal probe can identify the intrauterine sac earlier than pelvic ultrasound can.
   a. The intrauterine sac can be detected at hCG levels of 1500 to 2000 mIU/ml, which correlates with a 6-week gestation.
   b. An ectopic pregnancy can, therefore, be ruled out 4 to 6 days earlier with vaginal ultrasound than with pelvic ultrasound.

4. **Culdocentesis.** This test is useful in patients presenting acutely with pelvic pain, abnormal bleeding, syncope, or shock to determine whether there is free blood in the peritoneal cavity.
   a. An 18-gauge needle is inserted behind the uterus into the cul-de-sac.
   b. Aspiration of the cul-de-sac should produce fluid material.
   c. The **normal contents** are slightly yellow and clear, with a volume of 3 to 5 ml. The **presence of nonclotting blood in the syringe** is diagnostic of free blood in the peritoneal cavity and supports the diagnosis of ectopic pregnancy.

5. **Laparoscopy.** If the diagnosis is in doubt, laparoscopy should be performed. It allows for the direct visualization of the tubes and ovaries. The risk to the patient associated with performing a laparoscopy is far less than the risk associated with an undiagnosed ectopic pregnancy.

6. **Endometrial histology.** When a patient is undergoing a dilation and curettage for abnormal uterine bleeding, such as in a suspected spontaneous abortion, the finding of decidua in the endometrial sample without chorionic villi indicates an ectopic pregnancy until proven otherwise. An additional finding in such an endometrium may be the Arias-Stella reaction, which is an endometrial response to the hormonal stimulation of pregnancy, producing a patchy, hyperactive, often hypersecretory pattern.

V. TREATMENT OF ECTOPIC PREGNANCY

A. **Expectant management.** About 25% can be managed expectantly. Criteria include:

1. Falling hCG titer

2. Ectopic pregnancy definitely in the tube

3. No significant bleeding or evidence of rupture

4. Ectopic mass not larger than 4 cm in greatest diameter

B. **Salpingo-oophorectomy.** Surgical management (removal of the affected ovary) was formerly advocated if the other adnexa appeared normal and pregnancy was desired.

1. The rationale for this management was that all subsequent ovulations would occur from an ovary with an adjacent tube, thereby increasing the patient's potential pregnancy rate per cycle.

2. **Removal of a normal ovary. This procedure is no longer justifiable**—despite the need for removing the ipsilateral tube—because of the possibility of in vitro fertilization at a later date and the need for maximum potential in terms of ovum production.

C. **Salpingectomy.** This procedure is the most common treatment for a ruptured ectopic pregnancy. The salpingectomy is performed by cross-clamping the broad ligament and removing the whole tube. This form of surgical management is most appropriate in the ruptured ectopic pregnancy because there usually is considerable bleeding.

D. **Unruptured ectopic pregnancy.** The frequency with which the diagnosis of unruptured ectopic pregnancy can be made has increased significantly with the combined use of serial testing of hCG, pelvic ultrasound, and laparoscopy. With the unruptured tubal ectopic pregnancy, a more conservative approach to the tube is possible.

1. **"Milking" procedure.** In the patient with an unruptured tubal pregnancy, the pregnancy can be "milked" from the end of the tube. **Because of the high rate of recurrent ectopic pregnancy after this procedure, it is not recommended.**
   a. This procedure can damage the tube because most tubal pregnancies are not within the lumen of the tube.
   b. The pregnancy grows in the space between the endosalpinx and the serosa.

2. **Salpingostomy.** If the pregnancy is at the **midpoint of the tube,** a linear salpingostomy, an opening in the tube, may be performed to remove the ectopic pregnancy; the salpingostomy is not usually closed after removal of the products of conception.

3. **Segmental resection of the tube.** The segment of the tube involved in the ectopic pregnancy may be removed and an anastomosis of the tubal ends performed. Alternatively, the cut ends of the tube can be ligated, with an anastomosis at a later date.

4. **Operative laparoscopy.** Almost any surgical technique for ectopic pregnancy that is performed by a laparotomy can now be accomplished through operative laparoscopy.
   a. **Thermocoagulation** and **transection** are techniques that can be used for either partial or total salpingectomies.
   b. **Linear salpingostomies** can be accomplished using several incising modalities—high-power density electrocautery, carbon dioxide laser, or fiberoptic lasers (Figure 28-2).
   c. The **advantages** of operative laparoscopy include shorter operating time, decreased postoperative course, and shortened hospital stay, with the patient able to return to normal function much earlier than after a laparotomy.

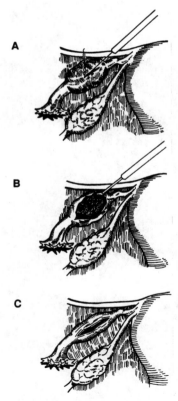

FIGURE 28-2. Laparoscopic salpingostomy for the management of ectopic pregnancy. (*A*) Salpingostomy, (*B*) removal of tubal contents, and (*C*) evacuated tube left to heal. (Reprinted with permission from Martin DC: *Intraabdominal Laser Surgery.* Memphis, Resurge Press, 1986, pp 568–617.)

5. **Medical treatment. Methotrexate chemotherapy with citrovorum factor (folinic acid) rescue** has been used successfully in treating small, unruptured ectopic pregnancies.

   a. **Methotrexate** is a folic acid antagonist that creates a block in folate metabolism and adversely affects the rapidly dividing (trophoblastic) cells.

   b. A **complication** in a small number of patients is acute bleeding from the site of the ectopic pregnancy 1 to 2 weeks after methotrexate therapy, at times requiring laparotomy.

   c. **Criteria for use of methotrexate** include an unruptured ectopic pregnancy of 4 cm or less in diameter; absence of cardiac activity; and hCG titers of less than 10,000 mIU/ml.

VI. PROGNOSIS. Patients with ectopic pregnancies must be told of the prognosis for future fertility (i.e., approximately 40% of patients never conceive again). Of the 60% who do achieve another pregnancy, 12% will have another ectopic pregnancy, and 15% to 20% will abort spontaneously. Because of the high risk of ectopic pregnancy in women with previous ones, the patient should be instructed to notify her physician as soon as she has missed her menses so that the location of the new pregnancy can be detected by serum hCG testing and ultrasound. If she has another tubal pregnancy, early surgical management to preserve the remaining tube is still a possibility at this early stage.

STUDY QUESTIONS

DIRECTIONS: Each of the numbered items or incomplete statements in this section is followed by answers or by completions of the statement. Select the ONE lettered answer or completion that is BEST in each case.

1. What percentage of women with a previous ectopic pregnancy can expect to have another ectopic pregnancy?

(A) 3%
(B) 6%
(C) 12%
(D) 20%
(E) 25%

2. A patient is admitted with a suspected diagnosis of ectopic pregnancy. She is unhappy with the prospects of either a tubal or an intrauterine pregnancy. Because of the patient's desire for termination of the pregnancy, a dilation and curettage with frozen section is performed before using the laparoscope. Which of the following pathologic findings on frozen section would obviate the need for laparoscopy?

(A) Decidua without villi
(B) Hypersecretory endometrial pattern
(C) Arias-Stella reaction
(D) Proliferative endometrium
(E) Chronic endometritis

3. What is the most accurate method of diagnosing an ectopic pregnancy?

(A) Culdocentesis
(B) Endometrial biopsy
(C) Laparoscopy
(D) Serial measurement of human chorionic gonadotropin (hCG) levels
(E) Pelvic ultrasound

DIRECTIONS: Each of the numbered items or incomplete statements in this section is negatively phrased, as indicated by a capitalized word such as NOT, LEAST, or EXCEPT. Select the ONE lettered answer or completion that is BEST in each case.

4. Which of the following sequelae of pelvic inflammatory disease (PID) does NOT enhance the possibility of ectopic pregnancy?

(A) Intraluminal fibrosis
(B) Altered cilia action
(C) Distal tubal closure (hydrosalpinx)
(D) Constriction of the tube
(E) False passage formation

5. Which of the following is NOT a likely reason for the establishment of an ectopic tubal pregnancy?

(A) Pelvic infection
(B) Peritubal adhesions
(C) Tubal anastomosis
(D) Assisted reproductive technology
(E) Uterine myoma

6. A patient is found to have a small, unruptured ectopic pregnancy in the midportion of the left fallopian tube. Which of the following is NOT appropriate therapy?

(A) Linear salpingostomy by laparotomy
(B) Linear salpingostomy through the laparoscope
(C) Left salpingectomy
(D) Segmental resection of the midportion of the left tube with anastomosis
(E) Methotrexate with citrovorum factor rescue

7. Which of the following is NOT a recommended therapeutic procedure for ectopic pregnancies?

(A) Salpingectomy
(B) Salpingo-oophorectomy
(C) Linear salpingostomy
(D) Segmental resection of the portion of the tube containing the ectopic pregnancy
(E) Milking of the tube

8. Which of the following has NOT been associated with an increased incidence of ectopic pregnancy?

(A) Endometriosis
(B) Chronic salpingitis
(C) Adenomyosis
(D) Use of the intrauterine device
(E) Tubal diverticula

ANSWERS AND EXPLANATIONS

1. The answer is C [VI]. There is significant infertility in patients who have had an ectopic pregnancy. Approximately 40% will never again be pregnant. Of the 60% of women who do get pregnant again, 12% will have another ectopic pregnancy, and 15% to 20% will abort spontaneously.

2. The answer is D [II C; IV C 6]. The finding of a proliferative endometrium would mean that the patient was preovulatory and therefore could not be pregnant; with such a finding, laparoscopy would be unnecessary. In an ectopic pregnancy, there are no products of conception (i.e., villi) in the endometrial cavity. Decidual tissue and a hypersecretory endometrial pattern (the Arias-Stella reaction) without evidence of chorionic villi are common. A chronic endometritis is found in the uterus of an intrauterine device user and might suggest implantation in the tube rather than in the uterus. When an endometritis is found, laparoscopy is indicated to rule out an ectopic tubal pregnancy.

3. The answer is C [IV C 5]. Laparoscopy allows direct visualization of the pelvis, including both tubes and ovaries, and a tubal pregnancy would be obvious. None of the other tests are absolutely diagnostic of an ectopic pregnancy. For example, a culdocentesis that reveals nonclotting blood could indicate a bleeding corpus luteum, and human chorionic gonadotropin (hCG) levels that do not rise at the expected rate could indicate an impending abortion.

4. The answer is C [II A 1, 2]. Pelvic inflammatory disease (PID) leads to fibrosis and scarring of intraluminal structures, which, in turn, result in transport dysfunction because of constriction of the tube, false passage formation, altered cilia action, and abnormal tubal muscular action. These intraluminal impediments to the passage of the fertilized ovum cause both arrest of migration and implantation in the tube. Distal tubal closure (hydrosalpinx) does not cause ectopic pregnancy formation because the egg cannot enter the tube to be fertilized.

5. The answer is E [II A 1, B 3–6, D]. Pelvic inflammatory disease (PID) with scarring and fibrosis of intraluminal structures is a predisposing factor in 50% of ectopic pregnancies. Peritubal adhesions, the result of appendicitis, pelvic surgery, or pelvic infection, have also been associated with ectopic pregnancies. Assisted reproductive technologies have increased the incidence of heterotopic pregnancies (an intrauterine pregnancy plus an ectopic pregnancy). Surgical repair of the tube, especially anastomosis of previously ligated tubes and narrowing of the tubal lumen, is a significant cause of tubal pregnancy. Uterine myomas rarely cause infertility or tubal blockage; this entity is more likely to be associated with a pregnancy loss than an ectopic pregnancy.

6. The answer is C [V C, D 1–5]. Salpingectomy is no longer justified in the presence of an unruptured tubal ectopic pregnancy; in most cases, the tube can be saved by conservative operative techniques. Linear salpingostomy by either laparoscopy or laparotomy is the treatment of choice. Segmental resection of the tubal pregnancy is acceptable, but this procedure then requires anastomosis, probably at a later date, which means another laparotomy. Methotrexate therapy is starting to be used at times for small unruptured tubal ectopic pregnancies; occasional heavy intraperitoneal bleeding is a serious risk with methotrexate therapy.

7. The answer is B [V B 2, C, D 1–3]. The goal in treating an ectopic pregnancy is to conserve as many of the reproductive organs as possible. Linear salpingostomy, segmental resection of the tube, and "milking" of the tube all preserve potential future tubal function. The salpingectomy removes the damaged tube but preserves the nearby ovary. The salpingo-oophorectomy is rarely used today because that procedure removes an ovary that might be of use at a later date as a source of ova for in vitro fertilization or other assisted reproductive technology.

8. The answer is C [II A 1–2, B 1–4, C]. Adenomyosis has no association with ectopic pregnancies because it has no effect on the tube. This uterine lesion is characterized by the presence of ectopic foci of endometrial glands and stroma in the myometrium. Chronic salpingitis leads to fibrosis and scarring of intraluminal structures so that a fertilized egg can become trapped in the tube.

Conditions that cause narrowing of the tube—diverticula, sacculations, benign tubal tumors and cysts, and endometriosis of the tube—increase the incidence of ectopic tubal pregnancies. A disproportionate number of pregnancies that occur with an intrauterine device in situ are ectopic.

Chapter 29

Sexually Transmitted Diseases

Kavita Nanda

I. **INTRODUCTION.** With the advent of the sexual revolution in the 1960s, there has been a broadened focus beyond the five classic sexually transmitted diseases (STDs) of gonorrhea, syphilis, chancroid, lymphogranuloma venereum, and granuloma inguinale. With the exception of the human immunodeficiency virus (HIV), the spectrum of "new" STDs has expanded with the recognition of the venereal nature of these infectious agents by means of sophisticated epidemiologic and diagnostic techniques. Despite screening, prevention and treatment programs, STDs remain a major health problem—in 1995, the World Health Organization (WHO) predicted 333 million new cases of curable STDs.

II. **SEXUALLY TRANSMITTED DISEASES**

A. **Bacterial STDs.** This group includes *Neisseria gonorrhoeae, Hemophilus ducreyi, Calymmatobacterium granulomatis,* and *Gardnerella vaginalis.*

1. *N. gonorrhoeae.* Caused by a gram-negative diplococcus, gonorrhea is the **second most commonly reported communicable disease** in the United States. Humans are its only natural host. The organism has a predilection for **columnar and transitional epithelium.** It causes cervicitis, urethritis, pelvic inflammatory disease (PID), and acute pharyngitis in women. In **men,** it causes urethritis, prostatitis, and epididymitis. Disseminated gonococcal arthritis occurs in both men and women. In the **newborn, gonococcal ophthalmia neonatorum** is a known consequence of maternal infection.
   a. **Epidemiology.** Although decreased since 1975, there were still 418,068 cases reported in the United States in 1994. At least an additional 400,000 cases are believed to be unreported. **Over 80% of reported cases occur in the 15- to 29-year-old age group.** In annual screening programs for non-STD clinics, the average gonorrhea detection rate is 2.7%. Transmission by sexual contact from the man to the woman is likely to result in infection after a single exposure. **Risk factors** include:
      (1) Young age
      (2) Multiple sexual partners
      (3) Failure to use barrier contraception
      (4) Early sexual activity
   b. **Clinical presentation.** *N. gonorrhoeae* has a short incubation time of 3 to 5 days. About 40% to 60% of women with gonorrhea have onset of symptoms at the end of menstruation (particularly with gonococcal PID). Symptoms include:
      (1) Mucopurulent cervical discharge, as occurs in acute cervicitis
      (2) Lower abdominal pain, anorexia, and fever, as is characteristic of acute PID
      (3) Dysuria
      (4) Bartholin's gland abscess
      (5) Infection of other sites:
         (a) Arthritis
         (b) Septicemia
         (c) Pharyngitis
         (d) Perihepatitis
         (e) Chorioamnionitis/endometritis
         (f) Endocarditis
   c. **Diagnosis.** Tests commonly used include:
      (1) Thayer-Martin culture medium (80%–90% sensitive; this is the gold standard)
      (2) Gram's stain of cervical secretions, looking for gram-negative diplococci or polymorphonuclear cells (50%–70% sensitive, 97% specific)

(3) The Gonozyme test, a solid-phase immunoassay for detecting gonococcal antigens (relatively insensitive)

d. Treatment

(1) Considerations

(a) **Single-dose efficacy** is a major concern.

(b) **Coexisting chlamydial infection,** which can occur in up to 45% of patients with gonorrhea in some populations, should be considered.

(2) Ceftriaxone (250 mg for PID, 125 mg for cervicitis) intramuscularly (IM), plus **doxycycline,** 100 mg orally (po) twice daily for 7 days, should be given. Ceftriaxone has the advantage of being effective against incubating syphilis.

(3) Alternative regimens include:

(a) **Ciprofloxacin,** 500 mg po

(b) **Ofloxacin,** 400 mg po

(c) **Spectinomycin,** 2 g IM

(4) Patients with acute PID may require hospitalization and broad-spectrum antibiotics.

e. Patients infected with gonorrhea should be screened for other STDs, including HIV and hepatitis B. Sexual partners should be referred for evaluation and treatment. Follow-up test-of-cure cultures are not required with the recommended treatment regimens for uncomplicated gonorrhea. **Rescreening for reinfection** in high-risk women should be considered at 3 to 6 months.

2. *H. ducreyi* (chancroid). The cause of one of the ulcerative genital diseases, *H. ducreyi* is a small, nonmotile, gram-negative rod that has a characteristic "chaining" appearance on Gram stain.

a. Epidemiology. Chancroid is rare in the United States but common worldwide. There were only 773 cases reported in 1994 in the United States, where this STD is seen most frequently in young, sexually active men who visit prostitutes. Trauma facilitates entry into mucosal vulvar tissues in women. The incubation time is 3 to 5 days. It is a known cofactor for HIV transmission. Ten percent of patients with chancroid may also be infected with syphilis or herpes.

b. Clinical presentation. The classic lesion of chancroid is a soft sore or chancre with a superficial, necrotic ulcer base surrounded by a red halo. The lesion is tender and, in nearly 50% of cases, is accompanied by inflammatory inguinal adenopathy (bubo).

c. Diagnosis. Culture is not commercially available. The most common diagnostic techniques, which demonstrate "school of fish" or "chaining" of gram-negative rods, are:

(1) Gram's stain of exudate from the chancre

(2) Gram's stain of the aspirate of the bubo

d. Treatment should include the partner. Treatment regimens include:

(1) Azithromycin, 1 g po

(2) Ceftriaxone, 250 mg IM

(3) Erythromycin base, 500 mg po four times a day for 7 days

3. *C. granulomatis* is a pleomorphic, gram-negative rod that is responsible for granulomatous and ulcerative lesions of the lower genital tract, also known as granuloma inguinale.

a. Epidemiology. This STD is rarely reported in the United States—only three cases were reported in 1994. Although predominantly sexually transmitted, an intestinal reservoir for *C. granulomatis* has been suggested. The incubation time is 1 month.

b. Clinical presentation

(1) The **initial lesion** is an indolent, irregular ulcer with a pink to beefy-red base.

(2) The **secondary phase** of the disease involves beefy-red, exuberant granulation tissue with scar formation. Inguinal swelling and suppurative abscess may occur secondary to granulomatous tissue formation.

(3) Advanced lesions become markedly hypertrophic. Fistulas of the adjacent structures of the vagina, bladder, and rectum may occur. Elephantiasis of the external genitalia may occur. Hematogenous spread to distant sites has been demonstrated.

c. **Diagnosis**
   (1) **Gram's stain of the lesion** reveals the pathognomonic cells—the mononuclear cells with intracytoplasmic inclusion cysts containing the pleomorphic rod-like organisms. These inclusion cysts are called **Donovan bodies.**
   (2) **Tissue biopsies** demonstrate Donovan bodies on Wright's or Giemsa stains.
d. **Treatment. Tetracycline,** 500 mg orally four times per day for 3 weeks, is effective therapy. Reconstructive vulvar or pelvic surgery may be required in advanced cases.

4. **Bacterial vaginosis (BV)** results from the replacement of the normal H_2O_2-producing *Lactobacillus* with high concentrations of anaerobic bacteria such as *Gardnerella vaginalis, Mobiluncus* sp, *Bacteroides* sp, and *Mycoplasma* sp.
   a. **Epidemiology.** BV is the most common cause of vaginal discharge and odor, but 50% of women who meet criteria for diagnosis have no symptoms. Although included in this chapter, BV is not considered exclusively an STD. It has also become increasingly associated with pregnancy complications.
   b. **Diagnosis.** BV may be diagnosed by the use of clinical or Gram's stain criteria. Clinical criteria require three of the following:
      (1) Homogenous, grayish, noninflammatory discharge that adheres to vaginal walls
      (2) Saline preparation of vaginal secretions that reveals squamous cells whose borders are obscured by coccobacillary forms, known as **clue cells**
      (3) **pH** of secretions greater than 4.5
      (4) Fishy odor after addition of **10% potassium hydroxide ("whiff" test)**
   c. **Treatment.** When not pregnant, only women with symptomatic disease require treatment. Effective treatments include:
      (1) **Metronidazole,** 500 mg po twice a day for 7 days
      (2) Metronidazole gel, 0.75%, one applicator, intravaginally, two times daily, for 5 days
      (3) **Clindamycin** cream, 2%, one applicator, intravaginally, at bedtime, for 7 days

B. **Spirochetal STDs.** The predominant member of this group is *Treponema pallidum,* which causes **syphilis,** a venereal disease that is disseminated by sexual intercourse or intrauterine transmission **(congenital syphilis).** Disease stages include **primary, secondary,** and **tertiary syphilis.**

1. **Epidemiology.** Approximately 80,000 new cases of syphilis are reported each year in the United States. It has been estimated, however, that there are four- to tenfold more new cases, many of which occur in the male homosexual population. The incubation period ranges from 10 to 90 days.

2. **Clinical presentation**
   a. The **initial lesion** of primary syphilis is a painless, ulcerated, hard **chancre,** usually on the external genitalia, although vaginal and cervical lesions are also detected. The primary lesions resolve in 2 to 6 weeks.
   b. In **untreated patients,** this chancre is followed in 6 weeks to 6 months by a **secondary or bacteremic stage** in which the skin and mucous membranes are affected. A **maculopapular rash** of the palms, soles, and mucous membranes occurs. **Condyloma latum** and **generalized lymphadenopathy** are seen as well. These lesions usually resolve within 2 to 6 weeks.
   c. Approximately 33% of untreated patients progress to **tertiary syphilis** with **multiple organ involvement.** Endarteritis leads to aortic aneurysm and aortic insufficiency, tabes dorsalis, optic atrophy, and meningovascular syphilis.

3. **Diagnosis. Dark-field examination** of fresh specimens detects spirochetes in the primary and secondary stages of the disease. **Serologic tests** are helpful in diagnosing syphilis in patients who have progressed beyond primary disease. In the primary stage, the infected person has not had sufficient time to mount an immune response that can be serologically detected. The **two types of serologic tests** are:
   a. Nonspecific reagin-type antibody tests:

   (1) RPR (rapid plasma reagin)
   (2) VDRL (Venereal Disease Research Laboratories)
   b. Specific antitreponemal antibody tests, which remain positive for life:
   (1) FTA-ABS (fluorescent treponemal antibody absorption test)
   (2) MHA-TP (microhemagglutination assay for antibodies to *T. pallidum*)

4. **Treatment.** Patients with either a history of sexual contact with a person with documented syphilis, a positive dark-field examination, or a positive FTA-ABS test should be treated. A fourfold rise in a quantitative antitreponemal test implies reinfection, and these patients should also be treated. Treatment regimens are based on duration and severity of the disease. Sexual contacts should be treated.
   a. **Early disease**—primary, secondary, or early latent (less than 1 year's duration):
      (1) Benzathine penicillin G, 2.4 million units IM in a single dose
      (2) Doxycycline, 100 mg po twice daily, or **tetracycline,** 500 mg po 4 times daily for 2 weeks in nonpregnant patients with penicillin allergy
   b. **Late disease**—late latent or tertiary syphilis
      (1) Benzathine penicillin G, 2.4 million units IM weekly for 3 weeks
      (2) Doxycycline, 100 mg po twice daily, or **tetracycline,** 500 mg po 4 times daily for 4 weeks in nonpregnant patients with penicillin allergy
   c. **Neurosyphilis** should be suspected in those patients who are HIV positive, fail initial treatment, have an initial titer in excess of 1:32, have neurologic or ophthalmic signs or symptoms, or are diagnosed with aortitis or gummas. Diagnosis is made by testing of the cerebrospinal fluid, and recommended treatment is **penicillin G,** 12 to 24 million units intravenously every 4 hours for 10 to 14 days.
   d. All **penicillin-allergic pregnant patients** should undergo skin testing followed by **penicillin desensitization** because tetracycline and doxycycline are contraindicated in pregnancy, and only penicillin has been proven to prevent fetal infection.

5. **Follow-up.** Patients should be tested by VDRL or RPR at 3 months and at 6 and 12 months. Patients with early syphilis should have a fourfold decline in titer by 3 months posttreatment.

C. **Chlamydial STDs.** There is a broad spectrum of sexually transmitted disorders caused by this genus of obligatory intracellular bacteria. The major pathogen is *Chlamydia trachomatis.*

1. *C. trachomatis,* serotypes D, E, F, G, H, I, J, and K, is responsible for acute urethritis, cervicitis, and acute PID. It may also cause neonatal conjunctivitis and pneumonia, and endometritis.
   a. **Epidemiology.** From 1984 to 1994, there has been a dramatic rise in the incidence of this STD, making it the leading STD in the United States. There were 448,984 cases reported in the United States in 1994. Because chlamydial infection is not a reportable communicable disease, it is estimated that there are at least 4 million new cases per year, most of which are unreported. Coexistence of *C. trachomatis* with gonorrhea is common. *Chlamydia* is frequently recovered in women whose partners have nongonococcal urethritis. Women at risk have risk factors similar to those in women who contract gonorrhea.
   b. **Clinical presentation**
      (1) Many women are asymptomatic.
      (2) In symptomatic women, **mucopurulent cervicitis** can be demonstrated.
      (3) Symptoms of **urethritis** and **pyuria** and a **negative urine culture** in sexually active women are suggestive of a chlamydial infection.
      (4) Fever and **lower abdominal pain** suggest PID. These may be more insidious and protracted in duration than those associated with gonococcal PID.
   c. **Diagnosis.** The **enzyme-linked immunosorbent assay (ELISA)** is the rapid diagnostic test of choice. The test is 90% sensitive and 97% specific. Screening of all young, sexually active women is recommended. Recently, the polymerase chain reaction has been shown to increase the yield of detection.
   d. **Treatment** for PID is detailed in Chapter 23. Treatment for uncomplicated cases of urethritis and cervicitis includes:
      (1) Doxycycline, 100 mg po twice daily for 7 days

      (2) Azithromycin, 1 g po
      (3) Ofloxacin, 300 mg po twice daily for 7 days
      (4) Erythromycin base, 500 mg po 4 times a day for 7 days
  e. Follow-up. Patients do not need to be retested for *Chlamydia* if treatment is with doxycycline, azithromycin, or ofloxacin. Patients treated with erythromycin should be retested in 2 to 4 weeks for a test of cure. Sexual partners should be referred for treatment. Rescreening for reinfection in high-risk women may be considered at 3 to 6 months.
  f. Sequelae include PID, ectopic pregnancy, and infertility.

2. *C. trachomatis,* serotypes L$_1$, L$_2$, and L$_3$, are responsible for **lymphogranuloma venereum,** which produces a wide variety of local and regional ulcerations and destruction of genital tissues.
  a. Epidemiology. More commonly seen in tropical countries, there are less than 500 cases each year reported in the United States, with most of the new cases found in men. The disease progresses through **primary, secondary, and tertiary stages. Incubation time** is between 4 and 21 days.
  b. Clinical presentation
      (1) The most common clinical manifestation in heterosexuals is unilateral tender inguinal lymphadenopathy.
      (2) In **women,** there may be a lesion that occurs on the vulva as a painless vesicle or papule, which generally resolves in 1 week. The secondary stage involves the development of **inguinal adenopathy,** which occurs 2 to 4 weeks after the resolution of the primary lesion.
         (a) The inguinal nodes enlarge and can create a linear retraction of the overlying subinguinal skin, creating a linear groove or **"groove" sign.**
         (b) Suppuration of the nodes with sinus tract formation ensues and is accompanied by generalized symptoms of fever, myalgias, and arthralgias.
      (3) In both women and homosexual men, there may be proctocolitis or inflammatory involvement of perirectal tissues, resulting in fistula formation.
  c. Diagnosis is usually made serologically or by exclusion of other causes of inguinal lymphadenopathy. **Complement fixation** is the test of choice. Complement fixation titers greater than 1:64 are indicative of active infection.
  d. Treatment
      (1) Doxycycline, 100 mg po twice a day for 21 days
      (2) Erythromycin, 500 mg po four times a day for 21 days
      (3) Sulfisoxazole, 500 mg po four times a day for 21 days
      (4) Surgical reconstruction may be required for those patients with considerable tissue destruction in the tertiary stage.

D. **Viral STDs.** The principal viruses associated with STDs include HIV, human papillomavirus (HPV), herpes simplex virus (HSV), and the pox virus that causes molluscum contagiosum.

1. Human immunodeficiency virus. Originally diagnosed in 1981, this unique retrovirus is believed to be responsible for severe deficiencies in cell-mediated immunity, leading to unusual opportunistic infections, malignancy, and, eventually, death. The diseases caused by the HIV are known as acquired immunodeficiency syndrome **(AIDS).**
  a. Epidemiology. The WHO estimates that 40 million men, women, and children will be infected with HIV by the year 2000.
      (1) Exhaustive epidemiologic studies have demonstrated male homosexuals and bisexuals, intravenous drug users, female heterosexual consorts of infected men, recipients of tainted blood or concentrated blood products, and neonates born to infected women are the predominant populations at risk. In addition, African-Americans and Hispanics are more likely to be HIV positive than whites.
      (2) Transmission is both horizontal and vertical. **Incubation or latency time** is between 2 months and 5 years. The **prevalence in the general population** is estimated to be 22/100,000 people. Men are affected more frequently than women, but the prevalence in women is increasing.

b. Clinical presentation. Approximately 80% to 90% of infected people are asymptomatic carriers. The median time between infection with HIV and the development of AIDS among adults is 10 years, ranging from a few months to longer than 12 years. Symptomatic disease develops in approximately 10% to 20% of carriers each year, and of these, 80% to 90% will die within 2 years of the onset of symptoms.

  (1) **Initial exposure to HIV** results in an acute mononucleosis-like syndrome in about 70% of patients.
  (a) The **usual incubation period is 2 to 4 weeks.**
  (b) **Symptoms** include febrile pharyngitis, fever, sweats, myalgia, arthralgia, headache, and photophobia.
  (c) **Lymphadenopathy** is usually generalized and starts in the second week.
  (2) Later, a **more severe form of the disease** may occur.
  (a) **Symptoms** are generalized lymphadenopathy, night sweats, fever, diarrhea, weight loss, and fatigue.
  (b) Infections such as **herpes zoster virus** and **oral candidiasis** can occur.
  (c) Within 4 to 5 years, 30% of cases progress to AIDS.
  (3) **AIDS is the final stage in HIV infection**
  (a) It is manifested by **severe alterations of cell-mediated immunity** (reversal of the T4-helper cell to T8-suppressor cell ratio).
  (b) The **result** is lymphadenopathy, Kaposi's sarcoma, opportunistic infections, malaise, diarrhea, weight loss, and death.

c. Diagnosis
  (1) Serologic screening with **ELISA** for people at risk detects greater than 95% of patients within 6 months of infection.
  (2) A positive ELISA is confirmed by a repeat ELISA, and then a **Western blot analysis,** which is more specific.
  (3) Many states require pretest and posttest counseling and written informed consent for HIV testing.

d. Management of HIV-positive patients. Development of appropriate care involves:
  (1) A thorough history and physical examination, including gynecologic examination and Pap smear
  (2) Evaluation for associated diseases such as STDs and tuberculosis (TB)
  (3) Identification of patients in need of immediate medical care and antiretroviral therapy or prophylaxis for opportunistic infections
  (4) Determination of need for referral
  (5) Administration of recommended vaccines
  (a) Pneumococcal
  (b) Influenza
  (c) Hepatitis B if susceptible
  (d) Measles if needed
  (e) *Haemophilus influenzae* B
  (6) Psychosocial and behavioral evaluation and counseling
  (7) A complete blood count and CD4+ T-lymphocyte count
  (a) **The CD4+ count** is the best laboratory indicator of clinical progression, and management strategies are stratified by CD4+ count. Patients with CD4+ counts greater than $500/\mu l$ are usually not clinically immunosuppressed.
  (8) **The purified protein derivative test** and **anergy panel** should be administered to all HIV-positive patients.
  (a) HIV may cause cutaneous anergy.
  (b) An area of induration larger than 5 mm in HIV-positive patients is considered indicative of TB infection, and preventive therapy with isoniazid should be considered after excluding active TB.
  (9) **Additional studies** may include chest radiogram, serum chemistry, and antibody testing for toxoplasmosis and hepatitis B and C.
  (10) **Antiretroviral therapy** may delay progression to advanced disease, but evidence for increased long-term survival is inconclusive.
  (a) **Zidovudine (AZT),** 500 to 600 mg/day, has been recommended for

asymptomatic patients with CD4+ counts of less than 300 or symptomatic patients with CD4+ counts less than 500.

(b) Side effects include pancytopenia, pancreatitis, peripheral neuropathy, vomiting, and headaches.

(11) *Pneumocystis carinii* **pneumonia (PCP) prophylaxis** with one of the following should be given to patients with CD4+ counts under 200 or with constitutional symptoms or previous PCP infection:

(a) **Trimethoprim-sulfamethoxazole,** one double-strength tablet po daily

(b) **Aerosolized pentamidine,** 300 mg once a month

(12) Nutritional evaluation and counseling

e. Pregnancy. Pregnant patients who are HIV positive should be evaluated as above. Without treatment, the risk of transmission to the fetus is 15% to 39%. ZDV prophylaxis should be offered to decrease the risk of perinatal transmission.

2. Human papillomavirus. The genital virus in this double-stranded DNA family is responsible for a variety of mucocutaneous genital lesions, affecting both men and women. It is also known to be associated with lower genital tract cancers.

a. Epidemiology. More than 40 million sexually active adults in the United States harbor these viruses.

(1) The predominant means of transmission is through sexual intercourse. The risk of contracting warts for women whose sexual partners have obvious genital warts is 60% to 85%. Incubation time is between 6 weeks and 18 months, with a mean time of 3 months.

(2) Recent evidence indicates that **transmission to the fetus may occur,** occasionally causing neonatal and juvenile respiratory papillomatosis. The risk is low, however, occurring in 1/1000 fetuses of infected mothers. Potential routes include transplacental, intrapartum, or postnatal. The presence of HPV infection is thus not an indication for cesarean section.

(3) Subclinical or latent papillomavirus lesions have been associated with an increased risk of preinvasive and invasive neoplastic lesions of the lower genital tract.

(a) HPV types 6, 11, 42, 43, and 44 are considered to be low-risk oncoviruses.

(b) HPV types 31, 33, 35, 51, 52, and 58 are intermediate-risk oncoviruses.

(c) HPV types 16, 18, 45, and 56 are believed to be high-risk oncoviruses.

b. Clinical presentation. Lesions include overt anogenital warts (condyloma acuminatum) and dysplastic lesions. Lesions can also be subclinical or latent, which are not visible to the naked eye. Visual inspection of overt warty disease of the lower genital tract detects obvious lesions, which are often multifocal in distribution.

c. Diagnosis

(1) Direct inspection discerns overt warts. If uncertain, their nature is confirmed by biopsy.

(2) Approximately 2% to 4% of **Pap smears** demonstrate the pathognomonic cell—the koilocyte (or halo cell). This exfoliated squamous cell has a wrinkled, somewhat pyknotic nucleus surrounded by a perinuclear clear zone or halo. Pap smears with this change are designated as low-grade squamous intraepithelial lesions.

(3) Colposcopy, the magnified inspection of lower genital tissues after staining with a weak acetic acid solution, is helpful in detecting latent or associated precancerous lesions caused by HPV. The lesions are flat, small, and acetowhite, with vascular punctation or mosaicism. Histologically, these lesions reveal koilocytosis, acanthosis, and variable nuclear atypia.

(4) Recently, **DNA hybridization techniques** have been used not only to detect HPV but to ascertain viral type. These are not used routinely, however.

d. Treatment does not eradicate the virus.

(1) For **overt genital condyloma,** there are a variety of acceptable treatment modalities, including:

(a) Chemical destructive techniques

(i) Podophyllin

(ii) Trichloroacetic acid

          (b) Cryotherapy
          (c) Electrocautery
          (d) Laser vaporization
          (e) 5-Fluorouracil cream
          (f) Interferon
      (2) For **HPV-related precancerous conditions,** treatment modalities include:
          (a) Loop electrode excision of the transformation zone
          (b) Laser vaporization
          (c) Cryotherapy
          (d) Cone biopsy of the cervix
          (e) Surgical excision of vulvar or vaginal lesions
      (3) The treatment of **latent HPV infections** without dysplasia is not recommended.

3. Herpes simplex virus. HSV-2, which is a double-stranded DNA virus, is the predominant genital pathogen, although HSV-1 is seen in approximately 13% to 15% of herpetic genital infections. These viruses have an affinity for **infecting mucocutaneous tissues of the lower genital tract.** The virus is maintained in pelvic ganglia as a latent reservoir for recurrent herpetic genital infection. It most commonly produces recurrent vesiculoulcerative genital lesions. It is responsible for the highly lethal neonatal meningitis in infants delivered through an actively infected cervix.

    a. Epidemiology. Estimates of the prevalence of HSV genital infections suggest that 30 million sexually active adults in the United States are afflicted with this disorder. Up to 50% of affected Americans are unaware that they have the virus. The predominant mode of transmission is sexual intercourse. The **incubation time** is between 3 and 7 days.

    b. Clinical presentation. Primary genital herpetic infections are both local and systemic diseases. Vulvar paresthesia precedes the development of multiple crops of vesicular lesions.

      (1) Primary lesions become shallow, coalescent, painful ulcers in a few days and can last for 2 to 3 weeks. These lesions can be accompanied by severe dysuria with urinary retention, mucopurulent vaginal discharge, painful inguinal adenopathy, generalized myalgias, headaches, and fever.

      (2) Recurrent lesions are similar but less severe in intensity, duration, and systemic side effects. **Menses** and **stressful life situations** are associated with recurrent outbreaks. Only 60% of patients have recurrent symptoms.

    c. Diagnosis. Herpes cultures obtained from the vesicular fluid or the edge of the ulcerative lesion give the best results. **Cytologic demonstration** of multinucleated epithelial cells with intranuclear inclusions is helpful in the diagnosis.

    d. Treatment

      (1) Primary herpes. Acyclovir, 200 mg po five times a day for 7 to 10 days, has been shown to decrease severity and duration of symptoms.

      (2) Recurrent herpes. Treatment is usually recommended only for those patients with more than six recurrences per year. Suppressive doses of **acyclovir,** 400 mg po twice daily, are used.

      (3) Topical acyclovir is not effective.

4. Molluscum contagiosum

    a. Epidemiology. Molluscum contagiosum is mildly contagious and is caused by a double-stranded DNA poxvirus. The incubation period is several weeks.

    b. Clinical presentation. This virus creates small (1–5 mm), umbilicated papules in the cutaneous genital region of sexually active individuals. It may also affect the nongenital skin.

    c. Diagnosis. The lesion itself is pathognomonic, but the diagnosis can be confirmed on histologic demonstration of a papule with a hyperkeratotic plug arising from an acanthotic epidermis. There are intracytoplasmic molluscum bodies noted on Wright's stain.

    d. Treatment. The disease is usually self-limited, with spontaneous resolution in 6 to 9 months. Local excision, cryotherapy, electrocautery, and laser vaporization are suitable treatment modalities to decrease the duration of symptoms.

E. **Protozoal STDs.** *Trichomonas vaginalis* infection is the most common sexually transmitted protozoal infection. This organism is responsible for **acute vulvovaginitis.**

1. **Epidemiology.** This protozoan is usually transmitted by sexual intercourse. Approximately 2.5 million infections are caused by this organism annually in the United States. Nearly one third of all office visits for infectious vulvovaginitis are made as a result of infection by *T. vaginalis.*

2. **Clinical presentation**
   a. Profuse, yellow-green, malodorous, frothy discharge of low viscosity
   b. Vulvar pruritus
   c. Vaginal erythema and intense erythematous mottling of the cervix **(strawberry cervix)** occasionally seen
   d. Male partner usually asymptomatic

3. **Diagnosis**
   a. Vaginal pH between 5 and 6
   b. Inflammatory response and motile, flagellated trichomonads on wet mount preparations. These organisms are twice the size of leukocytes.
   c. Cultures for *Trichomonas* are available but are usually reserved for resistant cases in which antimicrobial testing can be used.

4. **Treatment.** Both regimens have cure rates of >95%.
   a. **Metronidazole,** 2 g po
   b. Metronidazole, 500 mg po twice daily for 7 days, for recurrent or persistent cases
   c. Sexual partners must be treated to prevent reinfection

F. **Ectoparasites.** This group of STDs includes pediculosis pubis and scabies.

1. **Pediculosis pubis (*Phthirus pubis*).** The **crab louse** is a slow-moving insect approximately 1 mm long. It lays its eggs **(nits)** at the base of hair follicles. After 7 days, nymphs arise from the nits and progress to the adult stage in 2 to 3 weeks. Adult life expectancy of the pubic louse is 30 days.
   a. **Epidemiology.** Pediculosis pubis is **highly contagious.**
   b. **Clinical presentation.** Intense vulvar pruritus secondary to an allergic sensitization is the presenting symptom.
   c. **Diagnosis.** Identification of the crab louse or nits can be made with a **hand lens inspection** of the hair-bearing pubic region.
   d. **Treatment**
      (1) **Lindane** solution, 1%, applied to the infested area for 4 minutes and washed off is effective. Lindane is contraindicated in pregnancy and lactation.
      (2) **Permethrin** cream, 1%, rinse for 10 minutes

2. **Scabies (*Sarcoptes scabiei*).** This mite is 0.4 mm in length. Unlike the crab louse, it can be found anywhere on the skin, where it burrows a 5-mm-long tunnel to lay its eggs. Its life span is approximately 30 days.
   a. **Epidemiology.** Scabies can be transmitted by close sexual contact but also by nonsexual contact, such as sharing clothing or bedding.
   b. **Clinical presentation.** The predominant symptom is severe, intermittent itching. Hands, wrists, breasts, and buttocks are the most commonly affected sites.
   c. **Diagnosis.** Linear burrows are frequently seen with a hand lens. Microscopic slides prepared from scrapings of suspected lesions in mineral oil often demonstrate adult mites, eggs, and fecal pellets.
   d. **Treatment.** Decontamination of clothing and bedding is recommended, in addition to one of the following:
      (1) **Permethrin** cream, 5%, applied to the body from the neck down and washed off after 8 to 14 hours
      (2) **Lindane** solution, 1%, applied from the neck down and washed off after 8 hours (should not be applied after a bath, or in pregnancy or lactation)
      (3) **Crotamiton,** 10%, nightly for 2 consecutive nights, washed off 24 hours after the second application

STUDY QUESTIONS

DIRECTIONS: Each of the numbered items or incomplete statements in this section is followed by answers or by completions of the statement. Select the ONE lettered answer or completion that is BEST in each case.

1. Which of the following is a diagnostic test for *Hemophilus ducreyi* (chancroid)?

(A) Dark-field examination of specimens from the lesion
(B) Nonspecific reagin-type antibody test
(C) Gram's stain of the exudate from the ulcer base
(D) Thayer-Martin culture medium
(E) None of the above

DIRECTIONS: Each of the numbered items or incomplete statements in this section is negatively phrased, as indicated by a capitalized word such as NOT, LEAST, or EXCEPT. Select the ONE lettered answer or completion that is BEST in each case.

2. Which of the following is NOT a correct statement about *Phthirus pubis*?

(A) It is a slow-moving insect
(B) It is usually confined to hair-bearing regions of the body
(C) It has a tendency to burrow to lay its nits
(D) It causes a highly contagious disease
(E) It causes intense vulvar pruritus

3. Which of the following is NOT a correct statement characterizing human papillomavirus (HPV) infection?

(A) HPV types 16 and 18 are associated with cervical cancer
(B) Sexual intercourse is the only possible means of transmission
(C) The koilocyte (or halo cell) is pathognomonic
(D) Genital warts are caused by this virus
(E) Acetowhite flat lesions can be seen by colposcopy

4. Which of the following is NOT a correct statement concerning lymphogranuloma venereum?

(A) It is caused by *Chlamydia trachomatis*
(B) It can cause extensive anogenital destruction
(C) The "groove" sign is found in the secondary disease stage
(D) Lymphadenopathy is common
(E) The organism is exquisitely sensitive to penicillin

DIRECTIONS: Each set of matching questions in this section consists of a list of four to twenty-six lettered options (some of which may be in figures) followed by several numbered items. For each numbered item, select the ONE lettered option that is most closely associated with it. To avoid spending too much time on matching sets with large numbers of options, it is generally advisable to begin each set by reading the list of options. Then, for each item in the set, try to generate the correct answer and locate it in the option list, rather than evaluating each option individually. Each lettered option may be selected once, more than once, or not at all.

Questions 5–7

For each sexually transmitted disease (STD) or causative organism listed below, select the lesion that is most likely to be associated with it.

(A) Small umbilicated papule
(B) Condyloma acuminatum
(C) Condyloma latum
(D) Soft chancre
(E) Painless hard chancre

5. *Hemophilus ducreyi*

6. Molluscum contagiosum

7. Human papillomavirus (HPV), type 6 or 11

Questions 8–9

For each of the following clinical conditions, select the most appropriate diagnostic test.

(A) Gram's stain of the exudate
(B) Dark-field examination
(C) Saline wet mount preparation
(D) Enzyme-linked immunosorbent assay (ELISA)
(E) Culture on Thayer-Martin medium

8. The patient is a multiparous woman who comes to the office complaining of a vaginal discharge. Two weeks earlier she used an over-the-counter agent for a yeast infection. She also complains of a strong odor after she has intercourse.

9. A 19-year-old, sexually active woman complains of sporadic lower abdominal pain over the previous 3 weeks, accompanied by a low-grade fever (99.5°F). She has noted an increased amount of cloudy, nonirritating discharge and is having pain when she urinates.

ANSWERS AND EXPLANATIONS

1. The answer is C [II A 2 c]. Chancroid is best diagnosed by Gram's stain of the exudate obtained from the base of a chancre. The pathognomonic findings are gram-negative rods that form chains or a "school-of-fish" pattern. Dark-field examination and a nonspecific reagin-type antibody test diagnose syphilis. Thayer-Martin medium is the preferred culture medium in diagnosing *Neisseria gonorrhoeae* infection.

2. The answer is C [II F 1 a, b, 2]. *Phthirus pubis,* or the crab louse, causes a highly contagious sexually transmitted disease (STD) called pediculosis pubis in which a single exposure results in transmission 95% of the time. The crab louse is a slow-moving insect compared to the scabies mite. It is usually found attached to hair follicles, and it lays its nits at the base of the follicle without any burrowing. There is usually an intense pruritus secondary to an allergic sensitization.

3. The answer is B [II D 2 a–c]. Human papillomavirus (HPV), a double-stranded DNA virus, causes one of the most common viral sexually transmitted diseases (STDs), characterized by genital warts. HPV types 16 and 18 are associated with squamous cell cancer of the cervix. The koilocyte (or halo cell) is an exfoliated cell with a wrinkled, pyknotic nucleus surrounded by a perinuclear clear zone. After cleaning the cervix with acetic acid, acetowhite flat lesions characteristic of HPV infection can be seen through the colposcope. Although rare, this virus can be transmitted to the fetus from an infected mother, and is responsible for neonatal and juvenile respiratory papillomatosis.

4. The answer is E [II C 2 b–d]. Lymphogranuloma venereum is caused by *Chlamydia trachomatis,* serotypes L_1–L_3. The initial lesion is a painless vesicular or papular lesion in the genital region. The secondary stage is accompanied by lymphadenopathy of the inguinal lymph nodes, which become matted and retract the overlying subinguinal skin, creating the "groove" sign. In advanced or untreated states, ulceration, fistulization, and destruction

of recognizable anogenital structures occur. The treatments of choice are either erythromycin or doxycycline. *C. trachomatis* is resistant to penicillin.

5–7. The answers are: 5-D [II A 2 b], **6-A** [II D 4 b, c], **7-B** [II D 2 b]. The soft chancre is associated with *Hemophilus ducreyi* infection, or chancroid. The classic lesion of chancroid is a soft sore with a superficial ulcer crater surrounded by a red halo. This lesion is accompanied in nearly 50% of cases with flocculent inguinal adenopathy, or bubo.

The lesion of molluscum contagiosum is characteristic of the poxvirus infection. This virus creates small, umbilicated papules in the cutaneous genital skin. This lesion by itself is diagnostic.

Human papillomavirus (HPV) infection, usually by serotypes 6 and 11, is characterized by fig-like lesions (warts or condyloma acuminatum) in the anogenital region. In overt warty disease, visual inspection detects these obvious lesions, which may form in clusters. Genital condylomata develop in approximately 60% to 85% of women who have sexual intercourse with a male consort with overt warts.

8–9. The answers are: 8-C [II A 4 a, b], **9-D** [II A 1 b; C 1 b, c]. Because the multiparous woman continued to have symptoms of a vaginitis after treatment for a yeast infection, she must have a mixed vaginal infection, including *Gardnerella vaginalis.* The clue to the cause of the persistent infection is the strong odor after intercourse. This suggests bacterial vaginosis, which is diagnosed by using a saline wet mount and identifying the clue cell. Additional evidence for *G. vaginalis* is the "whiff" test, in which a 10% potassium hydroxide solution is added to the slide, generating a fishy odor resulting from the release of amines. The same thing happens during coitus, when the alkaline semen reacts with the bacterial vaginosis.

The 19-year-old woman has symptoms and findings suggestive of a chlamydial infection. The symptoms are mild and thus not suggestive of acute gonorrhea, in which there is much more pelvic pain and febrile morbidity. The dull, chronic lower abdominal pain, the low-grade fever, the discharge, and the dysuria are suggestive of chlamydial infection.

Examination of the urine would reveal white blood cells; the culture would be negative. With the suspicion of chlamydial infection in mind, the enzyme-linked immunosorbent assay (ELISA) is the diagnostic test of choice.

Chapter 30

Myomata Uteri
Michelle Battistini

I. INTRODUCTION

A. Definition. Uterine leiomyomas are proliferative, well circumscribed, pseudoencapsulated, benign tumors composed of smooth muscle and fibrous connective tissue; they are also referred to as **fibroids, myomas,** or **fibromyomas.**

1. They are the most common neoplasm found in the female pelvis and the most common uterine mass.

2. Leiomyomas may occur singly but most often are multiple; as many as 100 or more have been found in a single uterus.

3. Myomas also vary in size, ranging from 1 mm to 20 cm in greatest diameter.

4. They are present in 20% to 25% of women 35 years of age or older and are present in 40% of autopsy specimens.

5. Leiomyomas are the most common indication for hysterectomy in this country, accounting for 30% of hysterectomies on an annual basis.

6. Benign smooth muscle tumors may be found in organs outside the uterus, including the fallopian tubes, vagina, round ligament, uterosacral ligaments, vulva, and gastrointestinal tract.

B. Etiology. A leiomyoma is a benign neoplasm consisting of a localized proliferation of smooth muscle cells and an accumulation of extracellular matrix.

1. **Cytogenetic studies** suggest leiomyomas arise from a single neoplastic smooth muscle cell; myomas are monoclonal tumors resulting from somatic mutations.
   a. A variety of **chromosomal abnormalities** involving several chromosomes, particularly chromosome 12, have been identified, suggesting a genetic role in the pathogenesis of these tumors.
   b. The inciting event responsible for neoplastic transformation is unknown; **estrogen may be necessary** for expression of this mutation.

2. **Factors that affect growth** of leiomyomas appear to be distinct from etiologic mechanisms; estrogen, progesterone, and peptide growth factors play a role in regulation of growth.

3. Evidence suggests **estrogen is a promoter of leiomyoma growth.**
   a. Myomas are rarely found before puberty and stop growing after menopause.
   b. New myomas rarely appear after menopause.
   c. There is often rapid growth of myomas during pregnancy.
   d. Gonadotropin-releasing hormone (GnRH) agonists create a hypoestrogenic environment that results in a reduction in both tumor and uterine size that is reversible on cessation of treatment.

4. Recent investigations implicate **peptide growth factors**—epidermal growth factor (EGF), insulin-like growth factor-I, platelet-derived growth factor—in the regulation of leiomyoma growth.
   a. EGF induces DNA synthesis in leiomyoma and myometrial cells.
   b. Estrogen may exert its effect through EGF.

5. **Local factors** such as blood supply, adjacency to other tumors, and degenerative changes may account for variations in tumor volume and rate of growth.

II. CHARACTERISTICS OF MYOMATA UTERI

A. Classification of myomas according to location. Three types of leiomyomas occur based on their location within or on the uterus: intramural, submucous, and subserous.

1. **Intramural myomas** are the most common variety, occurring within the walls of the uterus as isolated, encapsulated nodules of varying size. As these tumors grow, they can distort the uterine cavity or the external surface of the uterus. These tumors can also cause symmetric enlargement of the uterus when they occur singly.

2. **Submucous myomas** are located beneath the endometrium. These tumors grow into the uterine cavity, maintaining attachment to the uterus by a pedicle. The **pedunculated myomas** may protrude to or through the cervical os. These tumors are often associated with an abnormality of the overlying endometrium, resulting in a disturbed bleeding pattern.

3. **Subserous myomas** are located just beneath the serosal surface and grow out toward the peritoneal cavity, causing the peritoneal surface of the uterus to bulge. These tumors may also develop a pedicle, become pedunculated, and reach a large size within the peritoneal cavity without producing symptoms. These potentially mobile tumors may present in such a manner that they need to be differentiated from solid adnexal lesions. When myomas extend into the broad ligament, they are known as **intraligamentary leiomyomas.** A pedunculated myoma may attach itself to an adjacent structure like the omentum, mesentery, or bowel; develop a secondary blood supply; and lose its connection with the uterus and primary blood supply. This occurs rarely and is known as a **parasitic leiomyoma.**

B. Pathology

1. **Gross pathology.** Leiomyomas are **pseudoencapsulated** solid tumors, well demarcated from the surrounding myometrium. The **pseudocapsule** is not a true capsule and results from compression of fibrous and muscular tissue on the surface of the tumor. Because the vasculature is located on the periphery, the central part of the tumor is susceptible to degenerative changes. On cut surface, the tumors are smooth, solid, and usually pinkish-white, depending on the degree of vascularity. The surface typically has a trabeculate, fleshy, whorl-like appearance.

2. **Microscopic pathology.** The leiomyoma is composed of groups and bundles of smooth muscle fibers in a twisted, whorled fashion. Microscopically, these appear as smooth muscle cells in longitudinal or cross section intermixed with fibrous connective tissue. There are few vascular structures; mitoses are rare.
   a. **Cellular leiomyomata** are tumors with mitotic counts of 5 to 10 per 10 consecutive high-power fields that lack cytologic atypia.
   b. **Leiomyosarcoma** is a distinct clinical entity and is based on a mitotic count of 10 mitotic figures per 10 high-power fields.

C. Degenerative changes. A variety of degenerative changes may occur in a myoma, which alter the gross and microscopic appearance of the tumor. Most of these changes lack clinical significance, with little effect on the clinical presentation. Degenerative changes occur secondary to alterations in circulation (either arterial or venous), postmenopausal atrophy, or infection, or may be a result of malignant transformation.

1. **Hyaline degeneration,** the most common type of degeneration, is present in almost all leiomyomas. It is caused by an overgrowth of the fibrous elements, which leads to a hyalinization of the fibrous tissue and, eventually, calcification.

2. **Cystic degeneration** may occasionally be a sequel of necrosis, but cystic cavities are usually a result of myxomatous change and liquefaction after hyaline degeneration.

3. **Necrosis** is commonly caused by impairment of the blood supply or severe infection. A special kind of necrosis is the **red,** or **carneous,** degeneration, which occurs most frequently in pregnancy. The lesion has a dull, reddish hue and is believed to be

caused by aseptic degeneration associated with local hemolysis. Clinically, carneous degeneration during pregnancy must be differentiated from a variety of acute accidents that occur within the abdomen involving the adnexa and other nongenital organs.

4. **Mucoid degeneration.** When the arterial input is impaired, particularly in large tumors, areas of hyalinization may convert to a mucoid or myxomatous type of degeneration; the lesion has a soft, gelatinous consistency. Further degeneration can lead to liquefaction and cystic degeneration.

5. **Infection** of a myoma most commonly occurs with a pedunculated submucous leiomyoma that first becomes necrotic and then secondarily infected.

6. **Calcification** of myomas is a common finding in the postmenopausal patient.

7. **Sarcomatous degeneration.** Malignant degeneration occurs in less than 1% (0.13%–0.29%) of leiomyomas. Controversy exists as to whether this represents a true degenerative change or a spontaneous neoplasm. Finding a leiomyosarcoma within the core of an apparently benign pseudoencapsulated myoma is suggestive of such a degenerative process. This type of sarcoma is usually of a spindle cell rather than a round cell type. The 5-year survival rates of a leiomyosarcoma arising within a myoma are much better than those for a true sarcoma of the uterus when there is no extension of the sarcomatous tissue beyond the pseudocapsule of the myoma.

III. SYMPTOMS AND SIGNS OF MYOMATA UTERI

A. **Symptoms** of leiomyomas vary greatly, depending on their size, number, and location. Most women with leiomyomas are asymptomatic; symptoms occur in 10% to 40% of affected women.

1. **Abnormal uterine bleeding** is the most common symptom associated with myomata uteri, occurring in up to 30% of symptomatic women. The typical bleeding pattern is **menorrhagia,** excessive bleeding at the time of menses, defined as greater than 80 ml. The increase in flow usually occurs gradually, but the bleeding may result in a profound anemia. The exact mechanisms of increased blood loss are unclear. Possible factors include necrosis of the surface endometrium overlying the submucous myoma; a disturbance in the hemostatic contraction of normal muscle bundles when there is extensive intramural myomatous growth; an increase in surface area of the endometrial cavity; and an alteration in endometrial microvasculature. In some cases, abnormal bleeding may be associated with anovulatory states. Frequently, myomas are associated with polyps and endometrial hyperplasia, which may produce the abnormal bleeding pattern.

2. **Pain.** Uncomplicated uterine leiomyomas usually do not produce pain. Acute pain associated with fibroids is usually caused by either torsion of a pedunculated myoma or infarction progressing to carneous degeneration within a myoma. Pain is often crampy in nature when a submucous myoma within the endometrial cavity acts as a foreign body. Some patients with intramural myomas experience the reappearance of dysmenorrhea after many years of pain-free menses.

3. **Pressure.** As myomas enlarge, they may cause a feeling of pelvic heaviness or produce pressure symptoms on surrounding structures.
   a. **Urinary frequency** is a common symptom when a growing myoma exerts pressure on the bladder.
   b. **Urinary retention,** a rare occurrence, can result when myomatous growth creates a fixed, retroverted uterus that pushes the cervix anteriorly under the symphysis pubis in the area of the posterior urethrovesicular angle.
   c. **Asymptomatic pressure effects of myomas** are usually caused by lateral extension or intraligamentous myomas, which produce unilateral ureteral obstruction and

hydronephrosis. A markedly enlarged uterus that extends above the pelvic brim may cause ureteral compression, hydroureter, and hydronephrosis.
   d. **Constipation and difficult defecation** can be caused by large posterior myomas.
   e. **Compression of pelvic vasculature** by a markedly enlarged uterus may cause varicosities or edema of the lower extremities.

4. **Reproductive disorders.** Infertility secondary to leiomyomata is probably uncommon. Infertility may result when myomas interfere with normal tubal transport or implantation of the fertilized ovum.
   a. **Large intramural myomas located in the cornual regions** may virtually close the interstitial portion of the tube.
   b. **Continuous bleeding in patients with submucous myomas** may impede implantation; the endometrium overlying the myoma may be out of phase with the normal endometrium and thus provide a poor surface for implantation.
   c. There are **increased incidences of abortion and premature labor** in patients with submucous or intramural myomas.

5. **Pregnancy-related disorders.** Uterine myomas, noted in 0.3% to 7.2% of pregnancies, are usually present before conception and may increase in size significantly during gestation.
   a. The **incidence of spontaneous abortion is higher** in women with myomas, but myomas are an uncommon cause of abortion.
   b. **Red degeneration,** more common during pregnancy, or **torsion of a pedunculated fibroid** may cause gradual or acute symptoms of pain and tenderness. These must be differentiated from other causes of abdominal pain in pregnancy because treatment is conservative with symptomatic relief and observation. Surgical intervention is rarely, if ever, indicated.
   c. **Premature labor** may be increased in women with leiomyomata.
   d. In the third trimester, leiomyomas may be a factor in **malpresentation, mechanical obstruction,** or **uterine dystocia.** Large myomas in the lower uterine segment may prevent descent of the presenting part. Intramural myomas may interfere with effectual uterine contractions and normal labor.
   e. **Postpartum hemorrhage** is more common with the myomatous uterus.

B. **Signs**

1. **Physical examination.** The diagnosis of myomata uteri can be made with confidence 95% of the time on the basis of physical examination alone. Uterine size is defined as the equivalent gestational size as determined by abdominal and pelvic examination.
   a. **Abdominal examination.** Uterine leiomyomas may be palpated as irregular, nodular tumors protruding against the anterior abdominal wall. Leiomyomas are usually firm on palpation; softness or tenderness suggests the presence of edema, sarcoma, pregnancy, or degenerative changes.
   b. **Pelvic examination.** The most common finding is uterine enlargement; the shape of the uterus is usually asymmetric and irregular in outline. The uterus is usually freely movable unless residuals of an old pelvic inflammatory disease persist.
      (1) In the case of **submucous myomas,** the uterine enlargement is usually symmetric.
      (2) Some **subserous myomas** may be very distinct from the main body of the uterus and may move freely, which often suggests the presence of adnexal or extrapelvic tumors.
      (3) The **diagnosis of cervical myomas or pedunculated submucous myomas** may be made on tumor extension into the cervical canal; occasionally a submucous myoma may be visible at the cervical os or at the introitus.

2. **Laboratory evaluation and diagnostic studies.** Additional diagnostic studies are based on individual presentation and physical examination. In the asymptomatic patient with a physical examination consistent with leiomyoma, it is not necessary routinely to obtain additional studies.
   a. **Hemoglobin/hematocrit** is obtained in the patient presenting with excessive vaginal bleeding to assess the degree of loss and adequacy of replacement.

b. **Coagulation profile** and **bleeding time** are ordered when a history suggestive of a bleeding diathesis is elicited.

c. **Endometrial biopsy** is performed in a patient with abnormal uterine bleeding who is thought to be anovulatory or at increased risk for endometrial hyperplasia.

d. **Ultrasonography** accurately assesses uterine dimension, myoma location, interval growth, and adnexal anatomy; however, routine ultrasound does not improve long-term outcome compared to clinical assessment alone. It is appropriate to obtain a pelvic ultrasound in situations when clinical assessment is difficult or uncertain; when physical examination is suboptimal, as in cases of morbid obesity; or adnexal pathology cannot be excluded on physical examination alone. Intrauterine infusion of sterile saline at the time of ultrasound examination can identify the presence of pedunculated submucous leiomyomas and endometrial polyps. Ultrasonography may be useful to detect hydroureter and hydronephrosis in the patient with marked uterine enlargement.

e. Evaluation of the endometrial cavity with **hysteroscopy** or a **hysterosalpingography** may be used in the workup of the patient with uterine myoma and infertility or repetitive pregnancy loss.

IV. **TREATMENT.** The treatment of myomas must be adapted to each patient, and includes nonsurgical and surgical options. Treatment decisions are based on symptoms, fertility status, uterine size, and the rate of uterine growth. Nonsurgical treatment includes expectant management and medical management with GnRH agonists. Surgical therapies include myomectomy and hysterectomy.

A. **Expectant management.** In the absence of symptoms, pain, abnormal bleeding, pressure symptoms, or large myomas, observation with periodic examinations is appropriate management. This is especially true if the patient is nearing menopause, at which time the myomas will atrophy as estrogen levels fall.

1. **Bimanual examinations** should be made every 3 to 6 months to determine uterine size and the rate of growth. After assurance of slow growth or stable uterine size, annual follow-up may then be appropriate. Rapid growth—a change of 6 weeks in size or greater during 12 months or less of observation—is an indication for surgical intervention.

2. Patients with **increased bleeding** should also receive a trial of conservative (nonsurgical) management; endometrial biopsy is performed as indicated. Patients should have regular blood counts; iron deficiency anemia is common with menorrhagia, and oral iron may be required to replace losses associated with the uterine bleeding. Nonsteroidal antiinflammatory drugs that inhibit prostaglandin synthesis, administered on a scheduled rather than as-needed basis, should be used to reduce menstrual blood flow. Low-dose oral contraceptives or progestin therapy are additional therapies that may reduce blood loss.

3. **Nonsteroidal antiinflammatory drugs** are also useful for treatment of pelvic discomfort or pressure.

B. **GnRH agonists.** Long-acting GnRH agonists suppress gonadotropin secretion and create a hypoestrogenic state similar to that observed after the menopause. They are administered, as a subcutaneous implant or intramuscular depot injection, every 4 weeks for 12—24 weeks.

1. Although there is a wide range of individual response, a median reduction in uterine size of 50% has been observed. Maximum response is seen after 12 weeks of therapy, with no added advantage to 24 weeks of therapy. Decreased size is secondary to a decrease in blood flow and cell size; cell death and a decrease in cell number are not observed.

2. Myomas rapidly regrow, returning to baseline size within 12 weeks after GnRH therapy is discontinued.

3. Use of GnRH agonist therapy is not recommended for longer than 24 weeks (6 months) because of the long-term effects of a hypoestrogenic state, most notably osteoporosis.

4. Long-term use of GnRH agonists with "add-back" hormone replacement therapy is under investigation.

5. For these reasons and because of the expense of these agents, GnRH agonists are recommended for short-term use and only in selected cases: the treatment of large submucous myomas to facilitate hysteroscopic resection; in the symptomatic perimenopausal patient who wishes to avoid surgery; and as presurgical treatment to decrease symptoms and size. The use of these agents to decrease uterine size to convert an abdominal hysterectomy to a vaginal procedure is being evaluated.

C. **Surgery.** Surgical interventions for leiomyomas include endoscopic resection, myomectomy, and hysterectomy.

1. **Indications for surgery.** Surgical intervention is indicated for the treatment of symptoms that fail to respond to conservative management.
   a. **Excessive bleeding** that interferes with normal life-style or leads to anemia and **chronic pelvic pain or pressure** are indications for surgery.
   b. **Protrusion** of a pedunculated submucous leiomyoma through the cervix requires excision.
   c. **Rapid growth** in a myomatous uterus at any age warrants exploration because this may represent a leiomyosarcoma as opposed to a benign leiomyoma. Most often leiomyosarcomas represent a distinct clinical entity rather than malignant degeneration within a leiomyoma. Because these malignancies occur primarily in women older than 40 years of age and their incidence increases with advancing age, any increase in uterine size in the postmenopausal woman warrants surgical exploration.
   d. When the **reproductive process is complicated** by repetitive pregnancy loss due to myomas, surgery is indicated. Other etiologies should be excluded before surgical intervention.
   e. Surgical intervention is indicated in the **infertility patient** with leiomyoma after evaluation and treatment of other causes, and the location or size of myoma indicates that it would be a probable factor.
   f. The designation of an **arbitrary uterine size,** greater than 12 weeks, in the asymptomatic patient, has traditionally been cited as an indication for surgery. This has recently come under scrutiny. There are no controlled data documenting that proposed benefits outweigh the risks of surgery; expectant management of the asymptomatic patient with uterine enlargement greater that 12 weeks' size with stable or slow growth is considered a reasonable treatment option. Surgical intervention is indicated if the patient is concerned regarding uterine size or is symptomatic.
   g. **Progressive hydronephrosis,** demonstrated by ultrasonography or intravenous pyelography, or **impaired renal function** are clear indications for surgery.

2. **Surgical procedures.** The type of surgery to be performed depends on the age of the patient, the nature of the symptoms, and the patient's desires regarding future fertility.
   a. **Myomectomy** involves the removal of single or multiple myomas while preserving the uterus; this procedure is usually reserved for women who desire future pregnancy and in whom pregnancy is not contraindicated. Myomectomy is a reasonable approach in symptomatic women unresponsive to conservative treatment who desire uterine conservation.
      (1) **Hysteroscopic resection** is an effective method of treatment of submucous leiomyomas; 20% of women require additional treatment within 5 to 10 years.
      (2) **Risks of abdominal myomectomy** include increased intraoperative blood loss, prolonged operative time, and increased postoperative hemorrhage compared

to hysterectomy. These are offset by a decreased risk of infectious morbidity and ureteral injury.

(3) Eighty percent of patients report subjective improvement of symptoms; 15% of patients experience symptom recurrence, and 10% require additional treatment.

(4) The recurrence of myomas after myomectomy depends on the race (higher in African-Americans) and age of the patient as well as the completeness of the original myomectomy; 10-year recurrence rates of 5% to 30% have been reported.

(5) At the time of abdominal myomectomy, it may be necessary to open the uterine cavity to remove intramural or submucous myomas completely; this is considered to be an indication for cesarean section in future pregnancies.

(6) Term pregnancy rates after myomectomy for infertility or repetitive pregnancy loss are 40%.

b. Hysterectomy. If the indications for surgery are present and if the patient's childbearing is complete, hysterectomy is definitive treatment for uterine myomata.

(1) With hysterectomy, both the leiomyomas and any associated disease are removed permanently, and there is no risk of recurrence.

(2) In the patient with abnormal bleeding, other causes such as anovulatory states should be detected and treated before hysterectomy. Hysterectomy should not be performed on the assumption that the bleeding is caused solely by the myomas. Curettage of the endometrial cavity is essential before hysterectomy to rule out endometrial neoplasia. The absence of cervical malignancy is ascertained before surgery.

(3) The patient's medical and psychological risks should be determined and addressed before surgical therapy.

(4) Ovaries should be retained in women younger than 40 to 45 years of age. The patient must play an important part in the decision concerning oophorectomy at any age; there is little evidence to support the contention that the residual ovary after a hysterectomy is at greater risk for development of ovarian cancer. The long-term consequences of estrogen deprivation—osteoporosis and cardiovascular risk—and implications of estrogen replacement therapy should be thoroughly addressed before surgical treatment.

STUDY QUESTIONS

DIRECTIONS: The numbered item or incomplete statement in this section is followed by answers or by completions of the statement. Select the ONE lettered answer or completion that is BEST.

1. Which of the following is a typical symptom associated with an abnormally enlarged 6- to 8-week myomatous uterus?

(A) Acute crampy pain
(B) Urinary frequency
(C) Constipation
(D) Urinary retention
(E) None of the above

DIRECTIONS: Each of the numbered items or incomplete statements in this section is negatively phrased, as indicated by a capitalized word such as NOT, LEAST, or EXCEPT. Select the ONE lettered answer or completion that is BEST in each case.

2. Submucous myomas may be associated with all of the following signs and symptoms EXCEPT

(A) abnormal bleeding
(B) reproductive failure
(C) anemia
(D) parasitic characteristics
(E) pedunculated characteristics

3. Abnormal uterine bleeding associated with myomata uteri is characterized by all of the following EXCEPT

(A) a gradual increase in the bleeding
(B) excessively long menstrual bleeding
(C) excessive bleeding during a menses of normal length
(D) the development of anemia
(E) irregular cycles with menorrhagia

4. Gross and microscopic features of myomas include all of the following EXCEPT

(A) a whorl-like appearance
(B) bundles of smooth muscle fibers
(C) a well-defined capsule of fibrous tissue
(D) central degeneration
(E) peripheral vascularity

5. A 46-year-old woman presents to the physician's office with known myomata uteri. She states that she has 30- to 50-day cycles with 7 days of heavy bleeding and 4 days of intermenstrual spotting every cycle. All of the following diagnostic techniques would be appropriate in the workup of this patient EXCEPT

(A) intravenous pyelogram
(B) pelvic ultrasound
(C) complete blood count
(D) endometrial sampling
(E) hysterosalpingogram

6. All of the following statements concerning uterine myomas are true EXCEPT

(A) malignant degeneration occurs in less than 1% of uterine myomas
(B) myomas can be found in the fallopian tubes and the vagina
(C) myomas rarely appear or grow after menopause
(D) hyaline degeneration is the least common form of myomatous degeneration
(E) although myomas appear encapsulated, no real capsule exists

7. Myomas are associated with all of the following clinical conditions EXCEPT

(A) anemia
(B) pyelonephritis
(C) urinary frequency
(D) dysmenorrhea
(E) amenorrhea

DIRECTIONS: The set of matching questions in this section consists of a list of four to twenty-six lettered options (some of which may be in figures) followed by several numbered items. For each numbered item, select the ONE lettered option that is most closely associated with it. To avoid spending too much time on matching sets with large numbers of options, it is generally advisable to begin each set by reading the list of options. Then, for each item in the set, try to generate the correct answer and locate it in the option list, rather than evaluating each option individually. Each lettered option may be selected once, more than once, or not at all.

Questions 8–10

For each of the following clinical situations involving a myomatous uterus, select the therapy that is most appropriate.

(A) Oral iron therapy
(B) Hormone suppression
(C) Endometrial biopsy
(D) Myomectomy
(E) Hysterectomy

8. A 50-year-old woman with a known myomatous uterus presents with the complaint of irregular bleeding. She states that her menses are heavy and occur every 5 to 6 weeks. She also mentions that she has had 5 to 7 days of intermenstrual spotting over the past three cycles.

9. A 32-year-old African-American woman with known myomas returns to the office after 3 years, complaining of mild left lower quadrant pain. Three years ago she had a tubal ligation. Physical examination reveals an irregular uterus the size of a 14-week gestation with an apparent 4-cm left fundal myoma.

10. A 28-year-old primipara presents with a uterine mass the size of a 14-week gestation, pain, and menorrhagia. A prominent posterior fundal mass is found on physical examination and seems to make up the bulk of the uterine mass.

ANSWERS AND EXPLANATIONS

1. The answer is E [III A 2, 3]. A 6- to 8-week myomatous uterus is not very big and should not cause the pressure symptoms of constipation, urinary frequency, or urinary retention, as would a grossly enlarged uterus that fills the pelvis. In addition, small, uncomplicated myomas, as exist in this case, that are not pedunculated, usually do not produce pain. Acute pain is usually associated with torsion of a pedunculated myoma.

2. The answer is D [II A 2, 3]. Submucous myomas are commonly associated with abnormal bleeding because of changes in the overlying endometrium that result in a disturbed bleeding pattern. Abnormal bleeding can lead to anemia. Reproductive failure, through poor implantation of the embryo in the abnormal endometrium overlying the myoma, may also occur. Submucous myomas can grow within the uterine cavity, remain connected to the uterus by pedicles, and become pedunculated with actual prolapse through the cervical os. These myomas, however, cannot become parasitic, as do some subserous myomas, because there is nothing to which they can attach and establish a secondary blood supply, as may happen within the abdominal cavity.

3. The answer is E [III A 1]. Abnormal menstrual bleeding is the most common characteristic associated with myomata uteri. Menorrhagia is common at the time of the menses, with excessive bleeding either in length or amount. The bleeding usually increases gradually and may eventually result in a significant anemia. Myomas are discrete objects and are not related to the hormonal aspects of the cycle. Therefore, irregular cycles are not characteristic because the length and regularity of the menstrual cycle are hormonally controlled.

4. The answer is C [II B 1, 2]. Myomas are made up of bundles of smooth muscle fibers that have a whorl-like appearance when cut on cross section. Degenerative changes within the myoma are common and may be caused by alterations in circulation, infection, or malignant transformation. The vascularity is on the periphery of the myoma, making the central part susceptible to degenerative changes.

Myomas behave as if they are encapsulated in the sense that they do not invade adjacent tissue, although no real capsule exists. The pseudocapsule is composed of fibrous and muscle tissue that has been flattened by the myoma and has the appearance of a capsule.

5. The answer is E [III A 1, B 2 a, c–e. This patient is in the perimenopausal age range and is having irregular, probably anovulatory bleeding. As such, her spotting could be secondary to endometrial neoplasia; endometrial sampling must be done to rule out neoplasia. Pelvic ultrasound would be appropriate to evaluate uterine size and structure and adnexal anatomy, and to rule out compression on the ureters and hydronephrosis. Intravenous pyelography could be obtained to evaluate the status of the ureters, although more information could be obtained with an ultrasound. Hemoglobin/hematocrit count is important to rule out anemia in a woman with heavy, irregular bleeding and known myomata uteri. There is no need to perform a hysterosalpingogram or hysteroscopy in this patient because she is not interested in fertility, and the presence of submucous myomas (as demonstrated by a hysterosalpingogram) would not matter or change the management plan in such a patient.

6. The answer is D [II C 1–7]. A leiomyoma is a localized proliferation of smooth muscle cells. Most of these occur in the uterus, but they also may occur elsewhere, including the fallopian tubes, vagina, round ligament, uterosacral ligaments, vulva, and the gastrointestinal tract. Myomas do not have a true capsule; the apparent capsule or pseudocapsule is composed of fibrous and muscle tissue that has been flattened by the tumor. It is believed that myomas depend on estrogen for growth because new myomas rarely appear and existing myomas stop growing after menopause. Hyaline degeneration is the most common form of degeneration, present in almost all leiomyomas. Malignant or sarcomatous degeneration occurs in less than 1% of leiomyomas.

7. The answer is E [III A 1–3]. Depending on the location of the myomas within the uterus, a number of different clinical conditions can exist. The submucous myoma can lead to menorrhagia, which results in anemia. The posterior subserous myoma can put pressure on the ureters, leading to hydronephrosis, stasis of urine, and pyelonephritis. An anterior subserous myoma, growing beneath the bladder, can compromise bladder capacity, leading to urinary frequency. Intramural myomas can result in the reappearance of dysmenorrhea after years of painless bleeding. Amenorrhea is not a feature of the myomatous uterus.

8–10. The answers are: 8-C [III B 2 c], **9-E** [IV C 1 a, 2 b (1), (4)], **10-D** [IV A 2, C 1 a, d, e, 2 a]. One cannot assume that abnormal bleeding in a 50-year-old woman is caused by the myomas simply because she has a myomatous uterus. At this age, the risk of endometrial disease, such as polyps, hyperplasia, or carcinoma, is significant and must be ruled out. Therefore endometrial sampling is indicated before considering any other therapy.

Hysterectomy is a consideration, if medical management fails to relieve symptoms, in the 32-year-old African-American woman who has had a tubal ligation. She has 15 to 20 years of ovarian activity remaining; ovaries would be conserved at the time of surgery. Surgery should not be based on size alone. Hysterectomy is definitive treatment of fibroids and is a therapeutic option for the patient with symptoms, who has completed childbearing and who has inadequate relief with medical management.

This patient is a young woman of low parity who is probably not finished with her childbearing. Physical examination suggests a single, large myoma in the uterus. The patient should be treated symptomatically. If surgery becomes necessary because symptoms fail to respond to medical management, or the patient experiences reproductive complications, myomectomy is the surgical treatment of choice.

Chapter 31

Female Urinary Incontinence

Jane Fang

I. INTRODUCTION

A. Epidemiology

1. Urinary incontinence affects women five times more frequently than men.

2. Ten to 25% of women 25 to 64 years of age suffer from incontinence.

3. Up to 40% of women older than age 65 have some form of incontinence.

4. Fifty percent of institutionalized women suffer from urinary incontinence.

B. Physiology of urinary incontinence

1. **Central nervous system**
   a. Loop I, the cerebral–brain stem loop, promotes storage.
   b. Loop II, the brain stem–sacral loop, promotes micturition.
   c. Loop III, the vesical–sacral loop, coordinates voiding.
   d. Loop IV, the cerebral–sacral loop, promotes storage.

2. **Autonomic nervous system**
   a. **Sympathetic (thoracocolumnar) nerves** promote storage
      (1) α-**Adrenergic receptors** in the bladder neck and urethra mediate **contraction.**
      (2) β-**Adrenergic receptors** in the bladder mediate **relaxation.**
   b. **Parasympathetic (sacral) nerves** promote micturition by relaxing the urethra and contracting the detrusor muscle.

II. TYPES OF URINARY INCONTINENCE

A. Stress urinary incontinence (SUI) is a loss of urine that occurs with increased abdominal pressure, such as coughing or straining.

1. **Genuine SUI (GSUI),** defined by urine loss as a result of an **anatomic defect of the urethrovesical junction,** most commonly follows pelvic floor muscle and nerve damage as a result of childbearing.

2. This category of SUI includes:
   a. **Urethral hypermobility.** This is the most common form and is usually surgically correctable with the anatomic restoration of the urethrovesical junction.
   b. **Intrinsic urethral sphincteric deficiency (ISD),** which is much less common, is caused by a defective urethral sphincter. It is a cause of surgical failure for procedures that correct GSUI.

B. Urge incontinence is defined by the symptom of urine loss that occurs when the patient experiences a strong desire to void, or when she feels that her bladder is full. This type of incontinence has traditionally been defined as having a separate etiology from GSUI, but many women with GSUI also experience urge incontinence symptoms. This type of incontinence includes the following subtypes:

1. **Detrusor instability (DI),** or unstable bladder, is defined when spontaneous bladder, or detrusor, contractions can be demonstrated during filling of the bladder. It is associated with the dysfunction of loop I, or loss of central inhibition. Its cause is unknown. DI can be treated with medications that relax the detrusor muscle.

2. In **urethral instability,** urine loss occurs with an involuntary loss of urethral pressure.

3. Detrusor hyperreflexia is defined by hyperactivity of the detrusor muscle associated with a central nervous system disorder. It is a common cause of incontinence in elderly and institutionalized women.

C. **Mixed incontinence** is classically defined by the demonstration of both GSUI and DI together. These patients usually are treated conservatively with medical and pharmacologic therapy for DI before a surgical approach is recommended.

III. EVALUATION OF URINARY INCONTINENCE

A. A **detailed history** is essential and should include:

1. A urinary questionnaire, including the presence of nocturia, urgency, precipitating events, and frequency of loss

2. A voiding diary, so the patient can document measured urine volumes and fluid intake during a 24-hour period

3. A history of urinary tract infections

4. Previous urologic surgery

5. Obstetric history: parity, birth weights, mode of delivery

6. Central nervous system or spinal cord disorders

7. Use of medications, including diuretics, antihypertensives, caffeine, alcohol, anticholinergics, decongestants, nicotine, psychotropics

8. The presence of other medical disorders (e.g., hypertension, hematuria)

B. **Physical examination** may detect:

1. Exacerbating conditions, such as chronic obstructive pulmonary disease, obesity, or intraabdominal mass

2. Uterine descensus, vaginal prolapse

3. Neurologic disorders

C. **Diagnostic tests**

1. A **midstream urine specimen** is collected for culture and sensitivity. Infection may aggravate urinary incontinence.

2. Urodynamic testing
   a. Uroflow. The patient voids into a commode connected to equipment that can calculate the flow rate of urine.
   b. Residual urine volume should be measured after the patient has voided. This should be less than 100 ml.
   c. Cystometrics are performed to evaluate bladder capacity, tone, and dynamics. The bladder is filled with sterile saline or water through a catheter in the supine position.
      (1) The following volumes are recorded:
         (a) First desire to void
         (b) Sensation of maximal fullness
      (2) When spontaneous detrusor contractions occur, this indicates DI.
      (3) During the evaluation, the examiner tries to reenact urine loss. If the patient leaks urine when coughing or straining, and there is anatomic descent of the bladder neck, this is indicative of GSUI.

3. The **Q-tip test** is an indirect measure of the urethral axis (angle of inclination). A Q-tip is inserted into the urethra with the patient in the lithotomy position. If the Q-tip moves more than 30 degrees from the horizontal, there is abnormal urethral mobility.

4. **Complex urodynamics.** These studies are performed when the cause of incontinence is confusing, if the results of simple cystometrics are conflicting, or if the patient has had a prior unsuccessful urologic procedure.

5. **Cystoscopy** is performed to examine the bladder and urethral mucosa for diverticula, or if neoplasia is suspected.

IV. TREATMENT

A. Nonsurgical treatment

1. **Infection** should be treated.

2. **Exercises of the pubococcygeus muscle (Kegel exercises)** can improve symptoms in 50% to 75% of patients.

3. **Weight reduction** in obese patients helps alleviate some of the symptoms.

4. **Chronic cough** should be evaluated and treated. Smoking should be stopped.

5. **Electrostimulators** can be used to strengthen pelvic floor musculature.

6. **Vaginal cones** can strengthen pelvic floor musculature by encouraging use of these muscles.

7. **Drug therapy**
   a. **Anticholinergics** (e.g., propantheline, imipramine) are beneficial in DI by relaxing the smooth muscle of the bladder, thus increasing bladder capacity.
   b. **Sympathomimetics** are useful for SUI; they work by elevating urethral pressure.
   c. **Estrogen** is beneficial in postmenopausal patients. Estrogens improve mucosal coaptation.

8. **Pessaries** can be used in patients who are not candidates for surgery to elevate the bladder neck.

9. **Collagen** can be injected in the periurethral tissues to improve mucosal coaptation for ISD.

B. Surgical treatment.
These procedures elevate the bladder neck and proximal urethra to the normal anatomic position, thus restoring the normal urethrovesical pressure differential. These procedures are indicated for SUI. The basic surgical approaches are listed here.

1. **Retropubic urethropexy** elevates the urethra and bladder neck by fixation of the paraurethral and paravesical structures to the pubis. The traditional Marshall-Marchetti-Krantz (MMK) procedure suspends the bladder neck to the pubic symphysis. Because of the risk of **osteitis pubis** as a late complication of the MMK procedure, the Burch modification has become more popular. The Burch procedure is the intraabdominal fixation of the paraurethral and paravesical tissues to the ileopectineal ligament (Cooper's ligament). Retropubic urethropexy is considered the gold standard procedure.

2. **Needle procedures** (e.g., Pereyra, Stamey, Raz) suspend the paraurethral tissues to the anterior aponeurosis of the abdominal wall, thus pulling up the urethrovesical angle to a retropubic position. They are performed from a vaginal or abdominal approach.

3. **Anterior colporrhaphy** with Kelly plication is performed from a vaginal approach and is the preferred method for cystocele repair with anterior vaginal wall prolapse. The Kelly plication tightens the paraurethral fascia to elevate the urethrovesical angle to a retropubic position.

4. **Hysterectomy** is often performed along with these procedures, especially when the pelvic support is poor.

5. **Sling procedures** are rarely used as primary procedures, but the cure rate is good. Because these procedures are very complicated and require additional materials (i.e., fascia lata), complications include infection and ulceration. They are often reserved for failed vaginal and retropubic procedures. This procedure is also indicated for ISD. Overcorrection with any of the sling procedures can lead to urinary retention.

STUDY QUESTIONS

DIRECTIONS: Each of the numbered items or incomplete statements in this section is followed by answers or by completions of the statement. Select the ONE lettered answer or completion that is BEST in each case.

1. The most important abnormality in the urethra and bladder that leads to stress urinary incontinence (SUI) is

(A) loss of estrogen in the postmenopausal period
(B) loss of the urethral sphincter
(C) prolapse of the uterus
(D) loss of the posterior urethrovesical angle
(E) rapid weight gain

2. Cystoscopy and cystometry are important in the evaluation of stress urinary incontinence (SUI) because

(A) urethral length can be measured
(B) the posterior urethrovesical angle can be measured directly
(C) the angle of inclination can be estimated
(D) there is no risk of infection
(E) causes of incontinence other than urethrovesical angle descent can be eliminated

3. Which of the following is true?

(A) Estrogens have no effect on the lower urinary tract
(B) Micturition is mediated entirely by the somatic nervous system
(C) β-Adrenergic receptors of the sympathetic nervous system promote storage of urine
(D) Urine storage is inhibited through the vesical–sacral loop (loop III)
(E) There is no interaction between the somatic and autonomic nervous systems during micturition

DIRECTIONS: The set of matching questions in this section consists of a list of four to twenty-six lettered options (some of which may be in figures) followed by several numbered items. For each numbered item, select the ONE lettered option that is most closely associated with it. To avoid spending too much time on matching sets with large numbers of options, it is generally advisable to begin each set by reading the list of options. Then, for each item in the set, try to generate the correct answer and locate it in the option list, rather than evaluating each option individually. Each lettered option may be selected once, more than once, or not at all.

Questions 4–6

For each result described below, select the procedure most likely to be associated with it.

(A) Marshall-Marchetti-Krantz procedure
(B) Burch procedure
(C) Sling procedure
(D) Pereyra procedure
(E) Anterior colporrhaphy

4. Associated with the complications of infection and ulceration

5. Suspends the urethra and vagina to the ileopectineal ligament

6. Associated with an excellent cure rate, but may be complicated by delayed postoperative osteitis pubis

ANSWERS AND EXPLANATIONS

1. The answer is D [II A 1]. The most important abnormality in the anatomy of the urethra and bladder that leads to stress urinary incontinence (SUI) is loss of the posterior urethrovesical angle. Uterine prolapse does not necessarily affect this angle. Loss of integrity of the urethral sphincter is an uncommon cause of stress incontinence.

2. The answer is E [III C 2, 5]. Cystoscopy and cystometry are important in the evaluation of stress urinary incontinence (SUI) because most causes other than urethrovesical angle descent can be eliminated. Cystoscopy permits internal visualization of the bladder to detect neoplasms, infections, stones, fistulas, and the ureteral orifices; cystometry allows assessment of bladder tone and dynamics and is essential for the diagnosis of detrusor instability.

3. The answer is C [I B]. β-Adrenergic receptors in the bladder wall cause detrusor relaxation, thus promoting the storage of urine. This is coordinated with α-adrenergic receptors in

the urethra and bladder neck that cause constriction, thus enhancing urine storage. The autonomic nervous system is coordinated with the somatic nervous system through loops I and IV to promote urine storage.

4–6. The answers are: 4-C [IV B 5], **5-B** [IV B 1], **6-A** [IV B 1]. Infection and ulceration are a problem with sling procedures because of the introduction of materials beneath the bladder neck in the retropubic space.

The Burch procedure, a retropubic urethropexy, fixes the paraurethral and paravesical tissues to the ileopectineal ligament, which corrects prolapse, something that is not routinely possible with other procedures.

All retropubic procedures have excellent cure rates, but when the adjacent bone periosteum is used, as it is in the Marshall-Marchetti-Krantz procedure, a reaction (osteitis pubis) may occur, which proves to be a serious delayed complication in some cases. The least complicated procedure is the Kelly plication procedure, which has an acceptable success rate for the first postoperative year.

Chapter 32
The Infertile Couple
William W. Beck, Jr.

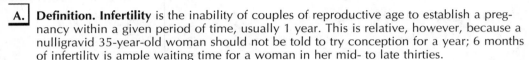

INTRODUCTION

A. **Definition. Infertility** is the inability of couples of reproductive age to establish a pregnancy within a given period of time, usually 1 year. This is relative, however, because a nulligravid 35-year-old woman should not be told to try conception for a year; 6 months of infertility is ample waiting time for a woman in her mid- to late thirties.

1. The monthly conception rate, or fecundability, among normal couples is about 20%.

2. Infertility increases with increasing age of the female partner. Age-related rates:
   a. 25 to 29 years: 9%
   b. 30 to 34 years: 15%
   c. 35 to 39 years: 22%

3. **Primary infertility** refers to couples who have never established a pregnancy.

4. **Secondary infertility** refers to couples who have conceived previously but are currently unable to establish a subsequent pregnancy.

B. **Incidence**

1. Approximately 10% of couples are infertile, using the criteria of at least 1 year of unprotected coitus.

2. **Etiology of infertility**
   a. Anovulation: 10% to 15%
   b. Pelvic factors (adhesions, endometriosis, infection, tubal occlusion): 30% to 40%
   c. Male factor: 30% to 40%
   d. Abnormal penetration of cervical mucus by sperm: 10% to 15%
   e. Idiopathic or unexplained: 10%

II. **PHYSIOLOGY OF CONCEPTION**

A. **Basic requirements for successful completion of the reproductive process**

1. Release of ova from the ovaries (**ovulation**) on a regular cyclic basis

2. Production of an ejaculate containing an ample number of motile spermatozoa

3. Deposition of spermatozoa in the female reproductive tract, usually at or near the cervical os

4. Migration of the spermatozoa through the female reproductive tract to the fallopian tubes

5. Arrival of the recently ovulated ovum capable of being fertilized in the fallopian tube

6. Patency of the fallopian tube

7. Normal intrauterine environment from the cervix to fallopian tube lumen to enable active movement of spermatozoa capable of fertilizing an ovum

8. Conditions appropriate for fusion of gametes (ovum and spermatozoon) within the fallopian tube

B. **Factors involved in fertility**

1. Spermatogenesis (the male factor)

2. Ovulation (the ovarian factor)

3. Mucus and sperm interactions (the cervical factor)

4. Endometrial integrity and cavity size and shape (the uterine factor)

5. Oviductal patency and anatomic relationships to the ovary (the tubal factor)

6. Insemination (the coital factor)

III. INFERTILITY EVALUATION

A. **Male factor.** The male gamete can be examined in its own environment, seminal fluid, as well as in its new environment, cervical mucus. The following tests are used to evaluate the male factor.

1. **Semen analysis.** The customary standards for normality include the following ranges:
   a. Volume: 2.5 to 6.0 ml
   b. Count: more than 20 million per milliliter
   c. Motility: more than 50% with forward progression
   d. Quality of motion: graded 1 to 4 going from poor to excellent (quality worsens with increasingly wobbly motion of spermatozoa as they progress across the microscopic slide)
   e. Morphology: more than 30% normal, with oval heads, an acrosomal cap, and single tails
   f. White blood cells: fewer than 1 million/ml

2. **Postcoital test.** Mucus is examined microscopically between 2 and 12 hours after coitus at midcycle for total number of sperm seen per high-powered field and percentage and quality of motility. A satisfactory test is one in which more than 10 motile spermatozoa are seen per high-powered field. An unsatisfactory test (no or few spermatozoa seen; nonmotile spermatozoa or those with a "shaking" movement) may be the result of:
   a. Azoospermia (no spermatozoa in the ejaculate)
   b. Poor inherent spermatozoa motility
   c. Hostile cervical mucus (e.g., infection, antibodies, or not enough estrogen priming)
   d. Poor coital technique
   e. Small ejaculate volume

3. **Sperm antibodies.** Occasionally, antibodies to sperm may be present in the man or woman and are responsible for fertility impairment.

4. **Tests of fertilizing capacity of spermatozoa** have been devised to assess the ability of sperm to fertilize an ovum.
   a. **Zona-free hamster ovum penetration test** measures the ability of spermatozoa to enter the ooplasm of the hamster egg compared with control spermatozoa (such as donor sperm).
   b. **Human zona binding assay.** The ratio of the number of the test spermatozoa bound to half a zona to the number of spermatozoa for a fertile control is the hemizona assay index.
   c. **Human ovum fertilization test** is rarely performed except at the time of in vitro fertilization. This procedure evaluates ability of sperm not only to penetrate the zona pellucida of a human egg but to initiate cell cleavage.

B. **Coital factor.** Details of coital frequency and technique can help to determine if coital dysfunction is a cause of infertility. **Coital dysfunction** can be studied by:

1. Taking a history of coital frequency, patterns, technique, satisfaction (a lack of sexual satisfaction dramatically diminishes coital frequency in some couples) and use of adjuvants (creams, jellies, or douches)

2. Anatomic evaluation of the position of the cervix with relationship to the vagina

3. Postcoital testing

C. **Cervical factor.** The cervix is the first major barrier encountered by sperm after arrival in the female reproductive tract. Spermatozoa migrate rapidly through the endocervical canal and have been demonstrated in the fallopian tube as early as 5 minutes after deposition at the cervix.

1. **Abnormalities in the cervix or the cervical mucus** that interfere with sperm migration include:
   a. Abnormal position of the cervix (prolapse of the cervix or uterine retroversion with anterior placement of the cervix)
   b. Chronic infection, which may produce an unfavorable mucus (e.g., *Streptococcus, Staphylococcus*, and *Gardnerella*)
   c. Colonization with organisms that are cytotoxic to sperm (e.g., *Ureaplasma*)
   d. Previous cervical surgery (e.g., conization), which may lead to mucus depletion
   e. Previous electrocautery, i.e. LEEP
   f. The presence of sperm antibodies in the cervical mucus

2. **Mucus quality** can be assessed by physical, biochemical, and physiologic parameters, including:
   a. pH, using Tes-Tape [an alkaline pH is optimum (pH 8.0)]
   b. Bacteriologic culture for microorganisms
   c. Crystallization (ferning) and spinnbarkeit (thread formation) of midcycle mucus
   d. Serologic tests for antibodies
   e. Postcoital testing
   f. Tests of sperm behavior in mucus (cross testing with donor sperm and mucus)
      (1) Examination of mucus (as in a postcoital test) after artificial placement of the partner's specimen
      (2) In vitro microscopic study of penetration of sperm through cervical mucus
      (3) In vitro cross-testing whereby the behavior of sperm in donor mucus is compared to the behavior of sperm in the patient's mucus, and the behavior of the partner's sperm is compared to the behavior of the donor sperm in the patient's mucus

D. **Uterine factor.** The uterus supports the journey of spermatozoa from the cervix to fallopian tube and performs many significant roles in reproduction.

1. **The roles of the uterus in reproduction** include:
   a. Retention of the zygote after arrival from the fallopian tube for several days before implantation
   b. Provision of a suitable environment for implantation
   c. Protection of embryo/fetus from the external environment

2. **Evaluation of the uterine factor** is done by the following methods:
   a. **Endometrial sampling by biopsy** to determine:
      (1) The occurrence of ovulation when evidence of progesterone secretion (i.e., secretory endometrium) is found on biopsy
      (2) The adequacy and maintenance of progesterone secretion during the luteal phase (i.e., inadequate luteal phase)
      (3) The presence of infection (e.g., endometritis)
   b. **Endometrial culture to identify bacterial organisms** in the presence of endometritis
   c. **Hysterography** to visualize the contour of the uterine cavity, using a radiopaque contrast medium with fluoroscopic radiography
   d. **Hysteroscopy** to visualize the uterine cavity to detect anomalous development, polyps, tumors, or adhesions (synechiae)

    e. Laparoscopy to detect and delineate anomalous uterine development or my-omata. (Laparoscopy permits visualization of the abdominal and pelvic cavities.) This procedure requires anesthesia and can be done at the time of hysteroscopy.

E. **Tubal factor.** The fallopian tube is responsible for efficient transfer of gametes and for fostering their approximation.

    1. Functions of the fallopian tube are twofold.
        a. Mechanical functions act to:
            (1) Convey recently ovulated ova into the fallopian tube
            (2) Permit spermatozoa to enter the oviduct
            (3) Effect transfer of the blastocyst into the uterine cavity
        b. Environmental functions provide for:
            (1) Fertilization of the ovum
            (2) Capacitation of spermatozoa
            (3) Early development and segmentation of the fertilized ovum

    2. Tests used to evaluate the function of the fallopian tube determine patency, location with respect to the ovary, and, to a lesser extent, function.
        a. Hysterosalpingography enables visualization of the lumen and patency of the fallopian tube using a radiopaque contrast medium.
        b. Laparoscopy allows direct visualization of the fallopian tube to identify abnormalities in structure or location and detect peritubal adhesions. This procedure is usually carried out in conjunction with transcervical lavage with a dye (usually indigo carmine) as a test of tubal patency.

F. **Ovarian factor.** The ovarian factor refers to the ability of the ovaries to release ova on a cyclic basis.

    1. Ovarian functions
        a. The ovaries serve as a repository for oocytes, and they release mature oocytes at regular intervals throughout reproductive life.
        b. The ovaries secrete steroid hormones that influence the structure and function of tissues in the reproductive tract, promoting fertility.

    2. Documentation of ovulation
        a. Direct means (impractical)
            (1) Observation of ovulation during laparoscopy or laparotomy
            (2) Recovery of an ovum from the fallopian tube or uterus
            (3) Establishment of pregnancy
        b. Indirect means (practical)
            (1) Basal body temperature records demonstrate a 14-day elevation of basal temperature beginning at or after ovulation, as a result of progesterone secretion, which has a thermogenic effect.
            (2) Elevated blood progesterone levels, between 6.5 and 10 ng/ml at midpoint of the luteal phase
            (3) Endometrial biopsy demonstrates the characteristic histologic changes of the endometrium achieved by circulating progesterone levels; namely, a secretory endometrial pattern.

    3. Corpus luteum production of progesterone must be sufficient to prepare the endometrium for implantation and maintenance of the pregnancy. Defects in luteal function can be reflected by:
        a. Short life span of the corpus luteum with a thermal shift of less than 12 days
        b. Reduced progesterone production during the luteal phase (i.e., values less than 5 ng/ml)

    4. Reasons for ovulatory defects
        a. Hypothalamic–pituitary insufficiency
            (1) Tumors or destructive lesions
            (2) Drugs that interfere with normal hypothalamic function
            (3) Hyperprolactinemia due to a pituitary adenoma

    b. Thyroid disease
       (1) Hypothyroidism
       (2) Hyperthyroidism
    c. Adrenal disorders
       (1) Adrenal insufficiency
       (2) Hyperadrenalism
         (a) Cortisol excess
         (b) Androgen excess
    d. Emotional disturbances
    e. Metabolic and nutritional disorders
       (1) Obesity
       (2) Malnutrition
    f. Excessive exercise (e.g., running, dancing)

IV. **THERAPY.** Treatment can be surgical or medical and is based on documentation of the abnormality or abnormalities leading to infertility.

A. **Correction of the male factor**

1. Medical
    a. Correction of underlying deficiencies (e.g., thyroid disorders, prolactin excess, dietary disturbances)
    b. Therapeutic donor insemination for azoospermic or severely oligospermic males

2. Surgical
    a. Reversal of sterilization
    b. Varicocele surgery

3. Assisted reproductive technologies
    a. **Intrauterine insemination of washed spermatozoa (IUI)** is used with cervical factors, male factors of oligospermia or poor motility, and unexplained infertility. It is usually used in conjunction with gonadotropin therapy (superovulation).
    b. **In vitro fertilization and embryo transfer (IVF/ET)** is the removal of oocytes from the ovary and the placement of the oocytes with sperm together in a dish in the laboratory to allow fertilization. After fertilization and cell division (in the 4- to 16-cell stage), the embryo is placed in the uterus.
    c. In **gamete intrafallopian transfer (GIFT),** the ovum and the spermatozoa are mixed together and are immediately placed into the distal fallopian tube, where fertilization then occurs. This procedure normally requires laparoscopy but has been accomplished transcervically under ultrasound guidance.
    d. **Assisted fertilization** is a technique of micromanipulation that thins the zona pellucida and injects sperm into the ovum in an effort to enhance fertilization.

B. **Correction of the coital factor**

1. Psychotherapy

2. Sexual therapy

3. IUI with washed spermatozoa

C. **Correction of the cervical factor**

1. Low-dose estrogen therapy (conjugated estrone 0.625 mg daily for a week before predicted ovulation)

2. Antibiotics

3. IUI with or without superovulation

4. Corticosteroids for antisperm antibodies

5. IVF/ET

D. **Correction of the uterine factor**

1. **Medical**
    a. Antibiotic therapy for endometritis
    b. High-dose estrogen or estrogen–progestin therapy for endometritis, after removal of intrauterine adhesions

2. **Surgical**
    a. Myomectomy for myomata by hysteroscopy or open laparotomy
    b. Metroplasty in certain anomalies (e.g., septate uterus)
    c. Removal of intrauterine synechiae, septum, or polyps by hysteroscopy

E. **Correction of tubal factor**

1. Tubal anastomosis for reversal of sterilization

2. Salpingoplasty for occluded distal or proximal fallopian tubes

3. Lysis of peritubal adhesions

4. IVF/ET when fallopian tubes are absent or irreparable

F. **Correction of the ovarian factor**

1. **Induction of ovulation**
    a. Correction of underlying endocrine disorders, such as thyroid disease
    b. Clomiphene citrate to correct hypothalamic dysfunction; patient must have estrogen levels; cannot be hypogonadal
    c. Human menopausal gonadotropins, which are the only source of follicle-stimulating hormone (FSH) and luteinizing hormone (LH) commercially, for pituitary insufficiency or when clomiphene citrate fails
    d. Bromocriptine for anovulation due to prolactin excess
    e. Glucocorticoids for androgen excess due to adrenal hyperplasia

2. **Correction of luteal phase defects**
    a. Clomiphene citrate
    b. Human chorionic gonadotropin
    c. Postovulatory progesterone supplementation
    d. Human menopausal gonadotropins (FSH and LH)

G. **Unexplained infertility.** Assisted reproductive technologies are used:

1. IVF/ET

2. GIFT

3. Zygote intrafallopian transfer and tubal embryo stage transfer

STUDY QUESTIONS

DIRECTIONS: The numbered item or incomplete statement in this section is followed by answers or by completions of the statement. Select the ONE lettered answer or completion that is BEST.

1. The most serious causative factor of infertility that can be reflected in the postcoital test is

(A) azoospermia
(B) poor cervical mucus
(C) tubal dysfunction
(D) poor coital technique
(E) luteal dysfunction

DIRECTIONS: Each of the numbered items or incomplete statements in this section is negatively phrased, as indicated by a capitalized word such as NOT, LEAST, or EXCEPT. Select the ONE lettered answer or completion that is BEST in each case.

2. Which of the following procedures is NOT diagnostic of a defect in corpus luteum function?

(A) Measurement of basal body temperature
(B) Endometrial biopsy and histologic dating
(C) Measurement of serum progesterone levels
(D) Determination of the length of the luteal phase
(E) Measurement of serum estrogen levels

3. Which of the following procedures is NOT appropriate for the evaluation of the endometrial cavity?

(A) Laparoscopy
(B) Endometrial biopsy
(C) Hysteroscopy
(D) Endometrial culture
(E) Hysterography

4. Which of the following would NOT be used in the correction of cervical factor infertility?

(A) Intrauterine insemination
(B) Low-dose estrogen
(C) Antibiotics
(D) Human chorionic gonadotropin injection
(E) In vitro fertilization and embryo transfer (IVF/ET)

5. Which of the following is NOT indicative of ovulation?

(A) A rise in the basal body temperature
(B) Pregnancy
(C) Progesterone level above 6.5 ng/ml
(D) Secretory endometrium
(E) The occurrence of menses

6. Which of the following is NOT reflected by a poor postcoital test?

(A) Blocked fallopian tubes
(B) Low sperm count
(C) Poor sperm motility
(D) Poor cervical mucus
(E) Poor coital technique

7. Which of the following does NOT contribute to abnormalities in the cervical mucus?

(A) Colonization of the cervix with cytotoxic organisms
(B) Uterine retroversion
(C) Chronic infection of the cervix
(D) Previous electrocauterization of the cervix
(E) Antisperm antibodies

DIRECTIONS: The set of matching questions in this section consists of a list of four to twenty-six lettered options (some of which may be in figures) followed by several numbered items. For each numbered item, select the ONE lettered option that is most closely associated with it. To avoid spending too much time on matching sets with large numbers of options, it is generally advisable to begin each set by reading the list of options. Then, for each item in the set, try to generate the correct answer and locate it in the option list, rather than evaluating each option individually. Each lettered option may be selected once, more than once, or not at all.

Questions 8–11

For the evaluation of the factors outlined below, select the best diagnostic test.

(A) Postcoital test
(B) Hysterosalpingography
(C) Semen analysis
(D) Endometrial biopsy
(E) Laparoscopy

8. The presence and patency of fallopian tubes

9. The occurrence of ovulation

10. Intrauterine malformation and pathology

11. The quantity and quality of cervical mucus and sperm interaction

ANSWERS AND EXPLANATIONS

1. The answer is A [III A 2]. Correction of azoospermia often requires artificial insemination with donor sperm. Poor cervical mucus and coital technique are correctable. The postcoital test does not yield the appropriate information to determine if tubal or luteal dysfunction is a cause of infertility.

2. The answer is E [III D 2 a, F 2 b (1)–(3), 3]. Measurement of serum estrogen levels is not useful when assessing a suspected inadequate luteal phase because progesterone is the hormone responsible for the luteal phase. The basal body temperature may show a slow rise and a short span of 10 days or less. Measurement of serum progesterone levels is helpful because progesterone levels are lower than normal in corpus luteum dysfunction. Endometrial biopsy shows a lag of at least 48 hours between the histologic dating and the cycle day of the biopsy.

3. The answer is A [III D 2 a–e]. Various clinical problems that contribute to infertility can occur within the endometrial cavity (e.g., chronic infection, inadequate hormonal preparation of the endometrium, submucous myomas, polyps, septum, and adhesions). Tests, such as endometrial culture and biopsy, hysteroscopy for direct visualization of the cavity, and hysterography for the radiographic outline of the cavity, are helpful in defining these problems. Laparoscopy is not helpful because the laparoscope cannot see into the uterine cavity; it merely reveals the external surface and is used to determine anomalous uterine development.

4. The answer is D [IV C 1–5]. Cervical mucus that is hostile to the penetration of spermatozoa can be a major factor in infertility. The poor cervical mucus may result from inadequate estrogen effects on the mucus or from infection. Therefore, low-dose estrogen or antibiotics could be used. With persistently poor cervical mucus despite therapy, the cervix may have to be bypassed with either intrauterine insemination (IUI) or in vitro fertilization (IVF), with implantation of the embryo. Human chorionic gonadotropin is not useful because it has no way of stimulating estrogen production. It could, however, be used at ovulation to help stimulate the secretion of progesterone from the corpus luteum.

5. The answer is E [III F 2 a, b]. Pregnancy is the best possible way to document ovulation. The secretory endometrium and the rise in the basal body temperature are reflective of progesterone secretion from the corpus luteum and, thus, ovulation, in that the corpus luteum does not exist in the absence of ovulation. The menses can occur in the absence of ovulation, as happens in dysfunctional uterine bleeding.

6. The answer is A [III A 1, 2, B 3, E 2 a]. A poor postcoital test means that there is some problem with the semen, the deposition of the semen onto the cervix, or the cervical mucus. If the sperm count is too low, the sperm motility is poor, or the coital technique does not provide adequate insemination of the cervix, few motile sperm will be seen in the cervical mucus. Hostile cervical mucus may not support the sperm so that none of them moves in the mucus. Patency of the fallopian tubes can be determined by hysterosalpingography, which enables visualization of the lumen of the tube using a radiopaque contrast medium.

7. The answer is B [III C 1 a–f]. Both conization and electrocauterization of the cervix destroy cervical endothelium and thus reduce or eliminate epithelium capable of producing mucus. Infection produces a viscous mucus that is hostile to spermatozoa. Antisperm antibodies also create a hostile mucus that inhibits sperm motility. Uterine retroversion has nothing to do with the cervical mucus. Because the cervix is anterior as a consequence of retroverted uterus, there can be an insemination problem.

8–11. The answers are: 8-B [III E 2 a], **9-D** [III F 2 b (3)], **10-B** [III E 2 a], **11-A** [III A 2 a–e]. Basic infertility evaluation should include some test of tubal patency. Hysterosalpingography offers this capability as well as information on tubal architecture. It is performed in the radiology department, requires injection of a radiopaque dye into the cervical os and uterus, and is associated with acceptable level of radiation exposure to a nonpregnant woman. The test is less invasive than laparoscopy and often provides valuable information regarding the genital anatomy.

Evaluation of the endometrium with an endometrial biopsy in the luteal phase, preferably cycle days 22 to 26, provides evidence of ovulation by observation of secretory endometrium, which results from the action of progesterone.

Hysterosalpingography enables the detection of müllerian anomalies and intrauterine pathology, which includes adhesions, polyps, septum, and myomas. Abnormalities secondary to in utero exposure to diethylstilbestrol can also be detected.

The postcoital test should be timed to coincide with ovulation, which is the time that cervical mucus should be of the best quality and in the greatest quantity. It allows for evaluation of cervical mucus, sperm numbers, and sperm viability and interaction with the cervical mucus, and also serves to confirm satisfactory coital technique.

Chapter 33

Amenorrhea

William W. Beck, Jr.

I. INTRODUCTION

A. **Amenorrhea is the absence of menses,** which may be **eugonadotropic, hypergonado-tropic,** or **hypogonadotropic.** It is important to realize that amenorrhea is not a diagnosis in and of itself, but is a symptom, indicating an anatomic, genetic, biochemical, physiologic, or emotional abnormality. The pathophysiology of amenorrhea must be understood in terms of the physiology of menstruation.

1. **Physiologic amenorrhea,** the absence of menses before or directly after menarche, during pregnancy and lactation, and after menopause, is not a manifestation of disease and does not need to be evaluated.
   a. A significant number of **teenage girls** have intervals of amenorrhea lasting 2 to 12 months during the first 2 years after menarche.
   b. **Spontaneous menopause** may occur in women as early as their mid-thirties.

2. **Pathologic amenorrhea** is suspected in the following situations:
   a. At 14 years of age, in the absence of both menstruation and secondary sexual characteristics
   b. At 16 years of age, regardless of whether there are secondary sexual characteristics
   c. At any age when menses have ceased in a woman who previously had normal menstrual function

B. **Menstruation depends on the following interrelated factors** that culminate in the visible discharge of menstrual blood. An interruption of any of these can result in amenorrhea.

1. An **intact outflow tract,** which assumes patency and continuity of the vaginal orifice, the vaginal canal, and the uterine cavity

2. An **endometrium that is responsive** to hormonal stimulation

3. An **intact hypothalamic–pituitary–ovarian axis,** allowing the sequential elaboration of steroid hormones from the ovary. The cascade begins in the hypothalamus with the secretion of **gonadotropin-releasing hormone,** which stimulates the pituitary to release the **gonadotropins: follicle-stimulating hormone (FSH)** and **luteinizing hormone (LH).**

4. **Secretion of estrogen from the ovary,** resulting ultimately in ovulation, with the secretion of progesterone as a result of FSH and LH stimulation

II. EUGONADOTROPIC AMENORRHEA.

The eugonadotropic causes of amenorrhea involve **congenital and acquired anomalies of the uterus and the outflow tract** as well as some forms of **androgen excess.** The ovaries are functional, producing normal levels of estrogen and progesterone, and the usual feedback to the pituitary results in normal gonadotropin levels.

A. **Congenital anomalies**

1. **Mayer-Rokitansky-Küster-Hauser syndrome,** the most common congenital anomaly of the uterus, is characterized by:
   a. Failure of fusion of the two müllerian ducts, vaginal agenesis, and normal ovaries; one third have urinary tract abnormalities

    b. Delayed menarche and the absence of the vagina

  2. Imperforate hymen and **transverse vaginal septum,** also causes for delayed menarche, are characterized by:

    a. Normal sexual development, pelvic pain, urinary frequency, and a perineal bulge (in patients with an imperforate hymen)

    b. Continued reflux of menstrual debris, which can lead to endometriosis and impaired future fertility, making these diagnoses relative emergencies

B. **Acquired anomalies**

  1. Asherman's syndrome is an acquired form of uterine dysfunction. The amenorrhea associated with this syndrome is caused by intrauterine adhesions that partially or completely obliterate the uterine cavity. The cause of these adhesions is traumatization of the endometrium and myometrium as a result of a vigorous curettage of the postabortal or postpartum uterus (because of bleeding), on which is superimposed an endometritis.

  2. Tuberculosis can lead to scarring of the endometrial cavity, causing amenorrhea, but this is now rare in the United States.

C. **Androgen excess** from either the adrenal gland or the ovary can cause amenorrhea.

  1. Androgen excess from the adrenal gland may be secondary to a virilizing tumor or congenital adrenal hyperplasia.

  2. Androgen excess from the ovary may be caused by a rare virilizing ovarian tumor or by the more common polycystic ovarian syndrome. The latter is characterized by hirsutism in a patient who is well estrogenized due to the conversion of excess amounts of the weak androgen androstenedione to testosterone and estrone.

III. **HYPERGONADOTROPIC AMENORRHEA,** or **primary amenorrhea,** involves gonadal, chromosomal, or genetic defects that inhibit the normal hormonal feedback mechanisms to suppress the secretion of gonadotropin.

A. **Chromosomal abnormalities.** Patients with sex chromosome abnormalities [45,XO (Turner's syndrome) or mosaicism] and absent or limited ovarian function are categorized as having gonadal dysgenesis. They usually express phenotypic differences, such as short stature. Identification of Y chromosomal material in these patients is essential because of the malignant potential of such a gonad (i.e., gonadoblastoma, dysgerminoma, yolk sac tumor, and choriocarcinoma).

B. **Normal chromosomes**

  1. Pure gonadal dysgenesis affects that group of women with ovarian failure who are phenotypically normal and who have 46,XX or 46,XY karyotypes. Receptor problems are evident in both karyotypes.

  2. Resistant ovary syndrome affects women with 46,XX karyotypes who present with amenorrhea and who have an ovarian membrane receptor defect. Gonadotropin levels are elevated because the ovaries do not:

    a. Respond to gonadotropin

    b. Secrete hormones

    c. Provide negative feedback to suppress the pituitary

  3. Premature ovarian failure might result from autoimmune disease.

  4. Androgen insensitivity syndrome, or **testicular feminization syndrome,** is characterized by patients who are gonadal males (46,XY) but phenotypic females. Other characteristics include the following:

    a. The **cytosol receptors for testosterone** are defective.

    b. The **testosterone level** is in the male range, but there is no biologic evidence of circulating testosterone, such as pubic and axillary hair.

    c. Patients have a **vaginal pouch with no uterine remnants** because of the active presence of testicular müllerian-inhibiting factor.

    d. **These patients should not have their gonads removed** until after full sexual development. (The risk of dysgerminoma or other gonadal neoplasms is minimal until the patient is older than 20 years of age.)

    e. **Pubescence** occurs normally in the presence of the patient's own endogenous hormones.

IV. **HYPOGONADOTROPIC AMENORRHEA,** or **secondary amenorrhea,** occurs after a menstrual pattern has been established. Most hypogonadotropic amenorrheas are acquired, resulting from a number of different causes: emotional stress, drugs, diseases of the pituitary, nutritional deficiencies, excessive exercise, and abnormalities of the adrenal and thyroid glands. These amenorrheas are both **hypogonadotropic** and **hypoestrogenic.**

A. **Kallmann's syndrome.** This is the **most common congenital form of hypogonadotropic amenorrhea.** There is both an irreversible defect in gonadotropin synthesis and an olfactory sensory defect.

B. **Emotional stress.** The **most common forms of acquired hypogonadotropic amenorrhea** are psychogenic in nature, occurring in association with either acute or chronic emotional stress.

C. **Nutritional deficiency.** Hypothalamic suppression in patients with classic **anorexia nervosa** is often manifested by secondary amenorrhea.

D. **Excessive exercise.** Women who are able to maintain a borderline body weight but who undergo strenuous physical activity, such as marathon running, swimming, gymnastics, or ballet, may present with secondary amenorrhea.

E. **Drugs.** Drug-induced amenorrheas include those associated with birth control pills, phenothiazine derivatives, reserpine, and ganglia-blocking agents.

    1. Less than 1% of women on birth control pills experience amenorrhea on discontinuation, and many of these had menstrual irregularities before using the pills.

    2. Phenothiazine derivatives, reserpine, and ganglia-blocking agents affect the **hypothalamus,** probably the **dopamine and norepinephrine balance,** and are sometimes associated with **galactorrhea.**

F. **Diseases of the pituitary.** Pituitary tumors and ischemia and necrosis of the pituitary can lead to amenorrhea.

    1. The pituitary tumors include **craniopharyngiomas** (in the younger age group), **chromophobe adenomas,** and **prolactin-producing adenomas.** These tumors may be accompanied by neurologic symptoms (blindness), galactorrhea, and signs of other tropic hormone deficiencies, including hypothyroidism, amenorrhea, and Addison's disease.

    2. **Ischemia and necrosis of the pituitary gland secondary to obstetric shock (blood loss)** are associated with varying degrees of insufficiency of all the pituitary tropic hormones.

G. **Other hormonal causes.** Amenorrhea is also seen **secondary to thyroid or adrenal hyperfunction or hypofunction;** the thyroid component of amenorrhea is the more common of the two.

V. EVALUATION OF AMENORRHEA

A. History. The first step in the workup of a patient with amenorrhea is a detailed history, which should include:

1. The age of the patient, the presence or absence of secondary sexual characteristics, and the time of the onset of the amenorrhea

2. A history of emotional stress, weight gain or loss, poor eating habits, a strenuous exercise program, use of medication, recent pregnancy, body hair growth, galactorrhea, or symptoms suggestive of thyroid or adrenal disease

3. A sexual history to rule out the possibility of pregnancy (discretion is necessary when eliciting sexual histories from young patients)

B. Physical examination. Either the presence or absence of findings can be informative.

1. In the case of **delayed menarche,** it is important to evaluate the status of the secondary sexual characteristics, to determine the presence or absence of a functional vagina, and to determine the presence of a palpable mass on rectal examination.

2. **Evidence of defeminization, masculinization, thyroid or adrenal dysfunction, and somatic abnormalities** can help to formulate a differential diagnosis.

C. Laboratory studies. The appropriate tests depend on whether a patient has ever had a menstrual flow and on her pelvic examination. If there has been previous menstrual function, the physician can assume that the ovaries have functioned and that there is a patent outflow tract.

1. **Previous menstrual function** (Figure 33-1)
   a. Measurement of **serum human chorionic gonadotropin levels** to rule out the possibility of pregnancy
   b. A **progesterone challenge** (medroxyprogesterone, 10 mg daily for 5 days) to determine the status of the hypothalamic–pituitary–ovarian axis
      (1) There will be **no flow due to progesterone withdrawal** in the **absence of estrogen priming** of the endometrium or **if the endometrium is nonfunctional.**
      (2) **Progesterone withdrawal** in the presence of amenorrhea indicates **anovulation** with estrogen secretion.
   c. **Evaluation of endometrial potential**
      (1) The evaluation is accomplished by the **sequential use of estrogen and progesterone** (a conjugated estrogen, 2.5 mg daily for 21 days, with medroxyprogesterone, 20 mg daily for the last 5 days of the estrogen therapy).
      (2) **Subsequent bleeding** suggests one of the hypogonadotropic or hypergonadotropic amenorrheas.
      (3) **Absence of bleeding** suggests either an abnormal outflow tract or a nonfunctional endometrium (as in Asherman's syndrome).
      (4) The **existence of a nonfunctional endometrium** can be confirmed by hysterosalpingography or hysteroscopy.
   d. **Measurement of prolactin levels**
      (1) A **normal level** (less than 20 ng/ml) in the presence of a progesterone withdrawal flow and the absence of galactorrhea essentially eliminates the possibility of a pituitary tumor.

FIGURE 33-1. Workup of amenorrhea for a patient with previous menstrual function. *hCG* = human chorionic gonadotropin; *TSH* = thyroid-stimulating hormone; *CAT* = computed axial tomography; *MRI* = magnetic resonance imaging; *IVP* = intravenous pyelography.

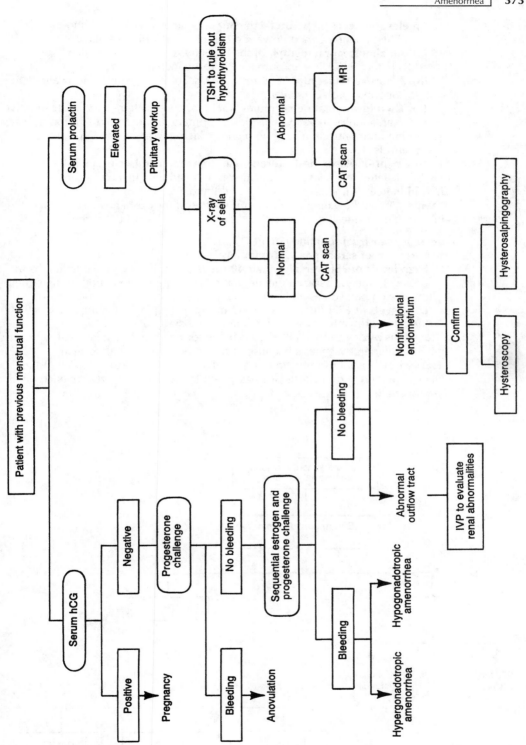

(2) An **elevated level (hyperprolactinemia)** demands a workup of the pituitary gland, including a coned-down radiographic view of the sella turcica.

    (a) An **abnormal radiograph** of the pituitary requires a computed axial tomography (CAT) scan or magnetic resonance imaging.

    (b) A **normal radiograph** requires a CAT scan of the pituitary to evaluate the abnormal prolactin level.

    (c) **Thyroid-stimulating hormone (TSH),** when elevated, is the most sensitive evaluation of hypothyroidism. The primary elevation of thyrotropin-releasing hormone stimulates the pituitary lactotropes, elevating prolactin levels.

  e. Measurement of plasma testosterone and dehydroepiandrosterone sulfate, which may be elevated in disease of the ovary and the adrenal gland

  f. Thyroid indices [triiodothyronine (T_3) and thyroxine (T_4)] to test for hyperthyroidism, morning and evening levels of cortisol to test for Cushing's disease, and a glucose tolerance test for diabetes to diagnose the cause of the amenorrhea

2. No previous menstrual function (Figure 33-2)

  a. Measurement of serum gonadotropin levels

    (1) **High levels of FSH (greater than 40 mIU/ml)** indicate gonadal failure as the cause of amenorrhea and dictate that a karyotype be done both to determine the sex chromosomes and to rule out the presence of a Y chromosome.

    (2) **Low levels of FSH (less than 5 mIU/ml)** indicate pituitary failure or inactivity, the latter probably caused by hypothalamic dysfunction.

  b. Intravenous pyelography (IVP) should be performed on all patients with any degree of müllerian dysgenesis because of the associated renal abnormalities.

  c. Laparoscopy. Visual examination of the pelvis may be necessary to determine the extent of müllerian dysgenesis or to ascertain the nature of the dysgenetic gonad (i.e., ascertain if it is a streak ovary).

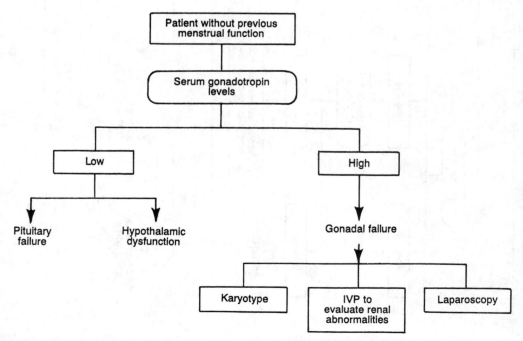

FIGURE 33-2. Workup of amenorrhea for a patient with no previous menstrual function. *IVP* = intravenous pyelography.

VI. TREATMENT OF AMENORRHEA

A. Eugonadotropic amenorrhea

1. Congenital anomalies

a. Incision of an imperforate hymen or a transverse vaginal septum to establish outlet patency and to release accumulated menstrual blood

b. Creation of an artificial vagina to correct the vaginal agenesis seen in some forms of müllerian dysgenesis

2. Acquired anomalies. Asherman's syndrome should be treated in the following ways:

a. Dilation and curettage with hysteroscopy

b. Insertion into the uterus of a pediatric Foley catheter for 7 days to keep the uterine cavity open

c. Broad-spectrum antibiotics for 10 days to prevent infection from the foreign body that has been inserted into the uterus

d. Sequential hormone therapy with high-dose estrogen (10 mg of conjugated estrogen daily for 21 days with 10 mg of medroxyprogesterone daily for the last 7 days of the cycle for 6 months) to help reestablish the endometrium

B. Hypergonadotropic amenorrhea. There is no curative therapy for these amenorrheas.

1. Estrogen replacement is administered to dysgenetic patients for the development of secondary sexual characteristics (2.5 mg of conjugated estrogen for 21 days with 10 mg of medroxyprogesterone daily for the last 7 days of the cycle).

2. Sequential hormone therapy is given as above (VI B 1) to maintain secondary sexual characteristics whenever a deficiency develops.

3. Surgical excision of gonads containing Y-chromosomal material should be undertaken:

a. Before puberty or at the time of discovery in dysgenetic patients with abnormal chromosomes

b. After puberty in dysgenetic patients with normal chromosomes (e.g., in the androgen insensitivity syndrome)

C. Hypogonadotropic amenorrhea. Therapy depends on the patient's desires regarding pregnancy or the presence or absence of regular menses, unless the situation is potentially life threatening, as it is with a pituitary tumor.

1. Patients not desiring pregnancy. Periodic progestin is administered to anovulatory patients who do not desire pregnancy (medroxyprogesterone, 10 mg daily for 5 days every 8 weeks).

2. Patients desiring pregnancy. Ovulation is induced with **clomiphene** or **gonadotropins** in women who desire a pregnancy.

3. Bromocriptine, a dopamine agonist that mimics dopamine inhibition of pituitary prolactin secretion, is recommended for patients with **hyperprolactinemia** accompanied by either a **normal pituitary** or **microadenomas.**

4. Surgery is recommended for **central nervous system tumors.**

5. Thyroid or adrenal medication is given as indicated.

STUDY QUESTIONS

DIRECTIONS: Each of the numbered items or incomplete statements in this section is followed by answers or by completions of the statement. Select the ONE lettered answer or completion that is BEST in each case.

1. Which of the following statements regarding the testicular feminization syndrome is correct?

(A) The testosterone level is in the male range, resulting in pubic and axillary hair
(B) The gonads should not be removed until after full sexual development
(C) The risk of dysgerminoma or other gonadal neoplasms is high until 20 years of age
(D) Pubescence is delayed because of the absence of endogenous hormones
(E) None of the above statements is true

2. Which of the following conditions is suitable for clomiphene citrate stimulation?

(A) Gonadal dysgenesis
(B) Asherman's syndrome
(C) Resistant ovary syndrome
(D) Psychogenic amenorrhea
(E) Kallmann's syndrome

3. In which of the following cases is it necessary to remove the gonads at the time the diagnosis is made?

(A) Androgen insensitivity syndrome (46,XY)
(B) Turner's syndrome (45,XO)
(C) Pure gonadal dysgenesis (46,XY)
(D) Kallmann's syndrome (46,XX)
(E) None of the above

4. Which of the following conditions is considered a relative emergency in a teenager with amenorrhea?

(A) Vaginal agenesis
(B) Turner's syndrome
(C) Uterine anomaly
(D) Imperforate hymen
(E) Androgen insensitivity syndrome

DIRECTIONS: Each of the numbered items or incomplete statements in this section is negatively phrased, as indicated by a capitalized word such as NOT, LEAST, or EXCEPT. Select the ONE lettered answer or completion that is BEST in each case.

5. Which of the following is NOT associated with the development of Asherman's syndrome?

(A) Delivery
(B) Endometriosis
(C) Dilation and curettage
(D) Postabortal hemorrhage
(E) Tuberculosis

6. Which of the following is NOT necessary for the establishment and maintenance of menstruation?

(A) Gonadotropin-releasing hormone
(B) An endometrium responsive to sex steroids
(C) Gonadotropins
(D) Patent fallopian tubes
(E) Ovarian steroidal hormones

DIRECTIONS: The set of matching questions in this section consists of a list of four to twenty-six lettered options (some of which may be in figures) followed by several numbered items. For each numbered item, select the ONE lettered option that is most closely associated with it. To avoid spending too much time on matching sets with large numbers of options, it is generally advisable to begin each set by reading the list of options. Then, for each item in the set, try to generate the correct answer and locate it in the option list, rather than evaluating each option individually. Each lettered option may be selected once, more than once, or not at all.

Questions 7–9

For each of the following clinical situations, select the laboratory study that would be most appropriate.

(A) Measurement of gonadotropin levels
(B) Measurement of serum prolactin levels
(C) Progesterone challenge
(D) Measurement of thyroid-stimulating hormone (TSH) levels
(E) Measurement of serum testosterone levels

7. A 24-year-old nulligravida stopped taking birth control pills to conceive. She had a menstrual flow after the last pack of birth control pills and then was amenorrheic for 6 months.

8. A 24-year-old primipara returns 6 months after delivery complaining of amenorrhea. Her pregnancy terminated with a cesarean section because of abruptio placentae and fetal distress, with an estimated blood loss of 2000 ml from a transient coagulation problem.

9. A 24-year-old woman with previously normal menstrual cycles begins to have irregular cycles and anovulation. Serum prolactin levels are elevated.

ANSWERS AND EXPLANATIONS

1. The answer is B [III B 4]. One of the entities associated with normal chromosomes in the group of diseases characterized by gonadal dysgenesis is the XY gonad found in the testicular feminization syndrome. That gonad has a much lower malignant potential than the dysgenetic gonad with Y material and abnormal chromosomes. Pubescence occurs normally in patients with testicular feminization; therefore, they should not have their gonads removed until after sexual development has occurred. In these patients, the risk of dysgerminoma or other gonadal neoplasms is minimal until the patient is older than 20 years of age.

2. The answer is D [IV B; VI C 2]. Women with amenorrheas associated with low gonadotropin levels are candidates for clomiphene therapy if they desire pregnancy; these include women with psychogenic (emotional stress) amenorrheas. Clomiphene citrate is an ovulation-inducing drug that stimulates the pituitary gland to secrete the gonadotropins necessary to induce the ovaries to ovulate. Therefore, clomiphene would not be useful in clinical conditions in which the gonadotropin levels are already high, such as gonadal dysgenesis or resistant ovary syndrome. The amenorrhea of Asherman's syndrome is caused by intrauterine adhesions, not low gonadotropin levels. There is a defect in gonadotropin synthesis in Kallmann's syndrome, so clomiphene would not help in that clinical condition.

3. The answer is C [III B 1; VI B 3 a, b]. Because of its malignant potential, the XY gonad of pure gonadal dysgenesis should be removed before puberty or at the time of diagnosis of the condition. It is not necessary to remove the gonads in a patient with either Turner's syndrome or Kallmann's syndrome because neither gonad has malignant potential; in Turner's syndrome, a chromosome is missing, and in Kallmann's syndrome, the chromosomes are normal. Androgen insensitivity syndrome is characterized by gonads that are XY; however, the gonads do not have to be removed until after full sexual development because the risk of gonadal neoplasms is low before age 20 years.

4. The answer is D [II A 2 a, b]. Transverse vaginal septum and imperforate hymen in a teenager with pelvic pain demand immediate attention. In both cases, the vaginal outlet, which is blocked, must be opened to prevent the continued reflux of menstrual material into the pelvis, with the potential for endometriosis and impaired fertility. Although vaginal agenesis and uterine anomalies result in reproductive failure, they are not medical emergencies. Turner's syndrome needs to be diagnosed and estrogen therapy started for the development of secondary sexual characteristics, but this is not an emergency. Likewise, the androgen insensitivity syndrome must be diagnosed, but the extirpation of those gonads should await the full development of the secondary sexual characteristics.

5. The answer is B [II B 1, 2]. Endometriosis plays no role in the establishment of intrauterine adhesions. Asherman's syndrome, characterized by intrauterine adhesions, which partially or completely obliterate the uterine cavity, is an acquired form of uterine dysfunction. A common history preceding the establishment of the adhesions involves the curettage of a postpartum or a postabortal uterus on which is superimposed an endometritis. Postabortal hemorrhage may be a component in the pathophysiology of Asherman's syndrome in that it may have been the reason for the curettage. Tuberculosis can lead to the scarring of the endometrial cavity and amenorrhea, but this disease is rare in the United States.

6. The answer is D [I B 1–4]. Menstruation depends on a series of interrelated events that culminate in the visible discharge of menstrual blood. It is a cascade phenomenon that involves the stimulation of the pituitary by gonadotropin-releasing hormone with secretion of gonadotropins. These gonadotropins stimulate the ovary to release steroidal hormones (estrogen and progesterone), which produce changes in a responsive endometrium. This whole process takes place with or without patent fallopian tubes because the tubes are not involved in menstruation.

7–9. The answers are: 7-B [IV E 1; V C 1 b, d], **8-A** [IV F 2; V C 2 a], **9-D** [V C 1 d (2) (c)]. The most important diagnosis to make in an amenorrheic woman coming off birth control pills is a pituitary adenoma. The patient could be amenorrheic because of the pills, but it is essential not to miss a pituitary lesion. Thus, measurement of serum prolactin should be the first test ordered.

From the clinical history of the 24-year-old primipara, the physician can assume that the patient was in shock and suffered ischemia or necrosis of the pituitary gland. In this situa-tion, there may be deficiencies of all the pituitary tropic hormones. Amenorrhea is the most obvious sign, so measurement of gonadotropin levels would be the appropriate test in this patient.

One cause of hyperprolactinemia is an elevated thyroid-stimulating hormone (TSH) level with stimulation of the lactotropes found in hypothyroidism. Thus, measurement of TSH levels would be indicated to rule out hypothyroidism as the cause of the hyperprolactinemia.

Chapter 34

Hirsutism

William W. Beck, Jr.

I. **INTRODUCTION. Increased hair growth in a woman** may be associated with normal or increased levels of **circulating androgens.** It is important to view hirsutism as a potential endocrine abnormality as well as a psychological and cosmetic problem.

A. **Definitions**

1. **Hypertrichosis** involves excessive growth of nonsexual hair, including eyebrows, eyelashes, and hair on the forearms and lower legs.

2. **Hirsutism** involves increased growth of male-like, pigmented, terminal hairs on midline portions of the body, including the face, chest, abdomen, and inner thigh. It may be associated with amenorrhea, anovulatory or dysfunctional uterine bleeding, or infertility.

3. **Virilization** involves hirsutism associated with increased muscle mass, clitorimegaly, temporal balding, voice deepening, and increased libido. There may also be signs of defeminization, such as decreased breast size and loss of vaginal lubrication.

B. **Etiology.** Cosmetically disturbing hirsutism is the result of:

1. The **number of hair follicles present** (e.g., hirsutism is rarely seen in Asian women, who have low concentrations of hair follicles)

2. The degree to which androgens are actively available to convert **vellus hairs,** which are finely textured and relatively unpigmented, to **terminal hairs,** which are coarse, thick, and pigmented, in the male sexual hair areas

3. The level of 5α-reductase activity in the skin

4. The ratio of growth to resting phases in affected hair follicles

5. The thickness and degree to which individual hairs are pigmented

II. **ANDROGENS.** Androgens are steroids that promote the development of masculine secondary sexual characteristics. In women, androgens are thought to be derived from three major sources—from the adrenal gland and the ovary as well as from the peripheral transformation of **androstenedione** to **testosterone.** This transformation is thought to occur in the **liver,** with extrahepatic conversion in tissues, such as **skin,** particularly in patients who manifest hirsutism. The **most important androgen is testosterone.**

A. **Total testosterone.** Blood testosterone levels are a function of blood production rates and metabolic clearance rates; thus, blood levels may not represent the actual state of androgenicity.

1. **Total testosterone levels** are as follows:
   a. **Normal women:** 30 ng/100 ml
   b. **Hirsute women:** 120 ng/100 ml
   c. **Men:** 600 ng/100 ml

2. **Circulating testosterone in women** is derived from the following sources:
   a. Ovarian origin (probably the stroma): 25%
   b. Adrenal origin: 25%
   c. Peripheral transformation of androstenedione to testosterone: 50%

3. **Free testosterone**

    a. Most testosterone in the blood circulates bound either to **albumin** (19%) or to a **binding globulin** (80%); only a small portion exists in the free form.
      (1) Normal women: 1.0%
      (2) Hirsute women: 2.0%
      (3) Men: 2% to 3%
    b. Androgenicity depends mainly on the unbound fraction of testosterone.

B. **Sex hormone binding globulin (SHBG)**

    1. Most circulating testosterone is tightly bound and is not biologically active.

    2. There is an inverse relationship between SHBG and the percentage of free testosterone. As SHBG decreases, the percentage of free testosterone increases; when SHBG increases, the percentage of free testosterone decreases.
      a. There is a **decrease in plasma SHBG** in:
        (1) Obesity
        (2) Increased androgen production
        (3) Corticosteroid therapy
        (4) Hypothyroidism
        (5) Acromegaly
      b. There is an **increase in plasma SHBG** with:
        (1) Estrogen therapy
        (2) Pregnancy
        (3) Hyperthyroidism
        (4) Cirrhosis

    3. Hirsute women in general have reduced serum concentrations of SHBG.

C. **5α-Reductase**

    1. 5α-Reductase converts testosterone to **dihydrotestosterone (DHT)** in androgen-sensitive tissues, such as hair follicles and skin.

    2. 5α-Reductase levels are significantly elevated in the skin of hirsute women compared to control subjects.

    3. DHT is thought to be responsible for stimulating hair growth and is two to three times as potent as testosterone.

    4. **3α-Androstanediol glucuronide (3α-AG)** is the peripheral tissue metabolite of DHT and has been used as a marker of target tissue cellular action.

D. **Pathophysiology of hirsutism** involves a combination of the following:

    1. Increased concentration of serum androgens, especially free testosterone

    2. Decreased levels of SHBG, resulting in an increase in the percentage of free or bioavailable androgen

    3. Increased activity of 5α-reductase

III. CLASSIFICATION

A. **Patients with regular menstrual cycles**

    1. Intrinsic factors
      a. Genetic: racial, familial, and individual differences
      b. Physiologic: premature pubarche, precocious puberty, puberty, pregnancy, and menopause
      c. Idiopathic

    2. Extrinsic factors
      a. Local trauma

     b. Drug-related factors
       (1) Without virilization
         (a) Phenytoin
         (b) Diazoxide
         (c) Hexachlorobenzene
         (d) Adrenocorticotropic hormone
         (e) Corticosteroids
       (2) With potential virilization
         (a) Progestins
         (b) Anabolic agents
         (c) Androgen therapy

  3. Hamartomas or nevi
    a. Pigmented nevi with hair
    b. Nevus pilosus
    c. Pigmented hairy epidermal nevus

B. **Patients with irregular menstrual cycles**

  1. Disorders of adrenal origin
    a. Congenital or adult-onset adrenal hyperplasia
    b. Androgen-producing tumors

  2. Disorders of ovarian origin
    a. Polycystic ovary disease (Stein-Leventhal syndrome)
    b. Androgen-producing tumors
      (1) Arrhenoblastoma
      (2) Granulosa–theca cell tumor
      (3) Luteoma of pregnancy
    c. Hyperthecosis
    d. Chronic anovulation associated with:
      (1) Hypothalamic amenorrhea
      (2) Emotional disorders
      (3) Thyroid disease

  3. Disorders of pituitary origin
    a. Cushing's syndrome
    b. Acromegaly

  4. Intersex problems
    a. Pseudohermaphroditism
    b. Gonadal dysgenesis (Turner's syndrome) with androgenic manifestations

IV. DIAGNOSIS

A. **History.** Important factors to note while taking a history include:

  1. The onset of hirsutism
    a. Gradual. A gradual onset of hirsutism is often associated with acne, weight gain, and increasing irregularity of the menstrual cycles, as is seen with polycystic ovary disease.
    b. Abrupt. An abrupt onset of hirsutism is often associated with signs of virilization, as is seen with androgen-producing tumors.

  2. The **presence or absence of other virilizing signs**

  3. Drug ingestion

  4. The **presence or absence of regular menstrual cycles.** Patients with regular menstrual cycles almost always have idiopathic, ethnic, or familial hirsutism; workup of these patients is unnecessary.

B. **Blood studies**

1. **Serum testosterone** is a marker of ovarian and adrenal activity.
   a. **Total testosterone levels of less than 200 μg/100 ml** (which decrease with birth control pills or prednisone administration) are usually associated with polycystic ovary disease.
   b. **Total testosterone levels of more than 200 μg/100 ml** suggest a tumor.
      (1) A **computed axial tomography scan** is indicated to define the location of the tumor.
      (2) **Laparoscopy** can be helpful in ruling out an ovarian neoplasm.

2. **Serum dehydroepiandrosterone sulfate (DHEAS)** is a marker for adrenal secretory activity.
   a. **A level above 700 μg/100 ml,** which can be suppressed with dexamethasone, suggests adrenal hyperplasia.
   b. Elevated DHEAS levels that cannot be suppressed suggest an adrenal tumor.

3. **Serum androstenedione.** Elevated levels of androstenedione suggest ovarian disease.

4. **Serum 3α-AG**
   a. **Increased levels of 3α-AG** indicate an increased activity of 5α-reductase in the periphery.
   b. 3α-AG is a measure of peripheral target tissue activity.

5. **Serum 17-hydroxyprogesterone**
   a. **17-Hydroxyprogesterone** is an intermediate metabolite in the steroidogenesis process in the adrenal.
   b. As an intermediate metabolite, it is elevated in the various enzyme deficiencies (i.e., 21-hydroxylase and 11β-hydroxylase deficiencies) seen in congenital adrenal hyperplasia (CAH). CAH can be an inherited disorder; it can be seen in other family members.

6. **Cortisol.** Elevated serum levels suggest Cushing's syndrome.

7. **Gonadotropins.** Levels of luteinizing hormone (LH) relatively elevated over those of follicle-stimulating hormone (FSH) suggest polycystic ovary disease.

V. TREATMENT

A. **Goal**

1. Patients should be told that the **goal of therapy,** because of the pathophysiology of hirsutism, is the **arrest of the virilizing process,** not the removal of hair.

2. Once terminal hair has been established in the area of sexual hair, withdrawal of the androgen does not affect the established hair pattern.

3. **Amelioration of a specific disease state** does not rid one totally of the excess hair growth, but it does help to slow the rate of growth.

B. **Elimination of specific causes**

1. Removal of ovarian or adrenal tumors

2. Elimination of drugs suspected to contribute to the abnormal hair growth

3. Suppression with prednisone or dexamethasone of the adrenal contribution to the androgen pool

4. Treatment for Cushing's syndrome, hypothyroidism, or acromegaly

5. Clomiphene induction for ovulatory cycles in patients with polycystic ovary disease; possible bilateral ovarian wedge resection for patients with ongoing hirsutism and anovulation who are resistant to clomiphene therapy

C. **Reduction of gonadotropins**

1. In most **idiopathic or ovarian-related hirsutism,** suppression of ovarian steroidogenesis is the goal.

2. The **combination oral contraceptives** have both a potent negative feedback effect on the pituitary and other effects that ameliorate peripheral androgen stimulation.
   a. Both **estrogen** and **progestin** in the oral contraceptives cause a decrease in gonadotropin secretion with a consequent decrease of ovarian steroidogenesis (i.e., ovarian production of androstenedione, and testosterone).
      (1) **Estrogen** causes increased binding of testosterone by stimulating the increase of SHBG.
      (2) **Progestin** can displace active androgens at the hair follicle level in the skin.
   b. Blood testosterone levels are effectively suppressed within 1 to 3 months of suppression therapy; this reduction has been associated with a clinical improvement in the progression of hirsutism.

3. **Medroxyprogesterone acetate,** 150 mg intramuscularly every 3 months, is effective in suppressing gonadotropin secretion in patients for whom oral contraceptives are contraindicated.
   a. There is decreased production of androgens.
   b. There is an increased clearance of testosterone from the circulation.

D. **Androgen antagonists**

1. **Spironolactone** may act at the cellular level by inhibiting 5α-reductase, thereby lowering the rate of conversion of testosterone to DHT.

2. **Cyproterone acetate** is a progestin that acts by blocking androgen receptors at the cellular level.

3. **Cimetidine** is a histamine receptor antagonist that blocks androgen action at the receptor level.

E. **Additional measures**

1. **Supportive therapy** is very important for the hirsute female.
   a. **Realistic goals** should be set, and the patient should understand that the therapy is a long-term process.
   b. **Treatment with the oral contraceptives** may be necessary for 6 to 12 months before an observable diminution of hair growth occurs.

2. Although **shaving** is often undertaken by hirsute women, they should be told that this eventually results in the need for daily shaving.

3. **Chemical depilatories** often produce skin rashes and may also have to be used daily.

4. **Wax depilatories** offer better long-term results than shaving and chemical depilatories.

5. **Bleaching** is often effective with mild cases and can be used early in the treatment.

6. **Plucking of terminal hairs** should be avoided, as it often causes pustule formation and scarring.

7. **Electrolysis,** which involves the destruction of hair follicles, is the main supportive measure; however, it is expensive, time consuming, and uncomfortable.

8. A **combination of hormonal suppression and supportive measures** offers the best long-term results for hirsute patients.

■ STUDY QUESTIONS

DIRECTIONS: Each of the numbered items or incomplete statements in this section is followed by answers or by completions of the statement. Select the ONE lettered answer or completion that is BEST in each case.

1. The least amount of hirsutism would be expected in women of which of the following nationalities?

(A) Italian
(B) Greek
(C) Chinese
(D) Irish
(E) French

2. Measurement of which of the following substances best demonstrates the ovary as the source of excess androgen?

(A) Androstenedione
(B) Dehydroepiandrosterone
(C) Dehydroepiandrosterone sulfate (DHEAS)
(D) 17-Hydroxyprogesterone
(E) Total testosterone

3. Which of the following is the most effective therapy for hirsutism in a young woman with irregular menstrual cycles?

(A) Chemical depilatories
(B) Plucking
(C) Electrolysis
(D) Birth control pills
(E) Bleaching

4. Androgen activity is blocked at the receptor level by which of the following substances?

(A) 5α-Reductase
(B) Spironolactone
(C) Cimetidine
(D) Prednisone
(E) Estrogen

5. The pathophysiology of hirsutism involves which of the following hormone or enzyme changes?

(A) Increased concentration of bound testosterone
(B) Decreased levels of sex hormone binding globulin (SHBG)
(C) Decreased 5α-reductase activity
(D) Increased levels of plasma progesterone
(E) Increased levels of luteinizing hormone (LH)

DIRECTIONS: The numbered item or incomplete statement in this section is negatively phrased, as indicated by a capitalized word such as NOT, LEAST, or EXCEPT. Select the ONE lettered answer or completion that is BEST.

6. Which of the following is NOT associated with a decrease in sex hormone binding globulin (SHBG)?

(A) Corticosteroid therapy
(B) Increased androgen productivity
(C) Hyperthyroidism
(D) Obesity
(E) Acromegaly

DIRECTIONS: The set of matching questions in this section consists of a list of four to twenty-six lettered options (some of which may be in figures) followed by several numbered items. For each numbered item, select the ONE lettered option that is most closely associated with it. To avoid spending too much time on matching sets with large numbers of options, it is generally advisable to begin each set by reading the list of options. Then, for each item in the set, try to generate the correct answer and locate it in the option list, rather than evaluating each option individually. Each lettered option may be selected once, more than once, or not at all.

Questions 7–9

For each of the following clinical presentations, select the laboratory test that would be most helpful in making a clinical diagnosis.

(A) Serum luteinizing hormone (LH) and follicle-stimulating hormone (FSH)
(B) Total serum testosterone
(C) Serum dehydroepiandrosterone sulfate (DHEAS)
(D) Serum 17-hydroxyprogesterone
(E) Serum cortisol

7. A 23-year-old woman gives a history of gradually increasing hair growth associated with an increasingly irregular menstrual pattern. In addition, she is concerned that she has not conceived over the last 18 months.

8. A 25-year-old woman gives a history of an abrupt onset of increased hair growth and amenorrhea. In addition, she complains of significant acne and a marked decrease in her breast size.

9. A 28-year-old woman gives a history of irregular menses over the past year and increased hair growth on her face, chest, and lower abdomen. When asked about her family history, she describes a first cousin who had the same problem and subsequently had a great deal of difficulty getting pregnant.

ANSWERS AND EXPLANATIONS

1. The answer is C [I B 1]. Hirsutism initially depends on the number of hair follicles present. Hirsutism is rarely seen in Asian women because of the low concentration of hair follicles in their skin.

2. The answer is A [IV B 3]. Androstenedione is a preandrogen that is secreted chiefly by the ovary; thus, measurement of androstenedione levels is a good screening test when the ovary is suspected of being the source of excess androgen. Elevated levels of dehydroepiandrosterone and dehydroepiandrosterone sulfate (DHEAS) suggest adrenal disease. Elevated levels of 17-hydroxyprogesterone suggest adrenal hyperplasia due to a 21-hydroxylase deficiency. Total testosterone is not specific enough to pinpoint the ovary as the source of excess androgen.

3. The answer is D [V C 1, 2]. The main goal in treating hirsutism is the elimination of the source of the excess androgens. Chemical depilatories, plucking, electrolysis, and bleaching are local treatments for hirsutism that do not affect the source of the androgens and, thus, the virilizing process. In a young woman with hirsutism and irregular cycles, the most likely source of the androgens is the ovary. By suppressing ovarian activity with birth control pills, ovarian steroidogenesis is decreased, and the secretion of the preandrogens is markedly reduced.

4. The answer is C [V D 3]. An androgen antagonist is often the only therapy that can be offered for the treatment of hirsutism for which there is no specific cause. Cimetidine is a histamine receptor antagonist that blocks androgen at the receptor level. Spironolactone inhibits the enzyme 5α-reductase, lowering the rate of conversion of testosterone to dihydrotestosterone. Prednisone, a corticosteroid, stimulates hair growth. Estrogen competes with androgen but does not block androgen activity at the receptor level.

5. The answer is B [II D 1–3]. Excessive hair growth depends on an increased availability of the biologically active androgen, testosterone. This can occur either by an increase in

the amount of free testosterone or an increase in the conversion of testosterone to dihydrotestosterone (DHT) within the cell. Thus, an increased amount of free, not bound, testosterone; an increase, not a decrease, in 5α-reductase activity; or a decrease in the concentration of sex hormone binding globulin (SHBG) with the consequent increase in free testosterone are expected in hirsutism. Plasma progesterone, a luteal phase component of the ovarian cycle, is not involved in the pathogenesis of hirsutism. Increased levels of luteinizing hormone (LH) may suggest polycystic ovarian disease, but this is not directly involved in the pathophysiology of hirsutism.

6. The answer is C [II B]. Sex hormone binding globulin (SHBG) is a key factor in determining androgen activity. As SHBG increases, there is an increased binding of testosterone and, thus, less free testosterone to exert biologic activity; with a decrease in SHBG, there is an increase in free testosterone. The conditions that decrease SHBG are increased androgen production, obesity, hypothyroidism, acromegaly, and corticosteroid therapy. Estrogen therapy, pregnancy, and hyperthyroidism tend to increase SHBG.

7–9. The answers are: 7-A, 8-B, 9-D [IV A 1, B 1–7]. The clinical picture of the 23-year-old woman with a history of gradually increasing hair growth is characteristic of polycystic ovary disease. Measurement of serum dehydroepiandrosterone sulfate (DHEAS), 17-hydroxyprogesterone, and cortisol would indicate adrenal disease. Total testosterone levels may be elevated, but the serum luteinizing hormone (LH) and follicle-stimulating hormone (FSH) would be more specific than total testosterone. In polycystic ovary disease, LH levels are constantly elevated over those of FSH.

The abrupt onset of both hirsutism and defeminizing signs (amenorrhea and decreased breast size) is suggestive of an androgen-producing tumor, such as arrhenoblastoma. In this case, the most definitive test would be measurement of total testosterone because testosterone would be the chief secretory product of the tumor, and levels would be markedly elevated.

The history of hirsutism developing in a woman with a family member having the same story suggests a late-onset or acquired congenital adrenal hyperplasia. In this abnormality, there is an enzyme deficiency (21-hydroxylase or 11β-hydroxylase), which leads to a decreased cortisol production from the adrenals. 17-Hydroxyprogesterone is an intermediate metabolite in the steroidogenesis process in the adrenal. If there is a block in that pathway, the intermediate metabolites will build up and can be measured. In this case, serum 17-hydroxyprogesterone level measurement would be diagnostic.

Chapter 35

Menopause
Michelle Battistini

I. DEFINITIONS

A. Menopause

1. **Menopause** is that point in time when there is a **permanent cessation of menses because of a loss of ovarian activity.**

2. The cessation of menses reflects the reduction of ovarian estrogen production to **levels insufficient to produce proliferation of the endometrial lining.**

3. Menses usually cease between the **ages of 50 and 52 years;** the median age of menopause is 51.3 years, with a range of 48 to 55 years.

4. **Premature menopause** is defined as the permanent cessation of menses occurring before age 40 years.

B. Perimenopause

1. The **perimenopause** refers to the period of time just before and after the menopause, usually spanning the age from 45 to 55 years.

2. The **transition** is a term used to describe the years leading up to and preceding the menopause.
   a. This period of time is marked by menstrual cycle irregularity, reflecting a gradual decline in and fluctuation of ovarian function.
   b. The median age of onset of menstrual irregularity is 47.5 years; the transition lasts an average of 4 years. Ten percent of women abruptly stop menstruating without preceding cycle irregularity.

C. Climacteric

1. **Climacteric** is a broad term encompassing the transitional years, the menopause, and the postmenopausal years.

2. This period of time reflects the decline and loss of ovarian function and the long-term consequences of reduced estrogen levels.

II. PHYSIOLOGY OF THE PERIMENOPAUSE

A. Ovarian function.
A period of waxing and waning ovarian function occurs before the menopause; it is a time of fluctuation in hormone production and reduced fecundability.

1. The **number of remaining follicles is reduced** and those remaining are less sensitive to gonadotropin stimulation.

2. Follicular function is variable not only among individual women but from cycle to cycle in each individual.

3. As follicular maturation declines, ovulation becomes less and less frequent as the menopause approaches.

4. Although fertility rates are markedly reduced, **conception** can occur during this time of fluctuating ovarian activity.

B. **Endocrinology**

1. **Inhibin** production by the ovary is dependent on the number of existing ovarian oocytes and therefore is reduced. Inhibin exerts a negative feedback on the secretion of follicle-stimulating hormone (FSH) by the pituitary.

2. An increase in **FSH** levels results from the decreased circulating levels of inhibin and the loss of negative feedback. This is the earliest evidence of a change in ovarian function. Elevated FSH levels can be seen with normal cycles as well as abnormal cycles.

3. **Luteinizing hormone (LH)** secretion escapes the negative feedback of inhibin; levels are not affected by the loss of inhibin production. LH levels rise much later in the transition than FSH levels; sustained elevations may not be seen until after the menopause.

4. **Estradiol** levels fluctuate but remain within the wide range of normal until follicular development ceases altogether.

5. **Progesterone** levels fluctuate depending on the presence and adequacy of ovulation and are frequently low during the transition.

6. **Androgen** levels steadily decline during the transitional period.

C. **Menstrual cycles.** Changes in the menstrual cycle reflect changes in ovarian function and circulating levels of ovarian steroids and pituitary gonadotropins.

1. Changes in menstrual cycle regularity occur as a woman progresses through her forties.
   a. Cycle length is determined by the length of the follicular phase.
   b. Cycle length is variable and may be normal, shortened, or prolonged.

2. **Shortening of cycle length** occurs early in the transition and is associated with ovulatory cycles, a shortened follicular phase, and elevated FSH levels.

3. **Anovulatory cycles** and **prolonged cycles** become more frequent as the menopause approaches, resulting in dysfunctional uterine bleeding (DUB) and oligomenorrhea.

III. PHYSIOLOGY OF THE MENOPAUSE

A. **Ovarian function.** Follicular reserve is depleted and is manifested by a permanent cessation in menses.

1. There are **few remaining follicular units present in the postmenopausal ovary,** and those present are no longer capable of a normal response despite stimulation by markedly elevated gonadotropins.
   a. **FSH receptors** are absent on a cellular level.
   b. **Estradiol** production by the ovary depends on FSH stimulation and is negligible in the postmenopausal ovary.
   c. **Estrone,** a less potent estrogen, is also produced in negligible amounts by the postmenopausal ovary.

2. **Ovarian stromal tissue** continues to produce androgenic steroid hormones for several years after the menopause.
   a. Although there is a lack of FSH receptors, ovarian stromal cells possess LH receptors and respond with the production of **ovarian androgens** [i.e., androstenedione, testosterone, dehydroepiandrosterone (DHA)].
   b. **Androstenedione** and **DHA** production continues, but at a decreased rate; **testosterone** production remains stable or may be slightly increased.

3. When menses have been absent for 1 year, conception is no longer an issue.

B. **Endocrinology**

1. **FSH levels** are elevated 10 to 20 times above premenopausal levels, reaching a plateau 1 to 3 years after the menopause, after which there is a gradual decline. This reflects loss of the negative feedback effects of both inhibin and estradiol. FSH levels never return to the premenopausal range even with estrogen replacement therapy, reflecting the influence of inhibin.

2. **LH levels** rise two- to threefold after the menopause, reaching a plateau in 1 to 3 years, after which there is a gradual decline. This reflects the loss of the negative feedback effect of estradiol. LH levels never reach those of FSH because of the shorter circulating half-life of LH (30 minutes as opposed to 4 hours).

3. Although there is negligible **ovarian estrogen production** after the menopause, there is individual variation in circulating estrogen levels as a result of peripheral conversion of androgenic precursors to estrone. Estrone, a less potent estrogen, is the principal estrogen after the menopause.
   a. **Androgens,** which serve as precursors for estrogen, continue to be produced by the postmenopausal ovary and the adrenal gland.
   b. **Aromatase enzymes** that convert androgens to estrone primarily, and estradiol to a lesser degree, are present in peripheral tissues but predominantly in adipose tissue.
   c. Estrogen levels vary with the degree of adiposity; **obesity** can lead to a state of relative estrogen excess.

4. **Peripheral testosterone levels** are decreased despite sustained or increased production rates by the ovary. Circulating testosterone levels are the net result of androstenedione and testosterone production by the adrenal gland and the ovary.
   a. Testosterone and androstenedione production by the adrenal gland does not decrease for several years after the menopause.
   b. Testosterone production by the ovaries does not decrease for several years after the menopause.
   c. Androstenedione production by the ovary is markedly reduced after the menopause and accounts for the fall in circulating testosterone levels characteristic of this time.

5. **DHA levels** are reduced after the menopause; dehydroepiandrosterone sulfate levels, which reflect adrenal gland activity, are unchanged.

C. **Menstrual cycles.** Menopause is the permanent cessation of the menses.

1. Menopause is a retrospective diagnosis and is said to have occurred when there is the absence of menses for 12 months in a woman older than 45 years of age.

2. The reduced level of estrogen is no longer sufficient to induce endometrial proliferative changes capable of producing menstruation.

D. **Premature menopause** or **premature ovarian failure** is the cessation of menses in a woman younger than 40 years of age.

1. The frequency of premature ovarian failure is 0.3%. This is the diagnosis in 5% to 10% of women with secondary amenorrhea (hypergonadotropic amenorrhea).

2. Most women with premature menopause undergo premature oocyte atresia and follicular depletion. This results from one of three mechanisms:
   a. Decreased initial germ cell number at birth
   b. Accelerated oocyte atresia after birth
   c. Postnatal germ cell destruction

3. A small number of affected women have abundant remaining follicles and elevated gonadotropins, suggesting a blockade of gonadotropin stimulation or biologically inactive gonadotropins.

4. Etiologies of premature ovarian failure and hypergonadotropic amenorrhea are diverse and fall under one of the following categories:

    a. Genetic and cytogenetic abnormalities
    b. Enzymatic defects
    c. Physical insults
    d. Autoimmune disturbances
    e. Abnormal gonadotropin structure or function
    f. Idiopathic

IV. CLINICAL MANIFESTATIONS OF THE PERIMENOPAUSE

A. **Manifestations of estrogen excess.** During the perimenopause, some women present with evidence of estrogen excess, rather than deficiency.

1. **DUB** is abnormal uterine bleeding that is excessive in amount, duration, and frequency secondary to prolonged exposure of the uterine lining to estrogen stimulation unopposed by progesterone.

   a. Anovulatory cycles, common to the perimenopausal transition, result in unopposed estrogen stimulation of the endometrial lining and result in DUB. DUB occurs with increased frequency in perimenopausal women.

   b. Increased endogenous estrogen can also be the result of increased peripheral conversion of androgen precursors to estrone and estradiol. This is most frequently seen in the obese perimenopausal woman.

   c. Less commonly, pathologic conditions are associated with increased estrogen production (ovarian tumors), or decreased metabolic clearance of estrogen (hepatic or renal disease), leading to elevated circulating estrogen levels.

2. **Endometrial neoplasia**

   a. Prolonged unopposed estrogen stimulation of the endometrial lining can lead to endometrial pathology, which manifests itself as **abnormal uterine bleeding.**

   b. Abnormal uterine bleeding that occurs in a woman older than 40 years of age, or in a younger woman as a result of prolonged anovulatory cycles, must be evaluated with sampling of the endometrium to rule out organic disease. **Endometrial biopsy** is usually sufficient; **dilation and curettage (D and C)** is performed when biopsy results are not conclusive.

   c. **Simple hyperplasia** has a low risk of progression to endometrial carcinoma and can be treated medically.

   d. **Complex hyperplasia without atypia** is a more advanced type of hyperplasia with a small but present risk of endometrial carcinoma. Complex hyperplasia can also be treated medically, including posttreatment biopsy.

   e. **Complex hyperplasia with atypia** is associated with an increased risk of an associated carcinoma; further evaluation with hysteroscopy and D and C is warranted before treatment. Because of a 25% risk of progression to endometrial carcinoma, surgery is the treatment of first choice for this condition.

   f. **Carcinoma of the endometrium** should be suspected in all women older than 40 years of age who present with abnormal bleeding and effectively ruled out with endometrial sampling; 20% of postmenopausal bleeding is secondary to a carcinoma.

B. **Manifestations of hormonal fluctuation**

1. **Menstrual cycle changes.** Some change in the character of the menstrual cycle is the most common manifestation of the perimenopause.

   a. **Menorrhagia** is increased blood flow (>80 ml) at the time of menses. Cycles are regular in timing and ovulatory in nature. Increased flow may result from a relative reduction in progesterone levels.

   b. **Polymenorrhea** is frequent menses. Shortening of cycle length is a common change reported early in the transition. Cycle length remains longer than 21 days but is typically shorter than cycles experienced during the reproductive years. Cycles are ovulatory with a shortened follicular phase.

    c. Midcycle spotting. With a drop in estradiol levels just before ovulation, mid-cycle estrogen withdrawal bleeding may occur.

    d. Oligomenorrhea. As the menopause approaches, missed periods are common and cycle length increases until a permanent cessation of menses occurs.

2. Other symptoms. Many women who are still menstruating experience a variety of symptoms traditionally attributed to the menopause. These symptoms are thought to result from the fluctuation of hormone levels that occurs from cycle to cycle.

    a. Hot flashes/flushes. Many women experience hot flushes before the menopause; frequently, their occurrence is not consistent from cycle to cycle.

    b. Headaches. Premenstrual migraines may appear or worsen during this time period.

    c. Premenstrual psychological symptoms. Some women report the onset or worsening of premenstrual symptoms, such as depression, anxiety, and irritability, during the transitional years.

    d. Sleep disturbances. Interrupted sleep, with or without hot flushes, is often reported by women during these years.

C. **Therapy**

1. Progesterone supplementation. Periodic administration of a progestin is used to treat conditions associated with estrogen excess.

    a. DUB is a result of anovulatory cycles and unopposed estrogen stimulation of the endometrium. Intermittent progestin therapy (medroxyprogesterone acetate) provides estrogen antagonism and allows for the orderly sloughing of the endometrium. This serves two purposes: to prevent uncontrolled uterine bleeding, and to prevent the development of endometrial hyperplasia.

        (1) Medroxyprogesterone acetate, 10 to 30 mg for 10 to 14 days each month, is administered for 3 to 6 months. Therapy may be continued for the long term until there is a lack of withdrawal bleeding. No further bleeding signifies a reduction of estrogen levels to the menopausal range.

        (2) Norethindrone acetate can be substituted for women who do not tolerate medroxyprogesterone acetate.

    b. Simple and complex hyperplasia can be treated effectively with progestin supplementation. Treatment with medroxyprogesterone acetate as described for DUB is prescribed. Follow-up biopsy is performed after 3 months of treatment to verify resolution of the hyperplasia.

    c. Complex hyperplasia with atypia can be treated with high-dose progestin if surgical therapy is not an option, after the presence of carcinoma has been effectively excluded. Follow-up biopsy after 3 months of treatment is mandatory to verify resolution.

        (1) Medroxyprogesterone acetate, 30 mg/day, is given daily for 3 months.

        (2) Megestrol, 20 to 60 mg, is given daily for 3 months.

2. Oral contraceptives are an attractive alternative in the woman older than 40 years of age who is a nonsmoker.

    a. Low-dose oral contraceptives (<35 μg) are effective treatment for abnormal bleeding associated with the perimenopause.

    b. Oral contraceptives often provide relief of other symptoms noted by women in this age group.

    c. Oral contraceptives are also an effective method of contraception for the woman older than 40 years, and carry no increased risk in the nonsmoker.

    d. Because oral contraceptives contain five to seven times the estrogen equivalent of postmenopausal hormone replacement therapy, it is desirable to change therapy with the onset of menopause. FSH levels are obtained annually after the age of 45 years on day 5 to 7 of the menstrual cycle. Oral contraceptives are stopped when the serum FSH level is greater than 30 IU/L.

3. Hormone replacement therapy

    a. Estrogen replacement therapy can be used to treat perimenopausal symptoms in the woman with oligomenorrhea before permanent cessation of menses.

      b. Progesterone is added sequentially or continuously to provide endometrial protection.

  4. Nonsteroidal antiinflammatory drugs (NSAIDs)
    a. NSAIDs can effectively reduce menstrual blood flow by 40% to 60% in women with ovulatory cycles.
    b. NSAIDs may be useful in the treatment of menstrual migraines.

V. CLINICAL MANIFESTATIONS OF THE MENOPAUSE

A. **Target organ response to decreased estrogen.** Estrogen-responsive tissues are present throughout the body. Chronic reduction of estrogen results in the following manifestations.

  1. Urogenital atrophy. The vagina, urethra, bladder, and pelvic floor are estrogen-responsive tissues; decreased estrogen levels after the menopause result in a generalized atrophy of these structures.
    a. There is a reduction in the height of **vaginal epithelium** and decreased vascular flow. The vaginal epithelium becomes pale, thin, and dry. Maturation of the vaginal epithelium is estrogen dependent. After the menopause, there is a shift (regression) in the maturation index, with a preponderance of immature cell types (basal and parabasal) over mature cell types (intermediate and superficial). There is a shift of the vaginal pH from acidic to alkaline.
    b. The vaginal walls lose elasticity and compliance; the **vagina becomes smaller,** and the size of the upper vagina diminishes.
    c. The **labia minora** have a pale, dry appearance, and there is a reduction of the fat content of the **labia majora.**
    d. The **pelvic tissues and ligaments** that support the uterus and the vagina **lose their tone,** predisposing to disorders of pelvic relaxation.
    e. The **epithelium of the urethra and bladder** mucosa becomes atrophic; there is a loss of urethral and bladder wall elasticity and compliance.

  2. Uterine changes
    a. The **endometrial tissue becomes sparse,** with an atrophic appearance.
    b. The **myometrium atrophies,** and the **uterine corpus decreases in size.** There is a reversal of the corpus–cervical length ratio compared to the reproductive years.
    c. The **squamocolumnar junction** relocates high in the endocervical canal; the cervical os frequently becomes stenotic.
    d. Fibroids, if present, reduce in size but do not disappear.

  3. Breasts
    a. There is progressive fatty replacement with atrophy of active glandular units.
    b. There is regression of fibrocystic changes.

  4. Skin. Skin collagen content and skin thickness decrease proportionately with time after the menopause.

  5. Bones. There is an accelerated loss of bone for the first 5 to 7 years after the menopause associated with decreased estrogen levels.
    a. The greatest effect is seen in **trabecular bone,** particularly in the spine.
    b. Excessive loss predisposes to the development of **osteoporosis** and increased fracture risk.

  6. Hair. With the loss of estrogen, there is a relative increase in circulating androgens with a tendency toward the development of increased facial hair and androgenic alopecia.

  7. Brain. Estrogen receptors are located throughout the brain. Reduced estrogen levels may affect cognitive function and moods after the menopause, although the precise contribution has not been fully defined.

8. **Cardiovascular system.** The incidence of cardiovascular disease increases after the age of 50 years in women coincident with the age of menopause.
   a. Estrogen favorably affects the lipid profile.
   b. Estrogen increases coronary and cerebral artery blood flow.
   c. Estrogen favorably affects atherogenic plaque formation.

B. **Symptoms related to estrogen reduction.** Symptoms are the manifestation of target organ response to declining estrogen levels.

1. **Vasomotor instability**
   a. The **hot flash, or flush,** is the most common symptom related to the menopause, occurring in 75% to 85% of perimenopausal women.
   b. The hot flush is the result of **inappropriate stimulation of the body's heat-releasing mechanisms** by the thermoregulatory centers in the hypothalamus. Although core body temperature is normal, the body is stimulated to lose heat. The onset of the flushes initially depends on a reduction of previously established estrogen levels; flushes do not occur in hypoestrogenic states, such as gonadal dysgenesis.
   c. The **flush is characterized** by progressive vasodilatation of the skin over the head, neck, and chest, accompanied by reddening of the skin, a feeling of intense body heat, and perspiration. Palpitations or tachycardia may accompany the flush. The flush may last a few seconds to several minutes and recur with variable frequency.
   d. Flushes appear to be more frequent and severe at night or during times of stress. They also can be precipitated by foods and beverages that are hot or spicy or contain methylxanthines.
   e. The vasomotor instability lasts for **1 to 2 years** in most women, but may last for as long as 5 years or more in up to one third of symptomatic women.
   f. **Estrogen replacement** reduces or eliminates hot flushes.
   g. **Progestins, clonidine, methyldopa, vitamin E, and herbal remedies** are used for the treatment of hot flushes in women in whom estrogen is contraindicated. Relief is not as complete as that seen with estrogen therapy.

2. **Altered menstrual function.** Oligomenorrhea is followed by amenorrhea.
   a. Menopause is defined as amenorrhea for 6 to 12 months in women 45 years of age and older.
   b. If vaginal bleeding occurs after 12 months of amenorrhea, endometrial disease (i.e., polyps, hyperplasia, or neoplasia) must be ruled out.

3. **Vaginal atrophy**
   a. **Dyspareunia** (painful intercourse) is another common symptom related to the menopause.
      (1) Changes in the vaginal epithelium and vaginal vasculature lead to decreased lubrication during sexual activity.
      (2) Decreased compliance and elasticity of the vaginal wall contribute to vaginal stenosis.
   b. **Atrophic vaginitis**
      (1) The postmenopausal vagina becomes more susceptible to pathogenic and nonpathogenic organisms.
      (2) Atrophy of the vaginal mucosa and changes in pH predispose to vaginitis, which presents with symptoms of discharge, pruritus, odor, and irritation.
   c. Symptoms related to vaginal atrophy respond to estrogen therapy.

4. **Urinary tract symptoms**
   a. Changes in the mucosal lining of the urethra and bladder may lead to symptoms of dysuria, nocturia, urinary frequency, urgency, and urgency incontinence.
   b. **Urinary stress incontinence** may progressively worsen after the menopause as a result of urethral changes and a loss of pelvic support.
   c. There is an increased incidence of bacteriuria in the postmenopausal woman compared to women in the premenopausal age group.

    d. Vaginal, urethral, and bladder symptoms improve with estrogen therapy.

5. Osteoporosis
    a. Osteoporosis is a systemic skeletal disease. It is characterized by **low bone mass** and **microarchitectural deterioration of bone structure,** both of which result in fragile bones that are at an increased risk for fracture. Osteoporosis may be a primary disease state or may be secondary to other diseases that affect calcium and bone metabolism.

        (1) Osteoporosis results when **bone resorption outweighs bone formation.** Trabecular bone is at greater risk than cortical bone because it is more metabolically active and structurally more porous. The bones most commonly affected by fracture are the vertebrae, the distal radius, the hip, and the humerus; however, all bones are at risk.

        (2) Peak bone mass is reached in the late twenties for trabecular bone and the early thirties for cortical bone. Thereafter, there is a gradual loss of bone with aging. Bone loss is accelerated for the first 5 to 7 years after the menopause as a direct result of declining estrogen levels. Osteoporosis is more common in women than men because of lower peak bone mass and higher rates of bone loss.

        (3) Risk factors other than age and gender include inadequate calcium intake, sedentary life-style, smoking, alcohol use, premature menopause, genetic predisposition, white and Asian race, chronic glucocorticoid use, and hyperthyroidism, including excessive thyroid replacement.

    b. Osteoporosis has reached epidemic proportions in the United States, with an estimated 1.3 million fractures occurring annually.

        (1) Approximately 25% of white American women older than 60 years of age who are not treated with estrogen replacement have spinal compression fractures.

        (2) Approximately 32% of white American women older than 75 years of age suffer hip fractures; there is an excess mortality rate of 10% to 30% at 1 year after fracture. Thirty percent of survivors no longer live independently.

    c. Osteoporosis is diagnosed late in the course of disease, when fractures typical of the disease occur [e.g., spinal compression fractures (dowager's hump)].

    d. Imaging modalities can be used to detect bone loss and those at risk for fracture earlier in the disease.

        (1) Single photon absorptiometry, used very little today, was the first modality used to measure bone density at the wrist.

        (2) Dual photon absorptiometry also is used very little today because of the use of a radionuclide source and inability to differentiate cortical and trabecular bone.

        (3) Dual energy x-ray absorptiometry is the most popular technique used today to measure bone density. An x-ray tube has replaced the radionuclide source and independent measurements can be made at the hip, spine, and other bone sites.

        (4) Quantitative computed tomography gives the most precise measurement of bone density at specific sites. However, its use has been limited by expense and higher radiation doses.

    e. Prevention of osteoporosis is the key to management. Exercise and adequate calcium intake and estrogen replacement after the menopause play key roles in the prevention of this disease.

6. The menopausal syndrome. This term has been used to include a variety of symptoms, such as fatigue, headache, nervousness, loss of libido, insomnia, depression, irritability, palpitations, and joint and muscle pain.

    a. There is progressive improvement of some of these symptoms with estrogen replacement.

    b. Addition of low doses of androgen in addition to estrogen replacement may enhance the therapeutic response.

    c. The etiology of these symptoms may be multifactorial; underlying medical illness should be considered in the differential diagnosis.

VI. ESTROGEN REPLACEMENT THERAPY

A. Benefits and indications

1. **Treatment of menopausal symptoms**
   a. **Estrogen replacement** usually **eliminates or significantly reduces hot flashes** and night sweats.
      (1) Estrogen decreases the frequency and sensitivity of the flashes.
      (2) **Progestins** alone are less effective than conjugated estrogen, estrone, or estradiol, but may provide relief in women who have contraindications to estrogen use.
   b. Estrogen replacement can be used for relief of symptoms associated with **urogenital atrophy.**
      (1) **Atrophic vaginitis** requires continuous therapy with either systemic or topical estrogen cream.
      (2) **Dyspareunia** can be treated symptomatically with nonhormonal lubricating agents. Estrogen replacement therapy restores vaginal epithelium, vasculature, and tone. Systemic or topical agents can be used on a long-term basis; full response takes 3 to 4 months of use.
      (3) **Urinary symptoms** of urgency, frequency, urgency incontinence, nocturia, and cystitis improve with systemic or topical replacement.
      (4) **Urinary stress incontinence** may improve with estrogen replacement therapy, but usually does not resolve completely.
   c. **Affective symptoms**—depression, insomnia, irritability, and loss of concentration—may improve with estrogen therapy.
      (1) Other etiologies should be considered when little or no response is seen with estrogen replacement.
      (2) Addition of low-dose testosterone may achieve a better therapeutic response.
   d. **Decreased libido** may respond to estrogen replacement therapy.
      (1) Libido may improve after treatment for dyspareunia.
      (2) There are often other underlying factors affecting sexual desire in addition to the hormonal changes associated with the menopausal state.
      (3) Addition of low-dose testosterone may achieve a better therapeutic response than estrogen alone.
   e. **Vaginal relaxation** usually is not responsive to estrogen therapy alone.

2. **Prevention and treatment of osteoporosis**
   a. Estrogen replacement after the menopause is the primary method of **osteoporosis prevention.** Estrogen acts through an **antiresorptive effect.**
      (1) Accelerated bone loss that occurs after the menopause can be prevented with early estrogen replacement therapy. Transdermal and oral preparations are effective in the reduction of bone loss.
      (2) Estrogen replacement is associated with a 50% reduction in fracture risk.
      (3) **Adequate calcium intake** must also be ensured through diet or supplementation:
         (a) 1000 mg elemental calcium if estrogen replacement is also used
         (b) 1500 mg elemental calcium if no estrogen replacement is used
      (4) A regular program of **exercise** is necessary to stimulate bone formation and ensure maintenance of muscle tone.
   b. Estrogen replacement is also used in the **treatment of osteoporosis.** There is a reduction in fracture risk noted even when therapy is started remote from the menopause.
   c. **Other antiresorptive agents** are also used in the treatment of osteoporosis, and include calcitonin and the bisphosphonates.
   d. **Estrogen antagonists** (e.g., tamoxifen) also display an antiresorptive, bone-sparing effect.

3. **Prevention of cardiovascular disease**
   a. Estrogen replacement therapy is associated with a 50% reduction in cardiovascu-

lar disease risk, with a decrease in the incidence of fatal and nonfatal myocardial infarctions.

b. Estrogen replacement is associated with increased long-term survival in women with significant coronary artery stenosis demonstrated on angiography.

(1) Estrogen favorably affects the lipid profile; 30% of estrogen's protective effect is attributed to this.

(a) A 10% reduction in total cholesterol is noted.

(b) A 10% to 20% increase in high-density lipoprotein cholesterol is noted.

(c) A 10% reduction in low-density lipoprotein cholesterol is noted.

(2) Estradiol **dilates coronary arteries** and increases blood flow in both normal and diseased vessels.

(3) Estradiol **inhibits atherogenic plaque formation** in the vessel wall through an antioxidant effect.

c. The effect of **progestin,** added for endometrial protection in standard regimens, has not yet been determined in terms of cardiovascular benefit.

d. Estrogen replacement is associated with a **decreased risk of stroke.**

e. Estrogen replacement is not associated with an increased risk of thromboembolic events.

4. Effects on Alzheimer's dementia. Preliminary information suggests a beneficial effect of estrogen with regard to memory in women with Alzheimer's dementia.

a. Epidemiologic data reveal a decreased incidence of Alzheimer's dementia in women who use estrogen replacement after the menopause.

b. Estrogen is demonstrated to have an effect on metabolism of acetylcholine, a neurotransmitter involved with memory function.

c. Randomized clinical trials, involving small numbers of women with Alzheimer's dementia, demonstrate an **improvement in certain aspects of memory function** associated with estrogen replacement.

B. **Risks and contraindications**

1. Absolute contraindications. The use of estrogen replacement therapy is contraindicated in women with conditions that could potentially worsen with estrogen exposure or conditions that affect the metabolism and clearance of estrogen.

a. Medical conditions related to estrogen exposure

(1) Recent vascular thrombosis

(2) Neuroophthalmologic vascular disease

(3) Recent history of endometrial carcinoma

(4) History of breast cancer (except in certain circumstances)

(5) Undiagnosed vaginal bleeding

b. Conditions related to estrogen metabolism

(1) Acute hepatic disease

(2) Chronically impaired liver function

2. Relative contraindications. The following conditions may worsen with estrogen exposure and therefore are relative contraindications to replacement. However, with adjustments in dosage or route of administration, estrogen replacement therapy is used safely and successfully on an individual basis.

a. Seizure disorders

b. High serum triglycerides

c. Current gallbladder disease

d. Migraine headaches

3. Endometrial cancer. Estrogen therapy increases the risk of endometrial hyperplasia and carcinoma when used without progestin.

a. The **risk of endometrial cancer** and hyperplasia is raised 2- to 20-fold depending on the duration of exposure and dose of estrogen; risk is duration- and dose-dependent.

b. Addition of a progestin for at least 10 days a month reduces that risk to less than 1% to 2%.

c. There is actually a decreased relative risk of endometrial cancer in women who are on combined estrogen and progestin replacement therapy.

d. Estrogen replacement therapy can be considered in women who have been successfully treated for stage I endometrial carcinoma.

4. Breast cancer. The controversy surrounding the risk of breast cancer in women who use estrogen replacement therapy continues; fear of breast cancer is one of the most common reasons women choose not to use estrogen after the menopause.
  a. In the general aging population, the benefits of estrogen replacement therapy still outweigh the risks, including the risk of beast cancer.
    (1) Epidemiologic studies show a 40% decrease in mortality rates from all causes, including cancer, in estrogen replacement therapy users compared to nonusers.
    (2) Estrogen replacement therapy after the menopause is associated with a 50% reduction in fracture risk
  b. There does not appear to be an increased risk associated with estrogen use of short duration, defined as no more than 5 years of use.
  c. There does not appear to be an increased risk in women who have used estrogen replacement therapy in the past.
  d. There is a question of an increased risk in older women with longer duration of use (at least 10 to 15 years).
  e. Because of the significant protective effect in terms of cardiovascular disease, the benefits of long-term estrogen replacement therapy outweigh the risks, in the general population.
  f. The role of estrogen replacement therapy in breast cancer survivors is being investigated.
  g. The addition of progestin does not appear to have a protective effect in terms of breast cancer.

5. Uterine bleeding. The return of periods is another common reason women avoid estrogen replacement therapy after the menopause.
  a. Progestin is added to estrogen therapy to prevent endometrial hyperplasia and carcinoma. This results in withdrawal bleeding, when progestin is given sequentially, or breakthrough bleeding, when progestin is given continuously.
    (1) Progestin given sequentially on a monthly basis (see VI C 3 a) results in regular withdrawal bleeding. The duration and flow usually decrease with time and may cease altogether.
    (2) Progestin given continuously does not induce cyclic bleeding, but is associated with irregular spotting and bleeding, particularly during the first year.
    (3) Progestin is associated with other side effects as well, which are often poorly tolerated, and include depression, irritability, mastalgia, and bloating.
  b. Abnormal bleeding that occurs on estrogen replacement therapy must be evaluated with **endometrial sampling** to rule out endometrial disease.
  c. Abnormal bleeding that continues after sampling and appropriate management should be evaluated with **hysteroscopy** or **sonohysterography.**

C. Current standard regimens

  1. Unopposed estrogen. Estrogen is given unopposed and on a daily basis.
    a. This is the treatment of choice in **women who have undergone hysterectomy.**
    b. This regimen can be used in the woman who cannot tolerate side effects related to progestational agents, provided there is adequate surveillance of the endometrial lining. **Endometrial biopsy on an annual basis** is recommended.

  2. Cyclic combined therapy
    a. Estrogen is given on days 1 to 25 of the month; the progestin is given for the last 10 days of the cycle, days 16 to 25.
    b. This is the original combined regimen designed to **mirror most closely the natural menstrual cycle;** bleeding patterns are most predictable on this regimen.
    c. There is no advantage in terms of endometrial protection; patients often become symptomatic on the hormone-free days.

  3. Sequential combined therapy

a. Estrogen is administered every day; progestin is administered for 10 to 14 days every month. The duration of progestin increases with a decrease in the dose.
b. Bleeding occurs on completion of the progestin.

4. Continuous combined therapy
 a. Estrogen and progestin are administered on a daily basis. There are **advantages** to maintaining a constant hormonal environment.
  (1) There is no scheduled withdrawal bleeding or resumption of menstrual-like bleeding; this was the initial reason this therapy was introduced.
  (2) Symptoms that worsen with hormonal fluctuations are improved, and include mood disturbances, migraines, and cyclic mastalgia.
  (3) The regimen is easy for patients to remember.
 b. The **disadvantage** to this regimen is the occurrence of irregular spotting and bleeding in up to 40% of women during the first year. This becomes a source of concern for the patient and physician and an indication for biopsy.

5. Periodic progestin
 a. Progestin is administered for 14 days once a quarter for the purpose of reducing the number of withdrawal bleeds and progestin side effects.
 b. Long-term endometrial protection has not been documented.
 c. Withdrawal bleeding tends to be heavy when it does occur.

6. Local applications
 a. **Topical estrogen** is used intravaginally to treat symptoms of **urogenital atrophy.** There is unpredictable and unreliable systemic absorption. Long-term use should be accompanied by surveillance of the endometrium or periodic progestin administration.
 b. Estrogen-impregnated rings and pessaries are being developed.
 c. Progestin intrauterine devices are being used as a method of providing endometrial protection and avoiding the side effects of systemic progestin.

D. Current agents

1. Estrogens. Estrogens, for the purpose of replacement, are administered orally or transdermally. Doses are based on information regarding lowest dose associated with medical benefits, particularly bone protection. An increase in dose is then based on symptom response.
 a. **Conjugated estrogens** are the preparation that has been used for the longest time for hormone replacement. The most popular and standard dose is 0.625 mg administered according to one of the regimens outlined in VI C.
 b. **Estrone sulfate** is administered in dosages of 0.625 to 1.25 mg according to one of the regimens outlined in VI C.
 c. **Estradiol** can be administered through the oral or transdermal route.
  (1) Oral dosing is 1 to 2 mg, with the lowest being the most popular.
  (2) Two patches are available for use at doses of 0.05 to 0.1 mg. Patches are changed once or twice a week, depending on the particular patch.

2. Progestins. Progestins are administered according to the regimens described in VI C for the purpose of prevention of endometrial hyperplasia and endometrial carcinoma.
 a. The most common agent is **medroxyprogesterone acetate.** Starting doses depend on the regimen used.
  (1) 10 mg for 10 to 12 days is used for cyclic or sequential therapy.
  (2) 5 mg for 14 days is used for cyclic or sequential therapy.
  (3) 2.5 or 5 mg is used in the continuous regimens.
 b. Other progestins are used but are less popular for hormone replacement. Doses vary according to regimen.

VII. RECOMMENDATIONS FOR CARE OF THE MENOPAUSAL WOMAN

A. Health risk assessment and physical examination

1. Identification of risk factors for cardiovascular disease and cancer in medical, social, family, life-style history

2. Annual height, weight, blood pressure

3. Annual physical examination, including breast and pelvic examination

B. Age/risk appropriate screenings. Screening tests are done to detect risk factors and early disease in the asymptomatic patient.

1. Cholesterol screening according to age and prior values

2. Fasting blood sugar screening according to risk and age

3. Mammography every 1 to 2 years from 40 to 50 years, annually after age 50 and in the woman on hormone replacement

4. Pap smear every 1 to 3 years depending on age, risk, and previous results

5. Guaiac stool testing for occult blood annually after age 40 years

6. Sigmoidoscopy/colonoscopy according to age and risk factors

C. Healthy life-style promotion

1. Smoking cessation

2. Nutritional assessment and recommendations regarding fat, cholesterol, calcium, and calories

3. Exercise recommendations

4. Identification of physical abuse and substance abuse

D. Menopause management

1. Hormone replacement therapy counseling

2. Nonhormonal management of symptoms

3. Problem-related detection and management

STUDY QUESTIONS

DIRECTIONS: Each of the numbered items or incomplete statements in this section is followed by answers or by completions of the statement. Select the ONE lettered answer or completion that is BEST in each case.

1. The hot flash that is characteristic of menopause is thought to be caused by

(A) a surge of follicle-stimulating hormone (FSH)
(B) a surge of luteinizing hormone (LH)
(C) an acute drop in estrogen
(D) an acute drop in progesterone
(E) none of the above

2. Which of the following is a major health hazard related to changes associated with menopause?

(A) Cardiovascular disease
(B) Pelvic relaxation
(C) Endometrial cancer
(D) Depression
(E) Osteoporosis

DIRECTIONS: Each of the numbered items or incomplete statements in this section is negatively phrased, as indicated by a capitalized word such as NOT, LEAST, or EXCEPT. Select the ONE lettered answer or completion that is BEST in each case.

3. Which of the following menopausal symptoms is NOT responsive to estrogen replacement therapy?

(A) Vaginal relaxation
(B) Depression
(C) Atrophic vaginitis
(D) Insomnia
(E) Dyspareunia

4. Recommended treatment for osteoporosis includes all of the following EXCEPT

(A) estrogen
(B) progestin
(C) exercise
(D) calcium
(E) vitamin D

5. Physiologic characteristics of perimenopause include all of the following EXCEPT

(A) reduction in the number of ovarian follicles
(B) decreased menstrual cycle length
(C) fluctuation in the estrogen concentration
(D) decreased secretion of follicle-stimulating hormone (FSH)
(E) reduction in follicle sensitivity to FSH

6. A 52-year-old woman complains of insomnia and depression. She states that her last menstrual period was 2 years ago. Her physician suggests that she should begin estrogen therapy, which should provide all of the following benefits EXCEPT

(A) prevention of osteoporosis
(B) an elevation of high-density lipoprotein levels
(C) prevention of endometrial hyperplasia
(D) improvement of urinary frequency and stress urinary incontinence
(E) prevention of cardiovascular disease

7. All of the following are contraindications to postmenopausal estrogen replacement therapy EXCEPT

(A) recent deep vein thrombosis
(B) acute liver disease
(C) high serum triglycerides
(D) premenopausal mastectomy for breast cancer
(E) diabetes

DIRECTIONS: The set of matching questions in this section consists of a list of four to twenty-six lettered options (some of which may be in figures) followed by several numbered items. For each numbered item, select the ONE lettered option that is most closely associated with it. To avoid spending too much time on matching sets with large numbers of options, it is generally advisable to begin each set by reading the list of options. Then, for each item in the set, try to generate the correct answer and locate it in the option list, rather than evaluating each option individually. Each lettered option may be selected once, more than once, or not at all.

Questions 8–10

For each case presented below, select the treatment that would be most appropriate.

(A) Medroxyprogesterone acetate
(B) Estrogen cream
(C) Continuous combined estrogen and progestin therapy
(D) Endometrial biopsy
(E) Hysterectomy

8. A 55-year-old woman presents with complaints of hot flashes and night sweats. Her last menstrual period was 3 years ago. Her only other medical complaint is migraine headaches. Family history includes breast cancer in her maternal aunt.

9. A 49-year-old woman presents with irregular cycles, intermenstrual bleeding, and hot flashes. She is very bothered by the hot flashes and insists that she needs medication. She has had irregular bleeding for 18 months.

10. A 54-year-old woman complains of vaginal spotting, discharge, and dyspareunia. She has been menopausal for 3 years. She had an endometrial biopsy 3 months ago, which revealed an atrophic endometrium.

■ ANSWERS AND EXPLANATIONS

1. The answer is C [V B 1 b]. The hot flashes that are characteristic of menopause appear to be related to a reduction in previously established estrogen levels. The flush appears to coincide with a surge of luteinizing hormone (LH), not follicle-stimulating hormone (FSH), and is more frequent and severe at night and during times of stress. The LH surge does not cause the hot flash because flashes occur in the absence of pituitary gland and LH.

2. The answer is E [V A 8, B 5]. Because of the consequences of bone loss, osteoporosis is a major health hazard directly associated with menopause; the problem is more widespread than endometrial cancer. Cardiovascular disease is a more prevalent problem; premature menopause is associated with an increased risk, whereas natural menopause is not. Compression fractures of the vertebrae and fractures of the upper femur demand bed rest and inactivity. An average of 16% of women with hip fractures die within 4 months of the injury.

3. The answer is A [V B 3, VI A 1 a–e]. Estrogen replacement therapy has good results in atrophic vaginal conditions, such as atrophic vaginitis and dyspareunia. It is also helpful in improving the affective symptoms associated with menopause—depression, insomnia, irritability, and loss of concentration. Pelvic tissues and ligaments that support the uterus and the vagina lose their tone in response to decreased estrogen; however, vaginal relaxation is not responsive to estrogen therapy.

4. The answer is B [V B 5, VI A 2]. A coordinated program of estrogen replacement (0.625 mg of conjugated equine estrogen daily), calcium (1–1.5 g daily), vitamin D (400 IU daily), and exercise is an approach to both the prevention and treatment of osteoporosis.

5. The answer is D [II A 1, B 2–4, C 1, 2]. As women near menopause, their cycles begin to change. There is a reduction in the number of ovarian follicles, and these follicles become less sensitive to follicle-stimulating hormone (FSH). With a reduced concentration of

inhibin and estrogen from the ovaries, there is less of a negative feedback effect, and there is increased secretion of FSH. The limited follicle maturation often leads to either a decreased cycle interval or lapses of cycles of oligomenorrhea.

6. The answer is C [VI A 1–3, VI B 3]. One of the most important features of estrogen replacement therapy in postmenopausal women is the prevention of osteoporosis. In addition, symptoms such as depression, insomnia, hot flashes, emotional lability, and vaginal dryness can be helped with estrogen replacement. Estrogen improves atrophic changes in the urethra and the bladder and can improve urinary frequency and stress urinary incontinence. Estrogen replacement therapy leads to increases in the level of high-density lipoproteins and reductions in levels of low-density lipoproteins; these changes are protective and contribute to the reduction of cardiovascular disease risk. Unopposed estrogen can cause endometrial hyperplasia; progestin inhibits endometrial growth and prevents hyperplasia when added to estrogen replacement.

7. The answer is E [VI B]. Although estrogen replacement therapy after the menopause has not been associated with an increased risk of thromboembolic disease, recent vascular thrombosis is a contraindication to hormone replacement therapy. There are clinical conditions that are worsened by exogenous estrogen, such as familial hyperlipidemia with an elevation of serum triglycerides. Although estrogen replacement improves the serum lipoprotein profile, its use is associated with an elevation of serum triglycerides. Elevated triglycerides are a risk factor for cardiovascular disease in women and can be associated with pancreatitis. In conditions that involve the liver, such as acute disease or cirrhosis, the circulating estrogen is not metabolized as rapidly; thus, a given dose of replacement estrogen can have a sustained and prolonged effect on target tissues. Premenopausal breast cancer may be estrogen related; therefore, affected women should not be offered estrogen replacement therapy. Diabetes is not worsened by estrogen replacement.

8–10. The answers are: 8-C [V A 1, B 1, 2], **9-D** [IV A 1, B 2 a, C 1, 2], **10-B** [V A 1, B 3, VI C 6]. The 55-year-old woman described in the question has vasomotor instability and needs hormonal replacement. Her family history of breast cancer is not extensive and does not involve a first degree relative. The potential benefits of hormonal replacement therapy in improving this woman's quality of life outweigh the risks. Hormonal replacement therapy for less than 5 years' duration has not been associated with an increased relative risk of breast cancer. Migraine headaches are a relative contraindication to hormonal replacement therapy. Some patients do not experience a worsening and may experience an improvement when placed on a hormonal regimen that is constant. Continuous combined therapy is preferred to a sequential regimen.

The 49-year-old woman described in the question presents with signs of unopposed estrogen stimulation of the endometrium—namely, irregular cycles and intermenstrual bleeding. Even though she is symptomatic at this point, additional estrogen is contraindicated without first sampling the endometrium to rule out endometrial neoplasia. Therefore, an endometrial biopsy is indicated as treatment for this patient.

The 54-year-old woman described in the question presents with symptoms of atrophic changes of the vagina—an atrophic vaginitis and dyspareunia. Discharge and spotting are common with atrophic vaginitis. Because she had an endometrial biopsy 3 months previously, it is unlikely that the spotting is a result of endometrial disease. Because the vagina is the chief source of discomfort, local vaginal estrogen cream should correct the problem. Hormone replacement therapy could be offered for long-term control.

Chapter 36

Pelvic Malignancies

Jane Fang

I. **CERVICAL CANCER.** The introduction of the Papanicolaou (Pap) smear in 1941 can account for the decline in the incidence and death rates from cervical cancer.

A. **Epidemiology.** Epidemiologic factors point to associations between **early age of coitus** and **sexual promiscuity** (male and female) and the development of precancerous and cancerous lesions of the cervix.

1. **Increased incidence** is related to:
   a. First intercourse at a young age
   b. Marriage or conception at an early age
   c. Multiple sexual partners
   d. Cigarette smoking
   e. High-risk male consort (i.e., one whose previous sexual partners developed precancerous or cancerous conditions of the cervix)
   f. Immunosuppression (i.e., due to human immunodeficiency virus infection)

2. **Viral transmission.** Sexually transmitted viruses, such as **human papillomavirus (HPV)** and **herpes simplex virus type 2 (HSV-2),** have been implicated as potential causal agents.
   a. **HPV**
      (1) HPV is detected in up to 95% of all squamous cell cancers of the cervix.
      (2) There is a high incidence of HPV infection in women with cervical intraepithelial neoplasia and invasive cancer.
      (3) Certain HPV subtypes (i.e., 16, 18, 31, 35, 39, 45, 51, and 52) are associated with high-grade neoplasms and cervical cancers.
   b. **HSV-2.** HSV-2 DNA and messenger RNA sequences have been found in cervical cancer cells.

B. **Cervical transformation zone (TZ).** The region on the ectocervix between the original squamous epithelium and glandular epithelium of the endocervical canal is the site of most **squamous** preinvasive and invasive neoplasms.

1. This zone undergoes a transformation from mucus-secreting glandular cells to non–mucus-secreting squamous cells in a process called **metaplasia** (a change in growth).
   a. **Metaplastic change** is most active during adolescence and pregnancy, when elevated estrogen levels may be the stimulating impetus.
   b. **Active metaplasia** is most susceptible to viral infection and integration of viral DNA (particularly HPV) into the host's DNA, presumably altering the controls on cellular differentiation.

2. **By-products of cigarette smoke** are concentrated in cervical mucus and have been associated with a depletion of the **cells of Langerhans,** which are macrophages that assist in cell-mediated immunity in the TZ.

C. **Evaluation of the abnormal Pap smear**

1. **Efficacy of cytologic screening programs**
   a. **Invasive carcinoma of the cervix** is usually preceded by a spectrum of preinvasive disease, which can be detected cytologically (i.e., with the Pap smear). Detection and simple local treatments of preinvasive cervical disease can prevent invasive cancer.
   b. **Regular cervical cancer screening programs** have demonstrated a significant de-

crease in mortality from cervical cancer. Unscreened populations can have as high as a 10-fold or greater increase in mortality from cervical cancer.

2. **Frequency of cervical cytologic screening**
   a. Screening should be initiated at the onset of sexual activity or age 18 years.
   b. Women with high-risk factors should be screened annually.
   c. Women with low-risk factors and three consecutive negative annual Pap smears can be screened less frequently at the discretion of the physician.

3. **Management of the abnormal Pap smear**
   a. **Classification**
      (1) **The Bethesda System** has replaced the older classification system. It uses terms that are more descriptive and correlate better with histology.
      (2) The format includes three parts:
         (a) A statement regarding the adequacy of the sample
         (b) A general categorization statement (optional)
         (c) A descriptive diagnosis regarding benign or reactive changes, low- or high-grade intraepithelial cell abnormalities, glandular cell abnormalities, or the presence of malignant cells
   b. **Colposcopy.** The Pap smear carries a false-negative rate between 15% and 40% for invasive cancers, and colposcopy provides a more definitive diagnosis. Colposcopically directed biopsies carry an accuracy of 85% to 95%. This technique involves inspection of the TZ and the squamocolumnar junction under 7.5- to 30-power magnification, after the application of a 3% to 5% acetic acid solution. An **endocervical canal curettage (ECC)** is performed in conjunction with colposcopy to rule out dysplasia within the canal that is colposcopically inapparent.
   c. **Treatment recommendations** are based on the colposcopic findings as outlined below.
      (1) **Low-grade lesions** may be treated surgically or followed conservatively. There is a 60% incidence of regression of these abnormalities, but a 15% incidence of progression to a high-grade abnormality.
      (2) **Destruction or excision of the TZ** to the depth of 7 mm can be performed with a fully visualized low- or high-grade lesion and a negative ECC with the following methods:
         (a) Diathermy loop (LEEP, LLETZ)
         (b) Cryotherapy
         (c) Laser vaporization
      (3) **Cold knife conization** is the gold standard procedure because a pathologic specimen with clean margins is obtained; it is recommended for the following circumstances:
         (a) Cervical intraepithelial lesions with either a nonvisualized lesion, a squamocolumnar junction, or a positive ECC
         (b) A high-grade lesion that does not correlate with colposcopic findings
         (c) Microinvasive carcinoma
         (d) Premalignant or malignant glandular cell abnormalities
   d. **Cure rates** for one treatment range from 85% to 95%. Repeat treatment of the adequately evaluated persistent lesion effects a cure rate of 95%.
   e. **Posttreatment follow-up.** The risk of premalignant lesions persisting or recurring is 5% to 15%. Of these lesions, 85% are detected within 2 years of the initial treatment. Follow-up of the treated patient should include:
      (1) Cytologic evaluation every 3 months for the first year posttreatment
      (2) Repeat colposcopic evaluation for persistent or recurrent cell abnormalities
      (3) Hysterectomy for those patients who have persistent severe lesions despite repeated conservative local destructive techniques

D. **Invasive cervical cancer**

1. **Microinvasive carcinoma of the cervix.** Much controversy surrounds the exact definition of this "early" invasive cancer of the cervix. A commonly adopted definition in the United States is a depth of invasion of less than 3 mm, and a width no greater than 7 mm.

a. The **diagnosis** can be made only by means of a thoroughly examined cone biopsy specimen.

b. The **incidence of pelvic lymph node metastases** is less than 1%.

c. **Total abdominal hysterectomy** is the treatment of choice, although cervical conization with negative margins can be used in women who wish to preserve fertility.

d. The **cure rate** is 95%.

2. **Invasive carcinoma of the cervix.** These invasive lesions are either clinically inapparent and found on histologic inspection of a cone biopsy (depth of invasion more than 3 mm, width more than 7 mm) or are clinically obvious, in which case a simple biopsy confirms the diagnosis.

   a. Symptoms

   (1) Postcoital or irregular bleeding are the most common symptoms.

   (2) Malodorous, bloody discharge, sciatica, leg edema, and deep pelvic pain are seen in advanced disease.

   b. Age. The mean age at diagnosis is approximately 45 years. Primary cervical cancers diagnosed before age 30 or after the age of 70 years occur in about 7% and 16% of women, respectively.

   c. Histology. Squamous carcinomas (85%) and adenocarcinoma (13%) account for most invasive cervical cancer. There appears to be no difference in survival rates between women with these two groups of cancer when the lesions are matched for grade, size, and stage. Rare tumors of the cervix include small cell carcinomas, verrucous carcinomas, sarcomas, and lymphomas.

   d. Staging. Clinical assessment of the extent of disease includes the following:

   (1) Stage I: Carcinoma is confined to the cervix

       (a) Stage IA: Microinvasive carcinoma

           (i) Stage IA1: Invasion less than 3 mm in depth and less than 7 mm in width

           (ii) Stage IA2: Invasion more than 3 mm and less than 5 mm in depth, and less than 7 mm in width

       (b) Stage IB: All other cases of stage I

   (2) Stage II: Carcinoma extends beyond the cervix but not onto the pelvic sidewall. The cancer extends into the vagina but not the lower third.

       (a) Stage IIA: No obvious parametrial involvement

       (b) Stage IIB: Obvious parametrial involvement

   (3) Stage III: Carcinoma extends to the pelvic sidewall. On rectal examination, there is no cancer-free space between the tumor and the pelvic sidewall. The tumor extends to the lower third of the vagina. All cases of hydronephrosis and nonfunctioning kidney should be included in stage III diagnoses unless another cause for these conditions can be found.

       (a) Stage IIIA: Tumor extends to the lower third of the vagina, with no extension to the pelvic sidewall.

       (b) Stage IIIB: Extension onto pelvic sidewall, hydronephrosis, or nonfunctioning kidney

   (4) Stage IV: Carcinoma extends beyond the true pelvis or clinically involves the mucosa of the bladder or rectum.

       (a) Stage IVA: Spread to the mucosa of the bladder or rectum

       (b) Stage IVB: Spread beyond the true pelvis

   e. Pretreatment staging evaluations. The diagnostic workup of a woman with histologically confirmed invasive cervical cancer is designed to examine the known patterns of spread, such as direct extension, lymphatic involvement, or hematogenous spread.

   (1) Diagnostic evaluation

       (a) Pelvic examination under anesthesia

       (b) Chest radiography

       (c) Intravenous pyelography (IVP)

       (d) Barium enema

       (e) Cystoscopy and proctosigmoidoscopy

(2) Other diagnostic tests
  (a) Computed axial tomography (CAT) scan
  (b) Magnetic resonance imaging
  (c) Radiologically guided fine-needle aspiration
f. Treatment. Therapeutic measures are governed by the patient's age and general health and by the clinical stage of the cancer. Primary modalities include surgery and radiotherapy. Chemotherapy can be used as an adjunct to radiotherapy or for control of locally recurrent or distant metastatic disease.
  (1) Surgery involves **radical hysterectomy** with paraaortic and pelvic lymphadenectomy. This procedure involves an en bloc removal of the uterus, cervix, upper third of the vagina, the parametrium, and the uterosacral and uterovesical ligaments. In addition, the lymphatics of the lower paraaortic, common iliac, and pelvic regions are removed en bloc.
    (a) The best results are achieved in patients with a tumor volume of 3 cm or less with no lymph node metastasis.
    (b) Comparable cure rates between surgery and radiotherapy are the rule in the treatment of early stage (IB and IIA) disease.
    (c) Surgery alone is usually reserved for patients with low-volume local disease who are reasonably young and medically sound. **Ovarian preservation** is an important component of these operations.
    (d) Five-year survival rates with surgery
      (i) Stage IB: 84%
      (ii) Stage IIA: 75%
  (2) Radiotherapy. This treatment modality can be used for all stages of cervical cancer, either for curative or palliative intent.
    (a) It can be used in conjunction with surgery for bulky (4 cm or more, **barrel cervix**) stage IB and IIA tumors and with chemotherapy (i.e., 5-fluorouracil) for locally advanced stage IIB to IVA tumors to improve survival.
    (b) Tumor cells appear more sensitive to the effects of ionizing irradiation and are less capable of repairing lethal damage than normal tissue.
    (c) Five-year survival rates with radiotherapy
      (i) Stage IB: 85%
      (ii) Stage IIA: 84%
      (iii) Stage IIB: 67%
      (iv) Stage IIIA: 45%
      (v) Stage IIIB: 36%
      (vi) Stage IV: 14%
g. Follow-up evaluation. It is estimated that approximately 35% of patients with invasive cervical cancer have persistent or recurrent disease. Most of these (85%) have a recurrence of disease within 3 years of the initial treatment. Thus, frequent checkups are mandatory in the first 3 years.
  (1) Evaluations include:
    (a) Pelvic examinations
    (b) Pap smears
    (c) Periodic chest radiographs
    (d) IVP
  (2) Suspect signs or symptoms include:
    (a) Persistent cervical lesion
    (b) Unexplained weight loss
    (c) Unilateral leg edema
    (d) Pelvic or sciatic pain
    (e) Serosanguineous vaginal discharge
    (f) Progressive ureteral obstruction
    (g) Supraclavicular node enlargement
    (h) Persistent cough or hemoptysis
h. Treatment of recurrent disease. Treatment rests with determining whether recurrent disease is locally confined or metastatic.
  (1) Locally confined

(a) Of **patients treated primarily with surgery,** 25% are saved after recurrence of the disease with pelvic radiotherapy.

(b) In **patients treated primarily by radiotherapy** and in whom extensive presurgical and intraoperative evaluations reveal no evidence of metastatic tumor, partial or total pelvic exenteration (i.e., en bloc removal of the uterus, cervix, vagina, parametrium, bladder, and rectum) can be curative in up to 70% of cases.

(2) Metastatic recurrence. These patients are usually treated with chemotherapy. Cure rates are exceedingly rare, and response rates are variable and of limited duration. Radiotherapy can be used in the palliation of painful metastases.

II. ENDOMETRIAL CANCER

A. Epidemiology

1. **Incidence.** Two to 3% of women in the United States will have endometrial cancer. The incidence of this malignancy appears to be increasing slightly. It is the **most common gynecologic cancer.**

2. **Risk.** Increased risk of endometrial cancer has been associated with:
   a. **Early menarche**
   b. **Late menopause**
   c. **Obesity**
   d. **Chronic anovulation/polycystic ovarian disease.** The increased risk has been attributed to unopposed estrogen stimulation of the endometrium. Conversion of adrenal or ovarian androstenedione (an androgenic precursor to estrogens) in the peripheral adipose tissue to estrone (a weak estrogen) shuts off the normal cyclic function of the hypothalamic–pituitary–ovarian axis. As a result, ovulation and the subsequent production of progesterone, a potent "antiestrogenic" hormone, ceases. There is, then, a chronic, unabated stimulation of the endometrium by estrone, leading to endometrial hyperplasia (a premalignant lesion) and endometrial carcinoma.
   e. **Exogenous unopposed estrogen.** There is a significant correlation between use of exogenous oral estrogen and endometrial cancer when estrogen therapy is administered without the protective effects of a progestin.
   f. **Estrogen-secreting tumors.** Granulosa–theca cell ovarian tumors produce active estrogen and have been associated with a 25% incidence of a concurrent endometrial carcinoma.
   g. **Other factors.** A history of breast and ovarian cancers is associated with an increased risk of a concomitant endometrial carcinoma. A history of hypertension and diabetes mellitus is also associated with an increased risk, although these factors may be related to obesity.
   h. Factors associated with **decreased risk** are smoking, high parity, and oral contraceptives.

B. Pathophysiology. Estrogen stimulation of the endometrium, without the controlling effects of a progestin or progesterone, leads to endometrial hyperplasia and, eventually, endometrial cancer.

C. Endometrial hyperplasia is thought to be a precursor to endometrial carcinoma. There is a spectrum of glandular proliferation with varying degrees of architectural disarray (i.e., epithelial stratification with or without cytologic atypia). No invasion can be demonstrated. The risk of progression to endometrial carcinoma is 1% to 14% in untreated cases. This risk is greatest in postmenopausal women and in women with atypical hyperplasia.

1. Types of endometrial hyperplasia
   a. Simple hyperplasia
   b. Complex (adenomatous) hyperplasia
      (1) Adenomatous hyperplasia without atypia is a proliferation of glands and stroma, with focal crowding of the glands and a relatively decreased background stroma.
      (2) Atypical adenomatous hyperplasia is adenomatous hyperplasia with cellular atypia (i.e., nuclear enlargement, hyperchromasia, increased nuclear:cytoplasmic ratio). Atypical hyperplasia is further subtyped as mild, moderate, and severe. This type of hyperplasia has a great potential for malignant progression, especially in the severe subtype.

2. Treatment of endometrial hyperplasia. First, the diagnosis must be established with adequate sampling of the endometrium in at-risk patients.
   a. The **teenage patient** can be treated conservatively with cyclic estrogen with progestin for 6 months, after which time endometrial sampling should be repeated. If the patient continues to be anovulatory after medical treatment, oral estrogen with progestin (i.e., birth control pills) or cyclic medroxyprogesterone acetate (10 mg for 10 days every month) should be continued to induce stabilization of the endometrium and to control withdrawal bleeding unless ovulation resumes.
   b. Women desiring fertility can be treated with three courses of cyclic progestin followed by a repeat endometrial sampling.
      (1) If pregnancy is desired, ovulation can be induced.
      (2) If pregnancy is not desired, the woman should be evaluated as to the cause of anovulation and treated with either cyclic estrogen with progestin or cyclic progestin.
   c. Perimenopausal and postmenopausal women. For low-grade lesions, treatment is initially conservative. Proper sampling of the endometrium to ensure the proper diagnosis is essential.
      (1) Three to 6 months of cyclic medroxyprogesterone acetate (10–20 mg for 10–12 days every month) or a depot of medroxyprogesterone acetate
         (a) Repeat endometrial sampling at 3 to 6 months is mandatory.
         (b) Persistent endometrial hyperplasia after progestational therapy is associated with a risk for development of endometrial carcinoma. This occurs in approximately 6% of treated patients. The cure rate is approximately 60%.
      (2) Hysterectomy is warranted in women with either persistent hyperplasia after treatment with progestational agents or in women with severe atypical hyperplasia.

3. Prevention of endometrial hyperplasia. In women on estrogen replacement therapy, the addition of a progestational agent has dramatically reduced the risk of endometrial hyperplasia and carcinoma.

D. Endometrial carcinoma

1. Symptoms. The most common symptom of endometrial carcinoma is irregular menses or postmenopausal bleeding.

2. Age. The median age for endometrial cancer is 61 years. The largest number of patients are between 50 and 59 years of age.

3. Histology. The **principal histologic subtypes** of endometrial carcinoma are **adenocarcinoma** (60%–65%) and **adenoacanthoma** (22%). The remaining subtypes are papillary serous carcinoma, clear cell adenocarcinoma, adenosquamous carcinoma, and secretory carcinoma. Papillary serous and clear cell subtypes are associated with a poorer 5-year survival rate. Histologic differentiation correlates with depth of myometrial penetration, pelvic and periaortic lymphatic metastases, and overall 5-year survival.
   a. Grade 1: Well differentiated adenocarcinoma with less than 5% solid components
   b. Grade 2: Moderately differentiated carcinoma with 5% to 50% solid components

    c. Grade 3: Poorly differentiated carcinoma with more than 50% solid components

4. **Staging.** Histologic differentiation **(grade)** is assigned to all stages.
   a. **Stage I:** Confined to the corpus
      (1) **Stage IA:** Tumor limited to the endometrium
      (2) **Stage IB:** Tumor invades less than one half of the myometrium
      (3) **Stage IC:** Tumor invades more than one half of the myometrium
   b. **Stage II:** Involvement of the cervix
      (1) **Stage IIA:** Endocervical glandular involvement
      (2) **Stage IIB:** Cervical stromal invasion
   c. **Stage III**
      (1) **Stage IIIA:** Tumor invades the serosa or adnexa, or positive peritoneal cytology
      (2) **Stage IIIB:** Vaginal metastases
      (3) **Stage IIIC:** Metastases to pelvic or paraaortic nodes
   d. **Stage IV:** Mucosal involvement of the bladder or rectum or extension beyond the true pelvis
      (1) **Stage IVA:** Tumor invades the bladder or bowel mucosa
      (2) **Stage IVB:** Distant metastases, including inguinal lymph nodes

5. **Diagnosis and staging evaluation**
   a. **Dilatation and curettage.** This procedure is the formal method of diagnosis.
   b. **Alternative diagnostic tests** can include endometrial biopsy with endocervical curettage, and hysteroscopically directed biopsies of the endometrium.
   c. **Staging workup**
      (1) Chest radiograph
      (2) Barium enema or proctosigmoidoscopy
      (3) Cystoscopy
   d. **Additional studies** can include CA-125 and CAT scan of the abdomen and pelvis.

6. **Treatment.** A surgical staging evaluation includes total abdominal hysterectomy and a bilateral salpingo-oophorectomy with paraaortic lymph node sampling, peritoneal cytology, careful abdominal inspection, and a pathologic evaluation of the depth of myometrial penetration. The need for adjuvant postoperative radiotherapy or chemotherapy can be made for those patients at high risk for local recurrence.
   a. **Low-risk patients** comprise those with **stage IA, grade 1 carcinomas.** This group of tumors has few poor prognostic features. Surgery (total abdominal hysterectomy and bilateral salpingo-oophorectomy) alone is usually considered adequate treatment. Their disease-free survival rate is 96%. Lymph node assessment is controversial.
   b. **Intermediate-risk patients** are those with **grade 1 or 2 tumors with less than one-third myometrial invasion,** and **no extrauterine spread.** Studies do not demonstrate improved survival with postoperative radiation therapy, but there is improved local control.
   c. **High-risk patients** include those with **adnexal spread, pelvic node metastases, outer one-third myometrial invasion,** or **grade 3 tumors with any invasion.** Adjuvant radiotherapy may be of benefit. Five-year survival rate is 40%. With clinical involvement of the cervix, radical hysterectomy or preoperative radiotherapy may be preferred.
   d. **Stage III and IV adenocarcinomas.** Treatment in these patients must be individualized. In most instances, treatment programs involve surgery with chemotherapy, hormonal therapy, and radiation therapy.
   e. **Medically inoperable patients.** Clinically early-stage patients who have serious medical conditions may receive radiation therapy with careful follow-up. Five-year survival rates are about 50%.
   f. **Recurrent disease.** Treatment for recurrent disease must be individualized, depending on the extent and site of recurrence, hormone receptor status, and the patient's health. Treatment programs can include exenterative procedures, radiotherapy, chemotherapy, and hormonal therapy.

III. OVARIAN CANCER

A. Incidence

1. Ovarian cancer is the **leading cause of death attributable to gynecologic cancers in the United States;** approximately 1 in 70 women will contract ovarian cancer.

2. The **incidence** starts to rise in the fifth decade and continues to rise until the eighth decade.

B. Risks

1. **Low parity, delayed childbearing,** and **infertility** are risk factors.

2. **Oral contraceptives** have a significantly **protective effect.**

3. **Family history** can increase the risk for first-degree relatives as high as 50%. Specific genes have been identified in these families (e.g., *BRCA-1*).

C. Ovarian cancer is **silent in its early development.**

1. In over 70% of cases, the ovarian disease has spread beyond the pelvis before the diagnosis is made.

2. There is **no dependable serodiagnostic screening test.** The CA-125 (a cancer antigen) level **cannot** serve as a screening test. Other markers include:
   a. **α-Fetoprotein (AFP):** endodermal sinus tumors and embryonal cell carcinomas
   b. **Human chorionic gonadotropin (hCG):** ovarian choriocarcinomas, mixed germ cell tumors, and embryonal cell carcinomas
   c. **Lactate dehydrogenase:** dysgerminoma
   d. **Carcinoembryonic antigen:** mucinous epithelial ovarian carcinoma

3. No cytologic sampling from the cervix, vagina, or cul-de-sac has been useful as a screening tool. Transvaginal ultrasound improves the accuracy in detecting pelvic masses, but is not an acceptable screening tool.

D. Ovarian neoplasms are categorized according to the site of origin:

1. **Epithelial** [e.g., serous, mucinous, endometrioid, clear cell (mesonephroid), Brenner tumor]

2. **Germ cell** (e.g., teratoma, dysgerminoma, embryonal cell, endodermal sinus tumor, choriocarcinoma, gonadoblastoma)

3. **Stromal** (e.g., granulosa cell, Sertoli-Leydig tumors)

4. **Nonspecialized stromal** (e.g., fibroma, lymphoma)

5. **Metastatic:** most commonly from the breast or gastrointestinal tract (Krukenberg tumors)

E. The **initial spread** is to adjacent peritoneal surfaces and retroperitoneal lymph nodes; however, spread may be to any surface and to the omentum.

1. **Extraabdominal and intrahepatic metastases** occur late in the course of the disease and only in a small percentage of cases.

2. As a terminal event, **bowel obstruction** is caused by massive serosal involvement.

F. Staging

1. **Stage I:** Limited to the ovaries
   a. **Stage IA:** Limited to one ovary; no ascites with positive cytology; no tumor on external surfaces; capsule intact
   b. **Stage IB:** Limited to both ovaries; no positive ascites; no tumor on the external surface; capsule intact

   c. **Stage IC:** Tumor either stage IA or IB but with ascites present or with positive peritoneal washings or capsule rupture

2. **Stage II:** Involvement of one or both ovaries with pelvic extension
   a. **Stage IIA:** Extension or metastases to the uterus or tubes or both
   b. **Stage IIB:** Extension to other pelvic tissues
   c. **Stage IIC:** Tumor either stage IIA or IIB but with ascites present or with positive peritoneal washings or with capsule rupture

3. **Stage III:** Involvement of one or both ovaries with peritoneal metastases outside the pelvis or superficial liver metastases or positive retroperitoneal nodes
   a. **Stage IIIA:** Tumor limited to the pelvis with negative nodes but microscopic seeding of the peritoneum
   b. **Stage IIIB:** Peritoneal implants no larger than 2 cm in diameter with negative nodes
   c. **Stage IIIC:** Implants larger than 2 cm in diameter or positive retroperitoneal or inguinal nodes

4. **Stage IV:** Involvement of one or both ovaries with distant metastases; this can include a positive pleural effusion and intrahepatic metastases

G. **Categories of tumors**

1. **Epithelial tumors.** These tumors arise from the coelomic mesothelium, which is capable of differentiating into both benign and malignant tumors. The transition from benign to malignant is not abrupt; there is an intermediate, or **borderline,** category. Distinguishing benign, borderline, and malignant tumors is important in terms of treatment and prognosis. Epithelial malignancies represent most of the ovarian malignancies.
   a. The **predominant cell types** are:
      (1) Serous
         (a) One of three serous tumors is malignant.
         (b) Serous cancers are more than three times as common as the mucinous variety and seven times as common as the endometrioid variety.
         (c) **Serous cystadenocarcinoma,** the most common type of ovarian cancer, tends to be bilateral in 35% to 50% of cases.
      (2) **Mucinous**
         (a) One of five mucinous tumors is malignant.
         (b) Mucinous tumors are bilateral in 10% to 20% of cases.
      (3) **Endometrioid**
         (a) The microscopic pattern is similar to that of primary adenocarcinoma of the endometrium.
         (b) Areas of endometriosis in the ovary may be present.
   b. The **prognosis** for each stage of epithelial ovarian tumors is linked to the grade of the tumor; poorly differentiated tumors have a poor prognosis. The prognosis for endometrioid tumors is much better than that of the serous and mucinous carcinomas. Long-term survival of patients with borderline or well-differentiated cancers after primary surgery is common.

2. **Sex cord stromal neoplasms.** Granulosa–theca cell tumors, granulosa cell tumors, and Sertoli-Leydig cell tumors, which comprise 3% of all ovarian neoplasms, are derived from mesenchymal stem cells in the ovarian cortex. These tumors have the potential to secrete estrogen. Endometrial hyperplasia has been reported with more than 50% of these tumors, and cancer in 5% to 10%.
   a. **Granulosa cell tumors** that occur in premenarchal women induce abnormal bleeding and breast development.
   b. **Granulosa cell tumors** have the following characteristics:
      (1) They are bilateral only 10% of the time.
      (2) They vary in size from microscopic to tumors that fill the abdomen.
      (3) They are characterized histologically by **Call-Exner bodies** (i.e., rosettes or follicles of granulosa cells, often with a central clearing).

(4) Approximately 30% of these tumors recur, usually more than 5 years after removal of the primary tumor, with occasional recurrences after 30 years.

c. Sertoli-Leydig cell tumors (e.g., androblastoma and arrhenoblastoma) are rare tumors of mesenchymal origin.

(1) Their usual endocrine activity is androgenic.

(2) Defeminization is the classic feature of the androgen-secreting tumors, including breast and uterine atrophy, which is followed by masculinization, including hirsutism, acne, receding hairline, clitorimegaly, and deepening of the voice.

3. Germ cell tumors. Malignant germ cell tumors are believed to arise from primitive germ cells in the ovary, which give rise to either dysgerminoma or tumors of totipotential cells. The latter tumors can be differentiated into **extraembryonic structures,** such as endodermal sinus or choriocarcinoma, or embryonal structures, such as the malignant teratomas. These tumors represent 5% of all ovarian malignancies but account for over two thirds of all malignant ovarian neoplasms in women younger than 20 years of age.

a. Dysgerminoma. Histologically, there are sheets of round to oval cells with clear cytoplasm and a centrally placed nucleus with prominent nucleoli. There is a characteristic lymphocytic infiltrate within fibrous septa. Occasionally, there are syncytiotrophoblastic giant cells. Other **characteristics of dysgerminomas** include the following.

(1) They are the **most common germ cell tumor,** accounting for approximately 50% of this type of tumor.

(2) Ninety percent of dysgerminomas are found in women younger than 30 years of age.

(3) The propensity for lymphatic invasion is great.

(4) Tumors can secrete detectable amounts of hCG.

(5) Bilateral tumors occur in more than 20% of cases.

(6) Tumors are exquisitely radiosensitive.

b. Embryonal carcinoma. The histologic appearance consists of solid sheets of anaplastic cells with abundant clear cytoplasm, hyperchromatic nuclei, and numerous mitotic figures. Embryonal carcinoma is further characterized by the following:

(1) The **median age of patients** with embryonal carcinoma is 15 years.

(2) The tumor elaborates both AFP and hCG; these trophic hormones may be responsible for precocious puberty in the prepubertal girl.

(3) Most often, the tumor is unilateral with explosive growth tendencies, leading to large tumor masses and acute abdominal pain.

c. Endodermal sinus tumor. The histologic appearance consists of a glomerulus-like structure resembling the papillae of the endodermal sinus in the rat's placenta. This pathognomonic structure is known as the **Schiller-Duval body.** This tumor is further characterized by the following:

(1) The **median age of patients** with endodermal sinus tumors is 19 years.

(2) A primary tumor is unilateral 95% of the time; the right ovary is most commonly affected.

(3) AFP is a tumor marker.

(4) There is a tendency toward rapid expansion.

d. Choriocarcinoma. This primary tumor must be distinguished from metastatic disease to the ovary from a gestational choriocarcinoma. The histologic appearance is that of atypical to highly anaplastic cytotrophoblastic and syncytiotrophoblastic elements. This tumor is further characterized by the following:

(1) It commonly occurs in young women.

(2) It is rarely bilateral.

(3) It elaborates hCG.

(4) It can present as a pelvic mass and precocious puberty in prepubertal girls.

e. Malignant teratomas. This broad spectrum of tumors arises from embryonal elements, which have differentiated into the embryonal somatic structures of the ectoderm, mesoderm, and endoderm. These tumors can be either solid or cystic and can give rise to:

(1) Immature malignant teratoma. The principal tumor characteristics are the atypical neural epithelial elements.

(2) Monodermal tumors. These tumors involve highly specialized tumors of **thyroid tissue (struma ovarii)** or **neurosecretory tissue (carcinoid).**

(3) Mature teratoma with malignant transformation. The principal tumor characteristics that undergo malignant transformation in the mature teratoma are the squamous elements.

4. Gonadoblastoma. This is a rare ovarian tumor found in phenotypically female patients with dysgenetic gonads and a karyotype that includes a Y chromosome.

a. The tumors are composed of granulosa, theca, Sertoli, and Leydig cells.

b. They frequently contain calcifications.

c. They have a tendency toward dysgerminomatous overgrowth; therefore, in the presence of a Y chromosome, all dysgenetic gonads should be removed as soon as they are diagnosed, except in the case of androgen insensitivity syndrome. Removal of these gonads should wait until after puberty and development of secondary sexual characteristics.

H. **Diagnosis**

1. Signs and symptoms. Ovarian cancers usually produce few symptoms until the disease is advanced.

a. Abdominal distention caused by ascites is often the presenting complaint.

b. Lower abdominal pain, a pelvic mass, and weight loss are additional features.

2. Early diagnosis of ovarian cancer is rare, except by vaginal probe ultrasound, which has not been proven to be cost effective for screening.

3. Pelvic ultrasound is helpful in characterizing the size and architecture of the adnexal mass. Approximately 95% of ovarian cancers are larger than 5 cm. Multicystic and solid components and free fluid in the cul-de-sac are ultrasonic features suggestive of ovarian carcinoma.

4. CA 125 levels are elevated above the normal range in more than 85% of patients with ovarian cancer, but also should not be used for screening purposes.

5. Abdominopelvic CAT scan, barium enema, and **chest radiography** are helpful in the evaluation of the extent of disease in women suspected of having ovarian cancer.

6. Surgical staging evaluation

a. Exploratory laparotomy through a vertical abdominal incision, allowing a thorough evaluation of the upper abdomen

b. Peritoneal washings from the pelvis and upper abdomen

c. Inspection of all peritoneal and diaphragmatic surfaces

d. Sampling of pelvic and paraaortic lymph nodes

e. Omentectomy

f. Thorough evaluation of the contralateral ovary to exclude occult disease in young women who wish to preserve fertility, and who have an ovarian cancer apparently confined to one ovary

I. **Treatment**

1. Epithelial tumors

a. Complete surgical excision in the form of total abdominal hysterectomy, bilateral adnexectomy, omentectomy, and tumor debulking is the desired initial treatment approach. Adjuvant platinum-based combination chemotherapy is recommended. Taxol is being investigated as first-line therapy.

b. Second-look laparotomy after the completion of chemotherapy in patients with no clinically detectable disease can be performed to tailor subsequent treatment recommendations.

c. Five-year survival rates

   (1) **Stage I:** 73%
   (2) **Stage II:** 46%
   (3) **Stage III:** 17%
   (4) **Stage IV:** 5%

   d. **Borderline epithelial neoplasms (tumors of low malignant potential)** account for 15% of epithelial malignancies. Patients with these tumors have higher survival rates, and most are diagnosed in stage I.

2. **Sex cord stromal tumors**
   a. Total abdominal hysterectomy and bilateral salpingo-oophorectomy after adequate surgical staging constitute definitive therapy in most patients.
   b. In young women with early-stage disease who desire fertility, a conservative approach with uterine and contralateral adnexal preservation can be performed.
   c. Patients with advanced or recurrent disease should be surgically debulked. If residual tumor is less than 2 cm, radiotherapy or chemotherapy may be beneficial.

3. **Germ cell tumors**
   a. **Stage IA:** Conservative surgery
   b. **All other cases:** Staging laparotomy and chemotherapy

IV. VAGINAL CANCER

A. **Squamous cell carcinoma** is the most common histologic type. They are usually located in the upper half of the vagina.

1. **Symptoms**
   a. The most common symptom is a **vaginal discharge,** which is often bloody.
   b. **Urinary symptoms** occur because of the close proximity of the upper vagina to the vesicle neck, with resulting compression of the bladder.
   c. The **elasticity of the posterior vaginal fornix** allows lesions in that area to become quite large, especially in sexually inactive women, before they are detected.

2. **Age.** This rare malignant cancer occurs in women between 35 and 70 years of age.

3. **Lymphatic spread.** The upper vagina is drained by the common iliac and hypogastric (internal iliac) nodes, whereas the lower vagina is drained by the regional lymph nodes of the femoral triangle.

4. **Staging**
   a. **Stage I:** Limited to the vaginal mucosa
   b. **Stage II:** Involvement of the subvaginal tissue but no extension onto the pelvic sidewall
   c. **Stage III:** Extension onto the pelvic sidewall
   d. **Stage IV:** Extension beyond the true pelvis or involvement of the mucosa of the bladder or rectum

5. **Treatment.** Treatment of squamous cell carcinoma is primarily by radiotherapy. Large carcinomas of the vault or vaginal walls are treated initially with external radiation; this shrinks the neoplasm so that local radiation therapy will be more effective.

6. **Five-year survival rates**
   a. **Stage I:** 80% to 90%
   b. **Stage II:** 60%
   c. **Stage III:** 40%
   d. **Stage IV:** 0%

B. **Diethylstilbestrol (DES)-related adenocarcinoma (clear cell carcinoma).** DES was used in the 1940s and 1950s in high-risk pregnancies (i.e., diabetes, habitual abortion, threatened abortion) to prevent pregnancy wastage. In all documented cases of genital tract abnormalities, DES was begun before the eighteenth week of pregnancy.

1. **Age**
   a. The mean age for development of clear cell adenocarcinoma of the vagina is 19 years for patients with a history of DES exposure.
   b. The risk for development of these carcinomas through the age of 24 years in DES-exposed women has been calculated to be between 0.14 and 1.4/1000.

2. **Characteristics of clear cell carcinoma**
   a. Approximately 40% of the cancers occur in the cervix, and the other 60% primarily in the upper half of the vagina.
   b. The **incidence of lymph node metastases** is high—about 16% in stage I, and 30% or more in stage II.

3. **Treatment**
   a. If the cancer is confined to the cervix and the upper vagina, radical hysterectomy and upper vaginectomy with pelvic lymphadenectomy and ovarian preservation are recommended.
   b. Advanced tumors and lesions involving the lower vagina are treated more appropriately by irradiation, which should include treatment of the pelvic nodes and parametrial tissues.

4. **Five-year survival rates** are better than those for the squamous tumors of the cervix and upper vagina, probably because of earlier detection.

V. VULVAR CARCINOMA

A. **Epidemiology.** Factors associated with vulvar carcinoma include the following.

1. A history of vulvar condylomata or granulomatous venereal disease is common.

2. Vulvar carcinomas occasionally arise from areas of carcinoma-in-situ.

3. They occur more frequently in women who have been treated for invasive squamous carcinomas of the cervix or vagina.

4. More than half of the patients are between the ages of 60 and 79 years. Less than 15% are younger than 40 years of age.

B. **Etiology.** Little is known about causal factors in this disease. Recently, HPV types 16 and 18 have been detected in squamous cancer of the vulva.

C. **Symptoms.** Recognition of a lesion is often accompanied by a delay in diagnosis because of either self-treatment by the patient or lack of recognition by the treating physician. Vulvar cancer usually presents with:

1. A history of chronic **vulvar irritation** or soreness

2. A **visible lesion on the labia,** which is often sore

D. **Histology.** Squamous carcinoma comprises 90% of these tumors. The remaining 10% consist of malignant melanoma, Bartholin's gland adenocarcinoma, verrucous carcinoma, and Paget's disease.

E. **Patterns of spread**

1. **Local expansion** involves the contiguous structures of the urethra, vagina, perineum, anus, rectum, and pubic bone.

2. **Lymphatic spread.** Metastases follow the lymphatic drainage pattern of the vulva, which includes superficial inguinal nodes, deep femoral groups, and pelvic nodes.

3. **Hematogenous spread** occurs in the advanced or recurrent cases.

F. **Diagnosis.** Incisional or excisional biopsy of the suspect lesion under local or general anesthesia confirms the diagnosis.

G. **Pretreatment evaluation** includes a clinical assessment of:

1. **Tumor size (T)**
   a. **T1:** Tumor that is 2 cm or less in size that is confined to the vulva
   b. **T2:** Tumor that is greater than 2 cm in size that is confined to the vulva
   c. **T3:** Tumor of any size that spreads to the urethra, vagina, perineum, or anus
   d. **T4:** Tumor of any size that infiltrates the bladder and rectal mucosa or is fixed to the bone

2. **Node assessment (N)**
   a. **N0:** No regional nodes palpable
   b. **N1:** Unilateral regional lymph node metastases
   c. **N2:** Bilateral regional lymph node metastases

3. **Metastases (M)**
   a. **M0:** No metastases
   b. **M1:** Distant metastases, including pelvic nodes

H. **Staging**

1. **Stage I:** T1 N0 M0

2. **Stage II:** T2 N0 M0

3. **Stage III:** T3 N1 M0, T1 N1 M0, T2 N1 M0

4. **Stage IVA:** T1 N2 M0, T2 N2 M0, T3 N2 M0, or T4 any N M0

5. **Stage IVB:** any T, any N, M1

I. **Treatment.** Surgical treatment has become less extensive than the traditional radical vulvectomy with bilateral inguinal lymphadenectomy. Therefore, surgical approaches have become much more conservative and individualized.

1. **T1 lesions (tumor no more than 2 cm in size)**
   a. Radical local excision of the lesion with a 1-cm margin laterally and a depth down to the inferior fascia is indicated when:
      (1) Biopsy of the tumor reveals a depth of invasion less than 1 mm
      (2) Tumor is unifocal
      (3) Remaining vulva is normal
   b. No groin dissection is necessary.

2. **T2 and early T3 tumors without suspect inguinal nodes**
   a. Radical vulvectomy
   b. Bilateral inguinal and femoral lymphadenectomy

3. **Tumors with clinically suspect inguinal nodes** are treated with lymphadenectomy; if there are more than two histologically positive nodes, external beam radiation to the groin is given.

4. **Advanced disease.** Individualized treatment can include surgery, radiation, and chemotherapy. Pelvic radiotherapy is recommended for patients with involved nodes.

5. **Five-year survival rates**
   a. **Stage I:** 71%
   b. **Stage II:** 47%
   c. **Stage III:** 32%
   d. **Stage IV:** 11%

STUDY QUESTIONS

DIRECTIONS: Each of the numbered items or incomplete statements in this section is followed by answers or by completions of the statement. Select the ONE lettered answer or completion that is BEST in each case.

1. Colposcopic examination of the cervix of a 38-year-old woman with a high-grade lesion on Papanicolaou (Pap) smear yields a negative biopsy and a positive endocervical canal curettage (ECC). Which action is appropriate follow-up?

(A) Repeat the Papanicolaou (Pap) smear in 3 months
(B) Repeat the colposcopic examination in 3 months
(C) Perform conization of the cervix
(D) Perform a vaginal hysterectomy
(E) No follow-up required

2. A patient presents with a gross lesion on her cervix, which appears to involve a small portion of the adjacent vagina. Biopsy of the lesion reveals invasive squamous cell carcinoma. Pelvic examination reveals thickening of the right parametrium but not out to the pelvic sidewall. What is the stage of this cancer?

(A) Stage IA
(B) Stage IB
(C) Stage IIA
(D) Stage IIB
(E) Stage III

3. The correct stage for a T2 N1 M0 carcinoma of the vulva is

(A) stage I
(B) stage II
(C) stage III
(D) stage IV
(E) stage V

4. Which of the tumors listed is most sensitive to radiation therapy?

(A) Serous cystadenocarcinoma
(B) Endometrioid cancer
(C) Gonadoblastoma
(D) Arrhenoblastoma
(E) Dysgerminoma

5. Endometrial hyperplasia could be expected in which one of the following conditions?

(A) Endodermal sinus tumor
(B) Cystic teratoma
(C) Polycystic ovary disease
(D) Sertoli-Leydig cell tumor
(E) Dysgerminoma

DIRECTIONS: Each set of matching questions in this section consists of a list of four to twenty-six lettered options (some of which may be in figures) followed by several numbered items. For each numbered item, select the ONE lettered option that is most closely associated with it. To avoid spending too much time on matching sets with large numbers of options, it is generally advisable to begin each set by reading the list of options. Then, for each item in the set, try to generate the correct answer and locate it in the option list, rather than evaluating each option individually. Each lettered option may be selected once, more than once, or not at all.

Questions 6–7

For each of the following pathologic findings, select the appropriate tumor

(A) Psammoma body
(B) Schiller-Duval body
(C) Call-Exner body
(D) Hobnail cell
(E) Rokitansky's protuberance

6. Granulosa cell tumor

7. Endodermal sinus tumor

Questions 8–9

For each of the following clinical presentations, select the procedure that would be most appropriate

(A) Endometrial biopsy
(B) Unilateral salpingo-oophorectomy
(C) Conization of the cervix
(D) Cyclic oral contraceptive agents
(E) Laser vaporization of the cervix

8. A 23-year-old woman underwent colposcopy for the evaluation of a high-grade lesion on Papanicolaou (Pap) smear. The squamocolumnar junction was seen in its entirety, and the endocervical canal curettage (ECC) was negative. A directed biopsy of the cervix revealed a 1-mm focus of invasion.

9. A 37-year-old woman has heavy, painless bleeding every 4 to 6 months. She is currently interested in contraception. Inspection of her cervix is negative, and her Papanicolaou (Pap) smear is negative.

ANSWERS AND EXPLANATIONS

1. The answer is C [I C 3 c (3) (a)]. An endocervical canal curettage (ECC) is performed with a colposcopy to rule out dysplasia within the canal that is colposcopically inapparent. With a negative colposcopic examination and a positive ECC, cervical dysplasia can be assessed adequately only by a cone biopsy and histologic inspection of the endocervical glands, which contain the abnormal epithelium. A repeat Papanicolaou (Pap) smear or colposcopic examination in 3 months leaves known disease in the canal unevaluated or untreated. Conization of the cervix is not only diagnostic, it is a minor procedure that is therapeutic in 85% of cases.

2. The answer is D [I D 2 d (2)]. Stage II cervical cancers involve the cervix and the vagina or the parametrium. Stage IIA involves the vagina without evidence of parametrial involvement. Stage IIB involves infiltration of the parametrium but not out to the pelvic sidewall.

3. The answer is C [V H 3]. Vulvar staging is based on the tumor size (T), regional node assessment (N), and metastatic assessment (M) system. A T2 N1 M0 tumor is a stage III tumor in which a tumor of 2 cm or more is confined to the vulva and is accompanied by palpable nodes that are not enlarged or mobile. There is no metastasis present.

4. The answer is E [III G 3 a (6)]. The dysgerminoma is the most common form of germ cell tumor. It has a favorable prognosis because of its radiosensitivity. Even though there is a 25% recurrence rate following conservative surgical treatment, most of these recurrent cases have complete remission after radiation therapy.

5. The answer is C [II A 2 d–f, B, C 1]. The etiology of endometrial hyperplasia appears to involve the secretion of estrogen that is unopposed by progesterone. Unopposed estrogen is characteristic of chronic anovulatory states, such as polycystic ovary disease, and

estrogen-secreting tumors, such as the granulosa–theca cell tumor. The cystic teratoma, the dysgerminoma, and the endodermal sinus tumor do not secrete estrogen, and the Sertoli-Leydig cell tumor secretes an androgen that would not produce endometrial hyperplasia.

6–7. The answers are: 6-C [III G 2 b (3)], **7-B** [III G 3 c]. There are certain pathologic findings that are indicative of specific tumors. Endodermal sinus tumors, also called mesonephromas, can be identified with the Schiller-Duval body, which is a characteristic invaginated papillary structure resembling a primitive glomerulus. Call-Exner bodies are characteristic of granulosa cell tumors and resemble follicles. Psammoma bodies are seen in papillary serous tumors. Hobnail cells are seen in the Arias-Stella reaction of gestational endometrium, and clear cell tumors of the ovary. Rokitansky's protuberance is seen macroscopically in benign dermoid cysts.

8–9. The answers are: 8-C [I D 1 a], **9-A** [II A 2 d, C 2]. In any woman whose colposcopically directed biopsy demonstrates microinvasion, an adequate histologic assessment in the form of a conization must be done to evaluate the extent of disease and the lymphovascular space involvement. The definition of microinvasive carcinoma of the cervix includes a depth of invasion of less than 3 mm and a width no greater than 7 mm. If the patient no longer desires fertility, the appropriate treatment is total abdominal hysterectomy. If the patient desires preservation of fertility, therapy with cone biopsy alone may be performed with careful follow-up.

The woman with a normal-appearing cervix with negative cytology is unlikely to have a cervical malignancy. The pattern of bleeding (i.e., every 4–6 months) suggests anovulatory cycles, which places this patient at risk for endometrial hyperplasia or carcinoma. Thus, the endometrium of this woman with abnormal uterine bleeding must be evaluated to exclude endometrial cancer before initiating any therapy.

Chapter 37

Medicolegal Considerations in Obstetrics and Gynecology

William W. Beck, Jr.

I. **INTRODUCTION.** Law defines modes of behavior among the members of a society, and the groups within a society, such that conflicting interests may be resolved in a civilized fashion. Medicine is one such group. In medicine, the law permeates, defining and regulating the relationship between the physician and patient, the physician and hospital, and the physician and society at large. Moreover, legal issues dealing with access to medical care and consumer demands regarding health care are dominant in public policy discussions. Obstetrics and gynecology is at the cutting edge of these matters because the field involves the most critical aspects of life: conception, reproduction, and abortion. Thus, it is important for the student of medicine to understand, in a preliminary fashion, the legal issues that involve the practice of obstetrics and gynecology.

II. **MALPRACTICE**

A. **Definition.** Malpractice is **professional misconduct** whereby a physician departs from the standards of reasonable physicians, either through a lack of skill or a lack of knowledge in carrying out professional duties.

B. **Elements of negligence**

1. **Duty.** A physician has a particular duty or obligation to the patient. A **physician–patient relationship** exists when a patient comes to a physician, who agrees to undertake her care in a fiduciary manner. It is a form of **implied contract.** In this relationship, a physician must act:
   a. In accordance with standards established or accepted by a reasonable fraction of the profession practicing in a given area
   b. As a reasonable physician, taking reasonable care of a patient and not taking unreasonable risks

2. **Breach of duty.** When a physician fails to act on a specific occasion in accordance with professional norms, she or he has departed from the standard of care and has committed a breach of the duty owed to the patient. This breach must be substantiated by the testimony of an expert.

3. **Causation.** The breach of duty owed must be the proximate cause of a patient's injury for a malpractice action to exist.

4. **Damages.** Actual loss, injury, or damage must have occurred, although pain and suffering is a common complaint.

C. **Recovery.** The patient or plaintiff must prove that it is more probable than not that the elements of negligence are satisfied **(preponderance of evidence)** to recover compensation for the damage incurred.

III. **PRECONCEPTION ISSUES.** A constitutional right of privacy protects an individual's procreative choice from government intrusion. The **right to use contraception** was the earliest right to reproductive freedom (*Griswold v Connecticut,* 1965).

A. Oral contraceptives

1. Most lawsuits regarding oral contraceptives are **product liability** cases against the manufacturer.
   a. The general rule is that a manufacturer must provide patients with a written warning of all untoward side effects.
   b. A physician must inform patients of the possible side effects and explain the alternative methods of contraception. All of these discussions must be documented.

2. A physician has a duty to:
   a. Perform a thorough physical examination
   b. Perform relevant laboratory examinations
   c. Warn patients of possible adverse side effects
   d. Monitor closely patients in whom side effects develop

B. Intrauterine devices (IUDs) have been the center of legal and medical controversy regarding contraceptives ever since the Dalkon Shield was recalled in 1974.

1. All IUDs, except for the Progestasert and the ParaGard (a copper-containing device), have been withdrawn by the manufacturers because of litigation costs. Most lawsuits have been product liability cases, with claims that the IUD has caused:
   a. Uterine and pelvic infections
   b. Infertility
   c. Uterine perforation
   d. Ectopic pregnancy

2. A physician has a duty to:
   a. Inform patients of the risks involved with IUD insertion and use
   b. Explain alternative methods of contraception and their risks
   c. Perform a physical examination
   d. Perform a Papanicolaou (Pap) test and cervical cultures
   e. Examine patients in 3 months after insertion of an IUD and yearly thereafter

C. Sterilization. Sterilization is a surgical procedure undertaken for the express purpose of eliminating reproductive capacity.

1. **Voluntary sterilization**
   a. **Public hospitals** cannot refuse to perform sterilization procedures because it would abridge a woman's reproductive right of privacy.
   b. **Private physicians and hospitals** may, however, decline to perform this procedure on moral grounds.
   c. **Federal funding regulations** require that a Department of Health and Human Services consent form be signed 30 to 180 days before surgery. Consent cannot be obtained if the patient is:
      (1) Younger than 21 years of age
      (2) In labor
      (3) Under the influence of alcohol or drugs
      (4) Mentally incompetent
      (5) Having an abortion; federal regulation is such that tubal ligation and abortion cannot be performed at the same time because the federal government will not fund abortion
   d. A physician has a duty to inform patients that:
      (1) The operation will result in sterility.
      (2) The procedure is permanent.
      (3) There are alternative forms of contraception.
      (4) There is no guarantee of sterility; pregnancy occurs in 2 to 4/1000 cases, with ectopic pregnancy being the main concern.

2. **Involuntary sterilization.** Twenty states authorize involuntary sterilization of

genetically retarded wards of the state. However, it is generally required that the patients:
  a. Have permanent medical conditions
  b. Have adequate sexual capacity
  c. Have a high probability of transmitting a genetic disease
  d. Be unable to care for children
  e. Be unable to use alternative methods of contraception

IV. GENETIC COUNSELING. Five percent of all newborns are born with a congenital disorder.

A. Routine genetic screening

1. Legislation requires **phenylketonuria** testing in newborns.

2. There are centers for voluntary **screening of sickle cell** disease.

3. Prenatal **maternal serum α-fetoprotein (MSAFP)** testing to determine the risk for neural tube defects and Down syndrome is routinely recommended.

4. Semen donors are routinely screened for genetic and chromosomal disorders.

B. Particular genetic problems of which a physician must be aware include the following.

1. **Teratogens**
   a. Rubella
   b. Phenytoin
   c. Alcohol
   d. Nicotine
   e. Illicit drugs (e.g., cocaine)

2. **Autosomal dominant disorders**
   a. Neurofibromatosis
   b. Hereditary familial polyposis

3. **Autosomal recessive disorders**
   a. Cystic fibrosis
   b. Infantile polycystic kidney disease
   c. Congenital deafness
   d. Tay-Sachs disease
   e. Thalassemia

4. **X-linked disorders**
   a. Duchenne muscular dystrophy
   b. Hemophilia

C. Offer the pregnant woman referral to a genetic counselor if there is:

1. A genetic or congenital abnormality in a family member

2. A family history of a genetic problem

3. Abnormal development in a previous child

4. Mental retardation in a previous child

5. Maternal age 35 years or older

6. Specific ethnic background suggestive of a genetic abnormality (e.g., Tay-Sachs disease in Ashkenazi Jews, among others)

7. Exposure to drugs or teratogens

8. A history of three or more spontaneous abortions

D. **Amniocentesis** must be offered to pregnant women with:

1. Age of 35 years or more
2. A history of multiple miscarriages
3. A family history of genetic disease
4. An abnormal MSAFP

V. TERMINATION OF PREGNANCY

A. **Right of privacy.** A woman's right to abortion falls within a right of privacy interpreted by the United States Supreme Court to exist within the Constitution. This right was upheld in *Roe v Wade,* 1973.

B. **Trimester model**

1. **During the first trimester,** the decision to abort is a decision that is strictly between a woman and her physician.
2. **During the second trimester,** the state may impose regulations reasonably related to a woman's health.
3. **After the second trimester or after the fetus is viable,** the state may regulate abortion, except when necessary to preserve a woman's health.

C. **State restrictions.** Since 1973, the time of the abortion decision, states have formulated many laws to limit a woman's access to abortion. Most recently, in *Planned Parenthood v Casey,* 1992, the United States Supreme Court upheld a Pennsylvania statute.

1. **Restrictions on elective abortion imposed by the statute**
   a. Physicians are required to discuss the nature, risks, and alternatives to abortion, as well as the gestational age of the fetus.
   b. A 24-hour waiting period is required in between the time this information is given and the abortion is performed.
   c. Either parental consent or, alternatively, the use of judicial bypass procedure if parental consent is denied, is required for a minor.
2. The Court struck down the provision of the statute that required spousal notification.

VI. NEW REPRODUCTIVE TECHNOLOGIES.
New techniques, such as artificial insemination by husband or donor, in vitro fertilization and embryo transfer (IVF/ET), and embryo freezing, have created a change in society's concept of the family. A child may be born with as many as five parents: a genetic father, a social father, a genetic mother, a gestational mother, and a social mother. These technologies create legal issues of linkage, inheritance, legitimacy, adultery, confidentiality, the legal status of residual embryos, the particular "parental" responsibilities for a child's diseases and defects, and the legal status and rights of each "parent."

A. **Artificial insemination**

1. **Definition.** Inoculation of a husband's semen [artificial insemination by husband (AIH)] or a donor's semen [artificial insemination by donor (AID)] into the female genital tract is called artificial insemination.
2. **Consent of the husband.** When the husband of a child's mother consents to

artificial insemination by donor, the husband obtains the same legal right and obligations as a natural parent, including:
   a. The duty to support the child
   b. The right to visitation in case of divorce

3. **Right to privacy.** Given the United States Supreme Court's recognition of a right to privacy, when a single woman requests AID, a public institution providing these services cannot abridge this woman's right to privacy and, thus, would logically have to provide this service; however, a private practitioner could choose not to provide this service. To date, there has not been a case about this issue.

4. **A physician has a duty to explain** that there is:
   a. No guarantee of pregnancy
   b. A possibility of birth defects that may be attributable to unknown recessive genes of the donor
   c. Little chance of sexually transmitted disease (STD) transmission because of screening and the quarantined freeze preservation of semen

5. **Liability** may arise when:
   a. A physician has not adequately screened a donor for genetic defects or STDs, including human immunodeficiency virus.
   b. A husband's consent has not been obtained.

B. **In vitro fertilization**

1. **Definition.** In IVF, sperm and ova are obtained, incubated outside the body, and then the blastocyst is implanted into a uterus.

2. **Legal concepts**
   a. When a husband provides sperm, and a wife provides an ovum, traditional family principles apply. This is similar to AIH.
   b. When a donor provides sperm and a wife provides an ovum, legal concepts of AID and adoption apply.
   c. When the ovum comes from a female donor and is fertilized and then transferred into another woman's uterus, the legal relationships arising are complex and not clearly formulated. The essential question is whether genetic material, a contractual relationship, or carrying and giving birth determine the claim of motherhood.

C. **Surrogate motherhood**

1. **Definition.** When a wife is incapable of bearing a child, a couple enters into a contract with another woman (a surrogate mother), who agrees to be artificially inseminated with the husband's semen, to carry and bear a child, and to relinquish her rights to the child. In exchange, she receives payment for medical care, lost wages, clothing, and hospitalization.

2. **Arguments against surrogate motherhood** include the following.
   a. It undermines the traditional family model.
   b. It threatens the institution of marriage.
   c. It cheapens and destroys maternal bonding.
   d. It treats children as commodities.
   e. It exploits poor women as vehicles to fulfill the dreams of the rich.

3. **Problems arising in the surrogate contract** include the following.
   a. Surrogate mothers develop maternal feelings toward their infants and refuse to give them to the husband and his wife.
   b. Surrogate mothers decide not to honor the contract and terminate the pregnancy.
   c. Surrogate mothers expose the fetus to teratogens or addicting drugs.
   d. The infant is defective, and the contractive couple decides not to accept it.
   e. There is a multiple gestation.

D. **Embryo freezing**

1. **Definition.** Embryo freezing entails the freezing of unused fertilized ova for future implantation.

2. **Problems**
   a. Concerns have been raised as to the propriety of eugenic considerations and commercialism.
   b. The disposition of unused embryos has been deemed unethical by some critics.
   c. If the parents die, the rights and obligations of frozen embryos have yet to be decided.

VII. BIRTH-RELATED SUITS

A. **Wrongful conception**

1. **Definition.** Conception is deemed wrongful if it arises after:
   a. Failed sterilization
   b. Ineffective prescription of contraception
   c. Failure to diagnose pregnancy in a timely fashion
   d. An unsuccessful abortion

2. **Liability** arises secondary to a physician's negligence, resulting in the birth of an unplanned child. Negligence is based on:
   a. The improper performance of a sterilization procedure or an abortion
   b. The failure to ascertain the success of the procedure
   c. The failure to inform the woman about the possibility of procedural failures

B. **Wrongful birth and wrongful life**

1. **Wrongful birth** is an action brought by parents of a child, alleging that a child with a congenital defect was born because of negligent genetic counseling. Thus, a physician has failed to:
   a. Recognize a genetic problem
   b. Recognize a condition that places a fetus at risk for a genetic problem
   c. Inform the mother of the ability to detect genetic problems and to offer termination

2. **Wrongful life** is an action similar to wrongful birth; however, the **child brings suit against the physician,** alleging that no life at all would have been preferable to life with a congenital defect.

VIII. BIRTH INJURY

A. **Definition.** A birth injury results when an obstetrician's neglect results in injury to a child (e.g., birth trauma, brain or neurologic damage).

B. **Negligence** may arise from a failure to:

1. Monitor fetal heart rate adequately

2. Assess the degree of risk of a pregnancy

3. Perform expedient delivery, resulting in perinatal asphyxia that leads to brain damage

4. Monitor a pregnancy adequately

5. Use obstetric forceps properly

    6. Recognize possible macrosomia and the potential for shoulder dystocia and resulting Erb's palsy

C. **Brain damage.** Current studies indicate that it is impossible to isolate a single cause of brain dysfunction. The National Institutes of Health have stated that:

    1. **Mental retardation is multifactorial,** resulting from a combination of genetic, biochemical, viral, and developmental factors, and is not necessarily related to birth trauma.

    2. **Severe mental retardation and epilepsy** are possibly associated with birth asphyxia but only when accompanied by cerebral palsy, which is associated with birth asphyxia, prematurity, and intrauterine growth retardation.

IX. INFORMED CONSENT

A. **General definition.** "Every human being of adult years and sound mind has a right to determine what shall be done with his own body" (*Schloendorff v Society of New York Hospital,* 1914).

B. **Negligence theory of consent.** To sue successfully under this theory, the patient or plaintiff must show that:

    1. A physician was under a duty to disclose an adequate amount of material information.

    2. A physician disclosed an inadequate amount of material information.

    3. The patient agreed to therapy based on this inadequate information

    4. The patient was harmed.

    5. If the significant information had been given, the suggested therapy would have been refused.

C. **Disclosure rules** establish the appropriate standard of care in obtaining informed consent. States differ as to which standard is applicable.

    1. **Majority rule.** A physician needs to disclose only information that a reasonable physician would disclose and need not disclose information that would not customarily be disclosed. This rule operates from the physician's point of view.

    2. **Minority rule.** A physician needs only to disclose information that a reasonable patient in similar circumstances would wish to know to make a reasonable decision.

D. **General guidelines in obtaining informed consent**

    1. A physician must obtain a patient's informed consent before treating her.

    2. A physician must provide information concerning the probable benefits, risks, and nature of the suggested diagnostic or therapeutic interventions.

    3. A physician must provide an explanation of reasonable alternatives to the recommended intervention and the consequences of no intervention.

    4. Information must be:
        a. What a reasonable practitioner would reveal under similar circumstances
        b. What a reasonable patient would consider significant under similar circumstances

    5. **Exceptions to informed consent** include the following:
        a. If a risk is not reasonably foreseeable, it need not be disclosed.

    b. Disclosure may be partial if full disclosure would be detrimental to a patient's best interest.

    c. If the danger is commonly known, it can be assumed that the patient knows of the danger.

    d. The patient may request not to be told of risks.

    e. If the risk concerns improperly performing an appropriate procedure, it need not be disclosed.

    f. In an emergency, where delay would result in death or serious injury and where a patient is unable to reflect and give an informed decision, informed consent is not required.

    g. If a patient is declared either generally or specifically incompetent, informed consent cannot legitimately be obtained.

E. **Procedure for obtaining informed consent.** Informed consent is a process by which a physician imparts information to a patient who, by virtue of this information, may intelligently decide whether to submit to and participate in the physician's proposed intervention. Thus, the physician must do the following:

    1. Discuss the need for the intervention.

    2. Discuss the intervention honestly and explain it in layman's terms along with the reason for its necessity.

    3. Explain the risks inherent in the procedure.

    4. Explain alternatives and the probable result of no intervention.

    5. Allow the patient to ask questions.

    6. Document the conversation, listing the major risks and alternatives presented.

    7. Explain that it is the patient's right to know a reasonable amount about the proposed intervention and that this right is being forfeited if she refuses to discuss the intervention. Document this discussion.

    8. Inform the patient about the risks and the recovery time.

    9. Refrain from altering records.

    10. Personally obtain the consent, not relegating this duty to a nurse or staff member.

STUDY QUESTIONS

DIRECTIONS: Each of the numbered items or incomplete statements in this section is followed by answers or by completions of the statement. Select the ONE lettered answer or completion that is BEST in each case.

1. An obstetrician is called at home by a woman who is in labor. Although she has never been to see the obstetrician for a prenatal visit, she would like him to deliver her infant. The obstetrician refuses to attend to her because he is in the middle of dinner. She subsequently delivers a healthy infant at home. If this woman sues the physician for negligence, which of the following would be his best defense?

(A) Labor is not a disease, so it was not necessary to attend to this pregnant woman
(B) Because the woman did not come for prenatal visits, she is not entitled to a physician
(C) Because the woman gave birth to a healthy infant, no harm was done
(D) Because the physician never accepted the woman as a patient, no physician–patient relationship existed
(E) The patient was contributorily negligent in not calling the physician long in advance of active labor

2. Most intrauterine devices (IUDs) have been unavailable recently because of which of the following reasons?

(A) The materials used to manufacture them have become extraordinarily expensive
(B) They have been found to be unreasonably dangerous and cause multiple pelvic problems
(C) The cost of litigation to the manufacturers is too high
(D) The demand for this form of contraceptive has fallen

3. A physician has a long-standing relationship with a gynecology patient. Unbeknownst to the gynecologist, the woman becomes pregnant. One Saturday, she calls her gynecologist to complain of nausea and vomiting. The patient is unable to reach the physician because she is on vacation and has left no other physician to take care of her patients. Three months later the patient goes into preterm labor and delivers a premature infant. The infant ultimately dies 1 month later. In a lawsuit, which of the following statements is the physician's best defense?

(A) No physician–patient relationship existed
(B) She did not breach any duty owed to the patient
(C) Her negligence was not the proximate cause of the woman's premature delivery and fetal death
(D) A premature infant is not a viable human being
(E) The woman has not suffered any injuries

DIRECTIONS: The numbered item or incomplete statement in this section is negatively phrased, as indicated by a capitalized word such as NOT, LEAST, or EXCEPT. Select the ONE lettered answer or completion that is BEST.

4. Which of the following is NOT necessary for a physician to do in counseling a couple who wishes artificial insemination by donor (AID)?

(A) Obtain consent from both husband and wife
(B) Explain that there is no guarantee of pregnancy
(C) Explain that, despite screening, birth defects are possible
(D) Explain that there is little risk of transmitting sexually transmitted diseases (STDs)
(E) Explain that a divorce excludes the husband from access to the child

DIRECTIONS: The set of matching questions in this section consists of a list of four to twenty-six lettered options (some of which may be in figures) followed by several numbered items. For each numbered item, select the ONE lettered option that is most closely associated with it. To avoid spending too much time on matching sets with large numbers of options, it is generally advisable to begin each set by reading the list of options. Then, for each item in the set, try to generate the correct answer and locate it in the option list, rather than evaluating each option individually. Each lettered option may be selected once, more than once, or not at all.

Questions 5–8

For each legal term listed below, select the statement that defines it.

(A) An action brought by a child, alleging that because of a physician's negligence in genetic counseling, she was born with congenital defects of such magnitude that no life (through mother's choice of abortion) would have been preferable
(B) An action brought by a child, alleging that his cerebral palsy was proximately caused by the negligent monitoring of his mother's pregnancy by the obstetrician
(C) An action brought by parents of a normal child, alleging that because of a physician's negligence in the performance of a sterilization procedure or an abortion, an unwanted child was born
(D) An action brought by the parents of a congenitally defective child, alleging that because of inadequate or absent genetic counseling, the option of abortion was taken away from them; thus, they seek compensation for the harm arising from the child's defects
(E) An action brought by a woman against her obstetrician stating that if she had known that there was a possibility of cesarean section in the delivery of her child, she would have sought the assistance of another obstetrician

5. Wrongful conception

6. Wrongful life

7. Wrongful birth

8. Birth injury

■ ANSWERS AND EXPLANATIONS

1. The answer is D [II B 1–4]. For a physician to be sued for negligence, the plaintiff must clear four hurdles. These are that a duty existed; the duty was breached; that, because of the breach of duty, harm was directly caused; and real damage occurred. In this case, no physician–patient relationship existed because the physician refused to help a person who was not his patient. Although it might be argued that it would have been morally correct for the physician to attend to this woman, the law does not recognize a duty to rescue. A physician–patient relationship must be entered into voluntarily and cannot be coerced on either part.

2. The answer is C [III B 1]. Although the Dalkon Shield was responsible for many cases of pelvic infection, the risk for pelvic infection is only slightly higher than the normal risk with other intrauterine devices (IUDs), such as the Copper-7 and Lippes Loop. Because defending challenges to the safety of IUDs has proven too costly, manufacturers have simply stopped manufacturing these devices. The IUDs now on the market are available at high cost to the consumer and are inserted only after extensive explanations are given to the patient of the possible risks involved.

3. The answer is C [II B 1–4]. Although the physician was negligent in not having another physician cover for her while she was on vacation, her negligence did not proximately cause her patient's ultimate injury. Any relationship between the physician's negligence of not being present and the patient's premature delivery 3 months later is too remote to establish causation. Because a premature infant was born and lived for 1 month, it is a human being and a legal entity that can maintain a lawsuit. Also, the mother can maintain a lawsuit apart from her infant.

4. The answer is E [VI A 2, 4, 5]. The couple who wishes artificial insemination by donor (AID) must be told of the risks of acquiring birth defects and sexually transmitted diseases (STDs). There are some STDs for which screening is not routine (e.g., human papillo-

mavirus) or about which there is no information (e.g., screening was unavailable for the human immunodeficiency virus 5 years ago). In this process, it is essential that the husband give his consent, because in so doing he is accepting all responsibility for the child born from this AID process. In addition to that responsibility, the husband also maintains the right to visitation in case of a divorce.

5–8. The answers are: 5-C [VII A 1, 2], **6-A** [VII B 2], **7-D** [VII B 1], **8-B** [VIII A–C]. In cases involving wrongful conception, namely parents seeking compensation for a normal child resulting from a failed sterilization, willingness to compensate has been low. In cases where the resulting child was abnormal, medical expenses for the care of the infant have been granted. Important to the determination of wrongful conception is documentation of whether the mother was informed of the possibility of failure of the sterilization procedure.

Wrongful life actions brought by a child, alleging that no life would have been better than life with congenital defects, have generally been unsuccessful. Compensation prior to these injuries, however, may be granted on negligence theory.

Wrongful birth actions are brought by the parents of a child with a congenital defect, alleging that a physician was remiss in genetic counseling, and because of this, a defective child was allowed to be born. In general, these cases have been successful, especially in cases where testing would have been easy, such as in parental testing for Tay-Sachs disease.

Birth injury cases are one of the most common cases plaguing obstetricians. A child may bring suit until the age of majority, after which time he or she is dependent on the statute of limitations of the particular jurisdiction. Because children represent a great emotional investment, a child who is abnormal in any way may be suspected of being a victim of an obstetrician's malpractice. Although the association of cerebral palsy and fetal heart monitoring is a weak one, these cases often prevail on public sentiment and liability based on a preponderance of evidence.

CASE STUDIES IN CLINICAL DECISION MAKING

Case 1: Hormone Replacement Therapy

A 53-year-old woman comes to her physician for a routine gynecologic examination. Once in the office, she starts to cry and asks how she knows when she is through menopause and how long it will take. She explains that her life isn't the same anymore; it must be due to "the change." She hasn't been to the gynecologist for several years. Her friends and family encouraged her to come today to get help.

QUESTIONS

1. *What is the definition of menopause?*

2. *When does menopause normally occur?*

DISCUSSION

Menopause is the point in time marked by the permanent cessation of menses. The diagnosis of menopause is made retrospectively. Menopause is defined as the absence of a menstrual period for 6 to 12 months in a woman 45 years of age or older. The cessation of menses reflects a decline in ovarian function. The average age of menopause is 51.4 years, with a normal age range of 48 to 55 years. Perimenopause is the period of time just preceding and following the permanent cessation of menses. The few years preceding menopause, characterized by a fluctuation of ovarian function, are referred to as the transition. The average length of transition is 4 years. This patient could be anywhere along the spectrum of declining or reduced ovarian function. How a woman experiences menopause is related to the hormonal changes characteristic of this time as well as other factors such as psychosocial issues, the presence of medical illness, and general physical condition.

The patient states that her last period was about 14 months ago but she really hasn't been herself for the last 2 years. During this time, she has been experiencing what she thinks are hot flashes that have been getting progressively worse. They seem to occur most often at night, and she doesn't remember when she last had a full night of sleep. Before this she usually adjusted quite well to changes in her life. Now, she can't seem to cope. She is grateful that her husband is very patient with her; after years of a rewarding sexual relationship, she has very little interest or enjoyment in their sex life.

QUESTIONS

1. *What are the characteristic symptoms of menopause?*

2. *What is the endocrinology, physiology, and clinical course of hot flushes?*

3. *What vaginal changes are characteristic of menopause?*

4. *How does menopause affect sexual function?*

DISCUSSION

The most common symptom of the menopausal period is the hot flush. Seventy-five to eighty-five percent of women experience hot flushes to some degree; they are the most common reason women seek treatment during menopause. Many women notice the onset of hot flushes before the permanent cessation of menses. Hot flushes may occur during the transition, most typically during periods of amenorrhea when circulating estradiol levels are reduced. Hot flushes occur in response to a reduction of estradiol levels from previously established levels. Women with hypogonadism secondary to gonadal dysgenesis who have always had low estrogen levels do not experience hot flushes. It has been noted that there is a surge of luteinizing hormone (LH) just before the onset of the hot flush. However, it is unlikely that the LH surge plays a causative role because women with hypopituitarism and no LH surge still experience hot flushes. Hot flushes are the result of an inappropriate stimulation of the heat-losing mechanism in the thermoregulatory center of the hypothalamus. Core body temperature has been measured and noted to be normal when the body is stimulated to lose heat to reduce core temperature. There is a corresponding decrease in core body temperature after the hot flush occurs. There is usually a prodromal aura signaling that the hot flush is going to occur, followed by a increasing sense of warmth progressing from the waist and over the chest, neck, and face. This sense of warmth is accompanied by peripheral vasodilation with a flushing of the skin, perspiration, and at times, heart palpitations. Hot flushes last from seconds to minutes and may be repetitive. They tend to occur more frequently at night and may be a source of significant sleep disturbances. Chronic sleep deprivation can result in fatigue, depression, anxiety, and an overall decreased sense of well-being. Hot flushes tend to decrease in frequency with time, although they may persist for over 3 to 5 years in up to one third of women. The pattern of symptoms seen in this patient is typical of the menopause experience. Insomnia and depression are symptoms of the menopausal period that may occur independently of hot flushes. However, the mood disturbances experienced by this woman may be secondary to the disruption in her life from hot flushes.

Dyspareunia, painful intercourse, is another common symptom experienced after menopause. The vagina is an estrogen-sensitive organ. With a decline in circulating estradiol levels after menopause, the vaginal epithelium atrophies, the vagina loses elasticity and compliance, and lubrication is decreased. As discomfort with intercourse increases, enjoyment and interest decline. Women also complain of decreased libido during the perimenopause and beyond, unrelated to dyspareunia. The etiology of decline in interest in sexual activity is usually multifactorial with a complex interplay of hormonal, psychological, and social factors. Some women experience a new enjoyment of sexual activity after the menopause with children moving away and removal of the risk of pregnancy.

The role of estrogen replacement therapy for relief of menopausal symptoms is discussed with the patient. She is eager to experience relief of her symptoms but is concerned because she has read that a risk of breast cancer is associated with estrogen replacement therapy. Further history shows the patient has no history of breast biopsy or problems, and a negative family history for breast, ovarian, and colon cancers. She has not had a mammogram and does not do breast self-examination regularly. She has four children; she had her first when she was 23 years of age. She has no known medical problems and is not taking any medications. She does not take vitamins or calcium supplements. The patient works as a secretary, and she does not exercise regularly; she neither smokes nor drinks alcohol. She gets one serving per day of dairy products, does not pay attention to fat in her diet, and drinks 4 to 5 cups of coffee per day. The patient's father died from a heart attack at age 62; he had his first heart attack at age 47. Her mother is alive and well at age 78. The patient has never had her cholesterol measured.

QUESTIONS

1. *What are the benefits of estrogen replacement therapy?*

2. *What are the risks of estrogen replacement therapy?*

3. *What are the contraindications of estrogen replacement therapy?*

DISCUSSION

Estrogen is approved for use after menopause to treat menopausal symptoms and for the prevention and treatment of postmenopausal osteoporosis. Estrogen, compared with placebo, has consistently reduced the severity, frequency, and intensity of hot flushes. With improvement in hot flush frequency, an improvement in sleep and mood is also noted. Estrogen replacement also effectively relieves symptoms related to urogenital atrophy. After 3 to 4 months of use, women experience an increase in vaginal lubrication, decreased discomfort with intercourse, and an improvement in symptoms of urinary urgency and frequency. Estrogen replacement alone is often insufficient to improve decreased libido. If a lack of desire is related to vaginal discomfort, marked improvement is often noted with replacement therapy. Adding androgens, in a low dose, to the hormone replacement therapy regimen may provide further improvement in the level of sexual desire.

Osteoporosis is a systemic skeletal disease characterized by a decease in bone mass with micro-architectural distortion associated with increased fragility of bone and susceptibility to fracture. The sites most frequently involved with fracture include the vertebrae, the hip, and the wrist, although all bones are at risk. Risk factors for osteoporosis include advanced age, female gender, white or Asian race, tobacco use, alcohol use, inadequate calcium intake, sedentary lifestyle, high protein diet, and excessive caffeine use. Medications associated with an increased risk of osteoporosis include chronic corticosteroid use and excessive thyroid replacement. Peak bone mass is reached for both trabecular and cortical bone by age 30. Thereafter, there is continuous age-related bone loss. For the first 5 to 7 years after menopause, there is an accelerated rate of bone loss secondary to reduction of circulating estradiol levels. Estrogen replacement therapy prevents the accelerated bone loss associated with menopause and effectively reduces the risk of fracture by up to 50%. Effective protection requires at least 3 to 5 years of estrogen use; bone loss occurs after cessation of therapy. Other measures such as adequate calcium intake and exercise are important in the prevention and treatment of osteoporosis.

Another important medical benefit of estrogen replacement is a reduction of morbidity and mortality associated with cardiovascular disease. Estrogen replacement is associated with a 50% reduction in cardiovascular mortality. Because cardiovascular disease is the leading cause of death in women, this is a benefit of utmost significance. Studies have also shown that women with established coronary artery disease have an improved 10-year survival rate with estrogen replacement therapy. The mechanisms by which estrogen exerts a protective effect include an improvement in the lipoprotein profile with an increase in high-density lipoprotein cholesterol, a decrease in total cholesterol, vasodilation of the coronary arteries with an increased blood flow, and an anti-atherogenic effect through anti-oxidant properties.

Other benefits attributed to estrogen use after menopause include a maintenance of skin thickness, treatment of androgenic alopecia, and increased sense of well-being. There is preliminary evidence that estrogen use may be associated with a retardation in the progression of memory loss associated with Alzheimer's dementia. Ongoing research will further define this proposed benefit.

Unopposed estrogen replacement therapy in a woman who has not undergone hysterectomy is associated with an increased risk of endometrial hyperplasia and carcinoma. Risk increases with increasing dose and duration of use. Adding a progestin at currently recommended doses and duration to the replacement regimen effectively decreases the risk to less than 1%. The addition of progestin enhances the protective effect estrogen exerts on bone. The impact of progestin on the cardiovascular benefit has yet to be defined.

Short-term use of estrogen replacement, defined as less than 5 years' duration, is not associated with an increased risk of breast cancer. The risk of breast cancer associated with long-term use of estrogen replacement continues to be controversial; there have been reports of no associated increased risk and reports of a 40% increased risk. Because of the other benefits that impact on quantity and quality of life, it is currently thought that the benefits of hormone replacement therapy outweigh the risk in a woman with no contraindications to therapy. The addition of progestin does not exert a protective effect in terms of breast cancer risk; progestin should not be added in a women who has undergone hysterectomy.

Women who are not candidates for hormone replacement therapy are those with conditions that could be worsened by hormone use or conditions that would impair the metabolism of estrogen leading to unpredictable circulating estrogen levels. These risk factors are a history of one or more of the following: breast cancer, endometrial cancer (except stage I disease), recent thromboembolic disease, hormone-related thromboembolic disease, acute or chronic hepatic disease. Other conditions are relative contraindications in that they are not life-threatening but could be worsened with hormone use. These include the presence of a seizure disorder, history of migraine headaches, cholelithiasis, and hypertriglyceridemia. Adjustment of the regimen or route of administration often allows safe effective use of hormones in women with these conditions.

This patient certainly will benefit from hormone replacement therapy for symptom management. Her history does not contain any absolute or relative contraindications to therapy. Because she has risk factors for both osteoporosis and cardiovascular disease, her risk profile indicates that the benefits of hormone replacement therapy outweigh the risks and she should be encouraged to comply with recommendations regarding therapy.

Physical examination reveals the patient to be normotensive and of average weight. Breast examination is normal, and breast self-examination was taught. Pelvic examination showed atrophic vaginal changes, a normal-sized uterus, and adnexae that were not palpable. Rectal examination was negative for masses and occult heme. A pap smear was obtained; mammography was ordered; and cholesterol and high-density lipoprotein (HDL) tests were ordered. Colorectal cancer screening with sigmoidoscopy was discussed.

QUESTIONS

1. What are the components of routine health maintenance that are important to include in the clinical encounter with a menopausal patient?

2. How should hormone replacement therapy be prescribed and how should the patient be counseled?

3. What follow-up should be recommended?

4. When would an endometrial biopsy be recommended?

DISCUSSION

Frequently, the only encounter the postmenopausal woman has with the health care system is for gynecologic care. It is of utmost importance to take full advantage of this opportunity to provide counseling regarding healthy lifestyle recommendations and obtain appropriate screenings according to the patient's age and risk profile. Blood pressure, weight, and height should be obtained on an annual basis. Breast self-examination should be reviewed and recommended to be done monthly by the patient. Clinical breast examination should be done annually; mammography should be obtained annually after the age of 50. Before age 50, mammographic screening should be obtained every 1 to 2 years beginning at age 40. A normal mammogram should be documented before initiation of hormone replacement therapy. A pelvic examination is recommended on an annual basis. A pap smear should be obtained annually; longer screening intervals can be used in the low-risk patient with a history of normal pap smears. After 50, cholesterol screening should be obtained every 2 to 3 years, if normal, and more frequently if abnormal. Before age 50, levels should be obtained every 5 years. Smoking cessation should be initiated when indicated. Recommendations regarding adequate calcium intake should be made, including a total of 1000 mg for the woman receiving hormone replacement therapy and 1500 mg when not receiving hormone replacement therapy. This total is the sum of both dietary and supplemental intake. Counseling regarding daily physical activity and an aerobic exercise program should be provided. Screening for colorectal cancer includes annual rectal examination and guaiac testing. Sigmoidoscopy in the patient of average risk and colonoscopy in the high-risk patient are recommended at intervals (1–5 years) according to risk and previous findings. The role of routine bone density measurements to detect osteoporosis has yet to be defined. Bone density measurements are obtained in the postmenopausal woman when the results would impact therapy; in the woman with asymptomatic hyperparathyroidism; and in the woman with a history of chronic corticosteroid use.

Estrogen replacement therapy should be prescribed for symptom relief, osteoporosis prevention, and reduction of cardiovascular risk. Progestin is added either sequentially (10–14 days/month) or continuously to provide endometrial protection. Prescribing progestin in a sequential manner has the disadvantage of inducing menstrual-like bleeding on a monthly basis. Continuous progestin therapy avoids regular cyclic bleeding but is associated with a higher incidence of irregular bleeding that is unpredictable in terms of amount, frequency, and duration. The lowest recommended dose of estrogen should be the starting point; this varies with the type of estrogen prescribed. Increasing the dose of estrogen may be necessary to obtain maximum symptom relief; this should be done for the shortest duration possible. A patch can be prescribed for those women who prefer this route of administration; in women in whom there is an advantage to bypassing the first-pass hepatic effect; or in women in whom consistent bioavailability is critical. Avoiding the first-pass effect on the liver may be advantageous in women who have cholelithiasis, women taking anticonvulsant medication, and women with a history of thromboembolic disease. Consistent bioavailability may be a factor in women who have depressive symptoms and hormone-related migraine headaches; avoiding fluctuations in serum estrogen levels may enhance the response to hormone therapy. Women with skin sensitivities may not tolerate patch therapy.

Adequate counseling regarding the risk, benefits, and expected side effects of hormone replacement therapy is a critical component of the menopausal encounter. Compliance with hormone replacement therapy continues to be a significant problem. Only 10% to 25% of appropriate candidates opt to initiate hormone replacement. Only 30% of these women continue therapy after 1 year. The patient should be warned that breast fullness, tenderness, or enlargement is not unusual, initially, and usually subsides with continued use. Initial water retention and weight gain may occur. Substantial weight gain has not been demonstrated to be secondary to hormone therapy. Woman who wear contact lenses may experience an intolerance for previously comfortable lenses secondary to fluid retention and change in corneal shape. If the patient is placed on a sequential regimen, she should be informed that normal bleeding occurs on completion of the progestin component. Bleeding that occurs at any other time is considered abnormal. Bleeding may be similar in amount to previous menses; lighter bleeding or no bleeding is an acceptable pattern as well. Patients often equate the presence of withdrawal bleeding with adequate endometrial protection. The woman needs to be assured that endometrial shedding is not essential to obtain endometrial protection. If a woman is started on continuous combined therapy, she should be warned about the likely occurrence of irregular bleeding. There is no normal expected bleeding pattern with this regimen. What is important to define is what is abnormal. Heavy, persistent, or frequent bleeding should be considered abnormal. The patient should be instructed to call the physician should she experience abnormal bleeding or symptoms that are new, persistent, and bothersome. After initiation of therapy, patient should return in 3 months to review her response to therapy and any questions or concerns. Once the patient's response to therapy has stabilized, she can return to routine, annual follow-up.

Routine endometrial biopsies are not necessary before the initiation of hormone replacement therapy but should be obtained in women who experience postmenopausal bleeding and in women who experience abnormal bleeding while taking hormone replacement therapy. On a sequential regimen, abnormal bleeding is any bleeding that occurs at a time other than with progestin withdrawal. On a continuous regimen, bleeding that is persistent, heavy, or prolonged is considered abnormal.

Case 2: Secondary Amenorrhea

A 28-year-old woman presents to her physician's office with amenorrhea of 6 months' duration. Her medical history includes a spontaneous vaginal delivery 1 year ago. This delivery was followed by postpartum endometritis and bleeding, which necessitated a dilation and curettage and a blood transfusion. The patient nursed her infant for 4 months and stopped because of lack of milk. She had two spontaneous light bleeds 6 weeks apart before becoming amenorrheic. She states that she always had irregular cycles and actually took 1 year to become pregnant. She has lost 50 lb. since her pregnancy.

QUESTIONS

1. What is the differential diagnosis of secondary amenorrhea?

2. Do the events before or after the pregnancy help to narrow the diagnosis?

DISCUSSION

This is a clinical picture of secondary amenorrhea with a significant differential diagnosis. With the history alone, the etiology of the amenorrhea could be pregnancy or could be secondary to hypothalamic, pituitary, ovarian, or endometrial dysfunction. In this case, the secondary amenorrhea could be hypothalamic due to stress or the significant weight loss. Normally a 50-lb. weight loss might explain the amenorrhea; however, the patient may have lost the weight in an effort to reestablish her prepregnancy weight. Either a pituitary adenoma with increased levels of prolactin or Sheehan's picture (hypoactive thyroid, adrenal, and ovarian function because of decreased stimulating hormones) secondary to postpartum bleeding, hypotension, and pituitary necrosis could cause the amenorrhea. The ovary might be the cause because of either an ovarian tumor or polycystic ovaries (irregular menses and relative infertility) or premature failure. The tumor and the premature failure are rare possibilities. Finally, the endometrium could be replaced by scar tissue (Ascherman's syndrome) secondary to the postpartum endometritis and curettage.

Physical examination shows no significant abnormalities. Breast examination is normal without any galactorrhea. Pelvic examination shows a normal sized, firm uterus with no apparent adnexal masses. The result of a urine pregnancy test is negative. A 5-day course of oral progesterone produces no withdrawal bleeding within 10 days.

QUESTIONS

1. What is the significance of the absence of withdrawal bleeding?

2. Does the absence of withdrawal bleeding eliminate any of the compartments in the etiology?

DISCUSSION

The negative pregnancy test result rules out pregnancy. The absence of a progesterone withdrawal flow means either that the endometrium is unresponsive to hormonal stimulation (synechiae), that the ovary cannot produce estrogen (premature failure), or that the ovary is inadequately stimulated because of low gonadotropins (pituitary or hypothalamic causes). This clinical test does not, therefore, eliminate any of the compartments as possible causes of the amenorrhea.

The patient is given sequential estrogen and progesterone and has a withdrawal flow within 3 days. Her thyroid function studies and cortisol levels are within normal limits. There is no elevation of her prolactin level.

QUESTIONS

1. What does the bleeding following sequential estrogen/progesterone therapy indicate?

2. Why are the normal values of the pituitary target glands important?

DISCUSSION

The withdrawal bleeding following sequential estrogen/progesterone therapy establishes the fact that the endometrium can respond if properly stimulated. This finding rules out intrauterine synechiae and polycystic ovaries. With polycystic ovarian disease and its estrogenic state, the endometrium would have been proliferative and would have bled with the initial progesterone challenge. The normal thyroid function tests and cortisol levels effectively rule out Sheehan's syndrome, a panhypopituitary state with low levels of all pituitary hormones. The normal prolactin level rules out a prolactin-secreting microadenoma that could be the cause of the amenorrhea secondary to suppression of follicle-stimulating hormone (FSH) and luteinizing hormone (LH). What is not yet ruled out is either premature ovarian failure or hypothalamic amenorrhea (hypogonadotropic hypogonadism).

The final and definitive test in this clinical picture is a gonadotropin assay (FSH and LH) assay; both levels are reported back as very low.

QUESTION

1. How do the FSH and LH levels differentiate between premature ovarian failure and hypothalamic amenorrhea?

DISCUSSION

The low level of gonadotropins indicates that the etiology of the amenorrhea is most likely hypothalamic in nature. The fact that the thyroid and adrenal glands are functioning normally eliminates the possibility of a nonresponsive pituitary. The gonadotropins would have been high in premature ovarian failure because of the lack of ovarian estrogen and the lack of consequent negative feedback on the hypothalamus. Thus, the cause of this postpartum patient's secondary amenorrhea is hypothalamic in nature, possibly due to the large amount of weight loss, but most probably due to the stress of new motherhood; this condition was foreshadowed by her inability to nurse because of a decreased milk supply.

Case 3: Female Urinary Incontinence

A 46-year-old woman, gravida 4, para 4, presents to her physician's office with complaints of urinary incontinence.

QUESTION

1. What are the causes of urinary incontinence in women?

DISCUSSION

There are three general categories of female urinary incontinence. Genuine stress urinary incontinence (GSUI) is the most common and is generally caused by an anatomic defect of the posterior urethrovesical angle. GSUI usually is a result of pelvic floor muscle damage from childbearing.

Urge incontinence associated with detrusor instability (DI) is another common cause of female urinary incontinence. DI is defined by the onset of spontaneous detrusor contractions with bladder filling; it may also be caused by neurologic disease.

Mixed incontinence includes both stress and urge components in the cause of urine loss.

QUESTION

1. What questions might the physician ask this patient to further evaluate her urinary incontinence?

DISCUSSION

In evaluating a patient with urinary incontinence, it is essential to obtain a voiding diary. In the diary the patient should document the times and amounts that she voids, the times that she is incontinent, and the precipitating events.

The patient should also complete a thorough urologic questionnaire, which should inquire about how often she voids during the day and night, the amounts of urine voided or leaked, the presence of an urgency to void, whether she has a history of urinary infections or stones, and when her incontinence began. It should also include questions regarding what medications she takes and what precipitates her urine loss.

The patient tells the physician that she typically loses urine with coughing or sneezing and that she sometimes doesn't make it to the bathroom in time. She noticed that these symptoms began after the birth of her second child, improved for a time, but have since worsened. She has to wear a diaper, which becomes soaked from leaking urine. Her diary shows that she drinks a cup of coffee and a glass of orange juice in the morning and a glass of iced tea at lunch. She doesn't drink any liquids after dinner for fear that she may have to get up during the night. She usually gets up to void once during the night. Her voiding diary demonstrates more episodes of leakage in the mornings than at any other time of day. She presently takes hydrochlorothiazide and verapamil for her hypertension.

QUESTIONS

1. What kind of incontinence might this patient have?

2. What part of her history could be exacerbating her incontinence?

3. What might be done to improve her symptoms?

DISCUSSION

Because she first reported symptoms after childbirth, and because her urine loss typically occurs with an increase in abdominal pressure (i.e., with coughing or sneezing), the patient most likely has stress incontinence. However, a patient's history does not always correlate with the type of urinary incontinence. This diagnosis should be confirmed with the demonstration of urine loss with the Valsalva maneuver, accompanied by a descent of the posterior urethrovesical angle. Detrusor instability should also be excluded cystometrically.

Coffee and tea can irritate the bladder mucosa and can exacerbate incontinence. The patient should be advised to avoid caffeine and tea intake. Her use of hydrochlorothiazide, a diuretic, and verapamil, a calcium channel blocker, also may be exacerbating her incontinence; she might be switched to an alternative medication with fewer effects on the bladder. The patient should also be instructed on how to perform Kegel exercises, which strengthen the pubococcygeus muscles and can improve incontinence symptoms in up to 75% of individuals.

QUESTION

1. What elements of the physical examination are important to obtain?

DISCUSSION

The physical examination is necessary to exclude a neoplasia, diverticulum or fistula, and pelvic mass. The examination should assess the patient's hormonal status; check for the presence of a cystocele, rectocele, and uterine prolapse; and evaluate for pelvic floor muscle tone. A neurologic examination of the perineum and lower extremities should also be performed to exclude neuromuscular disorders such as multiple sclerosis.

The patient's physical examination demonstrates a moderate uterine prolapse and a moderate cystocele and rectocele. The result of her neurologic examination is normal.

QUESTION

1. What other evaluation can be performed to confirm the diagnosis?

Once a presumptive diagnosis of stress incontinence has been established, office cystometrics can be performed to confirm the diagnosis and to exclude detrusor instability or mixed incontinence as the cause of urine loss. The office evaluation should include a post-void residual test, which should be less than 100 ml; this catheterized sample should be sent for culture and sensitivities to exclude urinary tract infection. Simple cystometrics can be performed by filling the bladder through a catheter, noting the patient's first sensation to void, and when she senses a maximally full bladder. If the patient develops spontaneous bladder contractions with bladder filling, this is indicative of detrusor instability, and not stress incontinence. If leakage of urine can be demonstrated with a full bladder with straining, this is indicative of stress incontinence. In the presence of both, further studies must be performed to evaluate for mixed incontinence or other causes.

Case 4: Hypertension in Pregnancy

A 33-year-old African-American primigravid woman presents for prenatal care at 10 weeks' gestation by her last menstrual period. Her blood pressure taken in the office is 150/100.

QUESTIONS

1. How common is hypertension in pregnancy?

2. What is the most likely diagnosis?

DISCUSSION

Hypertensive disease occurs in 8% to 11% of all pregnancies. It is second only to embolism as a cause of maternal mortality. Hypertension during pregnancy is divided into pregnancy-induced hypertension (PIH) and chronic hypertension. PIH usually occurs in the second half of pregnancy. Hypertension that occurs before 20 weeks' gestation, even in the absence of a history of hypertension, is defined as chronic hypertension. The one exception is patients with gestational trophoblastic disease, who may develop PIH before 20 weeks' gestation. The most likely diagnosis in this patient is chronic hypertension, but gestational trophoblastic disease should be excluded by ultrasonography.

Further questioning provides a history of essential hypertension since age 25. The patient reports that she is currently taking enalapril for control of her blood pressure. The remainder of her history is noncontributory, and a routine gynecologic examination is remarkable only for a 10-week–sized uterus.

QUESTIONS

1. Should the patient's medication be continued?

2. How else should she be evaluated?

DISCUSSION

Enalapril and other angiotensin-converting enzyme (ACE) inhibitors should not be continued in pregnancy. Their use beyond the first trimester has been associated with fetal hypocalvaria, renal failure, oligohydramnios, and fetal and neonatal death. If the patient's blood pressure is persistently 150/100, she should be treated to prevent maternal morbidity. The antihypertensive of choice in pregnancy is alpha-methyldopa. Further evaluation of this moderately hypertensive woman should include a complete physical examination including cardiac and funduscopic evaluation. Laboratory evaluation should include a complete blood count, urinalysis, serum creatinine, 24-hour urine test for protein and creatinine clearance, and serum electrolytes. An electrocardiogram, a chest radiograph for cardiac contour, and an ophthalmologic evaluation should also be considered. An ultrasound should be performed to confirm the patient's dates and exclude a hydatidiform mole.

The patient should be seen every 2 weeks, and serial sonography for fetal growth is indicated. Once the patient is in the third trimester, fetal surveillance is indicated. The clinician should be alert to signs and symptoms of placental abruption and superimposed PIH, which are common in pregnant women with chronic hypertension.

The patient's physical examination and laboratory evaluation are normal. Her pregnancy remains uncomplicated until 35 weeks' gestation, when she calls the physician's office with a complaint of a headache.

QUESTIONS

1. What should the physician be concerned about?

2. What should the physician do next?

DISCUSSION

The patient should be instructed to come in immediately for evaluation. Symptoms such as headache, visual changes, and epigastric pain may indicate PIH in any pregnant patient. Patients with chronic hypertension are especially at risk for superimposed PIH and preeclampsia.

The patient is seen on the labor floor, and her blood pressure is persistently 180/120. Urine protein is noted to be +2. The patient complains of a persistent headache that is not relieved by Tylenol. Physical examination is unremarkable, and her cervix is noted to be 1 cm dilated and 90% effaced with the fetal vertex at −1 station. Fetal monitor demonstrates irregular contractions and fetal heart rate in the 140's and reactive.

QUESTIONS

1. What is the physician's diagnosis now?

2. What laboratory studies are indicated?

3. How should the patient be managed?

DISCUSSION

Based on the patient's blood pressure and symptoms, the patient meets criteria for the diagnosis of superimposed severe PIH. Laboratory evaluation should include a complete blood count to look for hemoconcentration and thrombocytopenia, a serum creatinine and uric acid test to identify renal dysfunction, and liver function tests to identify a transaminitis. If the platelet count is abnormal, or if the patient has clinical signs of abruption, complete coagulation studies should be ordered. Because the diagnosis of severe PIH has been made, the indicated treatment is delivery of the fetus to prevent both maternal and fetal morbidity and mortality. Vaginal delivery is preferred, and with a favorable cervix intravenous oxytocin may be given. The patient should also receive parenteral magnesium sulfate for seizure prophylaxis.

Case 5: Menopause

A 51-year-old woman presents to her physician's office complaining of mood swings, vaginal dryness, and hot flashes for the past several months. She had a total abdominal hysterectomy 4 years ago secondary to uterine myomas.

QUESTIONS

1. What are the potential causes of this patient's complaints?

2. What laboratory values would help confirm the diagnosis?

DISCUSSION

Given the patient's age and symptoms, she is most likely going through menopause. It must be considered that, as women age, their risk for thyroid disease increases. The most common complaints that will bring a menopausal woman to her physician are hot flashes, irregular menses, vaginal dryness, mood swings, and sleep disturbances. This patient has undergone a hysterectomy so has not experienced irregular menses. Most women will begin to experience menstrual irregularities as the first sign of impending menopause. The irregularities are quite similar to the menstrual irregularities experienced by adolescents. The cessation of menses defines menopause. When a woman has had her uterus removed, the physician relies on symptoms to make the diagnosis. Serum levels of follicle-stimulating hormone and luteinizing hormone increase due to the loss of negative feedback from estrogen and inhibin from the ovary. In this situation, these values help confirm the diagnosis of menopause. A maturation index from the vaginal mucosa may be obtained to determine if the vaginal symptoms are caused by atrophy.

On further questioning, the physician discovers that the patient's mother died from a pulmonary embolus after surgical pinning of a fractured hip.

QUESTION

1. How will this information impact patient management?

DISCUSSION

This patient's mother may have suffered a fractured hip secondary to osteoporosis. A family history of osteoporosis is the strongest risk factor for the development of osteoporosis. This patient should be advised of her increased risk of osteoporosis and instructed as to how she can decrease her risk and keep her bones healthy. The health cost of osteoporosis is great. Over 10 billion dollars are spent every year caring for men and women who have osteoporosis. For elderly patients who suffer a hip fracture, the rate of morbidity is high. The mortality rate approaches 25% for women who have a hip fracture. The most common cause of death for women undergoing hip replacement or pinning of a fracture is pulmonary embolus. These elderly patients commonly have multiple medical problems complicating their recovery.

The physician discusses the use of estrogen replacement therapy, calcium supplementation, weight-bearing exercise, and the avoidance of smoking and alcohol to decrease the patient's risk of osteoporosis. The patient refuses estrogen replacement therapy because she is afraid of increasing her risk of breast cancer.

QUESTION

1. What other therapy should the physician offer this patient?

DISCUSSION

If the patient has already developed osteoporosis, she can be treated with alendronate sodium (Fosamax). This is a new class of drugs that inhibits osteoclastic resorption of bone. It is approved for use in menopausal women who have documented osteoporosis. This diagnosis can be made by demonstrating osteoporosis on a dual-energy x-ray absorptiometry (DEXA) bone scan. Adequate calcium supplementation is mandatory with this therapy. The patient should be advised to continue weight bearing exercise and the avoidance of alcohol and smoking.

Before leaving the physician's office, the patient asks the physician to recommend an internist for her. The physician gives the patient the name of an internist, explaining to her that all the routine primary care screenings will be forwarded.

QUESTION

1. What other studies should be ordered before the completion of the visit?

DISCUSSION

This patient needs a screening blood pressure measurement, urinalysis, weight measurement, and a screening cholesterol test. Total cholesterol and high-density lipoprotein are satisfactory. In addition, the patient should have a rectal examination with stool guaiac. After the age of 50, all men and women should have screening sigmoidoscopies performed every 3 to 5 years. Starting at age 65 all women should be screened for thyroid disease with a thyroid-stimulating hormone. The patient should be reminded about the need for yearly pap smears and mammograms.

The patient returns 2 months later stating that she and her husband have not been able to have intercourse due to severe pain. She is distressed by this and would like to resume a normal sex life.

QUESTIONS

1. What should the physician tell this patient?

2. What are the patient's options?

DISCUSSION

Vaginal dryness is a common complaint in menopausal women. This dryness is due to a decrease or lack of secretions. The pain with intercourse is due to the lack of lubricant as well as vaginal atrophy from estrogen deprivation. Most patients will have significant relief from the use of a lubricant with intercourse. Patients must be advised that continued sexual activity is necessary or the pain with intercourse will worsen. A maturation index can be helpful to confirm vaginal atrophy. A careful examination to diagnose vaginitis is mandatory. For those patients with severe atrophy who do not respond to lubricant, a trial of oral or local premarin therapy is indicated. Although there is systemic absorption of premarin cream applied to the vagina, the levels are much lower than with oral therapy.

This patient was willing to try the local premarin and had complete resolution of her symptoms. The patient returned 1 year later for her annual examination and was doing quite well. She has had a normal sex life with her husband, and the hot flashes have tapered. The only complaint that she has is mild bone pain in her back.

QUESTION

1. What could the physician recommend for this patient?

DISCUSSION

Bone pain is common in menopausal women. These symptoms commonly abate with estrogen replacement therapy. The patient should be informed of this and should have a DEXA bone scan to check for osteoporosis. If osteoporosis is diagnosed, the physician should suggest that the patient begin estrogen replacement therapy. Because she has had a hysterectomy, the patient can take just estrogen daily.

Comprehensive Exam

DIRECTIONS: Each of the numbered items or incomplete statements in this section is followed by answers or by completions of the statement. Select the ONE lettered answer or completion that is BEST in each case.

1. The fetal cardiac output is defined as

(A) output of the foramen ovale and left ventricle
(B) output of the aorta and ductus arteriosus
(C) output from the left ventricle alone
(D) output from the right ventricle alone
(E) being equal to total umbilical blood flow

2. During the second stage of labor, an undelivered infant develops fetal distress. The infant's head is at −1 station, and the mother's cervix is completely dilated. The obstetrician decides to perform an expeditious forceps delivery. A forceps delivery is accomplished without any sequelae. A few months later, the mother learns that forceps should not be applied to a fetus' head at −1 station and thus sues the obstetrician for negligence. Which of the following is the physician's best defense?

(A) There was no departure from the standard of care
(B) There was no damage involved
(C) The lawsuit is untimely
(D) This is malicious prosecution
(E) A cesarean section would have taken much longer to accomplish delivery

3. A woman who has a long history of infertility finally becomes pregnant. At 6 weeks' gestation, she develops right lower quadrant pain and bleeding. A physician examines her and confirms the tenderness in the right lower quadrant. He obtains serial values of the β-subunit of human chorionic gonadotropin (hCG) that return as follows: 3000 mIU/ml on day 1, 3100 mIU/ml on day 4, 2600 mIU/ml on day 10. If the physician reassures the woman that she has nothing to worry about, and the woman ultimately suffers a fallopian tube rupture and dies, a lawsuit would likely

(A) be resolved in favor of the woman's family
(B) be settled because of the inherent sympathy this case would engender
(C) be resolved in favor of the physician
(D) be defended on the basis of lack of causation
(E) be defended on the basis of lack of breach of duty

4. The hormone produced in pregnancy 1000-fold compared with nonpregnancy is

(A) estradiol
(B) progesterone
(C) cortisol
(D) estriol
(E) thyroxine

5. A unilateral tubo-ovarian abscess is removed from the pelvis of a woman who uses an intrauterine device (IUD). Which of the following organisms is most likely to be cultured from that abscess?

(A) *Mycoplasma*
(B) *Chlamydia*
(C) *Actinomyces*
(D) *Bacteroides*
(E) *Peptococcus*

6. An infertility patient reports that her menses, which have been irregular for 2 years, occur anywhere from 30 to 50 days apart. She has been unable to conceive for 1 year. She is a healthy appearing, thin woman who states that she has been competing in distance running races for 18 months. Which of the following procedures are most likely to reveal information regarding her infertility?

(A) Laparoscopy
(B) Semen analysis
(C) Basal body temperature record
(D) Postcoital test
(E) Hysteroscopy

7. Which of the following findings would be unexpected in the progression of a normal pregnancy?

(A) A weight gain of 11 lbs at 20 weeks
(B) Fetal heart tones at 13 weeks detected by Doppler ultrasound
(C) The fundus of the uterus at the level of the umbilicus at 20 weeks
(D) The uterus as a pelvic organ at 12 weeks
(E) Real-time ultrasonographic evidence of fetal heart motion 4 weeks after the last menstrual period (LMP)

8. The level of human chorionic gonadotropin (hCG) at which vaginal ultrasound is useful is

(A) 1500 to 2000 mIU/ml
(B) 2500 to 3000 mIU/ml
(C) 3500 to 4000 mIU/ml
(D) 4500 to 5000 mIU/ml
(E) 5500 to 6000 mIU/ml

9. A woman presents with an invasive squamous cancer of the cervix, which extends to the lower third of the vagina. A metastatic workup reveals a right hydronephrosis on intravenous pyelography (IVP). The correct clinical stage of this woman's cancer is most likely to be

(A) stage IB
(B) stage IIB
(C) stage IIIA
(D) stage IIIB
(E) stage IVA

10. Which of the following screening tests should be used in evaluating a patient at risk for human immunodeficiency virus (HIV)?

(A) Venereal Disease Research Laboratories (VDRL) test
(B) Eastern blot analysis
(C) Southern blot DNA hybridization
(D) Gonozyme test
(E) Enzyme-linked immunosorbent assay (ELISA)

11. Dysfunctional uterine bleeding (DUB) during the perimenopausal period can be associated with which of the following hormonal situations?

(A) Exogenous estrogen therapy
(B) Imbalance in the estrogen to progesterone ratio
(C) Increased aromatization of androgen precursors
(D) An atrophic endometrium
(E) Increased levels of follicle-stimulating hormone (FSH)

12. A 36-year-old nulligravid woman comes to the office complaining of painful menstrual periods and failure to achieve a pregnancy after 1 year of unprotected intercourse. She states that she had an intrauterine device (IUD) for several years; it was removed because of continuous pain. She was treated with antibiotics after the removal of the IUD. She wonders if she could have endometriosis. Which of the following findings would suggest that diagnosis?

(A) Nodularity of the uterosacral ligaments
(B) Ovarian enlargement
(C) Fixed retroversion of the uterus
(D) Laparoscopic visualization of implants
(E) Dyspareunia

13. A woman with stage I, grade 1 adenocarcinoma of the endometrium is treated with a total abdominal hysterectomy and a bilateral salpingo-oophorectomy. Examination of the uterine pathology reveals myometrial invasion to a depth of 3 mm. Follow-up should involve

(A) no further therapy
(B) local vaginal cuff radiation
(C) external pelvic radiation
(D) para-aortic lymph node biopsy
(E) medroxyprogesterone acetate therapy

14. The luteal phase of the menstrual cycle is characterized by

(A) a variable length
(B) growth and development of ovarian follicles
(C) secretion of estrogen
(D) a low basal body temperature
(E) secretion of progesterone

15. A 23-year-old woman presents to the physician's office complaining of a mucopurulent vaginal discharge, lower abdominal pain, and a fever, which began toward the end of her menstrual period. Which sexually transmitted disease (STD) is she most likely to have?

(A) *Gardnerella vaginalis*
(B) *Chlamydia trachomatis*
(C) *Neisseria gonorrhoeae*
(D) Chancroid
(E) Lymphogranuloma venereum

16. A 35-year-old patient completed her treatment for endometriosis 6 months ago. Her chief complaint at this point is amenorrhea. She states that she had irregular bleeding, weight gain, and bouts of depression while she was being treated. She reports that dyspareunia was not a problem during her treatment. Which of the following was the method of treatment in this patient?

(A) Gonadotropin-releasing hormone (GnRH) agonists
(B) Danazol
(C) Progestins
(D) Oral contraceptives
(E) Corticosteroids

17. A mother brings her 5-year-old daughter to the emergency room and relates a 4-day history of sore throat and a painless but persistent serosanguineous discharge from the child's vagina. Pelvic examination confirms the discharge, and the saline/potassium chloride preparations are negative. The most likely etiology is

(A) *Candida*
(B) foreign body
(C) *Neisseria gonorrhoeae*
(D) *Streptococcus*
(E) *Trichomonas*

18. A 32-year-old woman is 12 weeks pregnant. She has no history of Down syndrome in her family, but she has decided that she could not live with an infant with Down syndrome. She requests an interview with a genetic counselor to talk about amniocentesis. The physician should do which of the following?

(A) Explain that he understands her concerns and will set up an appointment for her
(B) Explain that she has only a small risk of having a child with Down syndrome, and she should not be concerned
(C) Tell her that it is too risky to subject her infant to an amniocentesis given the small risk of having an infant with Down syndrome
(D) Explain that, although she understands her concerns, she cannot ethically use up a genetic counselor's time simply for reassurance
(E) Refer her to another physician who would be able ethically to fulfill her desires

19. Which of the following historical features or physical findings confirm the diagnosis of endometriosis?

(A) Bilaterally enlarged ovaries
(B) Cul-de-sac nodularity
(C) Increasingly severe dysmenorrhea
(D) Infertility
(E) None of the above

20. Which of the following factors is the most common cause of dysfunctional uterine bleeding (DUB)?

(A) Constitutional disease
(B) Anovulation
(C) Organic lesions
(D) Chronic endometritis
(E) Cervical malignancy

21. Which of the following is a prophylactic measure used to prevent aspiration during induction of general anesthesia?

(A) Corticosteroids
(B) Antibiotics
(C) Bronchoscopy
(D) Sodium citrate
(E) Suction

22. After birth, the intraabdominal portion of the umbilical vein becomes the

(A) lateral umbilical ligament
(B) ligamentum teres
(C) urachus
(D) right hepatic ligament
(E) ligamentum venosum

23. Elevated gonadotropin levels are expected with which of the following conditions associated with amenorrhea?

(A) Mayer-Rokitansky-Küster-Hauser syndrome
(B) Kallman's syndrome
(C) Gonadal dysgenesis
(D) Anorexia nervosa
(E) Pituitary adenoma

24. A 52-year-old woman complains of 4 days of vaginal bleeding in the previous month. She states that her last menstrual period (LMP) was 2 years ago. An endometrial biopsy is performed, which reveals adenomatous hyperplasia. Which of the following would explain the pathophysiology of the endometrial histology?

(A) Peripheral conversion of preandrogens in fatty tissue
(B) Secretion of estrogens from the ovarian stroma
(C) Increased levels of follicle-stimulating hormone (FSH)
(D) Decreased aromatization of preandrogens in hypothyroidism
(E) Secretion of androgens from the adrenal cortex

25. A woman states that her last menstrual period (LMP) was 7 weeks ago and that she has had several days of light bleeding and lower abdominal discomfort. She has previously had a positive home pregnancy test. Measurement of which of the following hormone levels would be appropriate at this time?

(A) Human chorionic gonadotropin (hCG)
(B) Human chorionic somatomammotropin (hCS)
(C) Progesterone
(D) Estriol
(E) Prolactin

26. A prolonged gestation is associated with which of the following fetal abnormalities?

(A) Meningomyelocele
(B) Spina bifida
(C) Anencephaly
(D) Omphalocele
(E) None of the above

27. A 24-year-old woman reports that it has been 7 weeks since her last menstrual period (LMP). She states that her menstrual cycles have always been irregular, but she is now experiencing some vaginal spotting and mild right lower quadrant pain. On examination, she has a normal-size uterus with a soft top and a mild tenderness in the right lower quadrant. A human chorionic gonadotropin (hCG) β-subunit level of 1000 mIU/ml from the day before the examination is reported. The physician should do which of the following?

(A) Recommend diagnostic laparoscopy
(B) Perform an abdominal ultrasound examination of the pelvis
(C) Perform a culdocentesis
(D) Repeat the hCG β-subunit measurement in 24 hours
(E) Repeat the hCG β-subunit measurement within 1 week

28. A fractional dilation and curettage (D and C) for postmenopausal bleeding in a 51-year-old woman reveals a uterine depth of 7 cm, negative endocervical curettings, and a well-differentiated adenocarcinoma. A metastatic workup is negative. Which of the following treatments would be most appropriate for this woman?

(A) Total abdominal hysterectomy and bilateral salpingo-oophorectomy
(B) Radical hysterectomy
(C) Pelvic exenteration
(D) Radiation therapy
(E) Chemotherapy

29. A patient presents in her thirty-second week of pregnancy with a below-average estimated fetal weight. Her only significant history is smoking over a pack of cigarettes a day. She is worried about fetal movement. Which of the following hormone levels should be measured at this time?

(A) Estriol
(B) Progesterone
(C) Prolactin
(D) Human chorionic somatomammotropin (hCS)
(E) Human chorionic gonadotropin (hCG)

30. Which of the following patients is best categorized as manifesting a drug dependence syndrome?

(A) A college student who has smoked marijuana twice weekly for the past 4 years and now desires to discontinue its use
(B) An attorney who has started smoking crack regularly over the past 2 months after initially celebrating achieving partnership in a major law firm
(C) An anesthesiologist who explains that, although she has always been able to control her alcoholic consumption, the past year has brought degeneration of her family relationships and a loss of occupational privileges at a nearby hospital, despite numerous attempts over the past few months to discontinue drinking
(D) A store manager who comes to the physician for repeated prescriptions of diazepam for anxiety because she says she cannot cope with daily activities without this drug
(E) A minister who comes to the physician for help in controlling her need for heroin because she feels that over the past year this need has surpassed her devotion to her congregation

31. Which of the following is appropriate therapy for a 21-year-old single college student with proven mild endometriosis and dysmenorrhea?

(A) Continuous oral contraceptives
(B) Danazol
(C) Long-acting intramuscular progestin
(D) Cyclic oral contraceptives
(E) Gonadotropin releasing hormone (GnRH) agonists

32. An α-fetoprotein of 0.44 times normal would predict the possibility of which of the following conditions?

(A) Omphalocele
(B) Trisomy 21
(C) Multiple pregnancies
(D) Trisomy 30
(E) Turner's syndrome

33. A 19-year-old woman comes to a physician for evaluation of sharp pain that occurs in her lower abdomen for 2 to 3 days every month since her menses began at 14 years of age. Approximately 2 weeks after she experiences this pain, she has her menses. The most probable etiology for her pain is

(A) endometriosis
(B) dysmenorrhea
(C) pelvic infection
(D) mittelschmerz
(E) ectopic pregnancy

34. Which of the following hemoglobins is found in greatest concentration in the third-trimester fetus?

(A) $\alpha_4\beta_4$
(B) $\alpha_2\gamma_2$
(C) $\alpha_2\gamma_4$
(D) $\alpha_2\beta_2$

35. A 25-year-old woman presents with 3 days of vaginal spotting. She states that her previous menstrual period was 6 weeks before the spotting and that she has had regular cycles prior to that. She is having no pain. Pelvic examination reveals a uterus that is at the upper limit of normal size, and there are no adnexal masses. The physician should

(A) perform a hysteroscopy
(B) order a dilation and curettage (D and C)
(C) chart a basal body temperature
(D) measure human chorionic gonadotropin (hCG) levels
(E) prescribe a progestin, such as medroxyprogesterone acetate

36. A 34-year-old woman in her second pregnancy presents at 8 weeks' gestation requesting information about prenatal testing. She had had a 9-pound infant and hydramnios in her previous pregnancy. She is advised to have which of the following tests?

(A) Triple screen test
(B) Maternal serum α-fetoprotein (MSAFP)
(C) Glucose tolerance test
(D) Genetic amniocentesis
(E) Ultrasound

37. A 35-year-old woman (gravida 1, para 0) presents to a physician at 35 weeks' gestation complaining of the abrupt onset of frequent, painful abdominal contractions, back pain, and moderate vaginal bleeding. On examination, a firm uterus, which is moderately tender, is noted. The physician should take which of the following actions?

(A) Administer 0.3 mg of ritodrine as an intravenous bolus
(B) Accompany the patient to labor and delivery to rule out a placental abruption and advise personnel of immediate delivery
(C) Assure the patient that this often happens toward the end of pregnancy
(D) Immediately send the patient for an ultrasound and a chest x-ray
(E) Advise the patient to rest in the examination room until the pain subsides while performing hematologic and coagulation studies

38. Estriol levels are an indicator of fetal well-being because the majority of estriol precursors are formed in the

(A) placenta
(B) fetal adrenal gland
(C) maternal adrenal gland
(D) amniotic fluid
(E) maternal liver

39. Oxygen delivery to fetal tissues is most dependent on which of the following factors?

(A) Blood flow
(B) Fetal blood
(C) Hemoglobin type
(D) Diphosphoglycerate
(E) Hydrogen ions

40. A woman accuses a man of rape, and the case goes to trial. The defendant is confident that he will be acquitted because of a lack of evidence. The woman had had coitus with her husband 48 hours before the alleged attack and had not bathed between then and the alleged assault. On which of the following can the defendant rely to prove his innocence?

(A) The presence of nonmotile sperm
(B) The presence of acid phosphatase
(C) The fluorescence of the alleged victim's vulvar area when exposed to Wood's light
(D) The presence of an intact hymenal ring
(E) None of the above

41. A 28-year-old woman with a history of placental abruption in her first pregnancy is admitted at 37 weeks of her second pregnancy complaining of bleeding, abdominal pain, and frequent contractions. Measurement of which of the following serum levels would be appropriate?

(A) Iron
(B) Calcium
(C) Folic acid
(D) Magnesium
(E) None of the above

42. A patient at 33 weeks calls reporting a gush of fluid from her vagina while she was sleeping. She reports no uterine contractions or bleeding. She comes to the labor floor for which of the following procedures?

(A) Urinalysis
(B) Fetal monitoring
(C) Ultrasound for amniotic fluid volume
(D) Nitrazine testing
(E) Induction of labor

43. Which of the following is the characteristic anatomic abnormality in type II stress urinary incontinence (SUI)?

(A) Loss of the posterior urethrovesical angle only
(B) Retention of the angle of inclination
(C) Loss of the posterior urethrovesical angle and the angle of inclination
(D) A posterior urethrovesical angle of 120°
(E) An angle of inclination of 40°

44. A woman presents to the emergency room complaining of left-sided lower abdominal pain. She states that her last menstrual period (LMP) was 6 weeks ago but that she has had light bleeding for the past 2 days. She uses an intrauterine device (IUD) for birth control. Her blood pressure in the emergency room is 110/70, and her hemoglobin is 12.4 g. Which of the following would be most helpful in establishing the diagnosis?

(A) Pelvic ultrasound
(B) Determination of a left-sided adnexal mass
(C) Culdocentesis
(D) Vaginal ultrasound
(E) Urine pregnancy test

45. Which of the following conditions is associated with prolonged use of birth control pills?

(A) Amenorrhea
(B) Hypertension
(C) Thromboembolism
(D) Myocardial infarction
(E) Diabetes

46. Exclusion of the diagnosis of ectopic pregnancy is supported by

(A) culdocentesis revealing unclotted blood
(B) proliferative endometrium on dilation and curettage (D and C)
(C) absence of an intrauterine sac at 6 weeks on pelvic ultrasound
(D) negative urine pregnancy test
(E) negative serum human chorionic gonadotropin (hCG) β-subunit levels

47. Most circulating testosterone in women is derived from which of the following sources?

(A) Fat
(B) Ovary
(C) Skin
(D) Adrenal gland
(E) Muscle

48. Acute pelvic inflammatory disease (PID) is most commonly associated with which of the following events?

(A) Intrauterine device (IUD) insertion
(B) Sexual intercourse
(C) Dilation and curettage (D and C)
(D) Endometrial biopsy
(E) A recent menstrual flow

49. Birth control pills have a positive effect on cancer prevention in which of the following organs?

(A) Vagina
(B) Fallopian tube
(C) Endometrium
(D) Cervix
(E) Large bowel

50. A patient has been on the labor floor for 3 hours having regular contractions. The contractions are very painful and occur every 4 minutes. Pelvic examination reveals no change in cervical dilation over the 3 hours. Which of the following is appropriate therapy?

(A) Oxytocin
(B) Secobarbital
(C) Epidural anesthesia
(D) Morphine
(E) Prostaglandin gel

51. Blood levels of which of the following substances correlate best with the excess androgen state?

(A) Free testosterone
(B) Androstenedione
(C) Total testosterone
(D) Dehydroepiandrosterone sulfate (DHEAS)
(E) 17-Hydroxyprogesterone

52. A previously unsensitized Rh-negative woman in her second pregnancy is seen in her twenty-sixth week. She complains of edema in her legs and some tingling in her left hand. The appropriate clinical activity at this time is

(A) analysis of the husband's blood type
(B) intramuscular Rh$_o$(anti-D) immune globulin
(C) ultrasound evaluation of amniotic fluid volume
(D) Rh antibody titer
(E) amniocentesis

53. In evaluating abdominal and pelvic pain, the correct order of examining the patient's abdomen is

(A) inspection, percussion, auscultation, palpation
(B) palpation, inspection, auscultation, percussion
(C) inspection, auscultation, percussion, palpation
(D) auscultation, inspection, palpation, percussion
(E) palpation, inspection, percussion, auscultation

54. Which of the following methods for induced abortion is no longer routinely practiced?

(A) Dilation and evacuation (D and E) after 12 weeks' gestation
(B) Extrauterine administration of abortifacients
(C) Hysterotomy
(D) Intrauterine administration of abortifacients
(E) Laminaria for cervical dilation

55. A 17-year-old woman (gravida 2, para 0100) has been treated for premature labor at 28 weeks' gestation with multiple tocolytic agents. After 48 hours in labor, she is sent to the antepartum unit. At 3:00 A.M., the physician is called because the patient is having difficulty breathing. The physician should take which of the following actions?

(A) Administer a corticosteroid, sensing imminent delivery
(B) Obtain a chest x-ray, electrocardiogram, arterial blood gases, and a complete blood count (CBC); administer oxygen; and elevate the head of the bed
(C) Increase her intravenous fluids to 150 ml/hr
(D) Perform a therapeutic amniocentesis to decrease her work of breathing
(E) Discontinue tocolysis and induce labor

56. Which of the following methods of contraception is associated with the lowest incidence of pelvic inflammatory disease (PID)?

(A) Condom
(B) Diaphragm
(C) Foam
(D) Intrauterine device (IUD)
(E) Oral contraceptives

57. Glucosuria in urine samples during routine prenatal visits indicates

(A) gestational diabetes
(B) an increased glomerular filtration of glucose
(C) a need for dietary control
(D) a need for a 3-hour glucose tolerance test
(E) a need for small doses of insulin

58. Endometrial hyperplasia is discovered in a 23-year-old nulligravid woman with irregular menstrual cycles. She is anxious to start a family. Appropriate first-step therapy includes which of the following?

(A) Cyclic combination oral contraceptive therapy for 3 months
(B) Repeat endometrial biopsy after 3 months without therapy
(C) Clomiphene stimulation to induce ovulation
(D) Cyclic progestin therapy
(E) Continuous progestin therapy

DIRECTIONS: Each of the numbered items or incomplete statements in this section is negatively phrased, as indicated by a capitalized word such as NOT, LEAST, or EXCEPT. Select the ONE lettered answer or completion that is BEST in each case.

59. A 40-year-old woman delivered an infant at 22 weeks' gestation after experiencing abdominal pressure but no cramping pain. When she arrived at the hospital, she was completely dilated, and both feet were palpable vaginally through the membranes. When advising the woman about future pregnancies, the physician should state all of the following EXCEPT

(A) she probably has an incompetent cervix
(B) she is likely to have another preterm delivery
(C) she may have a structural uterine abnormality
(D) hysterosalpinogography in 6 months could help identify structural and uterine problems
(E) she should consider adoption rather than another pregnancy

60. Falling levels of estriol could be anticipated in all of the following clinical presentations EXCEPT

(A) preeclampsia and eclampsia
(B) Rh isoimmunization
(C) intrauterine growth retardation
(D) maternal renal disease
(E) pregnancy-induced hypertension

61. A false-normal fetal scalp pH reflects a disparity between predicted good Apgar scores and fetal pH. One could expect a normal scalp pH and Apgar scores of 2 and 4 at 1 and 5 minutes, respectively, in all of the following clinical presentations EXCEPT

(A) prematurity
(B) sedation of the mother
(C) intrauterine growth retardation
(D) abruptio placentae
(E) fetal infection

62. Genetic counseling is advisable in each of the following clinical situations EXCEPT

(A) a 35-year-old woman who plans to begin a family
(B) a single, nonpregnant woman who is a carrier of the Tay-Sachs gene
(C) a 39-year-old divorced woman who has one child with a neural tube defect and would like to have more children
(D) a couple who has two children with unbalanced translocations
(E) a pregnant 21-year-old woman who has no family history of genetic disease

63. The menopausal vagina has all of the following characteristics EXCEPT

(A) a pale, dry epithelium
(B) a reduction in the size of the upper vagina
(C) the appearance of superficial cells
(D) a loss of vaginal tone
(E) an increase in parabasal cells

64. The patient is a 38-year-old woman who is pregnant for the fifth time. Because bleeding is present in the week 15, the physician performs an ultrasound of the uterus, which demonstrates the typical appearance of a molar pregnancy and enlarged cystic ovaries. The right ovary is 8 cm in diameter, and the left is 6 cm in diameter. All of the following procedures would be appropriate EXCEPT

(A) suction dilation and evacuation (D and E)
(B) intravenous oxytocin
(C) hysterotomy
(D) resection of the ovarian cysts
(E) hysterectomy

65. Atrophic vaginitis would be expected in all of the following clinical situations EXCEPT

(A) menopause
(B) lactation
(C) oral contraceptive use
(D) surgical castration in a young woman
(E) pseudomenopause during endometriosis therapy

66. Smoking during pregnancy is associated with all of the following factors EXCEPT

(A) functional inactivation of fetal hemoglobin (Hb F) by carbon monoxide
(B) a low-birthweight infant
(C) increased levels of carbon dioxide
(D) reduced perfusion of the placenta
(E) intrauterine growth retardation

67. A woman who is 3 days late for her menses presents with lower abdominal pain, a low-grade temperature, a tender uterus, and a left-sided adnexal mass. She is using an intrauterine device (IUD) for birth control. Early management should include all of the following EXCEPT

(A) pregnancy test
(B) laparoscopy
(C) pelvic ultrasound
(D) antibiotics
(E) removal of the IUD

68. When obtaining consent for a laparoscopic tubal ligation, the physician must do all of the following EXCEPT

(A) explain that the operation will result in an inability to have children
(B) call the patient's husband to be certain that he is aware of his wife's desire for sterility
(C) explain that there is no guarantee of sterility
(D) ask the patient to call if she should miss her menses or develop any pain after the procedure
(E) explain other forms of contraception, including a vasectomy

69. Myomata uteri have been implicated in a number of reproductive problems in terms of both infertility and pregnancy loss. In fact, these myomas have been implicated in all of the following EXCEPT

(A) recurrent abortion
(B) luteal phase defect
(C) poor implantation
(D) blocked fallopian tubes
(E) premature labor and delivery

70. A woman presents with uterine bleeding at 15 weeks' gestation. Her blood pressure is found to be 160/100 with 2+ proteinuria. Doppler ultrasound of the uterus reveals fetal heart tones. All of the following findings are compatible with her suspected diagnosis EXCEPT

(A) human chorionic gonadotropin (hCG) level of greater than 100,000 mIU/ml
(B) trisomy 14
(C) normal karyotype
(D) normal villi
(E) bilateral ovarian enlargement

71. Characteristics of secondary syphilis include all of the following EXCEPT

(A) palmar and plantar maculopapular rashes
(B) condyloma latum
(C) a positive fluorescent treponemal antibody absorption test (FTA-ABS)
(D) painless chancres
(E) generalized lymphadenopathy

72. Epidemiologic factors that are associated with cervical cancer include all of the following EXCEPT

(A) early age of marriage
(B) sexual promiscuity
(C) latent human papillomavirus (HPV) infection of the cervix
(D) use of birth control pills
(E) cigarette smoking

73. All of the following statements concerning the function of progesterone are correct EXCEPT

(A) it prepares the endometrium for nidation
(B) it relaxes the myometrium
(C) it elevates serum binding proteins
(D) it stimulates aldosterone production
(E) it has natriuretic actions

74. The appearance of late decelerations would not be a surprise in any of the following situations EXCEPT

(A) intrauterine growth retardation
(B) preeclampsia
(C) chronic abruptio placentae
(D) chronic hypertension
(E) placenta previa

75. Indications for surgery on a myomatous uterus include all of the following EXCEPT

(A) hypermenorrhea with anemia
(B) 1 year of infertility
(C) uterine enlargement to an 18-week pregnancy
(D) rapid enlargement of the myomas
(E) hydronephrosis

76. Pregnant women who are short in stature or underweight are at increased risk for all of the following complications EXCEPT

(A) thromboembolism
(B) perinatal morbidity
(C) perinatal mortality
(D) low-birthweight infants
(E) preterm delivery

77. All of the following factors are necessary for assault to be designated as rape EXCEPT

(A) genital contact
(B) manual contact with the victim's genitalia
(C) threat of physical harm
(D) force

78. Characteristics of the androgen insensitivity syndrome include all of the following EXCEPT

(A) an XY gonad
(B) a vaginal pouch
(C) breast development
(D) pubic hair
(E) the presence of müllerian-inhibiting factor

79. The dependence of myomas on estrogen is demonstrated by all of the following characteristics EXCEPT

(A) they stop growing after menopause
(B) they often grow rapidly during pregnancy
(C) they are associated with a luteal phase defect
(D) they are unusual before menarche
(E) they may be found along with endometrial hyperplasia

80. A 55-year-old postmenopausal woman complains of vaginal burning and dyspareunia. She has a thin, watery discharge. She has not been on estrogen replacement therapy, and the use of a lubricant has not helped. Characteristics of the vagina would be expected to include all of the following EXCEPT

(A) a thinned epithelium
(B) superficial cells
(C) decreased glycogen
(D) an alkaline pH
(E) leukorrhea

81. All of the following conditions can be found in a patient with a pituitary chromophobe adenoma EXCEPT

(A) amenorrhea
(B) hypothyroidism
(C) galactorrhea
(D) blindness
(E) Cushing's syndrome

82. All of the following signs and symptoms should be reported immediately as potential danger signals in a pregnant woman EXCEPT

(A) vaginal bleeding
(B) severe headache
(C) swelling of the ankles and feet
(D) blurring of vision
(E) escape of fluid from the vagina

83. A woman in active labor (4 to 5 cm dilated) requests pain relief. She is having regular contractions, and the vertex is at 0 station. All of the following would be adequate anesthesia EXCEPT

(A) paracervical block
(B) caudal anesthesia
(C) pudendal block
(D) lumbar epidural anesthesia
(E) epidural fentanyl

84. When obtaining a patient's informed consent regarding an operative procedure, a physician must do all of the following EXCEPT

(A) discuss the patient's diagnosis
(B) discuss the treatment needed
(C) explain the risks of the procedure
(D) Advise the patient to read a pamphlet regarding the procedure and to call with any questions
(E) explain the alternative forms of treatment

85. Characteristics of a hydatidiform mole include all of the following EXCEPT

(A) presence of villous blood vessels
(B) absence of fetal tissue
(C) proliferation of the lining trophoblast
(D) enlargement of the villi
(E) edema of the villi

86. Habitual abortion can result from all of the following conditions EXCEPT

(A) cervical incompetence
(B) hormonal dysfunction
(C) chromosome abnormalities
(D) bicornuate uterus
(E) subserous myomas

87. A pregnancy in which an intrauterine device (IUD) has been left in place can include all of the following complications EXCEPT

(A) congenital anomalies
(B) ectopic pregnancy
(C) pelvic infection
(D) prematurity
(E) spontaneous abortion

88. Normal vaginal health depends on all of the following factors EXCEPT

(A) a pH of 4.5
(B) Döderlein's bacilli
(C) estrogen
(D) *Escherichia coli*
(E) lactic acid production

89. A 24-year-old woman (gravida 1, para 0) presents to the labor and delivery floor at 30 weeks' gestation, complaining of frequent abdominal cramps and vaginal spotting. The fetal membranes are intact, contractions are occurring every 10 minutes, and her cervix is 3 cm dilated and 80% effaced. The plan of management should include all of the following EXCEPT

(A) intravenous tocolysis with magnesium sulfate
(B) urine culture
(C) ultrasound for estimated fetal weight
(D) cervical cerclage
(E) coagulation profile

90. All of the following substances are appropriate therapy for a luteal phase defect EXCEPT

(A) clomiphene citrate
(B) human chorionic gonadotropin (hCG)
(C) postovulatory progesterone supplementation
(D) low-dose estrogen
(E) follicle-stimulating hormone (FSH) and luteinizing hormone (LH)

91. Follicle-stimulating hormone (FSH) stimulates all of the following actions EXCEPT

(A) growth and maturation of granulosa cells
(B) aromatase activity
(C) luteinizing hormone (LH) release
(D) increase in FSH receptors on the follicle
(E) development of LH receptors

92. A woman comes to see an obstetrician after her recent move to a new area. Records received from her previous obstetrician show that she is 38 weeks pregnant. After examining the patient, the physician realizes that her fundal size is smaller than the gestational age. An ultrasound examination is scheduled for the following day, and the physician advises the patient that she will speak to her on the day of the ultrasound. That evening, the patient arrives at the labor and delivery suite in active labor. After the obstetrician arrives, she delivers a 2330-g infant precipitously. All of the following are true EXCEPT

(A) the low birth weight of the infant and the gestational age, if confirmed by previous clinical and laboratory data, support the diagnosis of prematurity
(B) the low birth weight and the gestational age of the infant, if confirmed by previous clinical and laboratory data, support the diagnosis of intrauterine growth retardation
(C) because the infant is of low birth weight, it is at risk for neonatal complications, despite being born at 38 weeks' gestation
(D) during labor, an infant of this size is likely to exhibit fetal distress

93. Amenorrhea in a 16-year-old girl may result from all of the following conditions EXCEPT

(A) imperforate hymen
(B) androgen insensitivity syndrome
(C) Turner's syndrome
(D) cystic fibrosis
(E) granulosa–theca cell tumor

94. Cesarean section is indicated in all of the following women EXCEPT

(A) a woman with active herpes lesions whose membranes ruptured 2 hours before admission
(B) a woman who had a positive herpes culture 1 week before the onset of labor
(C) a woman who had a negative herpes culture 2 weeks previously but now has active herpes lesions and is in labor
(D) a woman with active herpes lesions whose membranes ruptured 24 hours before admission
(E) a woman who had a positive herpes culture 10 days previously and is now in active labor even though her membranes have not ruptured

95. Abnormal luteal phase function in a non-pregnant woman can result from depression of all of the following factors EXCEPT

(A) follicle-stimulating hormone (FSH) stimulation of the cycle
(B) estradiol levels
(C) prostaglandin production
(D) progesterone production
(E) luteal cell mass

96. The parasympathetic nerves innervate all of the following structures EXCEPT the

(A) cervix
(B) lower uterine segment
(C) uterine fundus
(D) uterosacral ligaments
(E) cardinal ligaments

97. A 32-year-old woman is referred to the gynecologist with irregular cycles and suspected polycystic ovary disease along with infertility. She brings with her a hysterosalpingogram that shows a normal endometrial cavity. A grossly enlarged irregular uterus with a solid 4-cm left adnexal mass is found on pelvic examination. History and workup of this patient could reveal all of the following signs and symptoms EXCEPT

(A) anemia
(B) hydronephrosis
(C) pedunculated myoma
(D) constipation
(E) pelvic pain

98. A woman who is known to use cocaine presents with seizures, a temperature of 104°F, and a blood pressure of 180/120. She is 36 weeks pregnant. After a thorough evaluation, the physician excludes preeclampsia and intrauterine infection. The diagnosis is cocaine toxicity. Actions to be taken include all of the following EXCEPT

(A) delivering the infant expeditiously
(B) providing oxygen and considering intubation
(C) providing a cooling blanket
(D) treating with intravenous propranolol
(E) treating with intravenous magnesium sulfate

99. Endometriosis may involve the presence of all of the following signs or symptoms EXCEPT

(A) cul-de-sac nodularity
(B) endometriomas of the ovaries
(C) endometrial glands and stroma outside the uterine cavity
(D) functioning endometrium within the myometrium
(E) pelvic adhesions

100. Postpartum hemorrhage could be a reasonable possibility in all of the following situations EXCEPT

(A) transverse lie
(B) triplets
(C) long labor
(D) hydramnios
(E) thrombocytopenia

101. Luteinizing hormone (LH) stimulates all of the following actions EXCEPT

(A) luteinization of the granulosa cells
(B) reduction division in the oocyte
(C) progesterone secretion by the corpus luteum
(D) production of LH receptors on the granulosa cells
(E) androgen synthesis by the theca cells

102. Indications for delivery in an insulin-dependent diabetic at 36 weeks' gestation include all of the following EXCEPT

(A) a poor biophysical profile
(B) a lecithin to sphingomyelin (L/S) ratio of 1.8/1
(C) a positive contraction stress test
(D) decreased insulin requirements
(E) spontaneous contractions with late decelerations

103. All of the following statements about menopausal osteoporosis are true EXCEPT

(A) most bone loss occurs to trabecular bone
(B) bone loss is most rapid after bilateral oophorectomy in a 35-year-old woman
(C) estrogen therapy can retard osteoporosis
(D) osteoporosis is more common in black than in white women
(E) about one-third of American women can expect a hip fracture

104. A 25-year-old woman wants to become pregnant and decides to discontinue her contraception. She had irregular cycles before starting contraception. While she was using birth control, she had no menstrual bleeding. All of the following could have been her method of birth control EXCEPT

(A) birth control pills
(B) progesterone-releasing intrauterine device (IUD)
(C) medroxyprogesterone
(D) gonadotropin-releasing hormone (GnRH) agonists

105. A 23-year-old single graduate student has a history of irregular menses (4–5 per year) and presents with increased hair growth. She asks for help with the excessive hair growth. Gonadotropin studies reveal a luteinizing hormone to follicle-stimulating hormone (LH/FSH) ratio of 3:1. The appropriate therapy improves the hirsutism by all of the following actions EXCEPT

(A) decreasing ovarian androstenedione
(B) displacing androgens at the skin level
(C) increasing sex hormone–binding globulin (SHBG)
(D) decreasing blood levels of testosterone
(E) decreasing the 5α-reductase activity

106. Factors that are important in the pathophysiology of pelvic inflammatory disease (PID) include all of the following EXCEPT

(A) intrauterine device (IUD) use
(B) intercourse
(C) menstruation
(D) uterine contractions
(E) uterine fibroids

107. A class II cardiac patient who is 38 weeks pregnant presents to the hospital in labor with dysnea on exertion and chest rales. Proper management of this pregnant patient includes all of the following EXCEPT

(A) epidural anesthesia
(B) diuretics
(C) digitalis
(D) oxygen therapy
(E) cesarean delivery

108. When taking a history from a rape victim, all of the following information is relevant EXCEPT

(A) the last menstrual period (LMP)
(B) bathing since the assault
(C) the most recent intercourse before the assault
(D) previous pregnancies
(E) birth control status

109. Epidural anesthesia can produce fetal distress by decreasing all of the following EXCEPT

(A) maternal venous return
(B) maternal cardiac output
(C) uterine blood flow
(D) maternal heart rate
(E) maternal blood pressure

110. Ovulation is associated with all of the following processes EXCEPT

(A) reduction division in the oocyte
(B) depression of the follicle-stimulating hormone (FSH)
(C) luteinizing hormone (LH) surge
(D) prostaglandin synthesis
(E) progesterone secretion

111. A woman who took birth control pills for 6 years without a break decides to stop the pills so that she can become pregnant. Four months later she still has not had a spontaneous menses. All of the following are possible explanations of her amenorrhea EXCEPT

(A) pituitary adenoma
(B) previous oligomenorrhea
(C) pregnancy
(D) length of use
(E) ovarian failure

112. A 30-year-old woman has a 2-year history of infertility. During this time, the diagnosis of moderate endometriosis was made. She decides to have surgery. Requirements of conservative surgery for moderate endometriosis include all of the following EXCEPT

(A) reperitonealization of all raw surface areas
(B) suspension of the uterus
(C) meticulous hemostasis
(D) instillation of 32% dextran 70
(E) postoperative danazol

DIRECTIONS: Each set of matching questions in this section consists of a list of four to twenty-six lettered options (some of which may be in figures) followed by several numbered items. For each numbered item, select the ONE lettered option that is most closely associated with it. To avoid spending too much time on matching sets with large numbers of options, it is generally advisable to begin each set by reading the list of options. Then, for each item in the set, try to generate the correct answer and locate it in the option list, rather than evaluating each option individually. Each lettered option may be selected once, more than once, or not at all.

Questions 113–115

For each clinical presentation, select the diagnosis most likely to be associated with it.

(A) Ectopic pregnancy
(B) Torsion of an ovarian cyst
(C) A threatened abortion
(D) A bleeding corpus luteum
(E) Hydatidiform mole

113. A 25-year-old woman whose last menses were 6 weeks ago presents with acute left lower quadrant pain. Serum human chorionic gonadotropin (hCG) β-subunit levels are positive. Pelvic ultrasound reveals no sac in the uterus and a 3 $\times$ 3-cm left adnexal mass.

114. A 30-year-old woman whose last menses were 8 weeks ago presents with heavy vaginal bleeding and lower left quadrant pain. Serum β-hCG levels are low for dates. Pelvic ultrasound reveals an intrauterine sac without fetal parts.

115. A 35-year-old woman whose last menses were 6 weeks ago presents with acute lower left quadrant pain but no vaginal bleeding. Serum β-hCG is appropriate for dates. Culdocentesis reveals nonclotting blood. A tender left 3 $\times$ 4-cm adnexal mass is present on pelvic examination. Ultrasound reveals no gestational sac in the uterus.

Questions 116–118

Each laboratory value listed is diagnostic of a particular clinical condition associated with hirsutism. For each laboratory value, select the most useful therapy for suppressing the androgen excess associated with that condition.

(A) Spironolactone
(B) Prednisone
(C) Clomiphene
(D) Birth control pills
(E) Cimetidine

116. Elevated dihydroepiandrosterone sulfate (DHEAS)

117. Elevated serum androstenedione

118. Elevated 17-hydroxyprogesterone

Questions 119–122

For each clinical presentation that follows, select the therapy that would be most appropriate.

(A) Estrogens and progestins
(B) Hydrocortisone
(C) Progestational agents
(D) Prostaglandin inhibitors
(E) None of the above

119. Congenital adrenal hyperplasia

120. Isosexual precocious puberty

121. Dysfunctional uterine bleeding (DUB)

122. Dysmenorrhea

Questions 123–125

Match the descriptions of vaginitis with the therapy that would be most appropriate.

(A) Metronidazole
(B) Estrogen cream
(C) Polyene antifungal agent
(D) Vinegar douche
(E) Sulfonamide vaginal cream

123. A woman states that she has been on ampicillin for 1 week because of a urinary tract infection. Upon completing the antibiotics, she noted a thick, white vaginal discharge with severe vulvar itching.

124. A patient states that she has a malodorous discharge and intense itching. She adds that her partner also has a slight discharge. Pelvic examination reveals "strawberry spots" on the cervix.

125. A patient complains of a watery, malodorous discharge with very little itching or burning. A wet mount preparation in saline of the vaginal secretions reveals clue cells.

Questions 126–128

For each case history, select the type of amenorrhea described.

(A) Eugonadotropic amenorrhea
(B) Physiologic amenorrhea
(C) Hypergonadotropic amenorrhea
(D) Androgen excess amenorrhea
(E) Hypogonadotropic amenorrhea

126. A 24-year-old nulligravid woman had a normal menstrual history until 8 months ago when she began intensive long-distance running. She has not had a menstrual flow since her first marathon 4 months ago.

127. An 18-year-old woman with well-developed secondary sexual characteristics complains of amenorrhea. She has a vaginal pouch and XX chromosomes.

128. A 15-year-old adolescent with normal sexual development complains of 5 months of amenorrhea. She states that her first menses were 9 months ago, after which she had three menses.

Questions 129–132

Match each description with the appropriate incision or procedure.

(A) Kerr
(B) Shirodkar
(C) Sellheim
(D) McDonald
(E) Sanger

129. Performed in the lower (noncontractile) segment of the uterus

130. Simple and easy to perform; also produces minimal trauma to the cervix

131. Can obviate repeating the procedure in a subsequent pregnancy

132. Dehiscence is more likely secondary to the scar extending into the uterine corpus

Questions 133–135

For each case presented, select the treatment modality that is most appropriate.

(A) Monthly human chorionic gonadotropin (hCG) titers
(B) Chest x-ray
(C) Chemotherapy
(D) Pelvic ultrasound
(E) Quantitative hCG titer

133. A woman presents with vaginal bleeding and a positive serum pregnancy test. She states that she had a spontaneous abortion 4 months ago. Her uterus is at the level of the umbilicus, and the handheld ultrasound instrument picks up no fetal heart tones.

134. A woman with metastatic gestational trophoblastic neoplasia (GTN) has been on chemotherapy for 1 year. She had her third negative monthly hCG titer and a normal chest x-ray 3 months ago. Since then, her monthly hCG titers have been negative.

135. A woman had a suction dilation and evacuation (D and E) for a molar pregnancy. Her postoperative hCG titers dropped steadily until 3 weeks ago. For the past 3 weeks, her hCG titer has been around 6500 mIU/ml.

Questions 136–138

For each clinical presentation, select the appropriate diagnostic test.

(A) Cystourethrography
(B) Stress testing
(C) Q-tip test
(D) Cystometry
(E) Cystoscopy

136. The patient is a 32-year-old multiparous woman with a 6-month history of urinary urgency and frequency. She states that she almost always feels as if she has to urinate and then voids only in small amounts.

137. The patient is an active 35-year-old parous woman who complains about involuntary loss of urine while she is jogging or exercising. She says that the problem began with the birth of her second child. The only way to prevent the problem is to void just before she starts jogging.

138. The patient reports that she is embarrassed by the involuntary loss of urine she experiences when feeling nervous, when rolling over in bed, and occasionally while sitting at her desk. She states that she has recently seen her internist who ruled out any infectious, metabolic, and neurologic diseases.

Questions 139–142

For each clinical situation, select the most appropriate form of treatment.

(A) Progestin
(B) Nonsteroidal anti-inflammatory drugs (NSAIDs)
(C) Oral conjugated estrogen
(D) Dilation and curettage (D and C)
(E) Oral contraceptive agents

139. A 30-year-old woman presents with a chief complaint of menorrhagia. She states that her cycles are regular, 28 or 29 days apart. Physical examination reveals a blood pressure of 140/90 mm Hg and a uterus of normal size.

140. A 35-year-old woman presented to another physician 3 months ago with irregular (every 30–40 days) heavy menses and some intermenstrual spotting. The physician prescribed two packs of oral contraceptives. When talking to a new physician, she reports that she has bled almost every day for the past 2 months, during which time she was taking the birth control pills.

141. A 23-year-old nulligravid woman presents with a 3-week history of bleeding, the last 3 days of which were heavy bleeding with clots. She feels weak. Her previous menstrual period was 3 months before this bleeding episode. Her hemoglobin is 9.0 g.

142. A 47-year-old woman complains of menometrorrhagia. She states that this type of bleeding has been occurring for the past 18 months. Physical examination reveals a mildly obese woman with a blood pressure of 140/95 mm Hg and a uterus of normal size.

Questions 143–145

Match each case history with the appropriate therapy.

(A) Cyclic estrogen on days 1 through 25 each month
(B) Cyclic progestin on days 1 through 10 each month
(C) Cyclic combination oral contraceptives
(D) Cyclic estrogen and progestin on days 1 through 25 each month
(E) No hormonal replacement

143. The patient is 47 years old and had a tubal ligation 10 years ago. She states that she is having irregular menstrual cycles, which occur every 2 to 3 months. When they occur, the menses are heavy and last for 10 days.

144. The patient is 47 years old and complains of insomnia, dyspareunia, and hot flashes. She reports that she had a myomectomy 7 years ago for a large fibroid. On examination she is found to have a nonspecific vaginal discharge.

145. The patient is 47 years old and comes to the office because of frequent irregular bleeding. She states that her menses have occurred every 2 weeks for the previous 2 months. Before that time she had regular monthly menstrual cycles.

Questions 146–148

For each clinical presentation listed below, select the most likely cause of the excessive bleeding.

(A) Cervical laceration
(B) Atonic uterus
(C) Uterine rupture
(D) Retention of a succenturiate lobe
(E) Thrombocytopenia

146. A 26-year-old woman has just delivered her second 9-lb infant in 2 years, having had an oxytocin-induced labor. She is bleeding heavily despite the use of oxytocics, a well-contracted uterus, and no evidence of vaginal or cervical tears.

147. A 31-year-old woman is in the recovery room bleeding heavily after having delivered twins vaginally.

148. Following a spontaneous vaginal delivery, a 24-year-old woman continues to bleed despite the use of oxytocin. The uterus appears to contract well but then relaxes with increased bleeding.

Questions 149–151

For each congenital condition listed below, select the diagnostic procedure that would be most helpful in identifying it.

(A) Measurement of maternal serum α-fetoprotein (MSAFP)
(B) Chorionic villus sampling (CVS)
(C) Maternal chromosome analysis
(D) Amniocentesis
(E) Real-time ultrasonography

149. Meningomyelocele

150. Tay-Sachs disease

151. Sickle cell anemia

Questions 152–153

For each situation described in postdates pregnancy below, select the next indicated procedure.

(A) Contraction stress test (CST)
(B) Fetoscopy
(C) Amniocentesis
(D) Proceed with delivery

152. The nonstress test (NST) is nonreactive

153. The biophysical profile score is 4

Questions 154–155

For each clinical situation involving a primary infertility problem, select the most appropriate procedure to evaluate it.

(A) Laparoscopy
(B) Hysteroscopy
(C) Postcoital test
(D) Endometrial biopsy
(E) Hysterosalpingography

154. A woman states that she has been infertile for 3 years with the exception of a pregnancy 10 months ago that aborted between the fifth and sixth weeks. She says that she ovulates. She has a record of basal body temperatures, which shows an average luteal phase temperature rise of 9 to 10 days.

155. A woman states that she has been infertile for 3 years. An operation for acute appendicitis at age 16 was the only event of any significance in her medical history. Her postcoital test and her husband's semen analysis were good. Her basal body temperature charts show consistent 12- to 14-day luteal phases.

Questions 156–158

For each clinical presentation choose the indicated medical therapy.

(A) Penicillin
(B) Metronidazole
(C) Doxycycline
(D) Doxycycline and ceftriaxone
(E) Ceftriaxone

156. An 18-year-old woman presents to the office with acute lower abdominal pain, nausea, and a temperature of 101°F. She reports that her last coitus was 10 days ago and that her menses stopped 3 days ago. Physical examination reveals a purulent cervical discharge and bilateral adnexal tenderness.

157. A 28-year-old nulligravid woman comes to the office with a chief complaint of painful urination. She also states that she has had a dull lower abdominal pain for several weeks. Pelvic examination reveals a mucopurulent cervical discharge. Examination of the urine reveals many white blood cells, but the culture is negative.

158. A 35-year-old patient presents to the office complaining of a vaginal discharge and malaise. Physical examination reveals enlarged lymph nodes in her groin and a maculopapular rash on her palms and soles. She reports that she had a painless sore on her outer vagina 2 months earlier.

Questions 159–161

For each clinical presentation listed, select the postpartum clinical entity most likely to be associated with it.

(A) Pelvic thrombophlebitis
(B) Infected hematoma
(C) Urinary tract infection
(D) Parametritis
(E) Episiotomy breakdown

159. A woman spikes a temperature to 102.6°F (39.1°C) on her first postpartum day. She had ruptured membranes for 36 hours prior to delivery, and the cervical culture was group B β-hemolytic streptococci. She has lower abdominal tenderness.

160. A woman had a cesarean section for fetal distress 5 days previously. Her clinical course has been marked by a spiking fever for 4 days and has not responded to triple antibiotic therapy.

161. A woman had a vaginal delivery with epidural anesthesia. She had to be catheterized once in the recovery room for urinary retention. One day postpartum she complains of shaking chills and back pain.

Questions 162–163

For each clinical presentation listed below, select the condition that it is most likely to represent.

(A) Ruptured vasa previa
(B) Placenta previa
(C) Ruptured uterus
(D) Bloody show
(E) Cervical cancer

162. A woman presents in active labor with significant vaginal bleeding. She is incoherent, but the physician is told that she had had a previous cesarean section. The fetal heart rate (FHR) is heard at 60 beats per minute.

163. A 39-year-old patient who has had no obstetric care during her pregnancy presents to the labor floor at term with heavy vaginal bleeding. Her last pregnancy was 12 years ago. Examination of the abdomen with ultrasound reveals a fetal heart rate (FHR) of 145 beats per minute and a fundal placenta.

Questions 164–166

For each case presented, select the diagnosis that best describes the patient's clinical condition.

(A) False labor
(B) Hypertonic uterine dysfunction
(C) Hypotonic uterine dysfunction
(D) Active phase of labor
(E) Latent phase of labor

164. A woman presents to the labor floor complaining of painful contractions that occur every 2 minutes. She is 2 cm dilated. Two hours later, she continues to complain of frequent painful contractions, but she is still only 2 cm dilated.

165. A woman presents to the labor floor 3 cm dilated with contractions every 5–7 minutes. About 2 hours later she is having contractions every 3 minutes and is 6 cm dilated. She is 8 cm dilated 1 hour later.

166. A woman presents to the labor floor with contractions 8–12 minutes apart. She complains of lower abdominal discomfort with her contractions, which last for only 20 seconds each. Sedation causes the contractions to be spaced at intervals of 15–20 minutes.

Questions 167–169

For each of the drugs listed below, select the malformation most commonly associated with it.

(A) Chondrodysplasia punctata
(B) Central nervous system (CNS) defects
(C) Absence of toes
(D) Hypospadias
(E) Limb reduction

181. Progestins

182. Thalidomide

183. Isotretinoin

Questions 170–171

For each clinical presentation, select the most appropriate test or therapy.

(A) Weekly human chorionic gonadotropin (hCG) levels
(B) Repeat serum test for syphilis
(C) Elective abortion
(D) Diethylstilbestrol (DES) therapy
(E) Intrauterine device (IUD) insertion

170. A 21-year-old woman was raped approximately 2 weeks after her last menstrual period. She was not using any birth control because she was not sexually active. One week after her assault she went to the physician's office for help.

171. A 21-year-old woman was raped approximately 2 weeks after her last menstrual period. She was not using any birth control because she was not sexually active. She was taken to the emergency room immediately after the assault and started on DES prophylaxis therapy.

Questions 172–174

For each clinical situation listed below, select the most appropriate form of management.

(A) Intravenous hydration
(B) Nasal oxygen
(C) Fetal heart rate (FHR) monitoring
(D) Fetal scalp pH
(E) Cesarean section

172. A patient with chronic hypertension presents to the labor floor at term in active labor. Her blood pressure is 140/100 and she has 1+ urinary protein. She is 4 cm dilated.

173. FHR monitoring reveals persistent late decelerations in the fetus of a primigravida whose cervix is now 7 cm dilated.

174. Fetal scalp pH in a fetus having late decelerations with slow recovery over a 30-minute period is 7.19.

Questions 175–176

For each clinical presentation listed, select the type of anesthesia that is most likely to have been administered.

(A) General anesthesia
(B) Paracervical block
(C) Spinal anesthesia
(D) Lumbar epidural anesthesia
(E) Meperidine

175. A woman is in labor, and her cervix is 2 cm dilated. She is having regular contractions, which occur every 3 minutes. She requests pain relief, but she has informed her physician that she is allergic to meperidine. Within 10 minutes of receiving the anesthesia, the fetal heart rate (FHR) drops to 60 beats per minute.

176. A woman is in active labor, and her cervix is 5 cm dilated. She requests something for pain relief. Within 5 minutes of receiving the anesthesia, she is in respiratory arrest.

177. A multiparous woman presents at 33 weeks' gestation complaining of vaginal bleeding in the absence of both contractions and ruptured membranes.

178. A woman at term is admitted with a tender uterus and a tense abdomen and no audible fetal heart tones.

179. A woman presents with moderate vaginal bleeding and uterine contractions that do not completely relax between contractions.

Questions 177–179

For each obstetric situation listed, select the sign or symptom with which it is most likely to be associated.

(A) Breech presentation
(B) Oliguria
(C) Occiput posterior position
(D) Transient fetal distress
(E) Hyperreflexia

ANSWERS AND EXPLANATIONS

1. The answer is B [Chapter 9 II A 3, 4, B]. The ductus arteriosus blood flow and the aortic blood flow constitute the cardiac output of the fetal heart. This enables adequate tissue oxygenation despite the low oxygen saturation of fetal blood. The fetal cardiac output of 200 ml/kg/min is higher than that of the adult.

2. The answer is B [Chapter 37 II B 4]. Since there is no mention in the facts that the infant suffered any adverse consequences from a forceps delivery, the best defense would be that no damage occurred. Although it is probably below the standard of care to apply forceps at a high station, damages must result for a patient to establish all of the elements of negligence (i.e., duty, breach of duty, causation, and damages).

3. The answer is A [Chapter 28 III; Chapter 37 II B 1–4]. This patient has a high potential for an evolving ectopic pregnancy. The clinical history and the laboratory data of plateauing values of the β-subunit of human chorionic gonadotropin (hCG) confirm this. Based on this information, a physician would be remiss in not ruling out an ectopic pregnancy with its potentially devastating consequences. If the woman dies, the elements of negligence (breach of duty and causation) cannot be defended. Because of proven negligence in this case, it would be resolved in favor of the plaintiff; the sympathy aspect would not be enough to maintain a lawsuit since sympathy alone would not determine if a case should be settled.

4. The answer is D [Chapter 1 VII A 2 c, B 1]. Progesterone, estradiol, cortisol, estriol, and thyroxine are all markedly elevated in pregnancy. Estriol, however, is in the highest concentration; its synthesis involves integration of fetal, placental, and maternal metabolic steps, and levels increase until the end of pregnancy. Thyroxine and cortisol are elevated artificially because of the increase in their respective binding proteins.

5. The answer is C [Chapter 23 III A 6; VII A 3]. *Actinomyces israelii* can be found in the 15% of cases of pelvic inflammatory disease

(PID) that are associated with the use of an intrauterine device (IUD). This is especially true when a unilateral pelvic abscess is present. Microscopically, actinomycotic "sulfur" granules are present; in addition, there is a monocytic infiltration, and giant cells may be present. *A. israelii* is rarely found in women who do not use an IUD.

6. The answer is C [Chapter 32 III F 2 b (1), 4 f]. Laparoscopy, semen analysis, basal body temperature record, postcoital test, and hysteroscopy are important in an infertility workup, but only a basal body temperature record would be helpful in identifying a potential ovulatory problem. Well-trained female distance runners are known to have infrequent or absent menses. Cycles lasting between 30 and 50 days are suggestive of irregular or absent ovulations. A basal body temperature record would help to determine whether or not ovulation was occurring, as a thermal shift indicates ovulation.

7. The answer is E [Chapter 3 III B 2 b, C 1–3; V A 2]. It is not possible to see fetal heart motion by real-time ultrasonography until 6 to 7 weeks after the last menstrual period (LMP) or 2 to 3 weeks after the first missed menses. In a normal gestation, the uterus is still a pelvic organ at 12 weeks. Fetal heart tones can be detected by Doppler ultrasound at 12 to 14 weeks, and the fundus of the uterus is at the level of the umbilicus at 20 weeks. A weight gain of 20 to 30 lbs during a pregnancy is normal, and at least 10 lbs should be gained by 20 weeks.

8. The answer is A [Chapter 28 IV C 1–3]. Ultrasound has proved to be a useful tool in diagnosing normal and abnormal pregnancies. For pelvic ultrasound to demonstrate a gestational sac in the uterus, the human chorionic gonadotropin (hCG) titer should be about 6000 mIU/ml. Vaginal ultrasound can pick up the presence of a gestational sac 4 to 6 days before pelvic ultrasound, with an hCG titer in the 1500 to 2000 mIU/ml range. The presence of a gestational sac in the uterus at the expected time is helpful in ruling out an ectopic pregnancy. The absence of a gestational sac, depending on the hCG level, by either vaginal or pelvic ultrasound, is suggestive of an ectopic pregnancy.

9. The answer is D [Chapter 36 I D 2 d (3) (b)]. The lesion of invasive cervical cancer is either clinically inapparent and found on cone biopsy or is clinically obvious, in which case, a simple biopsy confirms the diagnosis. In stage III disease, the carcinoma extends onto the pelvic sidewall and to the lower third of the vagina. Hydronephrosis detected by intravenous pyelography (IVP) is a feature of stage IIIB disease for invasive cervical cancer.

10. The answer is E [Chapter 29 II D 1 c]. An enzyme-linked immunosorbent assay (ELISA) is the screening test of choice for human immunodeficiency virus (HIV). Western (not eastern) blot analysis is a more sensitive test that will differentiate the true-positive from the false-positive on the ELISA test. Venereal Disease Research Laboratories (VDRL) test is a nonspecific reagin-type antibody test for syphilis. The Gonozyme test is a solid-phase immunoassay for detecting gonococcal antigens. DNA hybridization techniques have recently been employed to detect human papillomavirus (HPV) and to ascertain the viral serotype.

11. The answer is C [Chapter 35 IV A 1, C]. The basic characteristic of the perimenopausal period is anovulatory or dysfunctional uterine bleeding (DUB). This irregular, often heavy bleeding, is associated with excess endogenous estrogen that is unopposed by progesterone. An additional source of estrogen during the perimenopause is the increased aromatization of androgenic precursors, especially in obese women. There is no imbalance of estrogen and progesterone because ovulation does not occur and progesterone is not present. The endometrium is at least proliferative and possibly hyperplastic because of the unopposed estrogen. Follicle-stimulating hormone (FSH) would be elevated only in the absence of estrogen. In a situation in which there is increased endogenous estrogen, there would be no reason to add any exogenous estrogen.

12. The answer is D [Chapter 24 III B 1–4]. The only way to diagnose endometriosis is by visualization at surgery or laparoscopy or by biopsy of an implant. History and physical examination are suggestive, but not diagnostic.

The physical findings of cul-de-sac nodularity, fixed retroversion of the uterus, and ovarian enlargement are compatible with endometriosis but can also be found in ovarian or bowel cancer and in chronic pelvic inflammatory disease (PID). Dyspareunia can be a symptom of pelvic disease, such as endometriosis and chronic PID.

13. The answer is A [Chapter 36 III D 6 a]. The patient described in the question has a low-grade endometrial cancer that is limited to the inner one third of the myometrium. Therefore, no therapy other than the hysterectomy and bilateral salpingooophorectomy is indicated, and a very high cure rate can be expected. If the tumor was of a higher grade or involved the outer one third of the myometrium, external pelvic radiation following the hysterectomy would be indicated.

14. The answer is E [Chapter 20 I C 1–4]. The luteal or secretory phase of the menstrual cycle extends from ovulation to the onset of the next menses. The length of the luteal phase is fairly constant at 12 to 16 days. Before ovulation, there is growth and development of the ovarian follicles with secretion of estrogen; the basal body temperature is low (under 98°F) during the preovulatory or follicular phase of the cycle. With ovulation, the corpus luteum secretes progesterone, which has a thermogenic effect on the body, raising the basal body temperature to above 98°F for the length of the luteal phase.

15. The answer is C [Chapter 29 II A 1 b]. The symptoms with which the woman described in the question presents are most commonly seen in *Neisseria gonorrhoeae*–related acute pelvic inflammatory disease (PID). *Gardnerella vaginalis* produces a thin, greyish vaginal discharge associated with symptomatic vulvovaginitis, but not acute PID. *Chlamydia trachomatis,* serotypes D–K, is associated with PID, but the clinical course is indolent and not distinctly related to the menstrual cycle. Chancroid and lymphogranuloma venereum are ulcerative genital diseases and are not associated with acute PID.

16. The answer is C [Chapter 24 IV B 1–4]. This patient has a number of symptoms that suggest she was treated with long-acting intramuscular progestins (medroxyprogesterone acetate, 100–200 mg/month). Irregular bleeding, weight gain, and depression are common with progestin therapy, as is the posttherapy amenorrhea; the infertility is secondary to the inactivity of the ovary, which is reflected by the amenorrhea. This patient has no dyspareunia, which occurs in the hypoestrogenic states induced by danazol and gonadotropin-releasing hormone (GnRH) agonists. Oral contraceptive therapy for endometriosis is not associated with posttreatment amenorrhea. Corticosteroids are not used in the treatment of endometriosis.

17. The answer is D [Chapter 19 II F 1 b (2)]. A streptococcal infection elsewhere is almost always the predisposing factor for streptococcal vaginitis. Infections with *Candida, Trichomonas,* and *Neisseria gonorrhoeae* are rarely associated with bloody vaginal discharge. A foreign body should always be suspected, but, in the absence of pain, it is an unlikely causative factor.

18. The answer is A [Chapter 37 IV]. All obstetricians must realize that the physician–patient relationship in the field of obstetrics and gynecology is one of collaboration. Thus, situations where a reasonable request on the part of a concerned patient should be denied are rare. All women are at risk for having an infant with Down syndrome; 35 years of age is the age at which this risk approximates the risk of fetal loss secondary to amniocentesis. An individual, however, may not want to take any risk of having an infant with Down syndrome, and prenatal testing grants her some security. Denying a woman access to this type of testing is not only cruel but also may be later challenged as breaching a duty to provide access to prenatal testing and infringing on a right to procreative privacy.

19. The answer is E [Chapter 24 III A, B]. The only way to diagnose endometriosis is by visualization (through the laparoscope) or biopsy of the disease. Cul-de-sac nodularity could be metastatic carcinoma. Any benign or neoplastic lesion can cause ovarian enlargement. Infertility and dysmenorrhea are symptoms associated with endometriosis, but neither is diagnostic because there are other reasons for each of those symptoms.

20. The answer is B [Chapter 19 VI B]. Dysfunctional uterine bleeding (DUB), when strictly defined, is bleeding in the absence of organic lesions. It is almost always due to a disturbance in hypothalamic-pituitary-ovarian function, leading to anovulation. It is seen most often in adolescents and in women in the perimenopausal years.

21. The answer is D [Chapter 17 IV B 1 c]. A potential problem with obstetrical anesthesia, especially general anesthesia, is aspiration of gastric contents. Gastric emptying is significantly delayed during labor, even if the last meal was many hours before the need for anesthesia. Before and with intubation during general anesthesia, the gastric contents are neutralized with antacids, such as sodium citrate, and cricoid pressure is used to compress the esophagus. Intubation, suction, and possibly bronchoscopy are used as management modalities once aspiration has occurred. Corticosteroids and antibiotics are also used after aspiration has occurred to control the often severe chemical pneumonitis that can develop.

22. The answer is B [Chapter 9 V B 4]. The umbilical vein is patent for some time after birth and is used for intravenous administration and exchange transfusions in the early neonatal period. The lumen never disappears entirely but is not normally functional and, thus, is termed the ligamentum teres.

23. The answer is C [Chapter 33 II A 1, III B 1, IV A, C, F 1]. Even though Mayer-Rokitansky-Küster-Hauser syndrome is characterized by müllerian deficiencies, the ovaries are normal and so are the gonadotropin levels. Because of hypothalamic suppression, gonadotropin levels are low in the nutritional deficiency that characterizes anorexia nervosa. Likewise, gonadotropin levels are low and prolactin levels are elevated in pituitary adenomas. Gonadotropin levels are low in Kallman's syndrome because there is a congenital defect in gonadotropin synthesis. Gonadal dysgenesis is characterized by sex chromosome abnormalities and absent or limited ovarian function. Because the ovaries do not secrete estrogen, there is no negative feedback on the pituitary, and, thus, the gonadotropin levels remain high.

24. The answer is A [Chapter 35 III A 2, B 1–4]. When excess estrogen is found in premenopausal or menopausal women, it can occur from a number of sources. There is an increased aromatization of preandrogens to estrogen associated with obesity, liver disease, and hyperthyroidism (not hypothyroidism). The main product of the ovarian stroma is androstenedione and not estrogen. Increased direct secretion of endogenous estrogen is seen with functional ovarian tumors, such as granulosa cell tumors. Even if the follicle-stimulating hormone (FSH) levels are elevated, FSH is not responsible for the increased peripheral conversion of preandrogens from the ovary to estrogen.

25. The answer is A [Chapter 1 II D 1]. Serum human chorionic gonadotropin (hCG) can be very helpful as a marker to evaluate the health or normalcy of a pregnancy because, in a healthy pregnancy, hCG levels rise at a predictable rate: The hCG value should double every 2 days. Therefore, a quantitative hCG value, when lower than normal for the expected gestational age, is often indicative of an abnormal pregnancy, such as a threatened abortion or an ectopic pregnancy.

26. The answer is C [Chapter 4 I B 3; Chapter 6 I C 2]. An anencephalic fetus often is associated with a naturally prolonged gestation. According to one theory, fetal cortisol is thought to play an important part in the initiation of labor. There is faulty brain-pituitary-adrenal function in anencephalic infants, and fetal cortisol levels are low. These low levels of cortisol may cause the naturally prolonged gestation of an anencephalic fetus. Meningo-myelocele, spina bifida, and omphalocele are not associated with low fetal cortisol levels.

27. The answer is D [Chapter 22 VI A 1 b (1)–(5)]. The patient described in the question presents a diagnostic dilemma. On the one hand, she has some gynecologic complaints and an associated low human chorionic gonadotropin (hCG) β-subunit level. On the other hand, she has an enlarged uterus and a history of irregular menses. The differential diagnosis includes a normal intrauterine gestation with an associated corpus luteum cyst, causing right lower quadrant pain, a threatened abortion, and an ectopic pregnancy. The woman should be informed of these possibilities and be told to notify the physician if the pain increases. The optimum management at this point is to repeat the hCG β-subunit measurement in 24 hours to see if it is rising appropriately. Pelvic ultrasound would not be helpful since its sensitivity begins at 5000 to 6000 mIU/ml for an abdominal ultrasound and 1500 to 2000 mIU/ml for a vaginal ultrasound. Diagnostic laparoscopy and culdocentesis are invasive procedures that

should be used only after more information is obtained. Repeating the hCG β-subunit measurement in 1 week may result in clinical catastrophe since an ectopic pregnancy may be missed, and tubal rupture may occur.

28. The answer is A [Chapter 36 II D 1, 3 a, 4 a (1)]. The 51-year-old woman described in the question who presents with postmenopausal bleeding has a stage IA, grade 1 endometrial cancer, which is characterized by a well-differentiated adenocarcinoma (grade 1) and a uterine depth of 8 cm or less (stage IA). There is a very low risk of deep myometrial penetration or pelvic lymph node metastasis. The incidence of recurrent disease following a total hysterectomy and bilateral salpingo-oophorectomy is very low, making this the treatment of choice for this woman.

29. The answer is A [Chapter 1 VII D 1–3, E 1–3]. In a woman who smokes heavily, the suspected diagnosis of below average fetal weight at 32 weeks' gestation must be intrauterine growth retardation. If the fetus is distressed, there may be an actual reduction in fetal movement. One way to assess and follow this situation is by serial estriol determinations.

30. The answer is C [Chapter 15 II B, C 1–8]. The *Diagnostic and Statistical Manual of Mental Disorders* (Third Edition—Revised) states that, in a dependence syndrome, three or more out of eight certain criteria must be present continuously in the previous month or repeatedly in the previous year. The anesthesiologist fulfills three criteria. She has lost her family and her occupational privileges and has attempted on numerous occasions to stop drinking alcohol. Anyone from any walk of life can abuse drugs; there is no "typical" profile. The continuum from use through dependence is a progression from a hazardous activity to the forging of a relationship with a mood-altering substance that crowds out the other relationships in a person's life.

31. The answer is D [Chapter 24 V A, B]. The woman described in the question has mild endometriosis. Because she is a young college student, it is assumed that she has no immediate plans for pregnancy. Therefore, using gonadotropin-releasing hormone (GnRH) agonists, danazol, long-acting intramuscular progestin, or continuous oral contraceptives is not appropriate therapy at this time; one of these would be indicated if a patient had been infertile for some time and required treatment for her endometriosis. The nonsteroidal anti-inflammatory drugs (NSAIDs) are helpful with the dysmenorrhea, and the cyclic oral contraceptives help to prevent further growth of the endometriosis by minimizing the amount of monthly endometrial shedding and therefore the growth or extension of the endometrial implants.

32. The answer is B [Chapter 12 III D 1 a]. An α-fetoprotein of 0.44 times normal suggests the possibility of a Down syndrome (trisomy 21) fetus as 15% to 20% of Down syndrome fetuses have low α-fetoprotein values. Values are considered low if the α-fetoprotein is 0.5 times normal or less. In omphalocele, multiple pregnancies, trisomy 30, and Turner's syndrome, the α-fetoprotein concentration is elevated.

33. The answer is D [Chapter 22 VI A 2 a, B 1 a]. Cyclic pain associated with menses indicates a gynecologic cause of the pelvic pain of the young woman described in the question. Given that the pain is sharp and occurs 2 weeks before menses, it is most likely due to ovulation, namely mittelschmerz. Although dysmenorrhea is cyclic, by definition it occurs during the menses. Endometriosis may be chronic or cyclic, but it occurs at irregular intervals. Pelvic infection and ectopic pregnancy are not cyclic types of pain, although they present acutely.

34. The answer is B [Chapter 9 IV B]. $\alpha_2\gamma_2$ is the fetal hemoglobin (Hb F) that appears in the first trimester and constitutes 70% of the hemoglobin in the term fetus. Hemoglobin AA (Hb AA), or adult hemoglobin, appears in the second trimester and increases toward term but is secondary to fetal hemoglobin.

35. The answer is D [Chapter 26 IV C 1]. In a woman of childbearing age, pregnancy or a pregnancy-related complication, such as an ectopic pregnancy, must always be ruled out when there is either amenorrhea or unusual bleeding (i.e., spotting). Therefore, measurement of human chorionic gonadotropin (hCG) levels is necessary to rule out or confirm a pregnancy. Hysteroscopy, dilation and curettage (D and C), and basal body temperatures are inappropriate ways of diagnosing a pregnancy. A pregnancy diagnosis should always be excluded in a woman of childbearing age

before prescribing a progestin, which should not be taken in early pregnancy.

36. The answer is A [Chapter 3 IV A 2–4]. For a 34-year-old woman, an appropriate screening test would be a triple screen to evaluate the possibility of a Down syndrome fetus. She is under 35 years of age and thus not an automatic candidate for a genetic amniocentesis. The maternal serum α-fetoprotein (MSAFP) would be included in the triple screen test, which gives more information than the MSAFP test alone. The woman certainly would need a glucose tolerance test because of the previous large infant, but this would not be done until 26 weeks' gestation.

37. The answer is B [Chapter 11 II B 5; V B 3 c; Chapter 13 II E, F]. Given the abrupt onset of symptoms with vaginal bleeding, a placental abruption is likely. Until the cause of the bleeding is clarified, it is important not to administer tocolytic agents, which may cause vasodilation with hypotension. Since this patient is 35 weeks pregnant, significant bleeding or fetal compromise is best treated by immediate delivery. Therefore, the patient should be accompanied to labor and delivery to rule out a placental abruption, and personnel should be advised to prepare for immediate delivery. When she has reached labor and delivery and has been quickly evaluated, a decision may be made whether to temporize, and further evaluate, or to proceed to delivery.

38. The answer is B [Chapter 1 VII B 2 c, d]. Under normal circumstances, estriol levels increase with advancing gestation. Estriol is derived from 16-α-hydroxydehydroepiandrosterone sulfate (16-α-OHDHEAS), whose primary source is the fetal adrenal gland. There is a maternal source (liver) of estriol, but this comprises less than 10% of the total. Thus, maternal urinary levels of estriol have long been recognized as a reliable index of fetoplacental function.

39. The answer is A [Chapter 9 IV]. The primary determinant of oxygen supply to the tissues is blood flow to the various organs. Hemoglobin F (Hb F), or fetal hemoglobin, does not appear until 3 months' gestation. Oxygen saturation of the blood as well as the hemoglobin concentration are important but secondary to blood flow. Diphosphoglycerate does not bind to fetal hemoglobin and thus does not affect saturation and delivery of oxygen.

40. The answer is E [Chapter 27 III C 2, D 1–2]. Acid phosphatase is found in vaginal fluid, urine, and semen; therefore, the presence of acid phosphatase is not specific. Large quantities, however, in the vagina, mouth, or anus are suggestive of recent ejaculation in those areas. Histone, which is found in semen and was picked up by the Wood's light, could have come from the semen of either the husband or the attacker, so that is not helpful. An intact hymenal ring is found in many sexually active women. Even if the defendant has had a vasectomy and has no spermatozoa in his ejaculate, and the presence of the nonmotile sperm had to be from another source (i.e., the husband), this fact is no proof that he, in fact, did not have coitus with the victim.

41. The answer is C [Chapter 3 V E 1 b]. Folic acid deficiencies have been implicated in such reproductive problems as pregnancy-induced hypertension, fetal abnormalities, and placental abruption, and this patient is presenting with the signs and symptoms of another placental abruption. There is no association of low or high levels of iron, calcium, or magnesium with placental abruption.

42. The answer is D [Chapter 4 IV A 1]. When a woman reports a gush of fluid from the vagina, it is important to determine whether or not the membranes have ruptured. The gush may represent loss of urine, but a urinalysis will not help that determination. The nitrazine test of the fluid in the vagina will identify the presence of amniotic fluid because of the alkaline nature of amniotic fluid. Fetal monitoring, evaluation of amniotic fluid volume, and induction of labor are all important, but only after the determination of ruptured membranes by the nitrazine test.

43. The answer is C [Chapter 31 II A 1]. Type II stress urinary incontinence (SUI) is an indication of significant weakness of the supporting tissues of the pelvic floor. There is a loss of both the posterior urethrovesical angle and the angle of inclination. Loss of the posterior urethrovesical angle only, retention of the angle of inclination, a posterior urethrovesical angle of 120°, and an angle of inclination of 40° are all characteristic of type I SUI, with the posterior urethrovesical angle being greater than normal (normal is 90°–100°) and the angle of inclination being normal (normal is less than 45°).

44. The answer is D [Chapter 28 III B; IV C 1–4]. At 6 weeks from the last menstrual period (LMP), a pregnancy is too early to be diagnosed by pelvic ultrasound. Vaginal ultrasound, on the other hand, may pick up the gestational sac at 6 weeks, or 4 to 6 days before pelvic ultrasound in helpful. The urine pregnancy test is not useful because it is often negative in an ectopic pregnancy; a serum human chorionic gonadotropin (hCG) test is always positive if there is an ectopic pregnancy. Since this clinical picture could represent a threatened abortion with a corpus luteum cyst, the left-sided adnexal mass would not confirm the diagnosis of ectopic pregnancy. Culdocentesis would not be useful at 6 weeks because few ectopic pregnancies are symptomatic or have ruptured by that time.

45. The answer is B [Chapter 21 IV D 1–4]. Hypertension and liver tumors are two complications associated with prolonged use (more than 5 years) of oral contraception. There is no relationship between the length of pill use and amenorrhea; thus, a "rest period" to prevent amenorrhea is unnecessary. Diabetes is not associated with length of pill use. Incidence of both superficial and deep vein thromboses is increased in all oral contraceptive users as antithrombin III levels fall within 10 days of starting the pill; thromboembolism is, therefore, not associated with prolonged use.

46. The answer is E [Chapter 28 IV C 1–6]. A serum human chorionic gonadotropin (hCG) β-subunit pregnancy test is positive for all (100%) ectopic pregnancies. Only 50% of urine pregnancy tests are positive. Unclotted blood on culdocentesis could represent a bleeding corpus luteum. A gestational sac on pelvic ultrasound cannot be expected before 7 weeks. The finding of a proliferative endometrium means only that ovulation has not occurred.

47. The answer is C [Chapter 34 II]. In women, androgens are derived from three major sources—the ovary, the adrenal gland, and the peripheral transformation of preandrogens, such as dehydroepiandrosterone (DHEA) and androstenedione, to testosterone. Most testosterone comes from the peripheral transformation in the liver and the skin.

48. The answer is E [Chapter 23 IV A 1–3]. Pelvic inflammatory disease (PID) is usually preceded by vaginal and cervical colonization of pathologic bacteria. The most common inciting event is a menstrual period; degenerating endometrium is a good culture medium, and two-thirds of acute PID cases begin just after menses. Intrauterine device (IUD) insertion, sexual intercourse, dilation and curettage (D and C), and endometrial biopsy can also be inciting events, if the pathogens are present at the cervix, but they are less likely to be associated with acute PID than the menses.

49. The answer is C [Chapter 21 IV F 1–4]. Because of the progestin component in the birth control pill, there is an antiestrogen effect on the normal proliferative, stimulatory influence of estrogen on the breast and endometrium; this is thought to be protective in lessening the chance of the development of cancer in those organs. Because the pill suppresses ovarian activity and the number of ovulatory cycles, there may be protection against the incidence of ovarian cancer. There is no positive effect of the pill on the cervix. Some of the carcinogenic influences on the cervix are viral in nature, and only a barrier method of contraception is a positive influence. The pill also has no protective effect on the vagina, the fallopian tube, or the large bowel.

50. The answer is D [Chapter 4 IV B 5 b]. A woman who is having painful, regular uterine contractions without cervical dilation is experiencing a dysfunctional labor. Any kind of uterine stimulation with prostaglandin gel or oxytocin would be contraindicated. She is far too early in her labor for epidural anesthesia. She needs strong sedation and pain relief that is far better provided with morphine than with secobarbital.

51. The answer is A [Chapter 34 II A 3 b]. Dehydroepiandrosterone sulfate (DHEAS) and androstenedione are preandrogens that measure activity from the adrenal and ovary, respectively; they are weak androgens, which do not accurately indicate androgen excess. Total testosterone includes testosterone bound to protein, much of which is inactive. It is the free testosterone, which is only a small portion of the total testosterone, that reflects a woman's androgen activity. 17-Hydroxyprogesterone levels are elevated in congenital adrenal hyperplasia because of enzyme deficiencies in the steroid pathway.

52. The answer is D [Chapter 3 IV A 5 c–d]. An Rh-negative woman must be tested for the presence of antibodies at the beginning of the third trimester so that the rare Rh sensitization of that pregnancy can be detected. She is given Rh_0 (anti-D) immune globulin if she is still unsensitized, and amniocentesis is performed to determine amniotic fluid bilirubin levels if Rh antibodies are detected at 26 weeks' gestation. Cases of Rh sensitization may eventually necessitate intrauterine blood transfusion to prevent erythroblastosis fetalis.

53. The answer is C [Chapter 22 IV B 1–4]. In evaluating abdominal and pelvic pain, the correct order of examining the patient's abdomen is inspection, auscultation, percussion, and palpation. The physician must be careful not to elicit further pain, which may confuse the evaluation. To put the patient at ease, the abdomen should be inspected while conversing with the patient. Next, the patient should be asked to identify the area of maximal tenderness, and the area must be avoided until more information has been gathered. Auscultation follows; the physician may gently press down on the abdomen and then release pressure. True rebound tenderness will be elicited if peritoneal irritation exists. Percussion localizes the pain further and determines its severity. Palpation determines the presence of a mass.

54. The answer is C [Chapter 16 V B 1 a (1)]. With the legalization of abortion, many medical and mechanical means are now available to terminate a pregnancy safely. Hysterotomy, popular many years ago, is no longer used in induced abortion. Procedures now widely practiced are safer than those used previously (e.g., sharp curettage, hysterotomy, and hysterectomy), particularly dilation and evacuation (D and E) via suction curettage.

55. The answer is B [Chapter 11 V B 2 c (3)]. The patient described in the question is most likely suffering from pulmonary edema, which is a rare but serious side effect of tocolytic therapy. Given an increase in the maternal blood volume, increased fluid administration, increased sodium absorption in pregnancy, and β_2-mimetic effects on pulmonary vessels, this condition is more common in the pregnant than the nonpregnant patient. Therapy must be centered on diagnosis, oxygenation, termination of tocolytic therapy, diuresis, and fluid restriction. Corticosteroids will actually exacerbate this condition. Although therapeutic amniocentesis may decrease premature labor in the presence of polyhydramnios and facilitate maternal respiration, nothing in the facts indicate that polyhydramnios is a possibility. Although tocolysis may need to be stopped, labor induction is too early and radical a step at this point.

56. The answer is E [Chapter 23 II C 1–4]. Women who are sexually active and use no contraception develop 3.42 cases of pelvic inflammatory disease (PID) per 100 woman years. An intrauterine device (IUD) is linked to a higher incidence of PID than any other method of contraception. Oral contraceptive use is linked to the lowest incidence of PID, even lower than the barrier methods, perhaps as a result of a decreased menstrual flow, a decreased ability of pathogenic bacteria to attach to endometrial cells, and the presence of progesterone.

57. The answer is B [Chapter 7 I A 1–3]. Glucosuria is most often secondary to the pregnancy-related increased glomerular filtration of glucose without an increased tubular reabsorption. The finding of glucose in the urine (glucosuria) of a pregnant woman does not mean that she has gestational diabetes. However, it is an indication to perform glucose testing because gestational diabetes is a distinct possibility. The initial test would be a 1-hour screening test and not the 3-hour test, which is only done if the 1-hour glucose tolerance test is abnormal. It is unnecessary to control dietary glucose intake strictly without a diagnosis of gestational diabetes. Likewise, small doses of insulin would be unnecessary in the absence of a diagnosis of diabetes.

58. The answer is A [Chapter 36 II C 2 b]. The hyperplasia is treated with cyclic combination oral contraceptives for three cycles, followed by endometrial biopsy at the conclusion of the therapy to see if the lesion has cleared. Since the young woman wants to become pregnant, and, since her cycles are irregular and probably anovulatory with unopposed estrogen, ovulation induction would be appropriate after treating the hyperplasia. Cyclic progestin therapy would make her have regular cycles, but she would not ovulate without stimulation with clomiphene. Continuous progestin therapy is unnecessary and would negate any possible ovulation.

59. The answer is E [Chapter 11 II A 1–8; IV B 1–4]. The woman described in the question

suffers from an incompetent cervix. The incompetent cervix may be acquired congenitally or may be secondary to a previous gynecologic procedure, such as dilation and evacuation (D and E). Once suspected, it should be ruled out by hysterosalpingography, which would show dilation of the internal os. This study would also serve to exclude an associated uterine anomaly, which may increase the risk for preterm delivery and abnormal presentation of the fetus. Although the woman is at risk for preterm delivery, it is not advisable to discourage her from considering another pregnancy.

60. The answer is B [Chapter 1 VII A–E]. In Rh isoimmunization, large quantities of estriol are produced. In such clinical situations as preeclampsia, eclampsia, hypertension in pregnancy, intrauterine growth retardation, and maternal renal disease, estriol production often declines due to placental and fetal compromise. Obtaining 24-hour urinary estriol values has been helpful in monitoring these high-risk pregnancies as they approach term.

61. The answer is C [Chapter 5 IV C 2 a–c]. With intrauterine growth retardation, pH values and Apgar scores are both low because of the chronic associated hypoxia. A false-normal fetal scalp pH value is seen in infants who are flaccid at birth with poor respiratory efforts in such clinical settings as prematurity, sedation or general anesthesia in the mother and fetal infection and in events such as placental abruption, which occur after the pH determination and before delivery.

62. The answer is E [Chapter 12 I A; Chapter 38 IV]. A normal, 21-year-old pregnant woman has a 1% to 2% chance of having a child with a chromosomal anomaly or a congenital anomaly. Genetic counseling, therefore, is not indicated in this low-risk age-group. The risk is the same in this group even with the birth of a prior child with Down syndrome, for instance. The risk for neural tube defect in this age-group, however, would change if the family has a history of the anomaly.

63. The answer is C [Chapter 35 V A 1 a,b]. One of the most sensitive end organs to estrogen is the vagina. Consequently, changes are seen in and around the vagina after menopause, with the natural decline in estrogen. The epithelium becomes pale, thin, and dry.

The vagina becomes narrower, with a diminution in the size of the upper vagina. A loss of muscle tone occurs and can predispose to prolapse. Because of the estrogen deficiency, a change takes place in the cellular maturation of the vaginal epithelium. The less mature parabasal cells increase and the most mature superficial cells are absent. Therefore, superficial cells would not be expected in a cytologic evaluation of the menopausal vagina.

64. The answer is D [Chapter 18 II D 1–3].
In some molar pregnancies, the high levels of human chorionic gonadotropin (hCG) stimulate the formation of theca lutein cysts in both ovaries. Surgery is contraindicated on these ovaries because the cysts will regress with the evacuation of the molar (trophoblastic) tissue and the subsequent drop in hCG secretion once its source is removed. Oxytocin and suction curettage are indicated in a molar pregnancy when the woman wants future pregnancies; hysterectomy is the treatment of choice in the woman who has completed her childbearing. Hysterotomy is still a therapeutic option, but it has essentially been replaced by suction curettage.

65. The answer is C [Chapter 25 VI D 1].
Healthy vaginal epithelium that is resistant to infection depends on estrogen stimulation. When an estrogen deficiency occurs, atrophic changes in the vulvovaginal epithelium occur with thinning and decreased resistance to infection. Menopause, lactation, surgical castration, and endometriosis therapy are associated with markedly reduced or absent circulating estrogen levels. Even though progesterone is the dominant hormone in oral contraceptives, enough estrogen is present to prevent atrophic vaginitis.

66. The answer is C [Chapter 3 VI E 1–3]. A smoking woman has increased levels of carbon monoxide, not carbon dioxide, which can affect fetal and maternal hemoglobin. Pregnant women who smoke are at risk for small infants, growth-retarded infants, or both. This risk may be due, in part, to the vasoconstrictive effects of nicotine, which cause reduced placental perfusion.

67. The answer is B [Chapter 21 III D 3 c].
With an intrauterine device (IUD) in situ, a low-grade temperature, and a tender uterus, one must suspect an IUD-related pelvic infection. Because of the late menses, the pain, and the presence of an IUD, an ectopic pregnancy is possible; therefore, a pregnancy test is indicated. The pelvic ultrasound is indicated because of the left adnexal mass and the known association of the IUD with a unilateral tubo-ovarian abscess. Treatment of the pelvic infection involves antibiotics and removal of the IUD. A laparoscopy is not needed at this stage; everything points to pelvic inflammatory disease (PID) and treatment with antibiotics, unless the pregnancy test comes back positive.

68. The answer is B [Chapter 37 III C 1 d]. It is not the physician's duty to call the patient's husband to be certain that he is aware of his wife's desire for sterility. When obtaining consent for sterilization, the physician must explain that the procedure is permanent, but failures do occur, and these failures may result in pregnancy. Thus, if a woman misses her menses after a tubal ligation, the physician must rule out pregnancy. If she complains of pelvic pain, it is imperative to rule out ectopic pregnancy. In addition, before a sterilization procedure, a patient must be informed about all of the possible contraceptive alternatives.

69. The answer is B [Chapter 30 III A 4 a–c].
A luteal phase defect is a hormonal problem and is not caused by the mechanical problems associated with intramural or submucous myomas. Because of the thinned, sometimes poorly vascularized, endometrium that can overlie a submucous myoma, poor implantation of an embryo is likely, as is the possibility of recurrent spontaneous abortion early in the first trimester. Myomas growing at or near the cornual regions of the uterus can put pressure on the interstitial parts of the fallopian tubes and block them. Patients with submucous or intramural myomas have an increased incidence of premature labor (and possibly delivery).

70. The answer is C [Chapter 18 II A 1–2, B 1–6, C 2]. This patient presents with bleeding and preeclampsia early in the midtrimester; this early preeclampsia is almost pathognomonic of a molar pregnancy. This patient has an incomplete or partial mole because of the presence of a fetus along with molar tissue. Other features of a partial mole can include human chorionic gonadotropin (hCG) levels of greater than 100,000 mIU/ml, normal villi, trisomy or triploidy, and bilateral ovarian enlargement (theca lutein cysts secondary to the high hCG levels). With the trisomy or triploidy the karyotype is abnormal.

71. The answer is D [Chapter 29 II B 2 b, 3 b]. A painless chancre is the initial lesion of primary syphilis. Palmar and plantar rashes are one of the pathognomonic mucocutaneous lesions of secondary syphilis. Condyloma latum is an exuberant fig-like lesion of the mucocutaneous tissue seen in secondary syphilis. Lymphadenopathy is also common in secondary syphilis. The fluorescent treponemal antibody absorption test (FTA-ABS) is a specific antitreponemal antibody test, which is positive in patients with secondary syphilis.

72. The answer is D [Chapter 36 I A 1 a–f]. Use of the birth control pill has not been associated with an increased incidence of cervical cancer. Epidemiologic studies associate an early age of first intercourse and sexual promiscuity with an increased incidence of cervical cancer. Cigarette smoking, a high-risk male consort (i.e., one whose previous sexual partners developed precancerous or cancerous conditions of the cervix), and marriage or conception at an early age are additional risk factors. Sexually transmitted viruses, such as herpes simplex virus (HSV) and human papillomavirus (HPV), have also been implicated as causal agents.

73. The answer is C [Chapter 1 I A 3 a; VI E 1–6]. Progesterone has a number of important functions during pregnancy. It prepares the endometrium for implantation of the embryo and maintains the uterus in a quiescent state during pregnancy by relaxing the myometrium. Progesterone also has natriuretic actions, which stimulate an increased production of aldosterone. It is the elevated levels of circulating estrogen, not progesterone, that cause an increase in the serum binding proteins, which, in turn, leads to falsely elevated levels of certain hormones, such as thyroxine and cortisol.

74. The answer is E [Chapter 5 III C 2 e, f]. Placenta previa is an acute bleeding event, which usually occurs in the absence of labor and, thus, is not associated with decelerations. Late decelerations are suggestive of a problem with uteroplacental perfusion, which is commonly seen in such clinical states as preeclampsia, chronic abruptio placentae, and chronic hypertension. Intrauterine growth retardation is a reflection of poor placental perfusion; late decelerations are seen during the labor of a growth-retarded infant.

75. The answer is B [Chapter 30 IV C 1, 2]. Since the bleeding associated with myomas is not hormonally controlled, the presence of a profound anemia that cannot be corrected with iron is an indication for surgery. Rapid enlargement may be an indication of a malignant change in the myoma, and the hydronephrosis caused by pressure of a myomatous uterus on a ureter can be dangerous. When a uterus the size of an 18-week pregnancy fills the entire pelvis and makes examination of the ovaries very difficult, surgery is indicated. However, 1 year of infertility would not be a reason for surgery because the infertility may have nothing to do with the myomas. Myomas are usually not associated with infertility but with problems in maintaining a pregnancy once it is established.

76. The answer is A [Chapter 10 IV A 1, 2]. Thromboembolism is a medical complication that is more likely to develop in an obese rather than a thin pregnant woman. Pregnant women who are short in stature or underweight are at increased risk for perinatal morbidity and mortality, low-birthweight infants, and preterm delivery.

77. The answer is B [Chapter 27 I A 1–3]. For an assault to be designated as rape, contact must take place between the genitalia of both the offender and the victim. Manual contact by the offender with the victim's genitalia, against the victim's will, is a form of sexual assault but is not rape. Rape is the coital form of sexual assault. An element of force or threat of physical harm must be present, but the victim no longer has to demonstrate resistance to prove rape. The act must be performed against the victim's will.

78. The answer is D [Chapter 33 III B 4]. The androgen insensitivity syndrome is characterized by a phenotypic female with an XY gonad and a vaginal pouch. The presence of müllerian-inhibiting factor inhibits uterine development. When the cytosol receptors for testosterone are defective, evidence of circulating testosterone, such as pubic and axillary hair, is not present.

79. The answer is C [Chapter 30 I B 3 a–d]. Observations of the appearance, growth, and disappearance of myomas during the life of a woman suggest that myomas depend on estrogen for growth. At times of low or absent estrogen secretion, such as the premenarchal or postmenopausal years, myomas are absent or they stop growing. At times of high estrogen secretion, such as pregnancy or conditions that lead to endometrial hyperplasia (e.g., polycystic ovary disease), myomas may grow rapidly or appear for the first time. Even if a myomatous uterus is present with the clinical condition of luteal phase defect, the myomas are not an example of cause and effect because the luteal phase defect has nothing to do with estrogen—it is the result of a progesterone deficiency.

80. The answer is B [Chapter 25 VI D 1–3]. The patient is a postmenopausal woman who has very little estrogen in her system and also has an atrophic vaginitis. Without sufficient estrogen, the vaginal epithelium becomes thin, with an absence of superficial cells; cytology would reveal mostly parabasal cells. A decreased amount of glycogen is present in the vaginal epithelium, and the pH changes to an alkaline state. Common complaints are pruritus, leukorrhea, burning, and dyspareunia.

81. The answer is E [Chapter 33 IV F 1]. Cushing's syndrome would not be found in a patient with a pituitary tumor because it is a disease of cortisol excess. The pituitary tumors can produce galactorrhea, neurologic signs (blindness because of the proximity of the optic nerve), and signs of other tropic hormone deficiencies, such as hypothyroidism, amenorrhea, and Addison's disease.

82. The answer is C [Chapter 3 III A 2; IV C 1–10]. Swelling of the ankles and feet is common in most pregnancies because of increased venous pressure in the lower extremities; however, generalized swelling, especially of the hands and face, may indicate preeclampsia. Severe headache and blurred vision may be signs of preeclampsia, which needs immediate attention. Vaginal bleeding could indicate abruptio placentae or placenta previa. Rupture of membranes usually involves the escape of a large or small amount of fluid from the vagina.

83. The answer is C [Chapter 17 III A–C, E 1–3]. The pudendal block is used for delivery because it provides for perineal anesthesia, and not because it relieves the pain of uterine contractions. The woman described in the question is in active labor and needs pain relief. She needs something that will take away the pain of cervical dilation (the parasympa-

thetic fibers of the second, third, and fourth sacral nerves) and the pain of uterine contractions (the eleventh and twelfth thoracic nerves). The paracervical block and epidural anesthesia (either lumbar or caudal) successfully block the pain fibers associated with labor. In addition, continuous epidural fentanyl and local anesthetic agents are effective in relieving the pain of the first stage of labor.

84. The answer is D [Chapter 37 IX D, E]. The use of pamphlets (and video recordings) is becoming widespread in the practice of medicine. Although they are useful and can supplement the information that a physician provides to a patient, they should not replace the communication that must take place between physician and patient. In addition, a physician must be sure to read every sentence before giving it to the patient. Any statement made within the pamphlet may be seen as a promise made by the physician should the patient bring a lawsuit against the physician. Communication is essential in obtaining informed consent.

85. The answer is A [Chapter 18 II A 1, 2]. The microscopic characteristics of a hydatidiform mole include marked edema and enlargement of the villi. In addition, the lining trophoblast of the villi proliferates and fetal tissue is absent. Another important feature is the disappearance of the villous blood vessels; therefore, their presence would not be compatible with the diagnosis of a mole.

86. The answer is E [Chapter 16 V A 5]. The myomas on the surface of the uterus (subserous) do not cause abortions; however, the myomas within the cavity of the uterus (submucous) can cause abortions. Cervical incompetence, luteal phase (progesterone) deficiencies, balanced chromosomal translocations, and abnormal uterine configurations can lead to repeated abortions.

87. The answer is A [Chapter 21 III E 1–3]. Whenever a pregnancy is associated with an intrauterine device (IUD) left in situ, the IUD should be removed immediately because of the increased likelihood of a spontaneous abortion. In addition, serious infection can result, causing a loss of reproductive capacity or death. The risk of ectopic pregnancy is higher in IUD users than in nonusers; and if the IUD remains throughout the pregnancy prematurity may result from its irritative influence on the endometrium in the third trimester. Since the IUD is always extra-amniotic in a pregnancy, it cannot cause pressure damage or anomalies of the fetus.

88. The answer is D [Chapter 25 II B 1–2]. The vagina is normally resistant to most infections because of certain environmental factors. Normal levels of estrogen generate a thick protective epithelium; an atrophic epithelium is present in the absence of estrogen. An acidic pH is also necessary. The acidity (i.e., a pH between 4.0 and 5.0) results from the production of lactic acid by Döderlein's bacilli and protects the vagina from infection. *Escherichia coli* is a natural inhabitant but does not contribute to vaginal health.

89. The answer is D [Chapter 11 IV B 1–4; Figure 11-1]. The pregnancy of the woman described in the question would be placed in jeopardy by cervical cerclage. Not only is this pregnancy her first (so she has no history of cervical incompetence) but also she is contracting regularly, and her cervix is effaced. A cervical cerclage is a foreign body that acts as a medium for bacterial growth. With such growth, the fetal membranes rupture and allow bacterial growth within the mother and fetus. Thus, a cervical cerclage would be very dangerous, possibly leading to maternal morbidity and fetal morbidity or mortality. In the evaluation of preterm labor, a urinary tract infection should be ruled out, an ultrasound to determine fetal weight would be useful for future management decisions, and tocolysis with magnesium sulfate or a β_2-agonist should be used when attempting to arrest the labor. A coagulation profile may be beneficial in ruling out placental abruption.

90. The answer is D [Chapter 32 IV F 2]. The luteal phase defect implies a deficiency in progesterone secretion from the corpus luteum, which is treated by either exogenous progesterone or increased endogenous progesterone. Progesterone suppositories during the postovulatory part of the cycle (the luteal phase) can help, and human chorionic gonadotropin (hCG) given once or twice during the luteal phase can stimulate the corpus luteum to produce more endogenous progesterone. Clomiphene citrate and human menopausal gonadotropins, consisting of follicle-stimulating hormone (FSH) and luteinizing hormone (LH), stimulate the entire ovarian cycle, and it is hoped that they create a more functional ovulation with a better quality corpus luteum.

Low-dose estrogen is used in the preovulatory period to stimulate the production of good cervical mucus.

91. The answer is C [Chapter 20 III A 1–4]. Follicle-stimulating hormone (FSH), a glycoprotein secreted by the pituitary, stimulates the growth and maturation of granulosa cells and aromatase activity, which are necessary for the synthesis of estradiol. In the follicular phase of the menstrual cycle, FSH and estrogen promote increased numbers of FSH receptors on the follicle, and FSH induces the development of luteinizing hormone (LH) receptors on granulosa cells. LH release is stimulated by elevated levels of estradiol, not by FSH.

92. The answer is A [Chapter 11 I A]. A 2330-g infant born at 38 weeks' gestation indicates intrauterine growth retardation of a term fetus. At any gestational age, a fetus that is under the tenth percentile by weight is considered small for gestational age or is prenatally designated to have intrauterine fetal growth retardation. The neonatal outlook for growth and mental development is directly dependent on the etiology of the problem causing the growth retardation. Prematurity denotes underdevelopment, which is clinically expressed by low birth weight and physical evidence of immaturity. In labor, many of these infants may exhibit fetal distress.

93. The answer is E [Chapter 19 II D; V E; VI C 1–6, E 2 e]. Imperforate hymen is a vaginal anomaly that does not allow menstrual blood to escape. The androgen insensitivity syndrome involves an absent uterus and a vagina that ends in a blind pouch. Systemic illnesses, such as cystic fibrosis, can be associated with amenorrhea. A person with Turner's syndrome has only one X chromosome and has associated amenorrhea. On the other hand, the granulosa–theca cell tumor, which may secrete estrogen, can present as precocious puberty with uterine bleeding as early as age 9.

94. The answer is D [Chapter 25 VI H 5 a (1)–(3)]. In the woman with active herpes lesions whose membranes ruptured 24 hours before admission, the fetus has already been infected, so nothing is gained by performing a cesarean section. With ruptured membranes and active herpes, it is important to deliver the fetus within 4 hours of the rupture.

95. The answer is C [Chapter 20 IV F 2 a–c]. Abnormal luteal phase function can be the cause of both infertility and pregnancy wastage. Since oogenesis is sequential, it is logical that poor follicle-stimulating hormone (FSH) stimulation of the follicle can result in depressed estradiol levels, which can affect the midcycle luteinizing hormone (LH) surge. The depressed LH surge can, in turn, affect the formation of the corpus luteum by production of a small luteal cell mass and low midluteal progesterone production. Prostaglandin has not been implicated in the luteal phase defect. Elevated levels of serum prolactin have been found in some luteal phase defects.

96. The answer is C [Chapter 22 II B 1 a–j, 2 a–g]. The parasympathetic nerves (S2, S3, and S4) transmit sensations to the spinal cord via the hypogastric plexus from the upper third of the vagina, cervix, the lower uterine segment, the uterosacral and cardinal ligaments, posterior urethra, the trigone of the bladder, the lower ureters, and the rectosigmoid. The uterine fundus is innervated by the thoracolumbar sympathetic nerves (T11, T12, and L1).

97. The answer is A [Chapter 30 II A 1–3; III A 1–3]. In terms of the three different types of myomas, each can cause specific symptoms. The submucous myomas are often associated with heavy menstrual bleeding and anemia. The normal hysterosalpingogram in this patient eliminates a submucous myoma and the anemia that often results from that type of myoma. The patient's enlarged, irregular uterus has multiple subserosal myomas. These myomas are on the surface of the uterus and can put pressure on nearby structures such as the ureters and rectum, resulting in hydronephrosis and constipation. The solid 4-cm adnexal mass on the left is probably a pedunculated myoma, which could twist on its pedicle (torsion) and cause pelvic pain.

98. The answer is A [Chapter 15 V D 2 f]. A pregnant patient with cocaine toxicity presents a diagnostic dilemma. On the one hand, she may be suffering from eclampsia; on the other hand, she may be suffering from chorioamnionitis. A patient's history and a urine toxicology screen are essential in determining the cause of the constellation of symptoms. Regardless of the diagnosis, stabilization is essential. Thus, intravenous fluids, oxygenation, and control of seizure activity are the primary therapeutic actions. Thereafter, hypertension can be controlled with intravenous propranolol. Treatment with magnesium sulfate is ap-

propriate because it does not have stimulating effects on the heart muscle. Under no circumstances should a woman be submitted to an operative procedure until she is fully evaluated and stabilized. Therefore, although a fetus may be in jeopardy, the stability of the mother must be assured before taking actions toward delivery.

99. The answer is D [Chapter 24 III A 1–5]. Functioning endometrium within the myometrium is called adenomyosis, not endometriosis. Endometriosis involves the presence of functioning endometrium, both glands and stroma, outside the uterine cavity. This endometrium can implant anywhere in the pelvis, causing nodularity of the cul-de-sac, pelvic adhesions, or endometriomas of the ovaries. All of these conditions are due to the monthly bleeding that occurs within the implants, which then creates the nodularity or cystic ovarian enlargement.

100. The answer is A [Chapter 2 IV C 1]. Transverse lie is not associated with postpartum hemorrhage. Any obstetric situation that overdistends the pregnant uterus can be responsible for postpartum hemorrhage. The bleeding occurs because the myometrium does not contract well after delivery, and the vessels in the placental bed continue to bleed. Thus, multiple gestation and hydramnios can cause such bleeding because of overdistention. A long labor also contributes to uterine atony after delivery because of the inability of the myometrial fibers to contract well due to fatigue. Thrombocytopenia can cause postpartum hemorrhage because of the faulty clotting mechanism inherent in that disease.

101. The answer is D [Chapter 20 III B; IV E 2]. Luteinizing hormone (LH), a glycoprotein secreted by the pituitary gland, stimulates germ cell maturation and completion of reduction division in the oocyte. LH stimulates the theca cells to produce androgens, which are subsequently converted to estradiol in the granulosa cells. LH effects luteinization of the granulosa cells with subsequent progesterone secretion. Follicle-stimulating hormone (FSH), not LH, induces the production of LH receptors on the granulosa cells.

102. The answer is B [Chapter 7 I F 3 a,b]. Because of the significant incidence of fetal demise in insulin-dependent diabetic pregnancies, it is essential to terminate the pregnancy when fetal compromise is evident. A poor biophysical profile and a positive contraction stress test are indications of fetal distress. Late decelerations with either induced or spontaneous contractions are signs of fetal distress and necessitate active intervention. A decreased need for insulin is also a dangerous sign, indicating that the pregnancy is no longer a healthy one. A lecithin to sphingomyelin (L/S) ratio of less than 2:1 (or 2.0) means that the fetal lung is immature, which is a contraindication for delivery; in the fetus of a diabetic woman, in contrast to a nondiabetic, lung maturity may take longer to occur.

103. The answer is D [Chapter 35 VI A 2a]. Osteoporosis is the main health hazard associated with menopause. Bone loss occurs in the axial skeleton, most of which involves trabecular bone, with thinning of the cortex. With the current low numbers of postmenopausal women on estrogen replacement, about 32% can expect a hip fracture at some time, and this fracture involves significant mortality in the postmenopausal population. Bone loss is most rapid in women under age 45 who undergo castration by surgical oophorectomy. At any time, estrogen can prevent or retard bone loss, depending on when the replacement is started with respect to menopause. Osteoporosis is more common in white than black women.

104. The answer is B [Chapter 21 III B 2 a–b, D 1; IV C 2; V A 1–4, B 2 a–b]. Women who use the progesterone-bearing intrauterine device (IUD) continue to have menses, which may be light at times because of the regressive action of the progesterone on the endometrium. Any medication that suppresses hypothalamic–pituitary function and, consequently, ovarian activity, can result in amenorrhea. When the ovary produces little or no estrogen, the endometrium is so minimally stimulated that little or no tissue can slough, thus no menses. Birth control pills, gonadotropin-releasing hormone (GnRH) agonists, and medroxyprogesterone all have the ability to shut down the hypothalamic-pituitary-ovarian axis.

105. The answer is E [Chapter 34 V C 2 a–b]. With a significantly increased luteinizing hormone to follicle-stimulating hormone (LH/FSH) ratio, irregular cycles, and increased hair growth, the diagnosis in this patient most likely is polycystic ovary disease. At this stage in her life, the patient wants help with the

hair growth and not her fertility. Therefore, oral contraceptives rather than clomiphene citrate would be the drug of choice for her. Use of oral contraceptives decreases gonadotropin secretion, with a consequent decrease in ovarian steroidogenesis and a decrease in secretion of ovarian preandrogens, such as androstenedione. As a consequence of the decreased ovarian steroidogenesis, blood levels of testosterone decrease. The estrogen component of the oral contraceptives stimulates an increased production of sex hormone–binding globulin (SHBG) from the liver, and the progestin component displaces active androgens at the hair follicle level. The oral contraceptives do not affect the 5α-reductase enzyme activity.

106. The answer is E [Chapter 23 IV A 1–3]. Uterine fibroids are not linked to pelvic inflammatory disease (PID). Degenerating endometrium provides a good culture medium, allowing bacteria to ascend the uterus to the tubal lumen; thus, two-thirds of acute cases of PID begin just after the menses. Sperm can act as mobile transporters of bacteria into the uterus and tubes, and uterine contractions during sexual intercourse may assist their ascent. Intrauterine devices (IUDs) have been linked to an increased risk of PID (5.21 cases/100 woman-years) as compared to no contraception used by sexually active women (3.42 cases/100 woman-years).

107. The answer is E [Chapter 7 VI C, 2, D 1 a–d, 2, 3]. The patient described in the question presents with cardiac failure due to the stress of the pregnancy on her cardiorespiratory system. She must be stabilized while preparations are made for delivery. The usual methods of therapy in a patient in cardiac failure include the administration of oxygen, diuretics, and digitalis. The delivery should be accomplished vaginally (unless there is an overriding reason for cesarean section) because of less morbidity and mortality with a vaginal delivery. Epidural anesthesia effectively relieves pain, allowing for a safe forceps or vacuum extraction delivery to shorten the second stage of delivery and to eliminate or minimize the stress associated with this stage. A cardiac patient should not be permitted to push in the second stage of labor.

108. The answer is D [Chapter 27 III B 1–4]. It is important to determine the exact time of the last menstrual period (LMP) and the method of birth control, if any, because of the possibility of pregnancy following rape. Questions about bathing and previous intercourse are important when collecting evidence that may be used in the prosecution of the rapist. A woman's reproductive history is not relevant.

109. The answer is D [Chapter 5 V C 1–2]. Epidural anesthesia creates a sympathetic blockade that allows the pooling of blood in the lower extremities. When this situation occurs, maternal hypotension can develop due to decreased venous return and reduced cardiac output. These two factors lead to decreased uterine blood flow, which may translate into fetal distress. With hypotension secondary to epidural anesthesia, maternal heart rate actually increases as a compensatory mechanism for decreased venous return.

110. The answer is B [Chapter 20 IV E 1–4]. The luteinizing hormone (LH) surge is central to the ovulation process; it is triggered by an estradiol peak, which exerts a positive feedback effect on LH secretion. Along with the LH surge is a similar but smaller rise in follicle-stimulating hormone (FSH) levels, a response that is progesterone-dependent. The LH surge stimulates completion of reduction division in the oocyte, luteinization of the granulosa cells, and synthesis of progesterone and prostaglandins within the follicle. Prostaglandins play a part in the actual discharge of the ovum from the follicle.

111. The answer is D [Chapter 21 IV D 4 a–b]. The incidence of postpill amenorrhea is very small (0.2%–3.1%). Length of use of birth control pills is not related to the occurrence of amenorrhea. Many of the women who experience postpill amenorrhea have preexisting menstrual abnormalities, such as oligomenorrhea. If the menstrual abnormalities are an early sign of premature ovarian failure, this condition can become manifest with amenorrhea when the birth control pills are discontinued. Any amenorrhea following cessation of contraceptive use should suggest pregnancy; it is the first cause to be ruled out. Since a pituitary adenoma occasionally develops in women who use oral contraceptives and since it is the most dangerous reason for the amenorrhea, it must be ruled out promptly through measurement of serum prolactin levels.

112. The answer is E [Chapter 24 IV C 1 a, b]. As with all infertility surgery, gentle handling of tissue, lysis of adhesions, and meticulous hemostasis are important. In the situation involving adhesions with endometriosis and the raw surface areas that remain after dissection, reperitonealization helps to prevent the adhesions from recurring. The dextran is a useful adjunct because it is slowly absorbed from the peritoneal cavity and actually separates surfaces long enough to allow mesothelial cells to reperitonealize the areas spontaneously. Uterine suspension prevents refixation of the retroverted uterus. Danazol is helpful after surgery for severe endometriosis, but not for mild to moderate endometriosis, particularly because the woman described in the question wants to attempt pregnancy as soon as possible after surgery.

113–115. The answers are: 113-D [Chapter 28 IV B 3, C2], **114-C** [Chapter 28 IV B 2, C 1 a, b], **115-D** [Chapter 28 IV B 3, C1 a, b, 2, 4]. The 25-year-old woman described in the question presents with no bleeding, which is unusual with an ectopic pregnancy. The adnexal mass is the corpus luteum, not an ectopic pregnancy. The fact that there is no sac in the uterus on pelvic ultrasound is of no significance because pelvic ultrasound does not pick up a sac until after 6 weeks' gestation.

With the low-for-dates human chorionic gonadotropin (hCG) levels, the diagnosis in this 30-year-old woman could be either a threatened abortion or an ectopic pregnancy. Both conditions present with vaginal bleeding, but more bleeding is likely with a threatened abortion. The diagnosis is made by ultrasound, which reveals an intrauterine sac that would be absent in an ectopic pregnancy.

In the 35-year-old woman whose last menses were 6 weeks ago, the hCG level is appropriate and there is no vaginal bleeding, suggesting an intrauterine pregnancy. Neither nonclotting blood on culdocentesis nor the absence of a sac in the uterus on pelvic ultrasound at 6 weeks is diagnostic of an ectopic pregnancy. Therefore, the normal hCG levels, the lack of external bleeding, the tender mass on pelvic examination, and the intra-abdominal bleeding all point to an intrauterine pregnancy with a bleeding corpus luteum.

116–118. The answers are: 116-B [Chapter 34 IV B 2; V B 3], **117-D** [Chapter 34 IV B 3; V C 1–2], **118-B** [Chapter 34 IV B 5; V B 3]. In congenital adrenal hyperplasia, an enzyme deficiency is present along the steroid pathway to cortisol. As a result, a deficiency of the end product, cortisol, and a buildup of the intermediate metabolites occur in front of the enzyme block. Increased levels of both dihydroepiandrosterone sulfate (DHEAS) and 17-hydroxyprogesterone result from these enzyme deficiencies. In each case, therefore, the appropriate therapy would be the administration of a corticosteroid, such as prednisone. Providing the end product decreases adrenocorticotropic hormone (ACTH) secretion, reduces stimulation of adrenal steroidogenesis, and decreases secretion of the androgenic substances along the steroid pathway.

Since elevated levels of androstenedione point to an ovarian source of the androgens, birth control pills would be an appropriate therapy to shut down ovarian steroidogenesis, thereby reducing the androgenic substance (androstenedione) coming from the ovary.

119–122. The answers are: 119-B [Chapter 19 V A 3], **120-C** [Chapter 19 VI E 1 b (2)], **121-A** [Chapter 19 VI B 3], **122-D** [Chapter 19 VI A 3 b]. Congenital adrenal hyperplasia occurs when the enzymatic regulation of the biosynthesis of cortisol and aldosterone is impaired. A 21-hydroxylase defect is the most common cause of distinct virilization of the female newborn (95% of all cases of congenital adrenal hyperplasia). Hydrocortisone is administered indefinitely to all patients.

Isosexual precocious puberty is the early development of secondary sex characteristics (before 9 years of age) consistent with genetic sex. Although 80% to 90% of those with isosexual precocious puberty have no obvious underlying cause, progestational agents and gonadotropin-releasing hormone (GnRH) analogues have been found to be effective in suppressing uterine bleeding.

Dysfunctional uterine bleeding (DUB) [bleeding unaccompanied by ovulation] in adolescent girls is usually self-limited; however, if symptoms persist, cyclic hormone manipulation with combination estrogens and progestins is recommended.

Although dysmenorrhea may be secondary to obstructive or anatomic causes, frequently no organic cause is found. Prostaglandins are present during the menses and are known to cause painful uterine contractions. Therapy includes antiemetics for the nausea and vomiting and prostaglandin inhibitors for the pain.

123–125. The answers are: 123-C [Chapter 25 VI A 4], **124-A** [Chapter 25 VI B 4], **125-A** [Chapter 25 VI C 4]. A thick, cheesy, white vaginal discharge is characteristic of a yeast infection, and antibiotic use is one of the pre-disposing causes. The treatment of the woman who has been taking ampicillin involves one of the antifungal medications. Vinegar douche is not an acceptable choice because it is used for prevention, not treatment.

The patient who presents with a malodorous green-grey frothy discharge and intense itching has the signs and symptoms of trichomoniasis. Approximately 70% to 80% of the male partners of infected patients harbor the organism. Characteristic "strawberry spots" can be seen on the cervix and vagina. The organism can be seen microscopically when saline is used to prepare a wet mount of the vaginal secretions. Metronidazole should be used to treat both the patient and her partner.

When clue cells are found on microscopic examination of a vaginal discharge, the diagnosis is *Gardnerella* vaginitis. The most effective therapy for this vaginitis is oral metronidazole, with treatment of the sexual partner to prevent reinfection.

126–128. The answers are: 126-E [Chapter 33 IV C, D], **127-A** [Chapter 33 II A 1], **128-B** [Chapter 33 I A 1 a]. Hypogonadotropic, or secondary, amenorrhea is the most common type of amenorrhea. It occurs after a menstrual pattern has been established and has a number of causes, including emotional stress, drugs, nutritional deficiencies, abnormalities of the hypothalamic-pituitary axis, and excessive exercise. The inadequate amount of pituitary gonadotropin secretion, in turn, does not stimulate the ovary, leading to low estrogen output and absent menses. Marathon runners are known to experience this reversible type of amenorrhea occasionally.

A key feature of eugonadotropic amenorrhea is functional ovaries, which secrete estrogen, ovulate, and have the normal feedback on the pituitary, resulting in normal gonadotropin levels. This type of amenorrhea is characterized by an abnormality of the outflow tract, either congenital or acquired, which prevents the egress of menstrual blood. In this particular case, the young woman has normal ovaries and a congenital defect of the müllerian ducts, resulting in an absent uterus and a vestigial vagina, as seen in Mayer-Rokitansky-Küster-Hauser syndrome.

Physiologic amenorrhea occurs quite normally at certain times in the lives of most women, such as after menarche, during pregnancy and lactation, and after menopause. The gonadotropin levels may be in the normal range (after menarche), low (during pregnancy and lactation), or high (after menopause). The adolescent described in the question had a normal menarche with three subsequent menses before becoming amenorrheic. It is not uncommon to have intervals of amenorrhea lasting 2 to 12 months within the first 2 years of menarche.

129–132. The answers are: 129-A [Chapter 16 I C 1], **130-D** [Chapter 16 IV B 2], **131-B** [Chapter 16 IV B 1], **132-C** [Chapter 16 I C 2]. The eponyms Kerr, Sellheim, and Sanger come from the physicians who pioneered procedures for cesarean section; McDonald and Shirodkar pioneered procedures for cervical cerclage.

The differences in the procedures for cesarean section are the type and location of the incision into the uterus. The Kerr incision, which is transverse, is performed in the lower (noncontractile) segment of the uterus. The Sellheim incision, which is low and vertical, extends into the corpus. Dehiscence is more likely secondary to the scar extending into the uterine corpus. The Sanger incision is a longitudinal incision that is entirely in the corpus.

The cerclage procedures differ in the technique of placing the encircling suture around the cervix. Because the Shirodkar suture is buried beneath the cervical mucosa, it can be left in place for a subsequent pregnancy if a cesarean section is performed. The McDonald suture incurs less trauma to the cervix and less blood loss than the Shirodkar suture. It is a simple purse-string suture of the cervix.

133–135. The answers are: 133-D, 134-B, 135-B [Chapter 18 II B 2, C 3 E; III D 2; III C, D]. The human chorionic gonadotropin (hCG) level is unimportant in the woman who presents with vaginal bleeding and no fetal heart sounds. Because the most recent pregnancy was 4 months ago, this pregnancy could be only 12 weeks at the most; however, the top of the uterus is at the level of the umbilicus (i.e., the size of a 20-week pregnancy) and, thus, is larger than expected. With a positive pregnancy test, bleeding, a large uterus, and no fetal heart tones, a molar pregnancy must be ruled out. Thus, a pelvic ultrasound examination is indicated to determine the uterine contents.

It appears that the woman with metastatic gestational trophoblastic neoplasia (GTN) has been successfully treated. The follow-up protocol suggests monthly hCG titers for 1 year after they have been negative every 2 weeks for 3 months. A chest x-ray is required every 3 months. This woman had her previous chest x-ray 3 months ago and needs another one to complement the monthly hCG levels and follow the course of the disease appropriately.

Following evacuation of a molar pregnancy, the hCG titer is expected to become negative over 2 to 3 months; this situation must be carefully followed with weekly and then monthly hCG titers. If the hCG values plateau or rise, metastatic or nonmetastatic GTN is a possibility. Therefore, a chest x-ray is indicated to rule out pulmonary metastatis.

136–138. The answers are: 136-E [Chapter 31 II B, C], **137-B** [Chapter 31 I A, B; II A 1, 2], **138-D** [Chapter 31 II B 1; III C 2 c]. With the long history of urgency and frequency, the suspected diagnosis is a chronic urinary tract infection. Certainly a urine sample for culture and sensitivity is indicated; however, the culture is often negative. Cystoscopy is necessary to look at the inside of the bladder, especially in the area of the trigone, for evidence of chronic inflammation.

The patient has the classic features of stress urinary incontinence (SUI). When she has a full bladder and increases her intra-abdominal pressure, she loses urine. A distortion of the normal anatomic relationships between the urethra and the bladder results in an increase in the intravesical pressure, which exceeds urethral pressure, causing incontinence. Stress testing reveals leakage of urine coincident with increased intra-abdominal pressure, which is diagnostic of SUI.

This patient describes a loss of urine that is not associated with an increase in intra-abdominal pressure, such as coughing or jogging; therefore, it is not SUI. The absence of diabetes and neurologic disease eliminates the possibility of a neurologic bladder. The diagnosis is detrusor instability or dyssynergia, and the diagnosis is made via cystometry.

139–142. The answers are: 139-B [Chapter 26 I B 2; V B 1], **140-D** [Chapter 26 IV A 4; D], **141-C** [Chapter 26 IV B 1, 2; V A 3 e], **142-D** [Chapter 26 I B 3; III B 1; IV D 2]. The 30-year-old woman with menorrhagia is experiencing excessive bleeding during her menses. Her cycles are regular, and she has no ongoing, heavy bleeding that must be controlled. Because her cycles are regular, she is probably ovulating and needs no diagnostic curettage. In addition, her bleeding is neither irregular nor continuous; thus, she does not need estrogen or protestin therapy. Nonsteroidal anti-inflammatory drugs (NSAIDs), however, can help lessen menstrual blood loss in women who ovulate.

The 35-year-old woman who presents with continuous uterine bleeding despite hormone therapy should not have been given any medication without a diagnosis. Because of the continuous bleeding, it is inappropriate to add either estrogen or progestin alone without first sampling the endometrium to rule out an endometrial pathology. The only management at this point is to perform a dilation and curettage (D and C), which should have been done before starting her on the oral contraceptives.

The 23-year-old woman who presents with a 3-week history of bleeding needs something immediately to control this uterine bleeding, because of the amount of blood she has lost. She is probably not ovulating as indicated by the long periods between her bleeding episodes. She is experiencing estrogen breakthrough bleeding associated with long periods of unopposed estrogen. The therapy that most quickly controls this type of bleeding is oral conjugated estrogen, which provides rapid growth of endometrial tissue. A progestin should be added after the bleeding is under control. A progestin or oral contraceptive is not as effective in controlling dysfunctional uterine bleeding (DUB) as estrogen alone.

The 47-year-old woman with menometrorrhagia presents with classic perimenopausal bleeding, which is characterized by irregular anovulatory bleeding and sustained unopposed estrogen. The combination of obesity, hypertension, and irregular perimenopausal bleeding demands that an endometrial neoplasia be ruled out. Because endometrial hyperplasia or carcinoma is a possibility in women of this age, no hormone therapy can be given without a diagnosis. Performing a D and C to sample the endometrium can provide this diagnosis.

143–145. The answers are: 143-B [Chapter 35 IV C 1 a], **144-D** [Chapter 35 V B 1, 3 a; VI D 1, 2], **145-E** [Chapter 35 VI B 2]. The first patient is experiencing irregular anovulatory cycles due to sustained levels of unopposed estrogen. The result is a proliferative, or hyperplastic, endometrium with periodic sloughing and prolonged, heavy bleeding. This patient needs regular intermittent progestin therapy to oppose the endogenous estrogen and allow for controlled, regular uterine bleeding.

The second patient is postmenopausal with several of the classic symptms that characterize the hypoestrogenic state of menopause. She needs estrogen replacement. With the uterus present, she must have both estrogen and progestin as replacement therapy. The progestin is used to oppose the estrogen to prevent endometrial hyperplasia.

The third patient is perimenopausal in that she is just beginning to experience the irregularity of occasional anovulatory cycles. Her anovulatory bleeding has occurred for 2 months, and she could resume regular cycles in the coming months. She is experiencing no menopausal symptoms. At this point she needs no hormonal therapy. Estrogen alone or estrogen and progestin as replacement therapy would be unnecessary and would compound the bleeding problem because the exogenous hormones would be added to endogenous estrogen. Irregular and bothersome bleeding could result from such intervention at this point in the woman's perimenopausal physiology.

146–148. The answers are: 146-C, 147-B, 148-D [Chapter 2 IV C 1, 2]. An important sign of a ruptured uterus is continued heavy bleeding in the presence of a well-contracted uterus and the absence of cervical or vaginal tears. A clue to the possibility of a ruptured uterus is the history of the use of oxytocin during the labor of a parous woman with a large infant.

Anything that overdistends the uterus during labor such as twins, hydramnios, or a large infant can lead to a hypotonic myometrium and an atonic uterus; the relaxed myometrium does not contract and close down the exposed open vessles in the placental bed.

The inability of the postpartum uterus to stay in a contracted condition with the use of oxytocin suggests that something (e.g., a piece of placenta or a succenturiate lobe) remains in the uterine cavity. This piece of tissue distends the cavity and does not allow compression of the vessels of the placental bed.

149–151. The answers are: 149-A [Chapter 12 III D], **150-D** [Chapter 12 III B], **151-B** [Chapter 12 IV C]. Maternal serum α-fetoprotein (MSAFP) measurement is the best screening test for a neural tube defect, such as meningomyelocele. If the α-fetoprotein concentration is 2.5 times normal or above, an amniocentesis is performed to see if the α-fetoprotein concentration is also elevated in the amniotic fluid.

The diagnosis of Tay-Sachs disease is made by demonstrating a deficiency of the enzyme β-D-hexosaminidase A in cultured amniotic fluid cells. These fetal cells are obtained via amniocentesis.

Chorionic villus sampling (CVS) supplies trophoblastic tissue for evaluation. Chromosome abnormalities and hemoglobinopathies, such as sickle cell disease, can be identified with this procedure.

152–153. The answers are: 152-A [Chapter 6 III A 1], **153-D** [Chapter 6 III A 2; IV C 1]. A nonreactive nonstress test (NST) is an indication of potential fetal compromise. Additional testing for fetal well-being is indicated. The contraction stress test (CST) should be performed with either intravenous oxytocin or nipple stimulation. Contractions provide more stress on the uteroplacental unit and, thus, are a good test of its reserve. If the CST is positive, delivery is indicated.

A biophysical score of 4 indicates that the fetus is not normal. In a postdates pregnancy, prompt delivery is indicated to prevent possible further fetal compromise or fetal death. Cesarean delivery is not always necessary but should be performed without hesitation if delivery is to be expedited.

154–155. The answers are: 154-D [Chapter 32 III D 2 a (2), F 3], **155-A** [Chapter 32 III E 2 b]. With persistent short luteal phases determined by a basal body temperature graph and a very early spontaneous abortion, the suspected diagnosis must be an inadequate corpus luteum. The best test for an inadequate corpus luteum is the endometrial biopsy, which shows whether the endometrial histology or the preparation of the endometrium is in phase with the luteal phase as seen on the temperature graph.

With apparently good sperm and mucus interaction and regular ovulations, but infertility for 3 years, the woman's tubal function must be evaluated. The acute appendicitis and appendectomy may be precursors of pelvic adhesions and poor tubal function. Direct observation of the pelvic structures via the laparoscope would be the indicated procedure at this point.

156–158. The answers are: 156-D [Chapter 29 II A 1 a, b, d (2)], **157-C** [Chapter 29 II C 2 b, d], **158-A** [Chapter 29 II B 2 a, b, 4]. The 18-year-old patient has signs and symptoms of an acute gonorrheal pelvic infection. She has lower abdominal pain, a fever, a purulent cervical discharge, and adnexal tenderness. The symptoms began just after her menses. The treatment of choice is ceftriaxone with doxycycline for the often coexistent chlamydial infection.

The 28-year-old woman has a chlamydial pelvic infection, much more subtle and less symptomatic than a gonorrheal infection. The lower abdominal pain is low-grade and persistent. The urinary symptoms are secondary to urethritis. The treatment of choice is doxycycline for 1 week.

The 35-year-old patient has the signs of secondary syphilis—a maculopapular rash on her soles and palms and lymphadenopathy. Also noteworthy is the history of a vaginal sore 2 months earlier; this was the painless chancre that is pathognomonic for primary syphilis. In untreated patients, the chancre is followed in 6 weeks to 6 months by the secondary or bacteremic stage of the disease. Penicillin is still the mainstay in the treatment of syphilis.

159–161. The answers are: 159-D, 160-A, 161-C [Chapter 2 IV D 1 b, c, 2, 3]. With the prolonged rupture of membranes and the *Streptococcus* organism in the vagina, a postpartum uterine infection must be suspected. The high temperature early in the puerperium and the lower abdominal tenderness, probably myometrial and parametrial in origin, are highly suggestive of a parametritis.

A spiking fever that does not respond to antibiotic therapy 5 days after cesarean section is a classic sign of pelvic thrombophlebitis, especially after pelvic surgery. There are no pelvic physical findings. The diagnosis is confirmed when heparin therapy is instituted, and the temperature curve gradually returns to normal.

Conduction anesthesia may result in postpartum urinary retention because of the effect of the anesthesia on the autonomic nervous system. When this happens, a woman often needs to be catheterized once or twice before the anesthesia has completely worn off. The catheterization can easily introduce bacteria and seed a urinary tract infection. The chills and back (kidney) pain are common symptoms of a urinary tract infection.

162–163. The answers are: 162-C, 163-E [Chapter 13 III A 3, B 3]. The key to the diagnosis of the woman in active labor is the previous cesarean section and her moribund condition. Such a picture is not typical of either placenta previa or vasa previa. There is usually not enough blood loss with placenta previa to affect both the patient and the fetus, and only the fetus is affected with vasa previa. This patient had a previous cesarean section, and the scar represents a potential weak spot. With a ruptured uterus, there can be a great deal of blood loss, much of it hidden if the bleeding is intra-abdominal. If the placenta is involved with the rupture, the fetus can become distressed very quickly. The hypotension by itself can lead to fetal distress.

The woman who presents with heavy vaginal bleeding does not have a placenta previa or vasa previa, as demonstrated by the ultrasound findings [ie., a normal fetal heart rate (FHR) and a fundal placenta]. There is no historical reason to suggest a ruptured uterus, and the bleeding is too heavy for bloody show. This patient has previously unattended advanced cervical cancer, which has locally eroded into a blood vessel and caused the bleeding. She had not been seen for a number of years, including during this pregnancy, and has had no Papanicolaou (Pap) smear for over 10 years.

164–166. The answers are: 164-B [Chapter 4 IV B 5 b], **165-D** [Table 4-1], **166-A** [Table 4-1]. The woman who is having frequent painful contractions that have no gradient and cause no change in the cervical dilation is experiencing hypertonic uterine dysfunction. Oxytocin will not help this situation, but strong sedation, such as morphine, will relieve the pain, relax the patient, and result in a normal labor pattern.

The woman who is experiencing progressive cervical dilation is in the active phase of labor. Contractions are at intervals of 2–4 minutes and are strong enough to effect the cervical change.

The woman with contractions at irregular intervals is in false labor. The intensity of the contractions remains the same and is chiefly in the lower abdomen. There is no change in the cervical dilation. The contractions are usually relieved and often stopped with a sedative.

167–169. The answers are: 167-D, 168-E, 169-B [Table 14-4]. There is continuing controversy about the teratogenicity of synthetic progestational agents. Indeed, if they are teratogenic, the risk is extremely small. Exposure during the first trimester is possibly related to a two- to threefold increase in cardiac defects (from 8/1000 to approximately 20/1000 live-births). Prenatal exposure to a progestin may double the incidence of hypospadias in offspring; the resulting incidence of 140/10,000 male births is extremely low. Though uncommon, fusion of the labia majora and clitorimegaly have been observed in the female fetus.

It was not until the early 1960s that prenatal exposure to thalidomide was identified as a cause of serious defects in structural development. Thalidomide was used all over Europe as a very effective sleeping medication. Unfortunately, the pregnant animals that were used to test the safety of thalidomide in pregnancy rarely developed limb defects when exposed to teratogens. It was only after humans had been born with limb hypoplasia that repeated experimental studies in species similar to humans revealed devastating limb reduction defects, which serves to exemplify the variation of genetic susceptibility among species.

A vitamin A analogue, isotretinoin, has proven to be a potent human teratogen, causing craniofacial, central nervous system (CNS), and cardiac defects. A specific pattern of abnormalities in affected infants has been termed the retinoic acid embryopathy.

170–171. The answers are: 170-A, 171-A [Chapter 27 IV B]. Because the first patient presented to the office more than 72 hours after the assault, pregnancy prevention, such as diethylstilbestrol (DES) therapy or intrauterine device (IUD) insertion, would be ineffective. An elective abortion is not indicated in the absence of a pregnancy diagnosis. Therefore, the physician should follow the patient with weekly human chorionic gonadotropin (hCG) tests until a period occurs or until the test becomes positive. If the latter occurs, an elective abortion would be indicated.

Once again, it would be important to follow the patient with hCG tests. Because she presented within 72 hours of the assault, she is a candidate for DES therapy; however, DES preventive therapy is not 100% successful. Because of the teratogenic effects of DES on the fetus, it would be important to determine whether the patient becomes pregnant since termination of the pregnancy is recommended because of the teratogenicity. IUD insertion would not be appropriate because DES has already been administered.

172–174. The answers are: 172-C, 173-D, 174-E [Chapter 5 II A, B; III C 2; IV B 1]. In a patient with chronic hypertension, the index of suspicion about fetal distress must be high. However, no therapy is justified without first making the diagnosis of fetal distress. Thus, the first step would be fetal heart rate (FHR) monitoring to see if there is any distress.

In a primigravida who is 7 cm dilated, delivery is still some time off. There must be an accurate assessment of fetal well-being to see if labor can continue. A fetal scalp pH would be indicated with further management dependent on its value.

Immediate delivery is indicated in the patient with FHR monitoring and fetal scalp pH indications of significant fetal distress and acidosis. No further intrauterine resuscitation is indicated at this point.

175–176. The answers are: 175-B [Chapter 17 III B], **176-D** [Chapter 17 III D 2 b, E 1 b, 3 a]. For women in early labor (2 cm dilated in this case), spinal anesthesia is out of the question because delivery is still hours away. Epidural anesthesia is also not advisable this early in labor because it is usually given when the cervix is 4 to 5 cm dilated. The woman described in the question is allergic to meperidine, the commonly used intravenous narcotic for pain relief in early labor. Paracervical block is perfect for such women because it helps with the pain of uterine contractions. However, one of the complications of paracervical block is a transient fetal bradycardia.

The woman in active labor who is 5 cm dilated is a perfect candidate for epidural anesthesia. Spinal anesthesia is not an option at this point because delivery is not in the immediate future. Paracervical block would be possible, but it would not last until delivery. The woman received lumbar epidural anesthesia, which became a spinal when the dura was in-advertently punctured. The larger dose of anesthetic agent used in epidural anesthesia (as opposed to spinal anesthesia) was injected and caused the equivalent of a high spinal block with respiratory paralysis.

177–179. The answers are: 177-A [Chapter 13 I E 1], **178-B** [Chapter 13 II D; Figure 13-1], **179-D** [Chapter 13 II D; Figure 13-1]. The picture of painless vaginal bleeding in the third trimester strongly suggests placenta previa. One of the associated findings of placenta previa is fetal malpresentation, such as a breech. In this case, the placenta occupies the lower uterine segment, which causes the fetal head to occupy the roomier fundus of the uterus.

The clinical picture of a woman at term who presents with a tender uterus, tense abdomen, and no audible fetal heart tones is one of severe abruptio placentae, in which there has been almost complete separation of the placenta, leading to a rigid uterus and a dead fetus. One of the complications of severe abruptio placentae is renal failure, the chief sign of which is oliguria.

The clinical picture of a woman with moderate vaginal bleeding and uterine contractions and a uterus that does not entirely relax between contractions is one of mild to moderate abruptio placentae in which there is usually fetal distress but not to the extent that the fetus is immediately in jeopardy.

Index